Pain Comorbidities

Mission Statement of IASP Press®

The International Association for the Study of Pain (IASP) brings together scientists, clinicians, health care providers, and policy makers to stimulate and support the study of pain and to translate that knowledge into improved pain relief worldwide. IASP Press publishes timely, high-quality, and reasonably priced books relating to pain research and treatment.

Pain Comorbidities
Understanding and Treating the Complex Patient

Editors

Maria Adele Giamberardino, MD
Department of Medicine and Science of Aging
G. D'Annunzio University of Chieti, Chieti, Italy

Troels Staehelin Jensen, MD, DMSc
Department of Neurology and Danish Pain Research Center
Aarhus University Hospital, Aarhus, Denmark

IASP PRESS® ♦ SEATTLE

Library of Congress Cataloging-in-Publication Data

Pain comorbidities : understanding and treating the complex patient / editors, Maria Adele Giamberardino, Troels Staehelin Jensen.
  p. ; cm.
Includes bibliographical references and index.
ISBN 978-0-931092-92-3 (alk. paper)
  I. Giamberardino, Maria Adele. II. Jensen, Troels Staehelin. III. International Association for the Study of Pain.
  [DNLM: 1. Pain--physiopathology. 2. Comorbidity. 3. Pain Management. WL 704]

  616'.0472--dc23
                              2012010025

Published by:
IASP Press®
International Association for the Study of Pain
111 Queen Anne Ave N, Suite 501
Seattle, WA 98109-4955, USA
Fax: 206-283-9403
www.iasp-pain.org

Contents

Contents

Preface

This book offers an in-depth analysis of complex clinical situations involving multiple concurrent diseases. The occurrence of multiple concomitant medical conditions in the same patient is common in the clinical setting and is becoming increasingly more frequent with the progressive aging of the population. Multimorbidity in the elderly is estimated to range from 55% to 98%. In most circumstances, a patient with multiple disorders will have one or more conditions that are painful.

Myofascial pain syndromes resulting from trigger points—with a mean prevalence among middle-aged adults of 37% in men and 65% in women—have a significant tendency to co-occur with headache, fibromyalgia, and a number of visceral pain diseases. In turn, headache disorders, estimated to affect nearly half the world's adult population, have a significant tendency to coexist with fibromyalgia, dysmenorrhea, endometriosis, or irritable bowel syndrome, with epidemiological findings suggesting that having comorbid pain conditions may influence the transition of episodic to chronic headache. An overlap is frequently seen among different visceral pain diseases, such as ischemic heart disease, biliary calculosis, and pelvic disorders. These comorbidities may significantly influence each other, with trigger points exacerbating headache and fibromyalgia, or two types of visceral pain enhancing one another.

In comorbidities involving medical conditions that are not necessarily painful, there may be important symptom interactions and implications for diagnosis and therapy. The presence of hypertension or diabetes can decrease or even cancel the perception of pain in a number of specific conditions that normally involve pain, such as myocardial infarction, thus delaying their identification and treatment. A concurrent cardiovascular disease in migraine patients may preclude the therapeutic use of vasoactive compounds for headache, and the presence of cardiac conduction disturbances or arrhythmias in neuropathic pain patients can limit the use of first-line drug treatments for this condition. Medical problems such as obesity represent important risk factors for the development of certain types of pain, especially osteoarthritis and low back pain, and the co-occurrence of pain and overweight/obesity will negatively affect quality of life. Affective dysfunctions such as depression or anxiety are often associated with pain, and they require careful evaluation in terms of both diagnosis and management. Comorbidity in pain may thus involve increased or decreased pain perception and can have a significant impact on the patient's diagnosis and treatment.

A comprehensive volume addressing the clinical presentation and management of multiple interactions among different medical conditions was urgently needed. This book contains valuable contributions from a number of distinguished scientists, which are described in more detail in the synopsis at the end of the book.

Regardless of their primary specialty, clinicians who read this volume can expect to gain a better understanding of the influence of comorbidities on the experience of pain and gain valuable insights to guide optimal patient care. We are also confident that the book will be of use to basic scientists in different fields—from neurophysiology to genetics—who are investigating the pathophysiology of interactions among painful conditions.

Maria Adele Giamberardino, MD
Troels Staehelin Jensen, MD, DMSc

Introduction

Harold Merskey

Professor Emeritus of Psychiatry, University of Western Ontario, London, Ontario, Canada

Numerous conditions can cause pain. Many different conditions may occur simultaneously, either by chance or through some shared etiology, such
as fibromyalgia along with either hypothyroidism or rheumatoid arthritis.
Synovial disorders of the shoulder may be found in combination with arthritis of more than one type. The table of contents of this volume displays
this variety. In clinical practice the most common complication of chronic
pain is probably depression or a combination of anxiety and depression.
Hence, the main theme of this introductory chapter is the extent to which
pain, and particularly chronic pain, causes emotional change. Emotional
change can also contribute to causing chronic pain, but the psychological
causes of pain are relatively limited in their effects and mostly involve anxiety or depression exacerbating existing physical conditions. The problem
of distinguishing severe chronic pain from its emotional effects permeates
all types of pain, but especially conditions such as musculoskeletal pain
and headache disorders, where it can be difficult to define organic causes.
In such cases there is a particular need for caution because the physical or
pathophysiological explanation is often overlooked. In the past, this caveat

Pain Comorbidities: Understanding and Treating the Complex Patient
edited by Maria Adele Giamberardino and Troels Staehelin Jensen
IASP Press, Seattle, © 2012

probably applied to abdominal and pelvic pain as well, although we now have improved categories and better identification of physical diagnoses for those disorders.

Acute Pain

Because pain is common among numerous diseases, comorbidity may be everywhere. The possibilities of comorbidity may be endless, but to provide a perspective that may be helpful to the reader and practitioner, we will first look at the evolution of ideas about pain and the mind. We can start by quoting from the Book of Lamentations in the Bible: "Is it nothing to you, all you that pass by? Behold and see, is there any pain like my pain which is done unto me, with which the Lord has afflicted me in the day of His fierce anger? From above he has sent fire into my bones and I am weary and faint all the day" (Lamentations, 1:12–13). These words of Jeremiah on witnessing the destruction of Solomon's temple serve as a starting point for consideration of the psychogenesis of pain. The author, lamenting the sack of Jerusalem by the Babylonians, describes himself as having pain located in the body that is linked with depression. A similar view on pain and anxiety is offered by Montaigne (in 1580), when he says: "We feel one cut of the surgeon's knife more than ten blows of the sword in the heat of battle" [26]. He continues: "The pains of childbirth considered so great both by doctors and by God are held of no account amongst entire nations ... the wives of our Swiss Infantry trudging after their husbands may be seen today carrying on the shoulder the infant which only yesterday was in the womb."

    Until the advent of anesthesia, surgery was considered to be one of the most terrible painful experiences any human being could endure. In 1798, Petit [28] spoke of pain in an address to medical students: "The eternal enemy of the human race ... that strikes with equal cruelty the child and the old, the weak and the strong, sparing neither talent nor rank, never put off by sex or age, who strikes down his victims amongst his friends in the bosom of his pleasures and without fearing the light of day any more than the silence of night. Against whom all foresight is in vain and defense uncertain, which appears to arm itself against us with all the forces of his nature." The introduction of anesthesia put an end to much of the immediate pain of surgery, but pain still remained an immense burden for many, eased only by the opioids of the apothecary, with or without the help of alcohol. Petit's lecture challenges our current view that pain can depend much less upon physical damage than on state of mind. His eloquence comes as a strong reminder of the limitations of that opinion, and, indeed, the popular view has usually been dominant—the belief that the causes of pain are primarily physical and are related to bodily damage.

Ancient views may not allow valid comparisons. Beecher [2], comparing battle injuries with civilian surgical wounds, argued in favor of differences related to the significance of the injury to the person. He provided evidence that for the same amount of tissue damage, the pain reported or experienced was less in the soldiers, who although wounded, knew they were out of danger and had fulfilled their obligations. In turn, that systematic evidence is open to question because, despite similar amounts of tissue being involved, differences in the extent of the surgical intervention, the time taken in operating, the need for clamping with forceps, and the number of ligatures, as well as the sites of injury, all may have varied among groups. Thus, while emotions can increase or decrease pain severity, we need to recognize that the evidence for the effect of the emotions in diminishing pain is largely anecdotal—even when it is quite striking—and the most striking evidence is primarily about acute or relatively acute pain. Many systematic studies of the effects of psychological management fail to show major gains in the relief of pain by psychological means. It is easy to find papers on chronic pain that show statistically significant improvements, but they are not usually impressive with respect to the reduction in pain scores, even though small benefits are well appreciated. The overall effects are significant but remain small, and the difference may be accounted for by a small group of specific responders within the study population.

The definition of pain published by the International Association for the Study of Pain (IASP) covers pain that may be of organic origin, but it equally covers pain of psychological origin. It was designed in order to meet just those needs: "Pain is an unpleasant sensory and emotional experience associated with actual or potential tissue damage and described in terms of such damage" [21]. The experience is described in terms of actual or potential damage, whether or not the precise cause is identified.

Organic features are the starting point and the model, but the etiology is deliberately left open.

Psychological Causes for Pain?

If we return to the Biblical quotation, the question arises: Was Jeremiah describing his experiences literally, or was he using a metaphor or an illustration? Similarly, with Montaigne, was it merely his fantasy to suppose that emotions can either cause or exacerbate pain? With respect to acute pain, we can accept that a muscle spasm caused by a surprise or by an involuntary movement might be painful. Occasionally, a muscle spasm is palpable and thus can give indirect confirmation of experiences being generated physiologically. Yet, in principle, it seems reasonable to accept that movements caused by being startled—such as occasional involuntary tightening of muscles in response to an alarming sound—might be counterproductive, producing a spasm where none existed before, and where the best response might be to escape rather than stay where you are and be overwhelmed.

Some sudden pains appear to be "psychogenic" but are in fact based on a physical mechanism such as muscle spasms. Others may be spontaneous physically based experiences, arising for example from the gastrointestinal tract, that are briefly unpleasant in a manner that suggests bodily harm, and so they meet the definition of pain and also are due to physiological responses. Startle responses can include pain arising on a physiological basis. Some sudden pains might be purely hallucinatory, although there is no proof. However, evidence that *persistent* pains occur purely from psychological factors is either unavailable or weak.

A prolonged "psychogenic" pain could be counterproductive biologically, and it seems unlikely that persistent peripheral pains have a psychological cause rather than a physical one. As long as they occur without other complications, such pains as brief cramps or minor discomforts are not usually important clinically. Frequent lightning pains are not a feature of any psychological illness, but they can have a physical origin in muscle spasms or nerve lesions and were formerly common with tabes dorsalis. Muscle spasm occurs fairly commonly as cramps, which certainly have at least a partly physical or pathophysiological basis. The syndrome of painful legs and moving toes (see the *Classification of Chronic Pain* of the IASP [21]) is an example of fairly sharp or stabbing pains that have an identifiable cause, in the form of nerve damage affecting peripheral nerves or the dorsal spinal cord.

It appears overall that recognizable psychological mechanisms for troublesome pain are not strong and have been overestimated by many clinical investigators, including myself.

Later Sources on Acute and Chronic Pain

Throughout the 19th- and 20th-century literature there are many reports dealing with psychological states affecting the body, as well as lengthy descriptions of hypochondriasis. Most often, even when called hypochondriasis, the complaints are later seen as having been physical in origin but modified by the patient's mood, being increased by anxiety or worry. In such cases, hypochondriasis is taken to be a physical disorder with many symptoms whose importance is perhaps overestimated by the patient. Hypochondriasis may occur as a specific diagnosis or as a hypochondriacal pattern of behavior. Some people worry more than others about lesser symptoms, and it is common for them to be concerned about physical symptoms and seek reassurance. Where reassurance is justified, it receives a good response in most individuals. However, another trend can be recognized, where a greater problem may exist. This second trend involves a minority of patients who are very difficult to reassure. The clinician should not spend too much time trying to persuade or convert them, but rather should take steps to limit the damage to their lives and encourage them when possible to continue normally. In a third group of patients, a depressive illness may produce hypochondriasis, and treatment for depression can provide impressive benefits.

The internist or general physician can see various patterns in patients who have a number of physical complaints, including pain. One pattern may be a minor transient physiological problem that is troublesome, or else more bothersome to the patient than the physician would ordinarily recognize. In such circumstances, the physician should be careful to understand that since the patient's experience can be of severe pain, a physical illness may indeed exist, although it is not fully explained and may not be harmful. Of course, physical illnesses should be investigated in these situations. Notoriously, dismissal of persistent complaints focused on a specific symptom can lead to misdiagnosis of organic disease, which may be rejected too readily in some cases because of the physician's lack of incentive to follow up a patient after negative investigations for organic disease. It is prudent to reexamine patients who have persistent physical complaints of pain, and to avoid being dogmatic in rejecting their experience.

Pain often occurs in patients who have a minor hypochondriacal illness, but in psychiatry, severe hypochondriacal pain is rare. The psychiatric diagnosis of hypochondriasis depends upon the patient fearing a serious physical disease while being convinced, at the same time, that it is present. The complaint is usually a physical symptom but sometimes a psychological one. The combination of fear and the illusory conviction of having a certain complaint characterizes the hypochondriacal patient. While pain often figures in the considerations of patients who have had injuries, it is very rarely the main focus of a hypochondriacal psychological disorder. Such disorders are relatively rare, and when they occur in nonpainful conditions they usually need psychiatric treatment. Some patients respond gratifyingly to antidepressants, on a somewhat unpredictable basis.

Classical hypochondriacal feelings or attitudes, or behavior, are more likely to be about nonpainful symptoms than about pain itself. As I described above, the essence of hypochondriacal symptoms for the psychiatrist is that the patient has a fear of having a symptom and a conviction that it is present. Gillespie [12] described these problems very clearly, and Pilowsky [29] developed an index based upon identification of these phenomena in patients with hypochondriasis. These severe psychological conditions are not usually difficult for the somatic specialties to identify. Pain is only rarely their principal feature. In such cases diagnosis is usually obvious, but internists and specialists in the organic disciplines need to be particularly careful to undertake all appropriate investigations, notwithstanding any irritation that the patient may generate by persistently complaining about an elusive physical symptom for which no organic cause can be demonstrated. In cases where there is doubt, diagnostic follow-up is obviously prudent.

Many symptoms in everyday life are brief and are never fully accounted for, but those that give rise to trouble are persistent and may involve misdiagnosis and subsequent regrets on the part of the attendant practitioner. Psychological complaints about a single organ by a patient who has no former well-established pattern of hypochondriasis in psychiatry will usually be diagnosed by the "organic" disciplines first and then by the psychiatrist. Pain is rare in this situation, but it may be severe when it occurs.

Chronic Pain

Following the Pearl Harbor attack in December 1941, the understanding and treatment of chronic pain was promoted by advances in treatment by the American medical services in the Pacific theater of World War II. Notably, John J. Bonica [4], almost single-handedly, led the further development and extension of nerve blocks for pain in the treatment of wounded soldiers from the Pacific theater. Seeking to achieve better pain management for his patients, Bonica recruited specialists from all the relevant disciplines he could find to work together as a group in order to reach accurate and effective diagnoses. This was the foundation of pain clinics throughout the world. Bonica always gave credit to F.A.D. Alexander for concomitantly developing pain clinics, but Alexander did not continue this work, whereas Bonica continued it with sustained devotion and skill in order to establish an international organization, the IASP, which encourages multidisciplinary work to resolve the problems of patients with chronic pain.

In the period of time from the 1930s (preceding Bonica) to the 1950s, overlapping with Bonica's work, psychoanalysts took to describing individual cases of patients with chronic pain whose pain was treated psychologically. These psychoanalysts described more than 30 individual cases of chronic pain that they attributed to issues in their patients' state of mind [23]. These cases are not particularly persuasive to a current reader, but an internist interested in psychoanalysis, George L. Engel, did have a major influence on the writing about, and treatment of, chronic pain for several decades. Claims like his, favoring psychological treatment, still linger.

Engel's patients led unsatisfactory lives. Their personal relationships were a mess, general dissatisfaction and unrewarding jobs were common, marriages broke up, as did second marriages, and social adjustment
was often poor. Continuing bad marriages and a background of childhood
misfortune and ill-treatment were recorded for many. In three papers, Engel [7–9] ascribed both facial pain and chronic pain in general to these
psychological causes. Other writers followed him, producing many papers
on facial pain and temporomandibular pain and dysfunction syndrome.
Later, this approach was argued to be misleading as it was based on uncontrolled and highly selective data [34].

Blumer and Heilbronn [3] also produced material concerning psychiatric changes in patients with diffuse pain, but like Engel's publications,
their views were based entirely upon an anecdotal series. Nor is there
any good evidence for the cure of chronic facial pain through the use of
prolonged psychotherapy or psychoanalysis. Contributions to the field of
orofacial pain were made by Marbach [16], with Raphael, a psychologist
investigating the background of patients with facial pain syndrome, supporting the view that the psychological phenomena were complications
rather than primary causal factors, although the notion of using surgery
was rejected for most cases.

Psychological theories were advanced for many years by Harold
G. Wolff [13,38] with regard to migraine, to the effect that a profound
psychological dysfunctional factor was causing the pain. The supporting
evidence was never of the systematic and controlled type currently held to
be necessary.

Salter et al. [32,33] criticized the lack of controls and selection in
the literature on the supposed psychogenesis of a common type of orofacial pain and demonstrated with concomitant simple psychological tests
that the patients did not have any marked psychological disturbance. The
best treatments other than surgery were physiotherapy and adjustment of
the bite by noninvasive methods and careful management.

Merskey and Hester [22] had previously noted that amitriptyline, the second tricyclic antidepressant on the market in North America
and the rest of the developed world, appeared to have an independent
analgesic action and attributed the improvement of patients' alleged "psychogenic pain" in some instances to the analgesic treatment of physical

causes of pain. The regular accompaniment of continuing severe pain seen clinically was minor or moderately severe psychological distress, and the response in pain patients treated with amitriptyline was interpreted as directly understandable in terms of the patients obtaining relief from their physical illness [37]. Studies by Watson et al. [36], Max et al. [17], and others provided cumulative evidence that the response of chronic pain, including facial pain, to antidepressants is regularly based on analgesic effects in patients, independently of the drugs' antidepressant action. The comorbid psychological changes are secondary, and experts agree today that amitriptyline and some other tricyclic antidepressants—but not all— have an independent analgesic action.

General practice studies have demonstrated that patients are highly selective in the items they bring to physicians for attention. They may suffer or accept considerable numbers of symptoms, especially pain, that they only present to general practitioners or specialists in circumstances that make the complaint more important than would otherwise be the case. For example, headaches in adults are often treated casually, whereas sore throats in children get prompt medical attention [1]. When headaches are present, they may be mentioned because they are new to the patient or unusually severe, or because they are causing emotional changes, or because the patient has a tendency to seek medical help at the earliest opportunity.

Diagnoses "in the Borderland"

Some pain syndromes may receive diagnoses of pain with a physical cause and depression. These syndromes include cervical sprains and other musculoskeletal complaints, chronic facial pain, migraine, "tension headache," and neuralgias. In current practice they are usually diagnosed reliably and only tend to raise doubts when compensation may be an issue. Thus, headache that follows "whiplash," i.e., cervical hyperextension injury, often or almost always follows damage to structures in the neck, but it is often rejected as exaggerated or purportedly "psychogenic" when it is associated with claims for financial compensation. Similarly, pain in the low back and related to the spinal column may be diagnosable, yet harder to prove as "genuine." This difficulty occurs particularly often with post-traumatic neck pain and headache, persistent migraine, and low back pain, when compensation may be an issue.

There are two typical variations in management with these conditions. Many cases are diagnosed by family practitioners, or by neurologists or specialists in musculoskeletal medicine, and receive appropriate medication and treatment. This is particularly true with any condition that has a discrete pattern such as classical migraine or the piriformis syndrome (when it is recognized!), and with almost any condition that has a specific defining feature that is acceptable as proof of an organic or pathophysiological process. However, many patients present problems because of chronic neck or back pain following injuries for which compensation may be available, and in these cases, if the complaint has no related symptoms or signs, there is often much dispute. Such dispute varies in intensity and importance from center to center depending on the experience and biases of physicians and the legal situation with regard to compensation, and on the financial and institutional ability to treat patients with physiotherapy, massage, and sometimes specific measures such as percutaneous rhizotomy [14].

Many patients who have well-established physical conditions and whose complaints correspond to an updated understanding are nevertheless denied compensation because the diagnostician fails to recognize—or chooses to ignore—relevant evidence. There is argument about whether the condition is (a) "real," i.e., clearly physical in origin; (b) psychological, i.e., due to an emotional condition for which the individual is not at fault but which nevertheless handicaps him or her; or (c) unfounded. I say "unfounded" or "unexplained" rather than the common allegations of malingering or hypochondriasis, or overstated claims, in order to use a fairly neutral term. In these cases we typically have a combination of psychological and physical complaints. Psychological complaints have been shown by Radanov et al. [31] to occur in patients who have significant physical changes giving rise to their whiplash complaints. Further, Bogduk and colleagues [14] have abundantly established that there are specific explanations for the occurrence of physical complaints that can be identified and successfully treated in carefully selected cases following whiplash.

Likewise, MacNab [15], an orthopedic surgeon based in Toronto, illustrated very clearly the physical injuries of the joints of the neck and also other injuries that may occur after whiplash-type events. He demonstrated that cervical hyperextension/flexion injuries induced in monkeys corresponded to the patterns that are observed with cervical whiplash in humans. On post mortem examination of the animals' spines, MacNab found damage to the facet joints plus disk lesions, partial disk lesions, and damage to the anterior longitudinal ligament.

There is no usual neurotic syndrome or psychological illness that will account for alleged psychogenic low back pain or neck pain. Despite many studies, there is no good evidence that psychological or psychiatric treatment per se will remove or greatly alleviate the common accompaniments of pain, unless the pain improves independently. However, some psychotropic medications may relieve pain through secondary independent analgesic effects. Counseling may assist the overall situation, and antidepressants may help relieve the depression itself, besides being independently analgesic in some cases (such as amitriptyline).

Concomitant States

What has been said so far points to the role of pain in causing emotional change. The important question remaining in regard to symptoms is to what extent comorbid emotional states require recognition as causes or consequences. The fundamental issue is the status of the patient's physical condition in relationship to his or her pain, work, domestic responsibilities, income, and overall ability to manage. The pain referred to in the historical quotations given above is acute pain, occurring within days of stress or injury to the body. It is said to be physical and originating from within. It is a bodily sensation, and the description is given in physical terms. It could be a pathophysiological response to stress or a symbol for a physical cause. Still, the primary notion is of the patient expressing concern over a change felt in the body. However, as one goes through historical accounts and modern reports of bodily complaints and psychological states, there are detailed descriptions of hypochondriasis.

The word "hypochondriasis" has a range of meanings varying through the centuries. Currently it means an excessive focus on any bodily complaint, despite valid reassurance. It is best seen in some cases as the way in which the patient treats the seriousness of the issue. In the literature in English on this subject I found no persuasive report showing that specific painful conditions that would be treated today by a pain physician would primarily require psychological treatment, except for some cases of headache or facial pain if they have been associated with ideas of a psychological etiology. Bradley [5] found in patients with depression that when the pain first occurred with depression, it responded to antidepressant treatment, but that when it preceded the depression it tended to persist afterwards. This series is small and selected, but it suggests that mood can exacerbate persistent pain that is present for other reasons, and that there is no reason to suppose that the pain was due to some mysterious additional factor.

Pain, Compensation, and Dual Diagnoses

Dual diagnoses occur particularly often in individuals seeking compensation. They are usually forms of depression and anxiety combined with the effects of a physical condition. Schmiedebach [35] traced arguments over compensation and post-traumatic conditions to the first Prussian laws passed in 1838 on workplace injuries. Patterns of compensation were developed for workers and soon also for passengers injured in collisions on railways; by 1871 mines, quarries, and factories were also covered in Germany. At first the workers' unions or associations had a significant influence upon the choice of physicians who would examine individuals and report on them with regard to their insurance. Then, a change in the law brought in an insurance liability bureau so that costs were controlled by employers. As this change occurred, insurance companies appointed physicians to examine for them, and more physicians were needed. Medical schools increased their intake and output for that reason. Arguments about feigned illness appeared, and estimates ranged from less than 1% to as high as 33%. Eugen Bleuler, a distinguished psychiatrist who was classed as a "moderate" in the argument, blamed workers' wives "for telling their husbands to feign severe nervous ailments" so that the husbands could stay at home with them at times and help out.

It appears that ever since insurance became available, there were always some physicians who were being paid—perfectly legally—by insurance companies to provide reports on patients. Those physicians provided a more negative view of pain than their colleagues who supported—and were paid by—the patients. Miller [25] provides a good example of a distinguished neurologist who took a very negative view of patients' pain, supporting a previous statement by another English neurologist who later worked in New York, Foster Kennedy, to the effect that "a compensation neurosis [in which pain was often included] is a state of mind born out of fear, kept alive by avarice, stimulated by lawyers, and cured by a verdict." This claim was rejected by Mendelson [19] on the basis of 10 follow-up articles in the literature, of which every one reported some claimants who remained ill after the settlement of their claims.

There is a sad recent history in Canada, along with Britain Germany, Norway, the United States, and Australia (and I presume other developed countries), of similar attitudes to compensable pain. The automobile insurance company of the Province of Quebec, a body appointed by the government of the province, commissioned a report [30] that was held to be heavily biased in favor of the insurer and unfair to many injured people [24]. The Province of Saskatchewan did likewise (with the help of two of the individuals who had assisted in producing the Quebec report [6]), and other provinces in Canada have taken a similar approach but slightly less vigorously, although currently Ontario has imposed severe restrictions on the amount of money that can be claimed for treatment purposes by injured individuals. (This happens not infrequently, and not only in Canada, before election times, when it seems that insurance companies may advise governments that they need to raise their fees before the election unless the level of compensation declines.) Conflicts over payments for injured workers are more muted in this jurisdiction, partly because the workers' organizations also tend not to support their members thoroughly because they do not like to see increases in workers' insurance fees that come out of their wages.

Compensation is not often mentioned in technical discussions of pain, but it is a very persistent factor that can be described as "the elephant in the closet," affecting the recognition of pain and its causes, associations with injury, and psychological changes. The arguments resemble patterns of warfare where new weapons are met with new defenses that are countered with further new weapons. The front over which the battle rages is the extent of identification between psychiatric illness and physical complaints.

My personal experience was that I started by attempting to follow up on Engel's ideas and identify patients resembling those he described and to compare them first with psychiatric patients seen in a similar setting who did not have pain. I found that the group with supposedly psychogenic physical complaints and possible psychiatric problems were somewhat similar in their degree of anxiety and depression to other psychiatric patients in a general hospital location and were also compatible with Engel's claims [7]. Later, comparing patients with and without identified neurological lesions in general hospital locations, I found that both groups had similar levels of "neurosis" [22]. Dual diagnoses appeared to reflect the influence of chronic pain on samples of the population that were experiencing both a physical illness and its emotional effects.

The issue of entitlement for pain in the 19th century in Britain and North America caused a long-running controversy over "railway spine." This term refers to injury to the spinal column and complaints of neck and back pain after collisions that occurred when one train ran into another. Controversy arose in Continental Europe as word spread along with the railroads. Patients' doctors argued that they were suffering significant physical injury called "concussion of the spine." Erichsen [10,11], Professor of Surgery at University College Hospital in London, England, argued that disturbance to the nervous system might be physically produced in railway accidents, without hemorrhage, either by temporary disablement of cells or perhaps by the disruption of their connection or "concussion of the spine." He had attributed the complaints of many of his patients to a physical impact, noting that the passengers with their backs toward the direction of impact in railway collisions were the worst affected. At that time many railway carriages had compartments in which passengers sat facing each other across the width of the carriage. If there was a collision, those experiencing the impact from their rear would be affected the most, having symptoms that can be seen to resemble whiplash. Erichsen's views were rejected by some physicians, particularly those working for railway companies, such as Paige [27]. It seems likely that the same mechanism of impact from behind that jerked the heads and necks of railway passengers is involved in the continuing issue of cervical sprain injury from motor vehicle collisions.

Despite the existence of some articles [e.g., 18], which have been much questioned because of a difference between the evidence and the conclusions [see 19], there is no basis to argue that the pattern of pain injury is due to depression causing the pain. Radanov et al. [31] are particularly relevant here because they studied whiplash patients promptly after injury and found that patients' depression emerged after their pain had become established.

The comorbid conditions that I have been considering have a strong relationship to psychiatry. Comorbid conditions exist relating to loss of use when the individual is less able to function generally. One comorbid condition that is common is post-traumatic stress disorder. Another comorbid condition, noteworthy for its production of a second organic disorder, is hypothyroidism, with the combination of—fortunately—wholly recoverable painful hypothyroidism and myxedema commonly presenting as a version of fibromyalgia. This brings me to the last condition needing description: fibromyalgia.

Fibromyalgia has been a subject of controversy, very much on the same basis as the controversy about musculoskeletal pain and psychiatry, because of suppositions, arguments, and misapprehensions that fibromyalgia is a psychological disorder. There is abundant evidence against this hypothesis (see the article by McLean and Clauw [18]; see also the chapter in this volume on comorbidities of fibromyalgia). There is abundant evidence that glial cells, previously regarded merely as supporting structures, make a valuable contribution to the neurochemical basis for conduction, showing widespread changes throughout regions of the brain in a nonsegmental pattern in response to noxious stimulation and when patients feel pain. This evidence makes nonsense of arguments that suggest that the syndrome of fibromyalgia has nothing to do with injury and is one that patients can readily control by managing their emotions, for which they have primary responsibility.

From the 19th century onward, the reality of pain has been the topic for discussion and perhaps—or indeed—a problem that tends to be minimized. The issue of entitlement for pain relief became notable in the same century, with the development of both anesthesia, which took a lot of the dread away from pain, and workers' compensation, along with the long-running controversy over railway spine.

In my view, there is a persistent tendency for patients' pain to be minimized and rejected. When that cannot be done, reasons tend to be found to change the law, as is happening currently in Ontario, before an election and apparently at the request of insurance companies who may advise the government and public that their motor vehicle premiums will need to increase if the insurance industry is to stay solvent. For further discussion of this topic, see Schmiedebach [35] and Merskey [20].

References

[1]   Banks MH, Beresford SA, Morrell DC, Waller JJ, Watkins CJ. Factors influencing demand for primary medical care in women aged 20–24 years: a preliminary report. Int J Epidemiol 1975;4:189–95.

[2]   Beecher HK. Relationship of significance of wound to the pain experienced. JAMA 1956;161:1609–13.

[3]   Blumer D, Heilbronn M. The pain-prone disorder: a clinical and psychological profile. Psychosomatics 1981;22:395–7, 401–2.

[4]   Bonica JJ. The management of pain. Philadelphia: Lea & Febiger; 1953.

[5]   Bradley JJ. Severe localized pain associated with the depressive syndrome. Br J Psychiatry 1963;109:741–5.

[6]   Cassidy JD, Carroll LJ, Côté P, Lemstra M, Berglund A, Nygren A. Effect of eliminating compensation for pain and suffering on the outcome of insurance claims for whiplash injury. N Engl J Med 2000;342:1179–86.

[7]   Engel GL. Primary atypical facial neuralgia. An hysterical conversion symptom. Psychosom Med 1951;13:375–96.

[8]   Engel GL. 'Psychogenic' pain. Med Clin North Am 1958;42:1481–96.

[9]   Engel GL. 'Psychogenic' pain and the pain prone patient. Am J Med 1959;26;899–918.

[10] Erichsen, Sir John E. On railway and other injuries of the spine and nervous system in their clinical and medico legal aspects (a new and revised edition). New York: William Wood; 1886.

[11] Erichsen, Sir John E. On concussion of the spine, nervous shock and other excessive injuries to the nervous system. Philadelphia: Henry C. Lee; 1866.

[12] Gillespie RD. Hypochondria. London: Kegan Paul; 1929.

[13] Hardy JD, Wolff HG, Goodell H. Pain sensation and reaction. Baltimore: Williams & Wilkins; 1952.

[14] Lord SM, Barnsley L, Willis BJ, MacDonald GJ, Bogduk N. Percutaneous radiofrequency neurotomy of the cervical medial branch. A validate treatment for chronic cervical zygapophyseal joint pain. N Engl J Med 1996;395:1721–6.

[15] MacNab I, McCulloch J. Neck ache and shoulder pain. Baltimore: Williams & Wilkins; 1994. p. 141–3.

[16] Marbach JJ. The "temporomandibular pain dysfunction syndrome" personality: fact or fiction? J Oral Rehabil 1992;19:545–60.

[17] Max MB, Schafer SC, Culnane M, Smoller B, Dubner R, Gracely RH. Amitriptyline, but not lorazepam, relieves postherpetic neuralgia. Neurology 1988;38:1427–32.

[18] McLean SA, Clauw DJ. Biomedical models of fibromyalgia. Disabil Rehabil 2005;27:659–65.

[19] Mendelson G. Not "cured by a verdict." Effect of legal settlement on compensation claimants. Med J Aust 1982;2:132–4.

[20] Merskey H. Pain in somatization disorders and psychiatric illness. In: Cervero F, Jensen TS. Handbook of clinical neurology, 3rd series. Edinburgh: Elsevier; 2006. p. 803–16.

[21] Merskey H, Bogduk N. Classification of chronic pain: descriptions of chronic pain syndromes and definitions of pain terms, 2nd ed. Seattle: IASP Press; 1994.

[22] Merskey H, Hester RN. The treatment of chronic pain with psychotropic drugs. Postgrad Med J 1972;48:594–8.

[23] Merskey H, Spear FG. Pain: psychological and psychiatric aspects. London: Baillière, Tindall & Cassell; 1967.

[24] Merskey H, Teasell RW. A troubling story: insurance and medical research in Saskatchewan. J Whiplash Rel Dis 2003;215–8. Reprinted from Pain Res Manage 2002;7:65–7.
[25] Miller HG. Accident neurosis. BMJ 1961;1:919–25, 992–8.
[26] Montaigne De ME. Essais (1580). Book I, Chap. 40, 374–5 (Le Clerc J-V, editor). Paris: Garnier; 1865. Book I, Chap. 14 (Trechmann EJ, translator). Oxford: Oxford University Press; 1927.
[27] Paige HW. Injuries of the spine and spinal cord, without apparent mechanical lesion and nervous shock in their surgical and medical legal aspects. London: J. & A. Churchill; 1883.
[28] Petit MA. Discours sur la douleur. Lyon: Reymann et al.; 1798.
[29] Pilowsky I. Dimensions of hypochondriasis. Br J Psychiatry 1967;113:89–93.
[30] Quebec Task Force on Whiplash-Associated Disorders. Whiplash-associated disorders (WAD): redefining "whiplash" and its management. Société Automobile du Quebec; 1995.
[31] Radanov BP, Di Stefano G, Schnidrig A, Ballinari P. Psychosocial stress in recovery from common whiplash. Lancet 1991;338:712–5.
[32] Salter M, Brooke RI, Merskey H. Letter to the editor. Re: TMPDS (Greene et al.) Pain 1984;20:209.
[33] Salter M, Brooke RI, Merskey H, Fichter GF, Kapusianyk DH. Is the temporomandibular pain and dysfunction syndrome a disorder of the mind? Pain 1983;17:151–66.
[34] Salter M, Merskey H, Brooke RI. Temporomandibular pain and dysfunction syndrome. The relationship of clinical and psychological data to outcome. J Behav Med 1986;9:97–109.
[35] Schmiedebach HP. Post-traumatic neurosis in 19th century Germany: a disease in political juridical and professional context. Hist Psychiatry 1999;10:27–57.
[36] Watson GD, Chandarana PC, Merskey H. Relationships between pain and schizophrenia. Br J Psychiatry 1981;138:33–6.
[37] Woodforde JM, Merskey H. Personality traits of patients with chronic pain. J Psychosom Res 1972;16:167–72.
[38] Wolff HG. In discussion of the relation of attitude and suggestion to the perception of and reaction to pain. In: Wolff HG, Goodell H, editors. Proceedings of the Association for Research in Nervous and Mental Disease, Vol. 23. Association for Research in Nervous and Mental Disease; 1943. p. 447.

Correspondence to: Harold Merskey, DM, FRCP, FRCPsych, FRCPC, Professor Emeritus of Psychiatry, University of Western Ontario, 72 Logan Avenue, London, Ontario, Canada N5Y 2P9.

Part I

General Aspects, Epidemiology, and Models

Epidemiology of Pain and Non-Pain Comorbidities

Clare H. Dominick[a] and Fiona M. Blyth[b,c]

[a]University of Sydney Pain Management Research Institute, North Shore Hospital;
[b]Centre for Education and Research on Ageing, Concord Hospital;
[c]Sydney School of Public Health, University of Sydney,
Sydney, New South Wales, Australia

The study of chronic pain and non-pain comorbidity requires insights from different scientific perspectives. The epidemiological approach offers insights about the distribution and determinants of chronic pain and non-pain comorbidity within population subgroups, and also about the factors that influence the whole population, such as socioeconomic status. Uniquely, epidemiologists can also use a life-course approach to examine how the interrelationship of chronic pain and non-pain comorbidity develops and changes over the human lifespan.

Whereas clinical epidemiology focuses on the application of epidemiology to clinical settings, population epidemiology considers a broader population, including those with health conditions who are doing well, and those who are in need of help but are not seeking care. As populations age, the impact on the health, well-being, and functional status of individuals experiencing multiple health problems, including chronic pain, is becoming more apparent, as is the effect on health care systems. The population burden of chronic pain, along with any incremental effects from non-pain comorbidity, therefore has potential implications for public health, health policy, and delivery of health services.

There are several reasons why we might be interested in the relationship between chronic pain and non-pain comorbidity: does the presence of non-pain comorbidity influence the reporting of pain? Does it influence the outcomes associated with having chronic pain (such as functional status)? In addition, combinations of specific conditions may have an amplified effect on outcomes, exceeding what would be expected by the additive effect of two conditions occurring together. For example, the risk of disability in older people with comorbid arthritis and hypertension has been shown to be much higher than the sum of the individual risks of disability when each condition occurs alone [24]. Such epidemiological findings point to the possibility of shared risk factors and shared etiological pathways and offer new directions for research and, possibly, treatments.

In Part II of the book, the relationship of pain to specific non-pain comorbidity is explored in detail. The purpose of this chapter is to provide an overview of epidemiological approaches to investigating the relationships between chronic pain and non-pain comorbidity. Two approaches are commonly found in the literature. One focuses on pain as the index condition, with additional health burdens, whether differentiated by condition or not, considered as comorbidity (Fig. 1). The other, a multimorbidity perspective, considers the influence of an individual's total health burden (of which one component is pain) and its relationship with health outcomes. Interactions among conditions can be considered within both approaches, and both direct and indirect influences on chronic pain and health outcomes have been established.

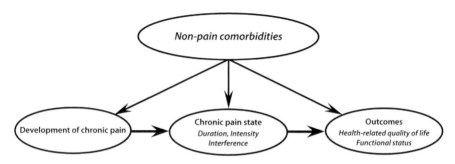

Fig. 1. Approaches to studying the influence of comorbidity on chronic pain.

Comorbidity and Multimorbidity: Concepts and Definitions

The empirical work on this topic to date uses a variety of implicit or explicit theoretical perspectives in framing questions about health burden. When health burden is viewed from a population perspective, environmental influences also need to be considered. This approach is congruent with the biopsychosocial models of pain, which explicitly acknowledge factors acting at different levels from the cell to the environment in the causes and expression of pain. Thus, we will provide a conceptual framework that can be used to underpin much of the work in this area.

Research on multimorbidity is a developing field. In recent years there has been growing recognition of the need for consistency in the definition and measurement of the terms "comorbidity," "multimorbidity," and related constructs such as burden of disease and frailty [9,16,43,59].

A simple definition of comorbidity is the "concurrent existence and occurrence of two or more medically diagnosed diseases in the same individual" [43]. However, increasingly the term "comorbidity" is used to refer to concurrent conditions, additional to a specific index condition under study [16,60]. In contrast, multimorbidity has a broader definition and does not refer to an index condition. For example, Valderas et al. [59] refer to multimorbidity as "the co-occurrence of multiple chronic or acute diseases and medical conditions within one person without any reference to an index condition," while Boyd and Fortin [9] define it as the "co-existence of two or more chronic conditions, where one is not necessarily more central than others."

Despite increasing agreement on definitions, differences are still apparent in several areas. On a broad conceptual level, definitions diverge in relation to the scope of factors that are included. Some definitions include, for example, disability as well as impairment [9]. However, other multimorbidity definitions exclude socioeconomic factors, lifestyle factors, and access to health care, as well as disability, because these factors are related to the environment [43].

Even definitions that focus on direct measures of poor health differ in terms of the "conditions" or "diseases" that are included, and the classification systems from which they are derived. Some definitions include both acute and chronic conditions [43], while others focus only on chronic conditions [9]. From a measurement perspective, there is no agreement on the number and type of diseases to be included in multimorbidity indices and how these indices account for the relative severity of the conditions that are included [16,43].

Although these factors have been organized differently at a conceptual level, most authors acknowledge that a broad set of factors needs to be taken into account when considering multimorbidity. The best way of doing so is under debate. Notions of load, such as "disease burden," "comorbid load," and "allostatic load" are also common in relation to multimorbidity and can be considered at population and individual levels. Models of allostasis and allostatic load take a multisystems perspective and delineate how social, psychological, and physical stressors can translate into physiological dysregulation. Allostatic load is the wear and tear on the body and brain resulting from chronic dysregulation (overactivity or inactivity) of physiological systems and is considered a broad spectrum risk factor for a range of diseases [26,41,49]. Measures of chronic condition load can be considered proxy measures of allostatic load because physiological measures of allostatic load are associated with a range of chronic conditions [40]. Accumulated load is being investigated as a contributor to a range of outcomes [41].

Conceptually, integrating the broad sets of factors included within the term "multimorbidity" and related concepts is very similar to the challenges of operationalizing the biopsychosocial model that underpins our understanding of chronic pain. To adequately account for the incidence, prevalence, associations, and consequences of chronic pain in the general population, interconnected physiological, psychological, and social models are needed. Ideally, these models would account for the full range of contributory factors across social, psychological, and biological domains and would explain their interaction in the context of a life-course perspective. Unsurprisingly, full articulation is rare, given the challenge of the task.

The development of chronic conditions, including chronic pain, is now often considered from a life-course perspective that identifies a range of possible interacting pathways in the development of chronic conditions [4]. Ben-Shlomo and Kuh [4] defined the life-course approach to chronic disease epidemiology as the "study of long-term effects on chronic disease risk of physical and social exposures during gestation, childhood, adolescence, young adulthood, and later adult life. It includes studies of the biological, behavioral, and psychosocial pathways that operate across an individual's life course, as well as across generations, to influence the development of chronic diseases." Models may include critical periods in development that may be associated with risk factors or effect modifiers later in life. Models may also identify the accumulation of risk through exposure to independent insults or correlated insults, resulting in clustering of risks or "chains of risk."

Evidence supporting the development of chronic diseases from a life-course perspective is increasing [33,34]; however, data informing a life-course perspective in relation to chronic pain remain sparse. Mac-Farlane [38] reports that developmental and life-course perspectives for chronic pain are in their infancy. Similarly, Walco [62] noted that developmental perspectives and longitudinal studies of pain are still relatively uncommon [29].

Chronic pain models incorporating biological and psychological factors are increasingly sophisticated and well articulated, whereas the psychosocial and social factors are less fully examined [7]. From biopsychosocial and life-course perspectives, many factors will interact to affect current experience of pain for people with multiple conditions. Some factors will have been the result of developmental processes, while others may be more closely related to features of the current biopsychosocial nexus and may be more responsive to intervention.

The potential interactions among factors engender a complex set of challenges for researchers and health service providers. Fig. 2 provides one perspective on the range of factors potentially influencing the experience of chronic pain across the life course and their impact on health-related quality of life and functional outcomes. Social, psychological, and biological pathways contribute to chronic pain and also to non-pain comorbidities. The diagram indicates that factors involved in these pathways may interact to exacerbate or mitigate a range of health outcomes. Some of the current evidence about the association of these factors with chronic pain and non-pain comorbidities and related outcomes is outlined later in this chapter.

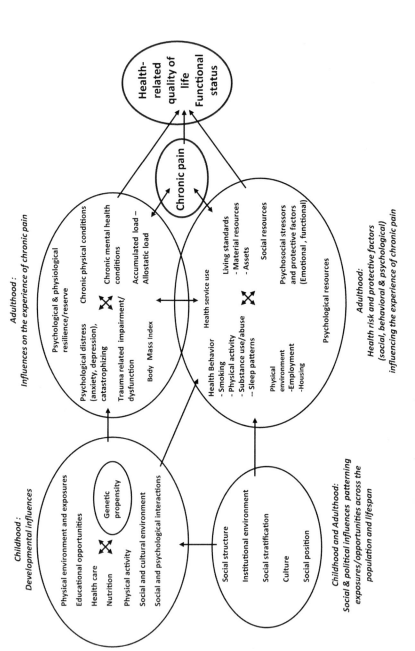

Fig. 2. Life-course influences on the development of chronic pain.

Epidemiological Approaches to Measuring Chronic Pain and Non-Pain Comorbidity

This section gives a brief overview of common approaches used in epidemiological studies of chronic pain and non-pain comorbidity. The list is not exhaustive, and there is still considerable heterogeneity in how both pain and comorbidity are measured.

Epidemiological Approaches to Measuring Chronic Pain

Epidemiological studies demonstrate considerable heterogeneity in their identification of participants with chronic pain. Some studies define chronic pain as a condition in its own right [50], and participants' pain status is ascertained with questions about duration of pain (e.g., [14,21]), which may be restricted to asking about pain in particular body sites (e.g., [53]). Other studies take a condition-specific approach to defining chronic pain, ascertaining first whether participants have conditions where pain is a common experience (for example, arthritis or a wider range of musculoskeletal conditions) and then asking about pain duration (e.g., [19,32]). A third approach is to explicitly define pain as a symptom, and then use symptom-based measures to define pain status [20,45].

Cross-sectional studies measure pain, non-pain comorbidity, and other factors of interest (for example, functional status) at one point in time. Such studies are unable to address causation and chronology, but they can identify strong or amplified associations between pain and non-pain comorbidity. Longitudinal studies follow individuals for a certain period, measuring risk factor exposures and outcomes over time. These studies can address chronology and provide some evidence of causal relationships by confirming the temporal relationship between exposures and outcomes. Life-course studies, as outlined above in the section "Comorbidity and Multimorbidity," offer the potential to examine cumulative and interacting risks for chronic diseases over many years.

Epidemiological Approaches to Measuring Comorbidity

There is no consensus on how best to measure comorbidity in epidemiological studies of pain, and different approaches have been taken, including the following:

1) Summed counts of conditions, which may be ascertained by self-report or sourced from records or based on criterion-based diagnostic interviews. For example, Eggermont et al. [19] used counts of self-reported doctor-diagnosed cardiorespiratory conditions, diabetes, and depressive symptoms in a study examining how pain characteristics such as pain location and pain severity were related to physical performance measures in community-dwelling older people.

2) Weighted counts that explicitly take into account dimensions such as disease severity. The best-known example of measures of this type is the Charlson Index [11]. For example, Singh and Lewallen [52] used a modification of the Charlson Index in a study identifying predictors of pain and medication use in a clinical cohort of patients who had total hip replacement surgery.

3) Approaches that use statistical simulation techniques to examine the potential impact of complex permutations of multiple interactions between comorbid conditions. For example, Merikangas et al. used statistical simulation to estimate the individual and combined effects of physical and mental health conditions on role disability using data from a large national survey [42].

4) Measures based on impairment of organ systems, such as the Cumulative Illness Ratings Scale [36], which also takes into account severity of impairment. For example, Leong et al. used this measure in a study that examined the relationship of medical comorbidity with aspects of pain experience in a cohort of patients attending a geriatric pain clinic [35].

5) Symptom-based rather than disease-based approaches, where pain is characterized as a symptom rather than as a condition in its own right, and the burden is symptom-based rather than condition-based. For example, Elliott et al. conducted a community-based descriptive study of 25 common health symptoms that included back pain, headache, and joint pain [20].

In a recent systematic review of the literature describing the development of weighted multimorbidity indices, more than half the studies included provided no explicit rationale for selecting the conditions included in the index [16]. In addition, there was variability in the populations studied, the sources of data on conditions, and the outcomes for which the measures were developed.

Context is very important here. If the primary focus of a population study is health in general, then frequently it is the case that information is collected on only a subset of health conditions, and the characterization of comorbidity is limited to those selected conditions. Generally speaking, the intent of measuring comorbidity here is to take into account its potential influence on the relationship between pain and outcomes such as functional limitations or health care use. In the study by Merikangas et al. given as an example above, musculoskeletal conditions and major depression were found to be most strongly related to the number of disability days, once the presence of comorbidity was rigorously taken into account using simulation methods [42].

Frailty measures in the elderly and measures of global self-rated health in populations of any age capture unique aspects of health burden that are not easily captured by measures based on condition counts. While there are several different measures of frailty that reflect differing perspectives on the components of frailty [47], the common core element is limited physiological reserves due to decline in function across multiple physiological systems. While frailty shares some overlap with comorbidity, it also has distinct dimensions [25,46]. Intrusive pain, experienced either as acute pain per se or as an acute exacerbation of persistent pain, can also be conceptualized as an additional challenge to the physiological reserves of older people. In a recent cohort study of older men, frailty was significantly associated with moderate to severe pain [8].

The global self-rated health measure is widely used to assess health-related quality of life. Self-rated health is measured with a single question asking respondents to rate their health on a scale from excellent to poor or very poor. There is some variation in how this question is framed (for example, asking respondents to rate their health now compared to a year ago, or compared to other people who are the same age as they are, or simply asking them to rate their health now). Self-rated health is a robust predictor of subsequent mortality [27]. Cohort studies have shown that self-rated health is strongly associated with a range of biomarkers in epidemiological studies [31] and is related to both physical and mental health [51]. Studies have shown a strong cross-sectional relationship between chronic pain and poorer self-rated health (e.g., [39]), as well as a prospective relationship between poorer self-rated health and incident pain conditions (e.g., [44]).

The Influence of Other Chronic Conditions on the Experience of Chronic Pain

A range of factors are associated with chronic pain, as outlined in Fig. 2. Comorbid physical and mental health conditions comprise an important set of factors contributing to the risk of chronic pain [13]. Recent analysis has started to clarify some of the relationships between concurrent conditions and chronic pain [18]. The nature of the relationships varies and may be direct or indirect. Evidence suggests that both accumulated comorbid load and several discrete chronic physical conditions are independently associated with chronic pain. That is, comorbid conditions do not need to have an independent association with chronic pain to increase the risk of chronic pain. Instead, they may contribute through an accumulation of load. Both specific conditions and accumulated comorbid load may contribute to the risk of chronic pain, either through the additional psychological, behavioral, and social demands and stress relating to the management of the conditions themselves and any associated disability [55], or more directly through dysregulated physiological mechanisms [26,28,50].

Risk of chronic pain appears to increase additively in relation to comorbid chronic conditions; that is, it appears to increase in line with the addition of risks associated with each comorbid condition. An exception may be arthritis and neck/back disorders, which may interact to increase risk beyond what would be expected from the addition of their individual risk [18].

Depression and anxiety are positively associated with physical conditions, although the association is stronger with some physical conditions than others [48,56]. Depression and anxiety are also strongly and independently associated with chronic pain [1–3,15]. Models of the relationship between chronic pain and depression are still under debate; however, more recent models consider that chronic pain and depression are distinct interacting conditions [56,61]. Recent research results indicate that arthritis and neck or back disorders may interact with anxiety or depression to increase the risk of chronic pain synergistically [18].

The Influence of Health Risk and Protective Factors on Chronic Pain

Particular health risk and protective factors such as smoking, physical activity, and body mass index are associated with the development of a range of chronic diseases [63]. These factors have also been found to be associated with chronic pain. The extent to which these factors are associated with an increased risk of chronic pain is yet to be established, as studies that control for a range of possible confounders need to be conducted.

The Association of Sociodemographic Factors with Multimorbidity and Chronic Pain in the General Population

Most of the information we have about chronic pain and multimorbidity has been derived from patient populations rather than from the general population. Patient populations provide an important focus in the clinical realm but potentially limit the conceptualization of relationships among the full range of factors and responses contributing to incidence, prevalence, and consequences. The association of the broader social environment with multimorbidity and chronic pain provides a public health perspective on the relationship between chronic pain and non-pain comorbidity and some insight on the social patterning of risk factors and conditions.

Both chronic pain and other chronic conditions are strongly associated with sociodemographic factors. Multimorbidity and chronic pain both increase in prevalence with age, but they are not confined to older age groups (e.g., [18,57]). People in lower socioeconomic groups have higher chronic pain prevalence estimates, whether measured from an individual or environmental perspective [e.g., 17,29], and are more likely to have multiple chronic conditions than those in high socioeconomic groups. Many studies, although not all, indicate that women are more likely than men to report chronic pain and are more likely to report multiple chronic conditions [e.g., 17,18].

Social relationships, including social networks and social support, are associated with the development of a range of chronic conditions and with mortality (e.g., [5,49,58]). However, the mechanisms are not well understood, although there is evidence for both direct and buffering (moderating) effects [54]. For chronic conditions, the influence of social relationships differs according to the type of support (including the quality of support over time) and the stage of the disease process [6,58]. In general, greater diversity of social relationships and perceived support appear protective, whereas social losses, negative interactions, and loneliness may be detrimental to health [12]. Social relationships are also associated with successful adjustment to chronic disease [55]. Similarly, the evidence base regarding the effects of social relationships on the development and maintenance of chronic pain is growing. Much research has been based on operant models, but other models are being proposed as potentially providing different insights on the positive and negative effects of social relationships on chronic pain and associated disability (e.g., [10,22,37]). As with chronic disease research, the complexity of the interrelationships among factors is evident.

Conclusions

With the increase in life expectancy and also in the prevalence of chronic conditions in both developed and developing countries, chronic pain and comorbid chronic conditions are important potential drivers of the population burden of poor health, reduced quality of life, and impaired functional status. Researching how chronic pain and non-pain comorbidity develop over the human lifespan and how each relates to the other offers the opportunity to understand the shared causal pathways of chronic pain with some comorbid conditions, and also the influence of non-pain comorbidity on chronic pain and vice versa. Progress in this regard will require a debate about how chronic pain and non-pain comorbidity should be conceptualized, and subsequently measured, in epidemiological studies.

As multimorbidity per se has a major impact on health outcomes and health care use [23], it is also critical that researchers and clinicians within the pain community think broadly about pain and non-pain comorbidity. Fortin et al. [23] have highlighted the limitations of using a condition-specific approach to patients with complex, intertwined health problems. This caution also extends to the incorporation of key social and psychological factors within this perspective, which will be critical for the development of nuanced models and interventions.

References

[1] Arnow BA, Hunkeler EM, Blasey CM, Lee J, Constantino MJ, Fireman B, Kraemer HC, Dea R, Robinson R, Hayward C. Comorbid depression, chronic pain and disability in primary care. Psychosom Med 2006;68:262–8.
[2] Asmundson GJ, Katz J. Understanding the co-occurrence of anxiety disorders and chronic pain: state-of-the-art. Depression Anxiety 2009;26:888–901.
[3] Bair MJ, Wu J, Damush TM, Sutherland JM, Kroenke K. Association of depression and anxiety alone and in combination with chronic musculoskeletal pain in primary care patients. Psychosom Med 2008;70:890–7.
[4] Ben-Shlomo Y, Kuh D. A life course approach to chronic disease epidemiology: conceptual models, empirical challenges and interdisciplinary perspectives. Int J Epidemiol 2002;31:285–93.
[5] Berkman LF, Glass T. Social integration, social networks, social support, and health. In: Berkman LF, Kawachi I, editors. Social epidemiology. New York: Oxford University Press; 2000.
[6] Birditt K, Antonucci TC. Life sustaining irritations? Relationship quality and mortality in the context of chronic illness. Soc Sci Med 2008;67:1291–9.
[7] Blyth FM, Macfarlane GJ, Nicholas MK. The contribution of psychosocial factors to the development of chronic pain: the key to better outcomes for patients? Pain 2007;129:8–11.
[8] Blyth FM, Rochat S, Cumming RG, Creasey H, Handelsman DJ, Le Couteur DG, Naganathan V, Sambrook PN, Seibel MJ, Waite LM. Pain, frailty and comorbidity on older men: the CHAMP study. Pain 2008:224–30.
[9] Boyd CM, Fortin M. Future of multimorbidity research: how should understanding of multimorbidity inform health system design? Public Health Rev 2010;32:1–18.
[10] Cano A, Williams AC de C. Social interaction in pain: reinforcing pain behaviors or building intimacy? Pain 2010;149:9–11.
[11] Charlson ME, Pompei P, Ales KL, MacKenzie CR. A new method of classifying prognostic comorbidity in longitudinal studies: development and validation. J Chron Dis 1987;40:373–83.
[12] Cohen S, Janicki-Deverts D. Can we improve our physical health by altering our social networks? Perspect Psychol Sci 2009;4:375–8.
[13] Croft P. Disease-related pain: an introduction. In: Croft P, Blyth FM, van der Windt D, editors. Chronic pain epidemiology: from aetiology to public health. Oxford: Oxford University Press, 2010. p. 203–8.
[14] Currow DC, Agar M, Plummer JL, Blyth FM, Abernethy AP. Chronic pain in South Australia: population levels that interfere extremely with activities of daily living. Aust N Z J Public Health 2010;34:232–9.
[15] Demyttenaere K, Bruffaerts R, Lee S, Levinson D, de Girolamo G, Nakane H, Mneimneh Z, Lara C, de Graaf R, Scott KM, Gureje O, Stein DJ, Haro JM, Bromet EJ, Kessler RC, Alonso J, von Korff M. Mental disorders among persons with chronic back or neck pain: results from the world mental health surveys. Pain 2007;129:332–42.
[16] Diederichs C, Berger K, Bartels DB, Diederichs C, Berger K, Bartels DB. The measurement of multiple chronic diseases--a systematic review on existing multimorbidity indices. J Gerontol A Biol Sci Med Sci 2011;66:301–11.
[17] Dominick CH, Blyth FM, Nicholas MK. Patterns of chronic pain in the New Zealand population. N Z Med J 2011;124:63–76.
[18] Dominick CH, Blyth FM, Nicholas MK. Unpacking the burden: understanding the relationships between chronic pain and comorbidity in the general population. Pain 2012;153:293–304.
[19] Eggermont LHP, Bean JF, Guralnik JM, Leveille SG. Comparing pain severity versus pain location in the MOBILIZE Boston Study: chronic pain and lower extremity function. J Gerontol A Biol Sci Med Sci 2009;64A:763–70.
[20] Elliott AM, McAteer A, Hannaford PC. Revising the symptom iceberg in today's primary care: results from a UK population survey. BMC Fam Pract 2011;12:16.

[21] Elliott AM, Smith BH, Penny KI, Smith WC, Chambers WA. The epidemiology of chronic pain in the community. Lancet 1999;354:1248–52.

[22] Evers AWM, Kraaimaat FW, Geenen R, Jacobs JWG, Bijlsma JWJ. Pain coping and social support as predictors of long-term functional disability and pain in early rheumatoid arthritis. Behav Res Ther 2003;41:1295–310.

[23] Fortin M, Soubhi H, Hudon C, Bayliss EA, van den Akker M. Multimorbidity's many challenges. BMJ 2007;334:1016–7.

[24] Fried LP, Bandeen-Roche K, Kasper JD, Guralnik JM. Association of comorbidity with disability in older women: the Women's Health and Ageing Study. J Clin Epidemiol 1999;52:27–37.

[25] Fried LP, Tangen CM, Walston J, Newman AB, Hirsch C, Gottdiener J, Seeman T, Tracy R, Kop WJ, Burke G, McBurnie MA. Frailty in older adults: evidence for a phenotype. J Gerontol A Biol Sci Med Sci 2001;56:M146–57.

[26] Ganzel BL, Morris PA, Wethington E. Allostasis and the human brain: integrating models of stress from the social and life sciences. Psychol Rev 2010;117:134–74.

[27] Idler EL, Benyamini Y. Self-rated health and mortality: a review of twenty-seven community studies. J Health Soc Behav 1997;38:21–37.

[28] Jones AKP, McBeth J, Power A. The biological response to stress and chronic pain. In: Croft P, Blyth FM, van der Windt D, editors. Chronic pain epidemiology: from aetiology to public health. Oxford: Oxford University Press; 2010.

[29] Jones GT. Pain in children: a call for more longitudinal research. Pain 2011;152:2202–3.

[30] Jordan KP, Thomas E, Peat G, Wilkie R, Croft P. Social risks for disabling pain in older people: a prospective study of individual and area characteristics. Pain 2008;137:652–61.

[31] Jylha M, Volpato S, Guralnik JM. Self-rated health showed a graded association with frequently used biomarkers in a large population sample. J Clin Epidemiol 2006;59:465–71.

[32] Kamaleri Y, Natvig B, Ihlebaek CM, Bruusgaard D. Does the number of musculoskeletal pain sites predict work disability? A 14-year prospective study. Eur J Pain 2009;13:426–30.

[33] Kuh D, Ben-Shlomo Y. Introduction. In: Kuh D, Ben-Shlomo Y, editors. Life course approach to chronic disease epidemiology, 2nd ed. Oxford: Oxford University Press; 2004.

[34] Kuh D, Hardy R, editors. A life course approach to women's health. New York: Oxford University Press; 2002.

[35] Leong IY, Farrell MJ, Helme RD, Gibson SJ. The relationship between medical comorbidity and self-rated pain, mood disturbance, and function in older people with chronic pain. J Gerontol A Biol Sci Med Sci 2007;62A:550–5.

[36] Linn BS, Linn MW, Guel L. Cumulative Illness Rating Scale. J Am Geriatr Soc 1968;16:622–6.

[37] Lopez-Martinez AE, Esteve-Zarazaga R, Ramirez-Maestre C. Perceived social support and coping responses are independent variables explaining pain adjustment among chronic pain patients. J Pain 2008;9:373–9.

[38] MacFarlane GJ. Life-course influences on chronic pain. In: Croft P, Blyth FM, Van der Windt D, editors. Chronic pain epidemiology: from aetiology to public health. Oxford: Oxford University Press; 2010.

[39] Mantyselka PT, Turunen JHO, Ahonen RS, Kumpusalo EA. Chronic pain and poor self-rated health. JAMA 2003;290:2435–42.

[40] Mattei J, Demissie S, Falcon LM, Ordovas JM, Tucker K. Allostatic load is associated with chronic conditions in the Boston Puerto Rican Health Study. Soc Sci Med 2010;70:1988–96.

[41] McEwen BS, Gianaros PJ. Central role of the brain in stress and adaptation: Links to socioeconomic status, health and disease. Ann NY Acad Sci 2010;1186:190–222.

[42] Merikangas KR, Ames M, Cui L, Stang PE, Ustun TB, Von Korff M, Kessler RC. The impact of comorbidity of mental and physical conditions on role disability in the US adult household population. Arch Gen Psychiatry 2007;64:1180–8.

[43] Nardi R, Scanelli G, Corrao S, Iori I, Mathieu G, Amatarian RC. Co-morbidity does not reflect complexity in internal medicine patients. Eur J Intern Med 2007;18:359–68.

[44] Palmer KT, Reading I, Linaker C, Calnan M, Coggon D. Population-based cohort study of incident and persistent arm pain: role of mental health, self-rated health and health beliefs. Pain 2008;136:30-37.

[45] Reyes-Gibby CC, Aday LA, Anderson KO, Mendoza TR, Cleeland CS. Pain, depression, and fatigue in community-dwelling adults with and without a history of cancer. J Pain Symptom Manage 2006;32:118–28.

[46] Rochat S, Cumming RG, Blyth FM, Creasey H, Handelsman DJ, Le Couteur DG, Naganathan V, Seibel MJ, Waite LM. Frailty and use of health and community services by community-dwelling older men: the Concord Health and Ageing in Men Project. Age Ageing 2010;39:228–33.

[47] Rockwood K. What would make a definition of frailty successful? Age Ageing 2005;34:432–4.

[48] Roy-Byrne PP, Davidson KW, Kessler RC, Asmundson GJ, Goodwin RD, Kubzansky L, Lydiard RB, Massie MJ, Katon W, Laden SK, Stein MB. Anxiety disorders and comorbid medical illness. Gen Hosp Psychiatry 2008;30:208–55.

[49] Seeman T, Epel E, Gruenewald T, Karlamangla A, McEwen BS. Socio-economic differentials in peripheral biology: Cumulative allostatic load. Ann NY Acad Sci 2010;1186:223–39.

[50] Siddall PJ, Cousins MJ. Persistent pain as a disease entity: implications for clinical management. Anesth Analg 2004;99:510–20.

[51] Singh-Manoux A, Martikainen P, Ferrie J, Zins M, Marmot M, Goldberg M, Singh-Manoux A, Martikainen P, Ferrie J, Zins M, Marmot M, Goldberg M. What does self rated health measure? Results from the British Whitehall II and French Gazel cohort studies. J Epidemiol Community Health 2006;60:364–72.

[52] Singh JA, Lewallen D. Predictors of pain and use of pain medications following primary Total Hip Arthroplasty (THA): 5,707 THAs at 2-years and 3,289 THAs at 5-years. BMC Musculoskelet Disord 2010;11:90.

[53] Smith BH, Elliott AM, Hannaford PC, Chambers WA, Smith WC, Smith BH, Elliott AM, Hannaford PC, Chambers WA, Smith WC. Factors related to the onset and persistence of chronic back pain in the community: results from a general population follow-up study. Spine 2004;29:1032–40.

[54] Stansfield S. Social support and social cohesion. In: Marmot M, Wilkinson RG, editors. Social determinants of health, 2nd ed. Oxford: Oxford University Press, 2006. p. 148–71.

[55] Stanton AL, Revenson TA, Tennen H. Health psychology: psychological adjustment to chronic disease. Annu Rev Psychol 2007;58:565–92.

[56] Steptoe A. Integrating clinical with biobehavioural studies of depression and physical illness. In: Steptoe A, editor. Cambridge: Cambridge University Press; 2007.

[57] Taylor AW, Price K, Gill TK, Adams R, Pilkington R, Carrangis N, Shi Z, Wilson D. Multimorbidity: not just an older person's issue. Results from an Australian biomedical study. BMC Public Health 2010;10:718.

[58] Uchino BN. What a lifespan approach might tell us about why distinct measures of social support have differential links to physical health. J Soc Pers Relat 2009;26:53–62.

[59] Valderas JM, Starfield B, Sibbald B, Salisbury C, Roland M. Defining comorbidity: implications for understanding health and health services. Ann Fam Med 2009;7:357–63.

[60] Van den Akker M, Buntinx F, Knottnerus JA. Comorbidity or multimorbidity: What's in a name? A review of literature. Eur J Gen Pract 1996;2:65–70.

[61] Van Puymbroeck CM, Zautra AJ, Harakas PP. Chronic pain and depression: twin burdens of adaptation. In: Steptoe A, editor. Depression and physical illness. New York: Cambridge University Press; 2007.

[62] Walco GA. Toward an integrated model of pain over the life course. Pain 2004;108:207–8.

[63] World Health Organization. Global health risks: mortality and burden of disease attributable to selected major risks. Geneva: World Health Organization; 2009.

Correspondence to: Fiona M. Blyth, MBBS, PhD, Centre for Education and Research on Ageing, Concord Hospital, Concord, NSW 2039, Australia. Email: fiona.blyth@sydney.edu.au.

Experimental Animal Models of Pain and Non-Pain Comorbidities

Anna P. Malykhina

Division of Urology, Department of Surgery, University of Pennsylvania,
Glenolden, Pennsylvania, USA

Comorbidity of painful and nonpainful disorders is commonly observed in the clinical setting. The presence of multisystem or multiorgan symptoms in the same patient significantly complicates diagnostic evaluation and limits the choices and effectiveness of therapeutic approaches. This problem is mainly due to unknown etiology and poor understanding of the mechanisms underlying comorbid disorders. Animal models have proven useful for mimicking human diseases, investigating disease mechanisms, and testing new pharmacological drugs. The challenge in creating an animal model for multisymptomatic disorders relates to how closely the model represents the human pathophysiology and related symptoms. The majority of animal models are designed to study a single pathophysiological condition, and very few are available for research on comorbid disorders.

An acute intervention (inflammation, infection, noxious distension, ischemia, or trauma) applied to healthy animals has often been used to study the effects on organs that are adjacent to or distant from the site of intervention. Procedures in which an initial acute stimulus is transient but

powerful enough to cause long-lasting hypersensitivity and hyperexcitability after full recovery from the initial intervention are of major interest
for studying pain-related disorders. In animal studies, acute peripheral
interventions and surgical manipulations allow investigators to test the
factors leading to concomitant dysfunctions. Application of known stimuli to genetically modified (knock-out or knock-in) animals is often used
to clarify the role of specific signaling pathways and their contribution to
the development of comorbidities. This chapter provides an overview of
the animal models currently available to study pain and non-pain-related
disorders, outlines the mechanisms underlying comorbidities, and discusses the potential clinical implications of translational and basic science discoveries.

Experimental Models of Systemic Dysfunctions and Related Comorbidities

Diabetes

Diabetes mellitus per se does not belong to a group of painful disorders;
however, it is associated with multiple complications related to pain perception and processing. Clinical studies provide evidence that diabetic
patients may have diminished pain sensitivity and "masked" pain-related
symptoms in a number of critical conditions, including myocardial infarction (Table I). Currently available animal models of type 1 and type
2 diabetes are used to clarify the mechanisms of diabetic complications
and comorbid conditions. Type 1 diabetes in rodents is usually induced by
intraperitoneal injections of streptozotocin, which selectively impairs beta
cells in the pancreas [29]. A type 2 diabetes model has been created by selective breeding of hyperglycemic rats with or without associated obesity
[38,53]. Multiple complications of diabetes are often linked to obesity in
type 2 diabetes patients.

Both type 1 and type 2 diabetes are significantly associated with
diabetic uropathies [29]. Voiding dysfunction associated with diabetes was
studied in female Zucker diabetic fatty (ZDF) rats. The investigators performed a histological evaluation of the urinary bladder, urethra, and vagina. The urinary bladder demonstrated significant edema and vasculopathy, and there was notable voiding dysfunction in both obese/nondiabetic

Table I
Animal models of systemic dysfunctions and related comorbidities

Method	Description/Procedure	Associated Conditions
Diabetes Models		
Genetic (selected breeding)	Zucker diabetic rats (ZDF), type 2	Edema, vasculopathy and voiding dysfunction [38]; increased atherosclerosis [53]
Chemical	Streptozotocin (type 1)	Diabetic uropathy [29]
	Streptozotocin (type 1) + intrapericardial capsaicin	Somatic hypersensitivity and reduction in cardiac nociception [61]
	Streptozotocin (type 1) + systemic inflammation	Increased level of inflammatory mediators in the heart and inhibited cardiac function [47,48]
Hypertension Models		
Genetic (selective breeding)	Spontaneously hypertensive rats (SHR)	Detrusor overactivity [50]; high propensity to depression [34]
	SHR + Freund's adjuvant in the hindpaw	Hypertension-associated hypoalgesia [79]
Genetic (chimeric renin-angiotensin gene)	Tsukuba hypertensive mouse	Osteoporosis with accelerated bore resorption [8]
Surgical	Renal artery ligation model+ Freund's adjuvant in the hindpaw	Decreased response to mechanostimulation and reduced expression of c-fos in the spinal cord [79]
Fibromyalgia Models		
Chemical	Systemic depletion of biogenic amines by reserpine	Tactile allodynia, a decrease in skeletal muscle response, increased immobility during a swim test [70]
Psychological	Unpredictable sound stress	Mechanical hyperalgesia in the muscle and skin; hyperalgesia in the masseter muscle; higher anxiety level [43]

and obese/diabetic rats [38]. Additionally, histology of the external ure-thral sphincter in obese diabetic rats showed increased fibrosis, leading to disruption of the skeletal muscle structure [38]. Another group studied the possible mechanisms of diabetes-induced atherosclerosis using the same ZDF model [53]. The results demonstrated that the endogenous response to ischemia was impaired in ZDF rats owing to downregulation of angiogenic factors such as hypoxia-inducible factor-1 (the master regulator of the transcriptional response to oxygen deprivation) [53].

Several studies have shown that cardiac function in streptozotocin-treated rats is affected by hyperglycemia and by treatment with insulin. The effects of systemic inflammation induced by intravenous lipopolysaccharide in diabetic rats included an increased level of inflammatory mediators in the heart and inhibited cardiac function [47,48]. One of the suggested mechanisms involved a downregulation of the cardioprotective enzyme aldehyde-dehydrogenase 2 that was associated with reduced contractility of the left ventricle [96]. Diabetic (streptozotocin-treated) rats also showed a reduced cardiosomatic reflex evoked by intrapericardial capsaicin, suggesting the development of somatic hypersensitivity (allodynia), with a concomitant reduction in cardiac nociception [61].

Hypertension

The spontaneously hypertensive rat is a useful model for studying related comorbidities and different complications of hypertension. Hypertensive animals show symptoms of detrusor overactivity; however, it is unclear how much of this effect is due to increased abdominal pressure resulting from hypertension [50]. Rats genetically prone to hypertension also have a very high propensity to depression, possibly because of a hyporesponsive hypothalamic-pituitary-adrenal axis [34]. One study investigated the correlation of hypertension with the occurrence of osteoporosis, both of which are age-related disorders. Using a chimeric renin-angiotensin model of transgenic Tsukuba hypertensive mice expressing both the human renin and human angiotensinogen genes, investigators demonstrated that activation of the renin-angiotensin system induces high-turnover osteoporosis with accelerated bone resorption [8].

In two rat models of hypertension (the spontaneously hypertensive model and the renal artery ligation model), chronic inflammatory pain was induced by injection of Freund's adjuvant, a model of monoarthritis. Systemic inflammation led to a decreased response to mechanostimulation with von Frey filaments, along with reduced c-fos expression in the spinal cord, suggesting reduced activity in the spinal neurons. These results provide evidence of hypertension-associated hypoalgesia in acute pain conditions [79].

Stress

Psychosocial stress is an established factor for exacerbating painful disorders and triggering concurrent affective and somatic disorders. Additionally, acute or chronic stress can serve as a pathophysiological factor itself. Experiments employing chronic or repeated stressors in rodents demonstrated the development of mechanical hyperalgesia in skeletal muscles [26], an increase in hyperalgesia evoked by local injections of prostaglandin E_2 or epinephrine [56], and increased colonic hypersensitivity [17]. These alterations could result from modulation of the hypothalamic-pituitary-adrenal axis and overactivity of corticotropin-releasing factor 1 (CRF1) signaling cascades in the brain and the gut [92]. Likewise, it was established that experimental gastritis modifies anxiety, the ability to cope with stress, and levels of circulating corticosterone in mice, with more prominent effects noticed in female animals [74].

The mechanisms of widespread hypersensitivity to nonpainful and painful skin stimuli (allodynia and hyperalgesia, respectively) were studied in a rodent model of migraine [21]. The results showed that transformation of headache into whole-body allodynia or hyperalgesia during a migraine attack is mediated by sensitized thalamic neurons that process nociceptive information from the cranial meninges, together with sensory information from the skin of the scalp, face, body, and limbs [21].

Fibromyalgia

The most common approach to creating an animal model of fibromyalgia includes repeated intramuscular injections of acidic saline or other chemical irritants to cause muscle pain and hyperalgesia [18]. However, very few animal models of fibromyalgia have been studied in association with complex comorbid symptoms (Table I). One recent experimental approach included depletion of the biogenic amines (serotonin, norepinephrine, and dopamine) throughout the body, including the peripheral and central nervous system, by subcutaneous injections of reserpine. In this model, animals developed tactile allodynia along with a significant decrease in the skeletal muscle pressure threshold [70]. These changes were accompanied by an increase in immobility time during the forced swim test, which was indicative of depression, a common comorbid symptom of fibromyalgia [70].

In another model of fibromyalgia, rats were exposed to unpredictable sound stress leading to a delayed enhancement and prolongation of cytokine-induced mechanical hyperalgesia in the muscles and skin [43]. Interestingly, this model also revealed multiple symptoms of conditions comorbid with fibromyalgia. Stressed rats developed both visceral sensitivity and hyperalgesia in the masseter muscles, mimicking temporomandibular disorder. Additionally, the elevated plus maze test caused a significantly higher anxiety level in rats exposed to sound stress. Thus, the unpredictable sound stress model produces a condition in rats that has several comorbid features—visceral and temporomandibular hyperalgesia and increased anxiety, in addition to cutaneous and muscle hyperalgesia—that are similar to the features observed in patients with fibromyalgia syndrome [43].

Animal Models of Viscerosomatic and Viscerovisceral Comorbidities

Thoracic Organ Models

Viscerovisceral convergence among thoracic organs has been studied in several animal species, including rats, cats, and primates (Table II). Experiments in cats have established that gallbladder distension alters neuronal activity in the upper thoracic spinal cord and increases blood pressure [6]. Studies on activation of gallbladder-responsive spinal neurons by intrapericardial bradykinin injections could partially explain why the chest pain of gallbladder origin may be confused with pain from angina pectoris [5].

Several rodent studies have investigated the clinically observed inability of patients to distinguish esophageal pain from cardiac pain [35]. In one study, 91% of spinal neurons activated by distension of the thoracic part of the esophagus and 98% of cells activated by distension of the cervical esophagus received somatic inputs from the chest, axilla, and upper back areas [81]. Eighty-four percent of spinal neurons at the T3 level receive convergent input from the heart and stomach [83]. Up to 88% of gastrocardiac convergent neurons also receive convergent somatic input from the chest, upper back, and triceps [52,83]. Gastroesophageal inflammation used as a model of human gastroesophageal reflux disease enhanced the number and duration of excitatory responses of thoracic spinal neurons to noxious cardiac stimulation with intrapericardial brady-kinin [87]. These results provide evidence that pain originating from the esophagus and heart might be difficult to distinguish because of visceroso-matic and viscerovisceral convergence onto the same spinal neurons [37].

Neurons in the thoracic spinal cord (T2–T4) receive input from the lower airways in addition to the extensive convergent input from the skin and the heart [49,84]. Interestingly, inhaled ammonia decreased the activ-ity of 52% of spinal neurons with lung input but increased the activity of the rest of the airway projecting neurons (48%), all of which responded to colonic distension [85]. Likewise, 23% of thoracic neurons (T3–T4) with cardiac input also responded to noxious urinary bladder distension [82]. The hypothesis that cervical headache might result not only from injured somatic structures in the neck but also occur from interactions with visceral organs was proven correct in rodents [36]. Results of another study sup-ported the concept that vagal or afferent activation of C1–C3 spinothalamic tract neurons might underlie referred pain that originates in the heart or other visceral organs but is perceived in the neck and jaw region [25].

Abdominal/Pelvic Organ Models

Both painful and nonpainful comorbidities among the abdominal-pelvic organs have been extensively studied in acute and chronic animal models of viscerovisceral and viscerosomatic interactions (reviewed in [10,20,62]) (Table II). In an in vivo preparation, pelvic nerve afferent fibers responded to a wide variety of mechanical stimulation applied to restricted regions of the vaginal canal, uterus, urinary bladder, ureter, colon, or anus [11].

Clinical data suggest a high prevalence of gastrointestinal and uri-nary tract dysfunctions in patients with chronic pelvic pain. Intracolonic application of 2,4,6-trinitrobenzene sulfonic acid (TNBS) is a well-estab-lished animal model of colonic inflammation [99] and an advantageous one for the study of colon/bladder interactions. In this model, inflamma-tion in the distal colon is induced by a single intraluminal administration of TNBS, with no requirements for previous sensitization of the animal [57]. This model is also histopathologically relevant to human inflammato-ry bowel disease because rats develop features similar to the human condi-tion, including mucosal thickening, preservation of goblet cells, and mast

Table II

Models of viscerosomatic and viscerovisceral cross-organ sensitization

Primary Organ	Model	Insult/Agent	Affected Organ	Changes Observed in Affected Organs [Reference]
Heart	Noxious stimulation	Intrapericardial bradykinin	Gallbladder	Increased activity of gallbladder spinal neurons [5]
Esophagus	Inflammation	Surgical manipulations to induce reflux	Heart	Enhanced number and duration of excitatory responses in spinal cardiac neurons [87]
Lungs	Irritation	Inhaled ammonia	Colon	Increased activity of the airway projecting spinal neurons with convergent colonic input [85]
Urinary bladder	Distension	Noxious mechanical stimulation	Heart	Increased activity of convergent cardiac and bladder neurons [82]
	Irritation	Protamine sulfate/ potassium chloride	Colon	Lower threshold of colonic afferents to colorectal distension [78]
		Overexpression of NGF	Colon	Lower threshold of colonic afferents to colorectal distension in mice [13]
		Zymosan	Perineum	Abdominal hypersensitivity [89]
	Inflammation	Injection of Bartha's strain virus	Colon	Increased mechanical sensitivity of colonic afferents [19]
		Cyclophosphamide	Colon	Colonic hypersensitivity [67]
		Acrolein	Hindpaw	Increased mechanical sensitivity [44,97]
		Turpentine oil	Uterus	Decreased amplitude and rate of uterine contractions [32]
	Infection	Intravesical E. coli	Hindpaw	Increased thermal sensitivity [14]

Organ	Condition	Agent	Site	Effects
Colon	Inflammation	Trinitrobenzene sulfonic acid	Urinary bladder	Increase in bladder contractility [78]; hyperactivity of bladder afferent fibers [94]; hyperexcitability of bladder projecting sensory neurons [63,64]; increased release of proinflammatory neuropeptides in the urinary bladder [75,95]; changes in detrusor contractility in vivo and in vitro [9,72,58]
		Dextran sulfate	Hindpaw	Increased allodynia [100]
		Sodium	Urinary bladder	Hyperexcitability of bladder projecting spinal neurons [86]
	Irradiation	Single dose	Urinary bladder	Detrusor overactivity [54]
	Irritation	Mustard oil	Urinary bladder	Increased vascular permeability [98]; increased external urethral sphincter reflex activity [76]
Ureter	Ureteral calculosis	Surgical implantation of a stone	Psychosomatic	Writhing behavior and hyperalgesia of the ipsilateral oblique musculature [40,41]
Uterus	Inflammation	Mustard oil	Colon	Increased number of substance P immunoreactive colonic DRG neurons [59]
Prostate	Irritation	Freund's adjuvant	Urinary bladder	Shortened intermicturition interval, decreased micturition threshold, and increased baseline pressure in the urinary bladder [27]

Abbreviations: DRG, dorsal root ganglion; NGF, nerve growth factor.

cell and lymphoid infiltration. The severity and persistence of damage can easily be reproduced, which allows investigators to study the events not only during the "acute" response but also after the recovery from initial inflammation. After recovery from inflammation (12–15 days later), neither the colon nor the urinary bladder has any detectable histological or biochemical changes. Studies using TNBS-induced colonic inflammation determined a significant increase in bladder contractility of almost 70% in the presence of acute colitis [78]. During experimental colitis, the bladder develops signs of neurogenic dysfunction, as shown by hyperactivity of bladder afferent fibers [94], hyperexcitability of bladder projecting sensory neurons [63,64] and spinal [86] neurons, increased release of proinflammatory neuropeptides in the urinary bladder [75,95], and changes in detrusor contractility in vivo and in vitro [9,72]. Acute TNBS-induced colitis also leads to early onset of micturition and decreased intermicturition interval in mice [58]. Local segmental irradiation of the colon was shown to induce detrusor overactivity, as detected by cystometric evaluations in rats [54].

In the model of colon irritation with intraluminal mustard oil in rats, vascular permeability in the normal bladder increased significantly after colonic treatment [98]. This effect was attenuated by transection of the hypogastric nerve [98], which suggests the importance of neural connections. Other studies also documented a reduction of colon/bladder cross-sensitization upon denervation of the urinary bladder [94]. Irritation of the descending colon with mustard oil sensitized the external urethral sphincter reflex activity evoked by pelvic afferent nerve stimulation [76]. Colon inflammation can also lead to significant somatic hypersensitivity at days 14–28 in response to von Frey filament testing of the hindpaw, suggesting viscerosomatic interactions [100]. Likewise, hindpaw incision in the rat produces persistent colonic hypersensitivity of longer duration than the hyperalgesia at the site of incision [22].

Inflammation or irritation of the urinary bladder leads to colon dysfunction in animal models of experimental cystitis. Bladder irritation induced by intravesical protamine sulfate/potassium chloride in rats [78] and overexpression of nerve growth factor in the urinary bladder of mice [13] lowered the threshold of colonic afferents to colorectal distension. Neurogenic cystitis induced by the injection of Bartha's strain of pseudorabies virus in female mice caused abdominal hypersensitivity that was significantly abolished by either intravesical (direct effect) or intra-colonic (cross-effects) application of lidocaine [89]. Similarly, cyclophos-phamide-induced cystitis in mice increased the mechanical sensitivity of colorectal afferents from the smooth muscle layer of the colon and also increased the proportion of chemosensitive colonic afferents [19]. Neo-natal cystitis induced at day 14 postpartum in mice resulted in colonic hypersensitivity in adult rats without significant histological changes in the colon or changes in the mechanosensitive properties of colonic af-ferents [67]. Bacterial cystitis induced by intravesical instillation of *E. coli* produced increased sensitivity to peripheral thermal stimuli in mice with competent toll-like receptor 4 [14]. Both acute and subacute cystitis in rats induced mechanical, but not thermal, referred hyperalgesia in the hind-paws that was attenuated by intravesical pretreatment with an antagonist of tyrosine kinase receptors [44]. Bladder inflammation induced by intra-vesical instillation of acrolein induced mechanical hyperreactivity in the bladder and increased mechanical sensitivity of the hindpaws in mice [97].

Animal models of pelvic organ dysfunctions and pelvic pain use surgical approaches to mimic human conditions such as ureteral calculosis or endometriosis. In a rat model of artificial ureteral calculosis, animals de-veloped writhing behavior and hyperalgesia of the ipsilateral oblique mus-culature [40,41]. Follow-up studies provided evidence that these changes were not associated with the spontaneous ureteral occlusion that frequently occurred in the implanted ureter [42]. Surgically induced endometriosis in rats increased the pain crises and muscle hyperalgesia associated with ure-teral calculosis, and ureteral calculosis revealed additional pain behaviors induced by endometriosis [39]. Experimental endometriosis also triggered an increase in myeloperoxidase activity in the colon and jejunum, followed by elevated tension in the colonic longitudinal smooth muscle [7]. In the lower urinary tract, endometriosis reduced the micturition threshold and produced signs of inflammation in the healthy bladder [68].

A series of experiments studied the effects of dysfunctions in the reproductive system on the activity of the urinary and gastrointestinal tracts. In female animals, uterine inflammation increased the number of substance P-immunoreactive dorsal root ganglion (DRG) neurons inner-vating either the colon or the uterus, as well as those innervating both organs [59]. These findings suggest that localized inflammation activates primary visceral afferents regardless of whether they innervate the affected organ. Similarly, bladder inflammation not only significantly reduced the micturition threshold but also decreased the amplitude and rate of uterine contractions [32]. The mechanisms underlying these cross-organ effects can involve the hypogastric nerve [32] and the endocannabinoid system [33], as was shown in a study in which close-arterial injections of a cannabinoid receptor agonist reduced bladder motility but simultaneously increased uterine motility [31]. In male animals, prostate irritation shortened the intermicturition interval, decreased the micturition threshold, and increased baseline pressure in the urinary bladder [27]. Pelvic pain along with hyperalgesia of the distal colon and urinary bladder was recorded in a murine model of autoimmune prostatitis. The pain was attenuated by lidocaine treatment administered into the prostate, but not into the bladder or the colon, suggesting that pain originated from the inflamed prostate [90].

Mechanisms Underlying the Development of Comorbid Conditions

Neural Mechanisms

The central and peripheral nervous systems coordinate the functions of all the organs and play the dominant role in modulating multisystemic dysfunctions. The phenomenon of sensitization of afferent nerves due to an initial acute intervention in one of the visceral or somatic organs is called cross-organ viscerosomatic or viscerovisceral sensitization [10,86]. Neural pathways are activated by an initial somatic or visceral stimulus, followed by the development of peripheral excitation or sensitization in afferent fibers and sensory neurons. Activation of peripheral neural pathways leads to central sensitization because the signaling is amplified in the spinal cord and brain. The efferent input from the brain may either facilitate or inhibit nociceptive transmission in the periphery [20,62].

The mechanisms of peripheral cross-organ sensitization have previously been discussed in several papers by our group [9,62,75] and by others [10,20,28,93]. Peripheral cross-sensitization includes convergence of sensory pathways at the level of the DRG and is caused by the following factors: (1) the existence of convergent DRG neurons with dichotomized peripheral axons, (2) cross-excitation between sensory neurons within the same DRG, and (3) activation of nonconvergent sensory neurons by the input from viscerosomatic or viscerovisceral convergent spinal neurons via dorsal root reflexes (reviewed in [20,62]) (see Fig. 1).

Tracing techniques with fluorescent dyes established the presence of convergent DRG neurons innervating two or more organs or structures. These neurons have been identified for the uterus and colon [23,59], colon and urinary bladder [28,55,64], urinary bladder and prostate [27], lumbar disk and groin skin [91], splanchnic and intercostal nerves [30], lumbar muscle and knee joint [73], and heart and left arm [66]. Activation of convergent

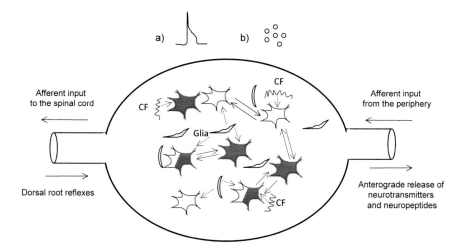

Fig. 1. Schematic presentation of interactions among primary sensory neurons within a dorsal root ganglion (DRG). There are distinct populations of sensory neurons receiving visceral inputs ("white" cells) or somatic inputs ("black" cells). A few cells receive convergent viscerovisceral or viscerosomatic input ("half black, half white" cells). Primary sensory neurons are electrically and chemically coupled (solid arrows) [1–4]. Electrical coupling includes cross-excitation of a silent neuron by stimulation of a neighboring neuron (a). Chemical coupling is a result of intraganglionic release of neurotransmitters and neuropeptides from sensory neurons activated by a peripheral experimental intervention (b). Excitability of sensory neurons could be influenced by substances released from surrounding glial cells and from the catecholaminergic fibers (CF) that form basket-like structures around the DRG cells (dotted arrows). Additionally, neuronal activity can be modulated by electrical processes conveyed via dorsal root reflexes from the second-order neurons in the spinal cord.

sensory neurons by peripheral stimuli may upregulate proinflammatory neurotransmitters and neuropeptides that could be anterogradely released in coinnervated organs via the axon-reflex mechanism and could lead to the development of neurogenic inflammation in an adjacent organ.

Another neural mechanism of cross-talk between sensory neurons occurs within a single DRG and results from electrical [1,3,4] and chemical [2] coupling (Fig. 1). Electrical "cross-depolarization" includes cross-excitation of a silent small-diameter neuron (with an unmyelinated C-type axon) by stimulation of a neighboring neuron [1]. Chemical coupling is usually a result of intraganglionic release (a paracrine mechanism) of neurotransmitters and neuropeptides from sensory neurons activated by a peripheral intervention [2]. For instance, colonic inflammation was shown to upregulate the expression of calcitonin gene-related peptide in bladder DRG neurons in rats [80].

Afferent inputs from distinct organs converge not only onto the same primary sensory neurons [28,64] but also onto the second-order neurons within the spinal cord [71,86] and in the brain [88]. Examples of convergence in the spinal cord between somatic and visceral structures (both thoracic and pelvic) were provided earlier in this chapter. The percentage of neurons receiving convergent input from two or more distinct structures increases with each level in the nervous system hierarchy, ranging from 3–20% in DRG to 35–85% in the spinal cord and more than 75% in various regions of the brain [10,88]. Convergence of sensory information in the spinal cord and brain contributes to the central mechanisms of cross-organ sensitization and plays a significant role in the development of pain and non-pain comorbidities in humans.

Endocrine and Immune Mechanisms

Although the development of cross-organ sensitization is conveyed predominantly via neural pathways, endocrine and immune mechanisms may significantly modulate neuronal responses. Interconnections and interrelationships among all the suggested pathways are currently not well established. The proposed existence of an estrous-stage-modifiable central nervous system substrate by which input from one organ can influence the functioning of other structures has been tested in several animal models. Hormonal factors (endocrine mechanisms) modulate the severity of changes caused by an initial experimental intervention and induce differential effects at low and high levels of estrogens, as was observed in female rats [15,51]. Response properties of peripheral afferent fibers supplying the vagina and uterus of the rat vary with estrous stage [16]. Additionally, estrogen may contribute to comorbidity of some pain syndromes by enhancing axon outgrowth by sensory DRG neurons [24].

Inflammation in one of the pelvic organs (the colon, uterine horn, or urinary bladder) was shown to produce estrous-stage-modifiable signs of inflammation in adjacent pelvic organs [98]. Rats in proestrus responded to colorectal distension with an increased visceromotor response compared with rats in metestrus or diestrus [46]. Pelvic-urethral reflex activity in rats caused by uterine capsaicin instillation revealed enhanced sensitization during proestrus when compared with metestrus [77].

Endometriosis-induced vaginal hyperalgesia correlates with estradiol levels during the estrous cycle, suggesting that hyperalgesia is modulated by estradiol [12]. Endometriosis increases sensitivity and decreases the pain threshold to vaginal distension, with the maximum response observed during proestrus [69]. The maintenance of vaginal hyperalgesia requires the continued presence of some ectopic endometrial tissue, and surgical treatment that fails to remove such tissue can exacerbate visceral sensitivity [65].

Female sex steroids might also influence the trigeminal nociceptive pathways activated in migraine. Downstream signaling, including extracellular signal-regulated kinase activation, calcium-dependent mechanisms, and cAMP response element-binding activation, are thought to be the major signaling events affected by sex hormones in migraine [45]. Psychological state (e.g., anxiety or persistent stress) could be as influential as hormonal status and may continue to modulate sensory processing long after the resolution of the initial peripheral damage.

Inflammation and infection are the most common triggering factors in cross-organ interactions; therefore, activation of immune cells (lymphocytes, macrophages, and mast cells) could be an additional modulatory mechanism in viscerosomatic and viscerovisceral cross-sensitization. Enhanced expression of mast cell growth factor and mast cell activation in the urinary bladder occurred following the resolution of TNBS-induced colitis in female rats [60]. Activated mast cells (containing <20% of cellular staining) contribute to the histological and biochemical changes in afferent and end-organ pathways that may be responsible for neurogenic inflammation and afferent cross-sensitization in the pelvis [60].

Conclusions

Animal models of concurrent dysfunctions are very limited, but they will continue to be of significant value in identifying the mechanisms underlying comorbidities of human disorders. Development of animal models in which the essential symptomatic and structural characteristics of comorbid disorders can be closely replicated is of the highest value. Additional comparative and translational studies are required to realize the full potential of findings obtained with these animal models and to develop innovative treatment strategies in order to improve clinical management of complex patients with multiple comorbidities.

Acknowledgments

The work in Dr. Malykhina's laboratory is supported by NIH/NIDDK grants DK077699, DK 077699-S2 (ARRA), and DK052620.

References

[1]   Amir R, Devor M. Functional cross-excitation between afferent A- and C-neurons in dorsal root ganglia. Neuroscience 2000;95:189–95.
[2]   Amir R, Devor M. Chemically mediated cross-excitation in rat dorsal root ganglia. J Neurosci 1996;16:4733–41.
[3]   Amir R, Kocsis JD, Devor M. Multiple interacting sites of ectopic spike electrogenesis in primary sensory neurons. J Neurosci 2005;25:2576–85.
[4]   Amir R, Michaelis M, Devor M. Burst discharge in primary sensory neurons: triggered by subthreshold oscillations, maintained by depolarizing afterpotentials. J Neurosci 2002;22:1187–98.
[5]   Ammons WS, Blair RW, Foreman RD. Responses of primate T1–T5 spinothalamic neurons to gallbladder distension. Am J Physiol 1984;247:R995–1002.
[6]   Ammons WS, Foreman RD. Cardiovascular and T2–T4 dorsal horn cell responses to gallbladder distention in the cat. Brain Res 1984;321:267–77.
[7]   Appleyard CB, Cruz ML, Rivera E, Hernandez GA, Flores I. Experimental endometriosis in the rat is correlated with colonic motor function alterations but not with bacterial load. Reprod Sci 2007;14:815–24.
[8]   Asaba Y, Ito M, Fumoto T, Watanabe K, Fukuhara R, Takeshita S, Nimura Y, Ishida J, Fukamizu A, Ikeda K. Activation of renin-angiotensin system induces osteoporosis independently of hypertension. J Bone Miner Res 2009;24:241–50.
[9]   Asfaw TS, Hypolite J, Northington GM, Arya LA, Wein AJ, Malykhina AP. Acute colonic inflammation triggers detrusor instability via activation of TRPV1 receptors in a rat model of pelvic organ cross-sensitization. Am J Physiol Regul Integr Comp Physiol 2011;300:R1392–400.
[10] Berkley KJ. A life of pelvic pain. Physiol Behav 2005;86:272–80.

[11] Berkley KJ, Hotta H, Robbins A, Sato Y. Functional properties of afferent fibers supplying reproductive and other pelvic organs in pelvic nerve of female rat. J Neurophysiol 1990;63:256–72.

[12] Berkley KJ, McAllister SL, Accius BE, Winnard KP. Endometriosis-induced vaginal hyperalgesia in the rat: effect of estropause, ovariectomy, and estradiol replacement. Pain 2007;132 Suppl 1:S150–9.

[13] Bielefeldt K, Lamb K, Gebhart GF. Convergence of sensory pathways in the development of somatic and visceral hypersensitivity. Am J Physiol Gastrointest Liver Physiol 2006;291:G658–65.

[14] Bjorling DE, Wang ZY, Boldon K, Bushman W. Bacterial cystitis is accompanied by increased peripheral thermal sensitivity in mice. J Urol 2008;179:759–63.

[15] Bradshaw HB, Berkley KJ. Estrous changes in responses of rat gracile nucleus neurons to stimulation of skin and pelvic viscera. J Neurosci 2000;20:7722–7.

[16] Bradshaw HB, Temple JL, Wood E, Berkley KJ. Estrous variations in behavioral responses to vaginal and uterine distention in the rat. Pain 1999;82:187–97.

[17] Bravo JA, Dinan TG, Cryan JF. Alterations in the central CRF system of two different rat models of comorbid depression and functional gastrointestinal disorders. Int J Neuropsychopharmacol 2011;14:666–83.

[18] Brederson JD, Jarvis MF, Honore P, Surowy CS. Fibromyalgia: mechanisms, current treatment, and animal models. Curr Pharm Biotechnol 2011; Epub Apr 5.

[19] Brumovsky PR, Feng B, Xu L, McCarthy CJ, Gebhart GF. Cystitis increases colorectal afferent sensitivity in the mouse. Am J Physiol Gastrointest Liver Physiol 2009;297:G1250–8.

[20] Brumovsky PR, Gebhart GF. Visceral organ cross-sensitization: an integrated perspective. Auton Neurosci 2010;153:106–15.

[21] Burstein R, Jakubowski M, Garcia-Nicas E, Kainz V, Bajwa Z, Hargreaves R, Becerra L, Borsook D. Thalamic sensitization transforms localized pain into widespread allodynia. Ann Neurol 2010;68:81–91.

[22] Cameron DM, Brennan TJ, Gebhart GF. Hind paw incision in the rat produces long-lasting colon hypersensitivity. J Pain 2008;9:246–53.

[23] Chaban V, Christensen A, Wakamatsu M, McDonald M, Rapkin A, McDonald J, Micevych P. The same dorsal root ganglion neurons innervate uterus and colon in the rat. Neuroreport 2007;18:209–12.

[24] Chakrabarty A, Blacklock A, Svojanovsky S, Smith PG. Estrogen elicits dorsal root ganglion axon sprouting via a renin-angiotensin system. Endocrinology 2008;149:3452–60.

[25] Chandler MJ, Zhang J, Foreman RD. Vagal, sympathetic and somatic sensory inputs to upper cervical (C1–C3) spinothalamic tract neurons in monkeys. J Neurophysiol 1996;76:2555–67.

[26] Chen X, Green PG, Levine JD. Stress enhances muscle nociceptor activity in the rat. Neuroscience 2011;185:166–73.

[27] Chen Y, Wu X, Liu J, Tang W, Zhao T, Zhang J. Distribution of convergent afferents innervating bladder and prostate at dorsal root ganglia in rats. Urology 2010;76:764–6.

[28] Christianson JA, Liang R, Ustinova EE, Davis BM, Fraser MO, Pezzone MA. Convergence of bladder and colon sensory innervation occurs at the primary afferent level. Pain 2007;128:235–43.

[29] Daneshgari F, Leiter EH, Liu G, Reeder J. Animal models of diabetic uropathy. J Urol 2009;182:S8–13.

[30] Dawson NJ, Schmid H, Pierau FK. Pre-spinal convergence between thoracic and visceral nerves of the rat. Neurosci Lett 1992;138:149–52.

[31] Dmitrieva N, Berkley KJ. Contrasting effects of WIN 55212-2 on motility of the rat bladder and uterus. J Neurosci 2002;22:7147–53.

[32] Dmitrieva N, Johnson OL, Berkley KJ. Bladder inflammation and hypogastric neurectomy influence uterine motility in the rat. Neurosci Lett 2001;313:49–52.

[33] Dmitrieva N, Nagabukuro H, Resuehr D, Zhang G, McAllister SL, McGinty KA, Mackie K, Berkley KJ. Endocannabinoid involvement in endometriosis. Pain 2010;151:703–10.

[34] Edwards E, King JA, Fray J. Hypertension and insulin resistant models have divergent propensities to learned helpless behavior in rodents. Am J Hypertens 2000;13:659–65.

[35] Euchner-Wamser I, Meller ST, Gebhart GF. A model of cardiac nociception in chronically instrumented rats: behavioral and electrophysiological effects of pericardial administration of algogenic substances. Pain 1994;58:117–28.

[36] Foreman RD. Integration of viscerosomatic sensory input at the spinal level. Prog Brain Res 2000;122:209–21.

[37] Garrison DW, Chandler MJ, Foreman RD. Viscerosomatic convergence onto feline spinal neurons from esophagus, heart and somatic fields: effects of inflammation. Pain 1992;49:373–82.

[38] Gasbarro G, Lin DL, Vurbic D, Quisno A, Kinley B, Daneshgari F, Damaser MS. Voiding function in obese and type 2 diabetic female rats. Am J Physiol Renal Physiol 2010;298:F72–7.

[39] Giamberardino MA, Berkley KJ, Affaitati G, Lerza R, Centurione L, Lapenna D, Vecchiet L. Influence of endometriosis on pain behaviors and muscle hyperalgesia induced by a ureteral calculosis in female rats. Pain 2002;95:247–57.

[40] Giamberardino MA, Dalal A, Valente R, Vecchiet L. Changes in activity of spinal cells with muscular input in rats with referred muscular hyperalgesia from ureteral calculosis. Neurosci Lett 1996;203:89–92.

[41] Giamberardino MA, Valente R, de Bigontina P, Vecchiet L. Artificial ureteral calculosis in rats: behavioural characterization of visceral pain episodes and their relationship with referred lumbar muscle hyperalgesia. Pain 1995;61:459–69.

[42] Giamberardino MA, Vecchiet L, Albe-Fessard D. Comparison of the effects of ureteral calculosis and occlusion on muscular sensitivity to painful stimulation in rats. Pain 1990;43:227–34.

[43] Green PG, Alvarez P, Gear RW, Mendoza D, Levine JD. Further validation of a model of fibromyalgia syndrome in the rat. J Pain 2011;12:811–8.

[44] Guerios SD, Wang ZY, Boldon K, Bushman W, Bjorling DE. Blockade of NGF and trk receptors inhibits increased peripheral mechanical sensitivity accompanying cystitis in rats. Am J Physiol Regul Integr Comp Physiol 2008;295:R111–22.

[45] Gupta S, McCarson KE, Welch KM, Berman NE. Mechanisms of pain modulation by sex hormones in migraine. Headache 2011;51:905–22.

[46] Gustafsson JK, Greenwood-Van MB. Amygdala activation by corticosterone alters visceral and somatic pain in cycling female rats. Am J Physiol Gastrointest Liver Physiol 2011;300:G1080–5.

[47] Hagiwara S, Iwasaka H, Hasegawa A, Asai N, Noguchi T. Hyperglycemia contributes to cardiac dysfunction in a lipopolysaccharide-induced systemic inflammation model. Crit Care Med 2009;37:2223–7.

[48] Hagiwara S, Iwasaka H, Kudo K, Hasegawa A, Kusaka J, Uchida T, Noguchi T. Insulin treatment of diabetic rats reduces cardiac function in a lipopolysaccharide-induced systemic inflammation model. J Surg Res 2011;171:251–8.

[49] Hummel T, Sengupta JN, Meller ST, Gebhart GF. Responses of T2–4 spinal cord neurons to irritation of the lower airways in the rat. Am J Physiol 1997;273:R1147–57.

[50] Jin LH, Andersson KE, Kwon YH, Park CS, Yoon SM, Lee T. Substantial detrusor overactivity in conscious spontaneously hypertensive rats with hyperactive behaviour. Scand J Urol Nephrol 2009;43:3–7.

[51] Johnson OL, Berkley KJ. Estrous influences on micturition thresholds of the female rat before and after bladder inflammation. Am J Physiol Regul Integr Comp Physiol 2002;282:R289–94.

[52] Jou CJ, Farber JP, Qin C, Foreman RD. Convergent pathways for cardiac- and esophageal-somatic motor reflexes in rats. Auton Neurosci 2002;99:70–7.

[53] Kajiwara H, Luo Z, Belanger AJ, Urabe A, Vincent KA, Akita GY, Cheng SH, Mochizuki S, Gregory RJ, Jiang C. A hypoxic inducible factor-1 alpha hybrid enhances collateral development and reduces vascular leakage in diabetic rats. J Gene Med 2009;11:390–400.

[54] Kanai A, Wyndaele JJ, Andersson KE, Fry C, Ikeda Y, Zabbarova I, De Wachter S. Researching bladder afferents-determining the effects of β_3-adrenergic receptor agonists and botulinum toxin type-A. Neurourol Urodyn 2011;30:684–91.

[55] Keast JR, De Groat WC. Segmental distribution and peptide content of primary afferent neurons innervating the urogenital organs and colon of male rats. J Comp Neurol 1992;319:615–23.

[56] Khasar SG, Burkham J, Dina OA, Brown AS, Bogen O, Alessandri-Haber N, Green PG, Reichling DB, Levine JD. Stress induces a switch of intracellular signaling in sensory neurons in a model of generalized pain. J Neurosci 2008;28:5721–30.

[57] Kim HS, Berstad A. Experimental colitis in animal models. Scand J Gastroenterol 1992;27:529–37.

[58] Lamb K, Zhong F, Gebhart GF, Bielefeldt K. Experimental colitis in mice and sensitization of converging visceral and somatic afferent pathways. Am J Physiol Gastrointest Liver Physiol 2006;290:G451–7.

[59] Li J, Micevych P, McDonald J, Rapkin A, Chaban V. Inflammation in the uterus induces phosphorylated extracellular signal-regulated kinase and substance P immunoreactivity in dorsal root ganglia neurons innervating both uterus and colon in rats. J Neurosci Res 2008;86:2746–52.

[60] Liang R, Ustinova EE, Patnam R, Fraser MO, Gutkin DW, Pezzone MA. Enhanced expression of mast cell growth factor and mast cell activation in the bladder following the resolution of trinitrobenzenesulfonic acid (TNBS) colitis in female rats. Neurourol Urodyn 2007;26:887–93.

[61] Liu XH, Qin C, Du JQ, Xu Y, Sun N, Tang JS, Li Q, Foreman RD. Diabetic rats show reduced cardiac-somatic reflex evoked by intrapericardial capsaicin. Eur J Pharmacol 2011;651:83–8.

[62] Malykhina AP. Neural mechanisms of pelvic organ cross-sensitization. Neuroscience 2007;149:660–72.

[63] Malykhina AP, Qin C, Foreman RD, Akbarali HI. Colonic inflammation increases Na+ currents in bladder sensory neurons. Neuroreport 2004;15:2601–5.

[64] Malykhina AP, Qin C, Greenwood-Van MB, Foreman RD, Lupu F, Akbarali HI. Hyperexcitability of convergent colon and bladder dorsal root ganglion neurons after colonic inflammation: mechanism for pelvic organ cross-talk. Neurogastroenterol Motil 2006;18:936–48.

[65] McAllister SL, McGinty KA, Resuehr D, Berkley KJ. Endometriosis-induced vaginal hyperalgesia in the rat: role of the ectopic growths and their innervation. Pain 2009;147:255–64.

[66] McNeill DL, Burden HW. Convergence of sensory processes from the heart and left ulnar nerve onto a single afferent perikaryon: a neuroanatomical study in the rat employing fluorescent tracers. Anat Rec 1986;214:441–7.

[67] Miranda A, Mickle A, Schmidt J, Zhang Z, Shaker R, Banerjee B, Sengupta JN. Neonatal cystitis-induced colonic hypersensitivity in adult rats: a model of viscero-visceral convergence. Neurogastroenterol Motil 2011;23:683–e281.

[68] Morrison TC, Dmitrieva N, Winnard KP, Berkley KJ. Opposing viscerovisceral effects of surgically induced endometriosis and a control abdominal surgery on the rat bladder. Fertil Steril 2006;86:1067–73.

[69] Nagabukuro H, Berkley KJ. Influence of endometriosis on visceromotor and cardiovascular responses induced by vaginal distention in the rat. Pain 2007;132 Suppl 1:S96–103.

[70] Nagakura Y, Oe T, Aoki T, Matsuoka N. Biogenic amine depletion causes chronic muscular pain and tactile allodynia accompanied by depression: a putative animal model of fibromyalgia. Pain 2009;146:26–33.

[71] Ness TJ, Gebhart GF. Characterization of neurons responsive to noxious colorectal distension in the T13–L2 spinal cord of the rat. J Neurophysiol 1988;60:1419–38.

[72] Noronha R, Akbarali H, Malykhina A, Foreman RD, Greenwood-Van MB. Changes in urinary bladder smooth muscle function in response to colonic inflammation. Am J Physiol Renal Physiol 2007;293:F1461–7.

[73] Ohtori S, Takahashi K, Chiba T, Yamagata M, Sameda H, Moriya H. Calcitonin gene-related peptide immunoreactive neurons with dichotomizing axons projecting to the lumbar muscle and knee in rats. Eur Spine J 2003;12:576–80.

[74] Painsipp E, Wultsch T, Shahbazian A, Edelsbrunner M, Kreissl MC, Schirbel A, Bock E, Pabst MA, Thoeringer CK, Huber HP, Holzer P. Experimental gastritis in mice enhances anxiety in a gender-related manner. Neuroscience 2007;150:522–36.

[75] Pan XQ, Gonzalez JA, Chang S, Chacko S, Wein AJ, Malykhina AP. Experimental colitis triggers the release of substance P and calcitonin gene-related peptide in the urinary bladder via TRPV1 signaling pathways. Exp Neurol 2010;225:262–73.

[76] Peng HY, Chen GD, Tung KC, Lai CY, Hsien MC, Chiu CH, Lu HT, Liao JM, Lee SD, Lin TB. Colon mustard oil instillation induced cross-organ reflex sensitization on the pelvic-urethra reflex activity in rats. Pain 2009;142:75–88.

[77] Peng HY, Huang PC, Liao JM, Tung KC, Lee SD, Cheng CL, Shyu JC, Lai CY, Chen GD, Lin TB. Estrous cycle variation of TRPV1-mediated cross-organ sensitization between uterus and NMDA-dependent pelvic-urethra reflex activity. Am J Physiol Endocrinol Metab 2008;295:E559–68.

[78] Pezzone MA, Liang R, Fraser MO. A model of neural cross-talk and irritation in the pelvis: implications for the overlap of chronic pelvic pain disorders. Gastroenterology 2005;128:1953–64.

[79] Pinho D, Morato M, Couto MR, Marques-Lopes J, Tavares I, Albino-Teixeira A. Does chronic pain alter the normal interaction between cardiovascular and pain regulatory systems? Pain modulation in the hypertensive-monoarthritic rat. J Pain 2011;12:194–204.

[80] Qiao LY, Grider JR. Up-regulation of calcitonin gene-related peptide and receptor tyrosine kinase TrkB in rat bladder afferent neurons following TNBS colitis. Exp Neurol 2007;204:667–79.

[81] Qin C, Chandler MJ, Foreman RD. Esophagocardiac convergence onto thoracic spinal neurons: comparison of cervical and thoracic esophagus. Brain Res 2004;1008:193–7.

[82] Qin C, Chandler MJ, Foreman RD. Effects of urinary bladder distension on activity of T3–T4 spinal neurons receiving cardiac and somatic noxious inputs in rats. Brain Res 2003;971:210–20.

[83] Qin C, Farber JP, Foreman RD. Gastrocardiac afferent convergence in upper thoracic spinal neurons: a central mechanism of postprandial angina pectoris. J Pain 2007;8:522–9.

[84] Qin C, Foreman RD, Farber JP. Characterization of thoracic spinal neurons with noxious convergent inputs from heart and lower airways in rats. Brain Res 2007;1141:84–91.

[85] Qin C, Foreman RD, Farber JP. Inhalation of a pulmonary irritant modulates activity of lumbosacral spinal neurons receiving colonic input in rats. Am J Physiol Regul Integr Comp Physiol 2007;293:R2052–8.

[86] Qin C, Malykhina AP, Akbarali HI, Foreman RD. Cross-organ sensitization of lumbosacral spinal neurons receiving urinary bladder input in rats with inflamed colon. Gastroenterology 2005;129:1967–78.

[87] Qin C, Malykhina AP, Thompson AM, Farber JP, Foreman RD. Cross-organ sensitization of thoracic spinal neurons receiving noxious cardiac input in rats with gastroesophageal reflux. Am J Physiol Gastrointest Liver Physiol 2010;298:G934–42.

[88] Rouzade-Dominguez ML, Miselis R, Valentino RJ. Central representation of bladder and colon revealed by dual transsynaptic tracing in the rat: substrates for pelvic visceral coordination. Eur J Neurosci 2003;18:3311–24.

[89] Rudick CN, Chen MC, Mongiu AK, Klumpp DJ. Organ cross talk modulates pelvic pain. Am J Physiol Regul Integr Comp Physiol 2007;293:R1191–8.

[90] Rudick CN, Schaeffer AJ, Thumbikat P. Experimental autoimmune prostatitis induces chronic pelvic pain. Am J Physiol Regul Integr Comp Physiol 2008;294:R1268–75.

[91] Sameda H, Takahashi Y, Takahashi K, Chiba T, Ohtori S, Moriya H. Dorsal root ganglion neurones with dichotomising afferent fibres to both the lumbar disc and the groin skin. A possible neuronal mechanism underlying referred groin pain in lower lumbar disc diseases. J Bone Joint Surg Br 2003;85:600–3.

[92] Tache Y, Million M, Nelson AG, Lamy C, Wang L. Role of corticotropin-releasing factor pathways in stress-related alterations of colonic motor function and viscerosensibility in female rodents. Gend Med 2005;2:146–54.

[93] Ustinova EE, Fraser MO, Pezzone MA. Cross-talk and sensitization of bladder afferent nerves. Neurourol Urodyn 2010;29:77–81.

[94] Ustinova EE, Fraser MO, Pezzone MA. Colonic irritation in the rat sensitizes urinary bladder afferents to mechanical and chemical stimuli: an afferent origin of pelvic organ cross-sensitization. Am J Physiol Renal Physiol 2006;290:F1478–87.

[95] Ustinova EE, Gutkin DW, Pezzone MA. Sensitization of pelvic nerve afferents and mast cell infiltration in the urinary bladder following chronic colonic irritation is mediated by neuropeptides. Am J Physiol Renal Physiol 2007;292:F123–30.

[96] Wang J, Wang H, Hao P, Xue L, Wei S, Zhang Y, Chen Y. Inhibition of aldehyde dehydrogenase 2 by oxidative stress is associated with cardiac dysfunction in diabetic rats. Mol Med 2011;17:172–9.

[97] Wang ZY, Wang P, Merriam FV, Bjorling DE. Lack of TRPV1 inhibits cystitis-induced increased mechanical sensitivity in mice. Pain 2008;139:158–67.

[98] Winnard KP, Dmitrieva N, Berkley KJ. Cross-organ interactions between reproductive, gastrointestinal, and urinary tracts: modulation by estrous stage and involvement of the hypogastric nerve. Am J Physiol Regul Integr Comp Physiol 2006;291:R1592–601.

[99] Yamada Y, Marshall S, Specian RD, Grisham MB. A comparative analysis of two models of colitis in rats. Gastroenterology 1992;102:1524–34.

[100] Zhou Q, Price DD, Caudle RM, Verne GN. Visceral and somatic hypersensitivity in TNBS-induced colitis in rats. Dig Dis Sci 2008;53:429–35.

Correspondence to: Anna P. Malykhina, PhD, Division of Urology, Department of Surgery, University of Pennsylvania School of Medicine, 500 S. Ridgeway Ave, #158, Glenolden, PA, 19036-2307, USA. Email: anna.malykhina@uphs.upenn.edu.

Experimental Human Models and Assessment of Pain in Non-Pain Conditions

Lars Arendt-Nielsen, Thomas Graven-Nielsen, and Laura Petrini

Center for Sensory-Motor Interaction, Department of Health Sciences and Technology, Faculty of Medicine, Aalborg University, Aalborg, Denmark

Chronic pain is common, causes suffering and disability, and is linked with high costs to society. Over the last four decades the number of research papers on nociception and pain has increased enormously, creating an impressive advance in basic knowledge. Studies in animals or healthy volunteers cannot be translated directly into clinical applications, but they have been highly successful in providing mechanistic information leading to a better understanding of clinical signs and symptoms and thus a more rational use of available treatments. Although some of this knowledge has been translated into improved treatment of chronic pain, the transfer of research findings to the clinic still remains generally insufficient.

There has been less focus on the status of the pain system in non-painful conditions, although pain mechanisms may also play a role in these conditions. A recent study examined the hypothesis that conditions with subjective symptoms elicited by odorous chemicals—multiple chemical sensitivity and eczema, in particular—may involve alterations such as central sensitization, similar to various chronic pain disorders. Intradermal injections of capsaicin evoked increased secondary hyperalgesia and facilitated the temporal pain summation response in patients as compared to controls. In addition, patients with either multiple chemical sensitivity or eczema who also had fibromyalgia, chronic pain, and chronic fatigue showed significantly enhanced temporal summation compared with patients without such comorbidities [76]. Another recent area receiving some attention is post-traumatic stress disorder (PTSD), a chronic and debilitating anxiety disorder in which some studies have shown altered pain processing, such as hypoalgesia in response to painful thermal stimulation [61]. However, patients also have enhanced responses to clinical pain [12], illustrating the complicated interaction between the pain system and nonpainful disorders.

This chapter will address the fundamentals of human quantitative pain assessment and its application in a variety of functional, neurological, psychiatric, and psychological nonpainful disorders.

Quantitative Pain Assessment

Studies of clinical pain and non-pain disorders are inevitably biased due to a variety of psychosocial factors involved. The great individual differences and concomitant symptoms in the clinical setting make it difficult to study basic pain manifestations without utilizing quantitative standardized assessment tools. Human experimental pain assessment tools overcome some of those biases because the location, quality, intensity, and modality of pain can be controlled precisely. Standardized experimental pain stimuli of different modalities can be applied to different tissues for mechanistic profiling and phenotyping of patients. The evoked responses can be quantified by subjective psychophysical measures (e.g., pain ratings, pain thresholds), electrophysiological tests (e.g., electroencephalography, evoked potentials, electromyography), or brain imaging methods (e.g., functional magnetic resonance imaging [fMRI], positron emission tomography).

Psychophysical methods are divided into response-dependent and stimulus-dependent methods. Response-dependent methods rely on the subject's evaluation of the stimulus intensity or unpleasantness on a given scale (a visual analogue scale [VAS], verbal rating scale, or numeric rating scale) or as a cross-modality match. Stimulus-dependent methods are based on the adjustment of stimulus intensity until a predefined response, typically a threshold, is reached. Stimulus-response functions are more informative than a threshold determination because suprathreshold response characteristics can be derived from the data.

In addition to various pain induction tools, the surrogate pain model may be used to study pain (Fig. 1). In this model, specific clinical symptoms (e.g., allodynia or hyperalgesia) can be induced to represent the alterations that may occur in the peripheral or central nervous system of patients with painful conditions. As the pain system may undergo changes not only in chronic pain, but also in nonpainful conditions, it is important to incorporate nonpainful stimuli such as brushing and stroking because they may elicit pain in sensitized conditions.

The following sections present examples of experimental pain assessment tools and describe how they may be applied in clinical nonpainful conditions. A variety of diseases (e.g., multiple sclerosis, diabetes, and pancreatitis) may begin without pain but develop into a painful condition, and hence a thorough assessment of the function of myelinated and nonmyelinated afferents may delineate subclinical differences in disease stage. Such early diagnosis may be useful for understanding and following disease progression. Different thresholds can be measured

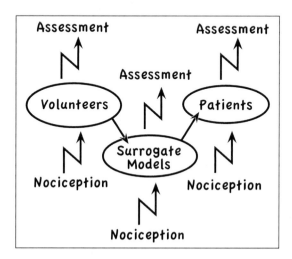

Fig. 1. An illustration of a standardized application of nociceptive stimuli to volunteers and patients and assessment of the responses provoked. The surrogate models mimic selected mechanisms that can occur in patients, and as such they constitute an intermediate translational step between volunteers and patients.

for different pain modalities, and they represent the activation of specific receptor populations (Table I). A number of different publications have shown the lack of correlation between thresholds assessed by different stimulus modalities [102], indicating that complementary information can be acquired by multimodal assessment.

Table I
The relation between individual thresholds and the somatic afferent fibers activated (the afferents activated by cold and cold pain are still controversial)

Stimulation	Fibers Activated
Thermal	
Warmth threshold	C
Heat pain threshold	Aδ
Heat pain tolerance threshold	Aδ + C
Cold threshold	Aδ
Cold pain threshold	Aδ + C
Cold pressor pain	Aδ + C
Mechanical	
Brush	Aβ
Touch threshold	Aβ
Pinprick threshold	Aβ + Aδ
Pressure pain threshold	Aβ + Aδ
Pressure pain tolerance threshold	Aβ + Aδ + C
Electrical	
Detection threshold	Aβ
Pain threshold	Aβ + Aδ
Pain tolerance threshold	Aβ + Aδ + C
Chemical	
Pain provocation	C

Mechanical Stimulation

Cutaneous Brushing

Brushing can be used for assessing the area and intensity of dynamic cutaneous allodynia, but the technique is generally difficult to standardize because a cotton swab is often used. Recently, we have developed a more standardized method, in which brushing speed, length and width of strokes, and application force can be controlled [79]. Stroking/brushing is a standard, clinical neurological test for assessing tactile Aβ-fiber function.

In a cohort of consecutive patients presenting with any symptomatic work-related disorder (involving upper limbs, low back, lungs, etc.) but without obvious pain complaints, a proportion showed mechanical allodynia as an indication of subclinical pain problems [80]. Similar findings have been reported in patients with restless genital syndrome [153].

Cutaneous Touch

Cutaneous mechanosensitivity and static mechanical allodynia may be assessed by applying light pressure with a finger or with a von Frey hair. Von Frey hairs were originally taken from horses' tails, and hairs of different diameters provided different stimulus intensities. Today, von Frey hairs are mainly calibrated nylon filaments of different diameters and hence with different bending force. A slight, but exact and reproducible, pressure can be applied, and the person reports when the touch sensation is first felt upon the application of hairs with different bending forces. A fibers mediate touch sensation [27]. Static mechanical hyperalgesia has been detected in patients with primary and secondary restless leg syndrome [139] or restless genital syndrome [153], to name a few examples.

Cutaneous Pinprick

Cutaneous pinprick stimulation consists of gently stimulating the skin with a needle, a safety pin, or a thick von Frey filament and is used for assessing pinprick hyperalgesia. Different bending forces are used until the sensation changes from touch to pinprick pain. Pinprick pain is mediated by Aδ fibers [27]. Pinprick hyperalgesia is found in patients with restless leg syndrome [17], for example.

Pressure Stimulation for Assessment of Deep-Tissue Sensitivity

Pressure pain can be induced by means of a handheld pressure algometer. The probe can be applied to a hard body structure, such as the periosteum or joints [8], or to soft tissue such as muscles and tendons [4]. Muscle pain sensitivity varies in different parts of a muscle and over a specific area [22]. To determine pressure pain threshold, the intensity of stimulation is increased, preferably by a fixed rate (measured in kilopascals per second) until the person defines the sensation as pain. The pressure can then be increased further until the pain tolerance threshold is reached. Both Aδ and C fibers mediate pain induced by pressure stimulation [3]. Automated pressure algometers are used in the most advanced laboratories because they are user-independent. The pressure is increased at a predefined rate for each assessment [104].

Pressure pain thresholds increase with age [97], and they are lower in females [32]. Pressure pain thresholds have been used for preoperative screening of non-pain patients because they can be indicative of postoperative pain intensity [77]. As an example of a non-pain condition, pressure pain thresholds are reduced in patients with insomnia [73].

Deep-Tissue Cuff Algometry

The different pressure pain devices are all designed to activate a relatively small area and a restricted structure. A cuff algometer designed to obtain a more general response from musculoskeletal structures has been developed and used in volunteers [118] and pain patients [81]. The standardized cuff is inflated at a predetermined rate, and the volunteer scores the pain on an electronic VAS and indicates when the pain detection and pain tolerance thresholds are reached. Pain ratings obtained with cuff algometry have been used preoperatively in non-pain patients and were found to be predictive for postoperative pain and analgesic request [122].

Barostat for Visceral Stimulation

Mechanical stimulation of the gastrointestinal tract, in particular balloon distension, has been widely used [26,41]. Most studies apply a method of measuring changes in the volume of air in a balloon at constant pressure levels (using a barostat), but new methods are based on impedance planimetry, which allows direct recording of the luminal cross-sectional area and estimation of the radius of the distended segment of the esophagus or intestine [44]. The technique has also been used in patients with nonpainful disorders such as grade B esophagitis [43] and systemic sclerosis [113].

Thermal Stimulation

Afferent somatic nerve fibers are activated by thermal stimulation, and so this modality has been widely used in clinical studies.

Cutaneous Cold and Cold Pain

Cold stimulation may be performed by applying ice [94], a wet alcohol sponge [124], or a cooling thermode [111] to the skin. Aδ and C fibers are assumed to mediate cold and cold pain sensations in humans [28,29], although there is no absolute consensus on which fibers play a prominent role. Cold thresholds have been used for diagnosing asymptomatic nerve damage [121], predicting postoperative pain [157], and phenotyping restless leg syndrome patients [17].

Ice Water (Cold Pressor Test)

Subjects immerse their hand or the foot into ice-saturated water (0–2°C) for 1 or 2 minutes for as long as they can tolerate the pain [99]. During this procedure, pain intensity is continuously rated on an electronic VAS. The nociceptors of cutaneous veins appear to mediate ice water pain in humans [85] via activation of both Aδ and C fibers [35].

      The cold pressor test has been particularly useful in psychological and behavioral studies investigating coping interventions [23] or anxiety [82], for example. The test has also been used diagnostically for clinical conditions such as dyspnea [165].

Cutaneous Warm Stimulation

A warm sensation can be evoked using the same thermode (a Peltier device) that can be used for cold stimulation, as the thermode can both cool and heat the skin. The warm sensation is mediated by C-fiber afferents [164].

      Warm stimulation has been widely used in neurology for diagnostic purposes, because its specificity for thin myelinated fibers is useful for separating patients with and without thin-fiber neuropathy [101]. Warm stimulation tests have also been used for predicting the outcome after surgery [75] and for diagnosing work-related disorders [107].

Cutaneous Contact Heat Pain

Heat pain can be induced by applying a heating thermode (Peltier device) to the skin or by using high-intensity lasers [7]. Heat pain activates nociceptors containing Aδ fibers (first pricking pain) or C fibers (second burning pain), depending on the heat intensity and whether the skin is heated at a rapid or slow rate during threshold determinations, respectively [166]. A heat foil-based thermal pain stimulator can be used to assess temporal and spatial summation of heat pain [105]. This stimulator has been developed into a commercial device for eliciting heat-pain-evoked potentials to assess the function of the Aδ fibers in various neurological conditions, such as amyotrophic lateral sclerosis [161], and for diagnosing thin-fiber neuropathies [14].

Cutaneous Laser Stimulation

Lasers can deliver fast and short-lasting stimuli with the advantage of not touching the skin and hence not coactivating tactile fibers. Lasers are useful for evoked potential studies. A laser pulse elicits a distinct pricking pain mediated by Aδ fibers [9] and a burning pain mediated by C fibers [11], along with the related brain potentials. The fiber activation pattern depends on the stimulus intensity. Lasers have been used to assess the nociceptive pathways in many nonpainful conditions such as Huntington's disease [38], Charcot-Marie-Tooth neuropathy [112], and nerve entrapments [147].

Thermal Stimulation of Deep Somatic and Visceral Structures

Although thermal stimulation of muscles is possible [71], no clinical studies have been performed. Thermal stimulation devices for the visceral structures have been developed for the gastrointestinal tract [44]. One example of their use is in a study of patients with esophagitis [43].

Electrical Stimulation

Electrical stimulation is a widely used technique because it is easy to deliver and control different stimulation patterns with different waveforms, frequencies, and duration. However, under normal conditions the stimulus is not nerve fiber specific, with C fibers having a higher activation threshold than Aδ fibers, which again have a higher threshold than Aβ fibers. Recent developments have refined the technique so that it may be nociceptive-specific under very standardized conditions [100]. Because the electrical pulses are short and generate synchronized afferent volleys, the technique is adequate for evoked potential studies.

Cutaneous Electrical Stimulation

Electrical pulses can be delivered to the skin via surface or intradermal electrodes. In recent years the intradermal approach has gained more acceptance because this technique seems to allow direct nociceptive activation [78]. As electrical stimulation is easy to use, pain thresholds have been widely applied for pre- and postoperative monitoring of patients [1,96,106,159] and for assessing the pain pathways in patients with infections [167].

Intramuscular Electrical Stimulation

Needle stimulation is an appropriate, but not nerve-selective, stimulation technique for eliciting muscle pain and assessing pain thresholds [62] or for inducing referred pain patterns [88]. Intramuscular pain thresholds have been used to assess how visceral conditions modulate the sensitivity in referred pain areas [63] and to characterize sensory disturbances in chronic fatigue syndrome [150].

Visceral Electrical Stimulation

The electrical stimuli have proven to be safe in all parts of the gastrointestinal system [42,55,95]. The major shortcoming is that electrical gut stimulation, as for the other tissues, bypasses the receptors and activates the nerve fibers directly. Visceral electrical stimulation has been used to profile the esophageal sensation in patients with disorders such as globus (a disorder causing a sensation of a lump in the throat) [31] or Barrett's esophagus [86].

Chemical Stimulation

Chemical provocation of various tissues is a way to selectively activate specific receptors, such as TRPV1 (transient receptor potential vanilloid 1), NMDA (N-methyl D-aspartate), or tyrosine kinase A receptors. The assessment parameter is normally the intensity or quality of pain rather than a threshold. Various chemical tests have been developed for provoking allergic reactions or coughing, but they are not specifically used for assessing pain reactions.

One example of chemical stimulation is capsaicin injected intradermally or applied topically to the skin to provoke pain. The capsaicin activates the TRPV1 receptors located on the C-nociceptive afferents [134]. The capsaicin test has been used for assessing specific genetic deficits [143] and diagnosing nerve disorders [16].

Assessing Specific Pain Mechanisms

A number of specific pain mechanisms can be provoked by specialized stimulation and assessment techniques, and a limited number of studies have applied those methods in nonpainful conditions. This chapter will address two mechanisms: temporal summation and descending inhibition of pain.

Temporal Summation (Wind-Up-Like Pain)

If a painful stimulus is repeated 1–3 times per second for 5–10 seconds, the pain will integrate and become more painful (temporal summation) and may cause a facilitated withdrawal reflex response [6]. This integration is assumed to be related to the initial process of wind-up measured in animal dorsal horn neurons following repeated stimulation. Temporal summation can be elicited by electrical [6], mechanical [103], and thermal [105] stimulation modalities and can be elicited from skin, muscle, or visceral structures [10].

An enhanced temporal summation pain response before surgery has been shown to predict post-thoracotomy pain intensity during the acute postoperative phase [156]. Wind-up-like pain is associated with the degree of catastrophizing in amputees with phantom limb pain [149]. Another study showed that patients receiving surgical treatment for breast cancer could be classified into different groups according to sensory testing, including tests of temporal summation [151].

Descending Inhibition

Descending control of spinal nociceptive neuronal excitability is manifested via inhibitory and excitatory circuits operating principally at the monoamine systems and via pathways that originate at higher levels. In animals, the mechanism is termed "diffuse noxious inhibitory control" (DNIC), and this term has been adapted into human research. More recently, the term "conditioning pain modulation" (CPM) has been suggested [162]. The technique requires a 1–2-minute application of a tonic conditioning pain stimulus (e.g., cold pressor pain, thermal stimulation, or mechanical pressure) and a test stimulus applied to a heterotopic location to determine a parameter such as pressure pain threshold, heat pain threshold, or pain ratings.

The potency of CPM is reduced in a number of chronic pain conditions, but only a limited number of studies have applied CPM testing in nonpainful conditions. Examples are preoperative monitoring of CPM as a predictor for the development of postoperative chronic pain [158,163], for genetic association studies [145], for phenotyping patients with polyneuropathy [101], for characterizing patients with insomnia [73], and for assessing psychological states such as the level of catastrophizing [69].

Nonpainful Functional Disorders

In this chapter, the functional disorders are characterized mostly by symptoms with no known etiology. Quantitative pain assessment has yielded abnormal findings in different conditions such as chronic fatigue syndrome [58] and restless leg syndrome [127].

In more recent years, there has been increased focus on the changes in pain processing in PTSD and in other disorders seen in war veterans, as such disorders have gained some acceptance. In general, pain assessments have shown abnormalities in PTSD [138]. In war veterans, the findings are more diffuse, with some veterans showing no sensory abnormalities [135] and others showing visceral hypersensitivity as well as cutaneous hyperalgesia [45].

Patients with functional abdominal pain syndrome have a different pain response profile to rectal distension as compared with irritable bowel syndrome (IBS) patients [108]. For some IBS cases, discomfort may be the prominent symptom rather than pain, and hence IBS can be characterized as a non-pain disorder. Sensory profiling in IBS has been able to phenotype up to four different subgroups [5]. Other studies have found that IBS patients show hyperalgesia in response to a large variety of pain tests [169] and generalized widespread hyperalgesia [115]. Functional dyspepsia is another visceral condition in which discomfort may be more prominent as compared with pain, and those patients have also shown abnormal responses to experimental pain stimuli [148]. Few pain assessment studies have been performed in children, but Faure et al. [52] showed abnormal responses to rectal distension in children with functional gastrointestinal disorders.

A number of studies have been performed in gastroesophageal reflux diseases (GERD). In erosive GERD, Fass et al. [51] found enhanced perception in response to acid perfusion but a normal response to me-chanical esophageal stimulation. In non-erosive reflux disease (NERD), Rodriguez-Stanley et al. [125] found decreased pain thresholds to dis-tension, similar to findings by Trimble et al. [146]. Patients with grade B esophagitis displayed hyposensitivity to mechanical esophageal stimula-tion, together with hyperalgesia to heat [43].

Patients with multiple chemical hypersensitivities are known to have a lowered cough threshold to capsaicin inhalation, but only recently has the pain system also been shown to be hypersensitive to capsaicin, in this case administered via intradermal injections [76]. This finding has changed our understanding of this functional disorder.

Nonpainful Neurological Disorders

A wide variety of neurological nonpainful disorders have pain as an im-portant comorbidity. This section provides examples of pain manifesta-tions in patients with Parkinson's disease and multiple sclerosis.

Parkinson's Disease

In Parkinson's disease, one of the major non-motor comorbid symptoms is pain [54]. Ford et al. [53] estimated that pain occurs in approximately 40% of patients with Parkinson's disease. The pain is frequently related to dysto-nia or muscle cramps [68], but the motor disease may also cause overload-ing of the musculoskeletal system (because of lack of mobility, stiffness, and atypical movements), and the neurodegenerative disease also may cause a central pain syndrome [54]. The neurodegenerative process result-ing in motor disorder in Parkinson's disease involves higher brain centers typically also involved in nociception, making it plausible for the pain sys-tem to be affected. A recent study demonstrated that the pain threshold and tolerance level to electrical cutaneous stimulation were significant-ly reduced in Parkinson's disease patients compared with age- and sex-matched healthy subjects; in contrast, the electrical tactile threshold was not affected [168]. Interestingly, the reduced pain thresholds were found in Parkinson's disease patients with and without pain complaints, although the thresholds were inversely correlated with the degree of motor symp-toms and with depression. That result may confound the interpretation of the results, however, because there is a potential influence of depression on pain thresholds. Reduced heat pain thresholds have also been reported in Parkinson's disease patients compared with control subjects [40], and a study using immersion of the hand in cold water showed increased cold pain sensitivity [92]. The threshold for eliciting the nociceptive withdrawal reflex was found to be reduced in Parkinson's disease patients compared with healthy control subjects, and levodopa administration in patients significantly increased their threshold [59]. Using the same model, Perrotta et al. [114] showed that temporal summation of pain was facilitated in Parkinson's disease patients compared with control subjects. The effect of levodopa on thermal pain thresholds in Parkinson's disease has also been demonstrated by investigators who reported less activation in the right insula and the prefrontal and left anterior cingulate cortices during heat stimulation compared with the activation pattern without levodopa administration [25]. In a more recent study, however, the effect of levodopa or deep brain stimulation did not increase the thermal and mechanical pain thresholds in Parkinson's disease patients [67], but these discrepant findings may be linked to the pain mechanisms involved, whether nociceptive or related to the central mechanisms in Parkinson's disease.

Multiple Sclerosis

Central pain is a key symptom for approximately 30% of multiple sclerosis patients [109]. In study participants who had multiple sclerosis associated with pain, pressure pain thresholds were significantly lower than those of sex- and age-matched multiple sclerosis patients without pain. Compared with matched healthy control subjects, subjects with multiple sclerosis (including those with and those without pain) had significantly lower pressure pain thresholds [141].

The pressure pain threshold in multiple sclerosis patients with comorbid pain did not differ according to whether the pain had central or musculoskeletal characteristics [141]. Moreover, in the same study, tactile, heat, and cold pain thresholds were not significantly affected in multiple sclerosis patients, but temporal summation evoked by repetitive mechanical pinprick stimulation on the skin was significantly more frequent in patients compared with control subjects (21% versus 6%). In a recent study, the location of demyelinations in multiple sclerosis patients with pain was comparable with their location in multiple sclerosis patients without pain [142]. These data suggest that pressure allodynia may precede the pain, and a quantitative assessment of the data may provide valuable information to improve diagnosis and treatment.

Nonpainful Psychiatric Disorders

Changes in pain experience are often reported in psychiatric disorders such as borderline personality disorders, major depression, and schizophrenia. For example, altered pain sensitivity is described in individuals with schizophrenia in numerous published studies [2,46,72,83,89,126]. Although the literature contains a number of observations, case reports, and clinical studies concerning patients with schizophrenia being relatively indifferent or insensitive to pain, there is a lack of empirical controlled studies in this area [120,119,137].

In fact, numerous papers published before the 1980s dealt with pain perception in patients with schizophrenia. These studies applied a variety of experimental methods such as thermal pain, electrical pain, cold-pressure pain, pressure pain, and imagined painful situations [47,89]. Unfortunately, the majority of these studies had methodological problems. As reported by Dworkin [47], the problems range from limitations of psychophysical methods and diagnostic reliability to inadequacies in formulating the precise hypothesis to test. Consequently, at present there is still a need for empirical, well-controlled studies to characterize and explain changes in pain responsiveness in individuals with schizophrenia.

Recent experimental studies have overcome these methodological shortcomings by using careful designs in controlled settings. This new literature has reported a consensus in finding reduced pain sensitivity in individuals with schizophrenia [15,24,36,37,120]. In one study [24], sensation thresholds, pain thresholds, and the perception of acute painful stimulation on the tooth were significantly higher in a group of psychiatric patients with schizophrenia as compared with age- and gender-matched healthy control subjects. Potvin and colleagues [120] used the temporal summation test (Peltier thermode) administered before and after activation of the diffuse noxious inhibitory control (DNIC) by means of a cold pressor test. Pain ratings increased during the temporal summation test among controls but not in schizophrenia patients. DNIC was similar in magnitude in both patients and controls.

Additionally, recent studies combined neuroimaging (fMRI) with psychophysical methods to obtain reliable objective measures of pain processing in individuals with schizophrenia [36,37]. Data from these studies showed that nonmedicated individuals with schizophrenia had higher pain tolerance to heat stimulation than healthy control subjects. Neuroimaging data have provided evidence for a decreased activation in affective and cognitive pain-processing regions (such as the insula, posterior cingulate cortex, and brainstem areas), along with overactivation of the primary sensory-discriminative pain-processing regions (such as the primary somatosensory cortex) [37].

An investigation of medicated schizophrenia patients (considered clinically stable) found that their pain tolerance was no different from that of healthy control subjects. Interestingly, the patients showed higher activation in the primary somatosensory cortex and superior prefrontal cortex and less activation in the posterior cingulate cortex and brainstem than the control group of healthy subjects. These findings suggest that the central processing of pain was not normalized when antipsychotic treatment was administered [36]. Certainly, additional studies are needed to determine whether these results reflect a generalized dysfunction of the neural pain perception circuit and whether these data can be further generalized to other modalities of experimental pain stimulation. Furthermore, particular attention must be paid to studies that have applied similar experimental measures across different groups of patients using age- and gender-matched control groups. For example, Atik and colleagues [15] compared pain sensitivity in subjects with schizophrenia, subjects with bipolar disorders, and control subjects by measuring pain thresholds and pain tolerance in a cold pressor task. This study showed a reduced pain threshold in subjects with bipolar disorders and an increased pain threshold in subjects with schizophrenia as compared with healthy control subjects. Pain tolerance was higher in subjects with schizophrenia and reduced in those with bipolar disorders when compared with healthy control subjects.

A lot of attention has also been devoted to understanding the close interaction existing between pain and depression. Pain is a common comorbidity in patients with depression [98], with the incidence of pain complaints reaching as high as 92% in patients with major depression [34,91]. Recent interest has been focused on the controversial relationship between depression and superficial pain sensitivity observed in experimental pain studies [155]. In fact, a number of empirical investigations using several pain induction stimulations (electrical, heat, and cold pain) have reported a reduced sensitivity to cutaneous pain, a phenomenon labeled as "the paradox of pain perception in depression" [89]. In contrast with this line of evidence, increased sensitivity to pain has been reported in other studies [84,110,140]. However, with regard to deep somatic pain, there seems to be consensus in the increase in pain responsiveness (such as ischemic muscle pain) observed in patients with major depressive disorders.

Consequently, at present we have a number of mixed findings that are not able to account for the controversial relationship between depression and superficial pain sensitivity observed in a number of empirical investigations. Recent literature has focused on this phenomenon. Recently, Weiss et al. [155] investigated the differences in Aδ- and C-fiber activation in response to laser heat stimuli. Depressed individuals showed elevated pain thresholds and significantly reduced C-fiber responses as compared with healthy control subjects. Furthermore, the subjects with depression failed to recognize noxious laser heat stimuli significantly more often. These findings mean that higher pain thresholds to experimental stimuli in depressed patients are not only associated with reduced perception of cutaneous Aδ-fiber input, but also with decreased perception of selective C-fiber input. Unfortunately, the reaction times based on the behavioral method used did not explain whether the low responses to C-fiber input were due to changes in peripheral or central processes. The study might have been biased because antidepressants are known to have antinociceptive effects [136].

To overcome some of these restrictions, a subsequent study [144] directly tested the involvement of central processes using laser evoked potentials (LEPs) in a group of depressed patients who were not taking antidepressants or analgesics. Similarly, this study reported higher laser pain thresholds in depressed patients as compared with control subjects. Furthermore, the data showed smaller Aδ-fiber LEP amplitudes and longer C-fiber LEP latencies in comparison with control subjects, suggesting that depressed individuals might have altered central processing.

Finally, an experimental study [18] investigated the influence of pharmacological treatment with an antidepressant (duloxetine) on pain perception in patients with major depressive disorders. This study showed differential pain changes from baseline to the treatment phase (measured 1 week and 6 weeks after the beginning of treatment). Interestingly, the study reported for the first time that at baseline the increased heat pain thresholds on the skin observed in the patient group were associated with augmented pain perception measured on a VAS. On the basis of these findings, the authors relabeled the term "hypoalgesia" as "pseudohypoalgesia" when referring to perception of heat stimuli in patients with depression. Furthermore, the results showed a decrease in heat pain thresholds during the course of treatment. However, no differences were found in measures of ischemic pain. Therefore, the differences observed between thresholds for heat and ischemic pain at baseline still showed that depressed patients respond differently according to the pain modality examined.

Nonpainful Cognitive Disorders

Pain in individuals with cognitive impairments is often unnoticed or inaccurately assessed. Due to the need for self-reporting, pain is difficult to study in the presence of cognitive impairment. Consequently, research has focused on developing objective tools to assess pain in vulnerable individuals. This section presents examples of recent experimental pain findings in individuals with dementia, the elderly, and individuals with cognitive disabilities.

A recent interest in experimental pain research is the investigation of nociception and pain processing in patients with dementia. Dementia involves an irreversible decline of cognitive abilities, which correlates strongly with age. In fact, age is the highest risk factor for both dementia and pain [132]. Neurophysiological and psychological studies suggest that with advancing age there is a small decrease in the early warning functions of pain. Age seems to have a small, but significant, effect on pain thresholds. Although most of the experimental findings support an increase in pain thresholds with age, a few studies have reported a decrease in pain thresholds. Many factors have been suggested to account for this variability, such as stimulus modality, duration, and site of stimulation as well as the methodological procedures adopted across studies [56,57,64,65]. In an empirical investigation [90], the effect of age on pain thresholds was demonstrated to be dependent on the type of pain induction adopted. The dependence on pain induction suggests that age induces a stimulus-specific change in pain perception where superficial (skin) and deep tissue (muscle) nociception are affected differently. Heat pain thresholds showed no age-related changes.

Several other investigations [49,97,116,160] have found pressure pain sensitivity to be markedly enhanced in the elderly. Furthermore, additional experimental findings support an age-related decline in the endogenous DNIC [48,154]. Thus, it has been hypothesized that the progressive degenerative changes involved in dementia can influence and consequently alter the processing of pain [50,133]. Several lines of evidence have indicated that pain perception is altered in different types of dementia such as Alzheimer's disease, which is currently the most widely investigated type of dementia [19,20,50,131,133]. In fact, reduced consumption of analgesic drugs has been observed in Alzheimer's patients [129]. The reason for this reduction is not clear. However, several factors might help to explain it. For example, these patients are less able to communicate their pain, and their memory of pain is impaired. They may also have fewer painful conditions, or perhaps they experience pain to a lesser extent [130], than healthy individuals. The question as to whether and how pain processing changes in these individuals still remains unanswered. Moreover, the way in which pain experience is altered depends on the type of dementia examined—for example, Alzheimer's disease, vascular dementia, frontotemporal dementia, or Parkinson's disease with dementia [132,133].

Noncommunicative demented patients present a greater challenge in pain assessment. Consequently, experimental investigations are lacking in these individuals. Recent experimental studies have investigated some of these aspects, but the authors are not reporting convergent results. Several studies have found that pain thresholds were not changed in patients with dementia, raising the hypothesis that the sensory-discriminative component of pain is preserved in these patients [19,20,66,123]. Conversely, pain tolerance has been shown to increase, thus suggesting that the affective-emotional dimension of pain is altered in individuals with dementia [20,128]. However, in a study that measured pain ratings and brain activity (recorded by fMRI) in response to mechanical pressure stimulation, the authors failed to find diminished pain-related brain activity in Alzheimer's disease patients [33]. In contrast, the authors found greater amplitude and duration of pain-related activity in both sensory and brain areas, which suggests that the central processing of nociceptive information might actually be facilitated in these patients. In another study [87], pain perception was addressed using multiple methods such as self-report ratings, facial responses, motor reflexes, and autonomic responses. The key finding of the investigation was that multiple components of pain should be used for assessing pain in patients with dementia rather than relying on subjective self-report ratings. This conclusion was based on the observation that dementia had differential effects on the different pain components.

Finally, an experimental pain study [30] that was the first to investigate pain perception in patients with frontotemporal dementia showed increased pain thresholds and pain tolerance in these patients. These findings suggest differences in pain processing in this distinct type of dementia.

Evidence based on several observational studies, personal interviews, or even nonvalidated self-report questionnaires indicates that individuals with cognitive disabilities show reduced pain behaviors in situations where pain behaviors would be expected [13,21,93]. Consequently, pain is often overlooked and goes undertreated in clinical situations. Nevertheless, recent experimental pain studies using quantification methods reported interesting new insights. For example, in one study [74], cold pain thresholds were measured in individuals with Down's syndrome compared with age- and gender-matched control subjects. The findings showed that individuals with Down's syndrome exhibited higher pain thresholds but were not insensitive to pain. They expressed pain and discomfort more slowly and less precisely than their counterpart control subjects. Even though this study used a pain control procedure for assessing pain, the methodology for obtaining pain thresholds was later criticized because the reaction time artifact may have biased the conclusions [39]. Defrin and collaborators [39] later developed an experimental pain protocol where individuals with cognitive disabilities (unspecified moderate or severe mental retardation and Down's syndrome) were trained in the use of heat pain threshold measurements applied to the hand. Measurement was performed using both the method of limits, which relies on reaction time, and the method of levels, which is independent of reaction time [60,70]. In this way the authors tested whether the elevation of pain thresholds was due to a decreased sensitivity to noxious stimuli or a methodological artifact. The results showed that individuals with cognitive disabilities were more sensitive to heat pain than were matched control subjects. These data suggest that computerized quantitative sensory testing of pain thresholds is a feasible tool that can be reliably adopted when testing individuals with cognitive disabilities. Furthermore, the authors suggested that the method of levels is preferable due to the lower reaction times and slower conduction velocity exhibited by these individuals. However, the differences observed in these studies could also have been due to the different pain modalities examined.

Conclusion

It is of obvious interest to study the status of the pain system by quantitative sensory testing in chronic pain conditions because of the potential implications for diagnosis and management. Assessing pain in nonpainful conditions with pain as a comorbidity has not been a major focus of research as it is less obvious how such research could affect management. In recent years, however, more studies have been conducted that have provided important new information on how the pain system can be affected in patients having pain as a comorbidity. Importantly, quantification of pain mechanisms and manifestations may be used to subgroup or differentiate patients with a "non-pain" diagnosis and thereby help us to understand the prevalence of symptoms, the progression of disease, and the nature of comorbidities in such patients.

References

[1]   Aasvang EK, Hansen JB, Kehlet H. Can preoperative electrical nociceptive stimulation predict acute pain after groin herniotomy? J Pain 2008;9:940–4.
[2]   Adler G, Gattaz WF. Pain perception threshold in major depression. Biol Psychiatry 1993;34:687–89.
[3]   Adriaensen H, Gybels J, Handwerker HO, Van Hees J. Nociceptor discharges and sensations due to prolonged noxious mechanical stimulation: a paradox. Hum Neurobiol 1984;3:53–8.
[4]   Andersen H, Arendt-Nielsen L, Danneskiold-Samsøe B, Graven-Nielsen T. Pressure pain sensitivity and hardness along human normal and sensitized muscle. Somatosens Mot Res 2006;23:97–109.

[5]   Arebi N, Bullas DC, Dukes GE, Gurmany S, Hicks KJ, Kamm MA, Hobson AR. Distinct neu-
       rophysiological profiles in irritable bowel syndrome. Am J Physiol Gastrointest Liver Physiol
       2011;300:1086–93.
[6]   Arendt-Nielsen L, Brennum J, Sindrup SH, Bak P. Electrophysiological and psychophysical quan-
       tification of temporal summation in the human nociceptive system. Eur J Appl Physiol Occup
       Physiol 1994;68:266–73.
[7]   Arendt-Nielsen L, Chen AC. Lasers and other thermal stimulators for activation of skin nocicep-
       tors in humans. Neurophysiol Clin 2003;33:259–68.
[8]   Arendt-Nielsen L, Nie H, Laursen MB, Madeleine P, Simonsen OH, Graven-Nielsen T. Sensitiza-
       tion in patients with painful knee osteoarthritis. Pain 2010;149:573–81.
[9]   Arendt-Nielsen L. First pain event related potentials to argon laser stimuli: recording and quan-
       tification. J Neurol Neurosurg Psychiatry 1990;53:398–404.
[10]   Arendt-Nielsen L. Induction and assessment of experimental pain from human skin, muscle and
       viscera. In: Jensen TS, Turner JA, Wiesenfeld-Hallin Z, editors. Proceedings of the 8th World
       Congress on Pain, Progress in Pain Research and Management, vol. 8. Seattle: IASP Press; 1997.
       p. 393–425.
[11]   Arendt-Nielsen L. Second pain event related potentials to argon laser stimuli: recording and
       quantification. J Neurol Neurosurg Psychiatry 1990;53:405–10.
[12]   Asmundson GJ, Coons MJ, Taylor S, Katz J. PTSD and the experience of pain: research and
       clinical implications of shared vulnerability and mutual maintenance models. Can J Psychiatry
       2002;47:930–7.
[13]   Astin M, Lawton D, Hirst M. The prevalence of pain in a disabled population. Soc Sci Med
       1996;42:1457–64.
[14]   Atherton DD, Facer P, Roberts KM, Misra VP, Chizh BA, Bountra C, Anand P. Use of the novel
       Contact Heat Evoked Potential Stimulator (CHEPS) for the assessment of small fibre neuropa-
       thy: correlations with skin flare responses and intra-epidermal nerve fibre counts. BMC Neurol
       2007;7:21.
[15]   Atik L, Konuk A, Akay O, Ozturk D, Erdogan A. Pain perception in patients with bipolar disor-
       der and schizophrenia. Acta Neuropsychiatr 2007;19:284–90.
[16]   Aykanat V, Gentgall M, Briggs N, Williams D, Yap S, Rolan P. Intradermal capsaicin as a neuro-
       pathic pain model in patients with unilateral sciatica. Br J Clin Pharmacol 2012;73:37–45.
[17]   Bachmann CG, Rolke R, Scheidt U, Stadelmann C, Sommer M, Pavlakovic G, Happe S, Treede
       RD, Paulus W. Thermal hypoaesthesia differentiates secondary restless legs syndrome associated
       with small fiber neuropathy from primary restless legs syndrome. Brain 2010;133:762–70.
[18]   Bär K-J, Terhaar J, Boettger MK, Boettger S, Berger S, Weiss T. Pseudohypoalgesia on the
       skin. A novel view on the paradox of pain perception in depression. J Clin Psychopharmacol
       2011;31:103–7.
[19]   Benedetti F, Arduino C, Vighetti S, Asteggiano G, Tarenzi L, Rainero I. Pain reactivity in Al-
       zheimer patients with different degrees of cognitive impairment and brain electrical activity de-
       terioration. Pain 2004;111:22–9.
[20]   Benedetti F, Vighetti S, Ricco C, Lagna E, Bergamasco B, Pinessi L, Rainero I. Pain threshold and
       tolerance in Alzheimer's disease. Pain 1999;80:377–82.
[21]   Biersdorff KK. Incidence of significantly altered pain experience among individuals with devel-
       opmental disabilities. Am J Ment Retard 1994;98:619–31.
[22]   Binderup AT, Arendt-Nielsen L, Madeleine P. Pressure pain threshold mapping of the trapezius
       muscle reveals heterogeneity in the distribution of muscular hyperalgesia after eccentric exer-
       cise. Eur J Pain 2010;14:705–12.
[23]   Blacker KJ, Herbert JD, Forman EM, Kounios J. Acceptance- versus change-based pain manage-
       ment: the role of psychological acceptance. Behav Modif 2012;36:37–48.
[24]   Blumensohn R, Ringler R, Eli I. Pain perception in patients with schizophrenia. J Nerv Ment Dis
       2002;190:481–3.
[25]   Brefel-Courbon C, Payoux P, Thalamas C, Ory F, Quelven I, Chollet F, Montastruc JL, Rascol
       O. Effect of levodopa on pain threshold in Parkinson's disease: a clinical and positron emission
       tomography study. Mov Disord 2005;20:1557–63.
[26]   Brock C, Arendt-Nielsen L, Wilder-Smith O, Drewes AM. Sensory testing of the human gastro-
       intestinal tract. World J Gastroenterol 2009;15:151–9.
[27]   Burke D, Mackenzie RA, Skuse NF, Lethlean AK. Cutaneous afferent activity in median and
       radial nerve fascicles: a microelectrode study. J Neurol Neurosurg Psychiatry 1975;38:855–64.

[28] Campero M, Bostock H. Unmyelinated afferents in human skin and their responsiveness to low temperature. Neurosci Lett 2010;470:188–92.

[29] Campero M, Serra J, Bostock H, Ochoa JL. Slowly conducting afferents activated by innocuous low temperature in human skin. J Physiol 2001;15:535:855–65.

[30] Carlino E, Benedetti F, Rainero I, Asteggiano G, Cappa G, Tarenzi L, Vighetti S, Pollo A. Pain perception and tolerance in patients with frontotemporal dementia. Pain 2011;151:783–9.

[31] Chen CL, Szczesniak MM, Cook IJ. Evidence for oesophageal visceral hypersensitivity and aberrant symptom referral in patients with globus. Neurogastroenterol Motil 2009;21:1142–e96.

[32] Chesterton LS, Barlas P, Foster NE, Baxter GD, Wright CC. Gender differences in pressure pain threshold in healthy humans. Pain 2003;101:259–66.

[33] Cole LJ, Farrell MJ, Duff EP, Barber JB, Egan GF, Gibson SJ. Pain sensitivity and fMRI pain-related brain activity in Alzheimer's disease. Brain 2006;129:2957–65.

[34] Corruble E, Guelfi JD. Pain complaints in depressed inpatients. Psychopathology 2000;33:307–9.

[35] Davis KD. Cold-induced pain and prickle in the glabrous and hairy skin. Pain 1998;75:47–57.

[36] de la Fuente-Sandoval C, Favila R, Gómez-Martin D, León-Ortiz P, Graff-Guerrero A. Neural response to experimental heat pain in stable patients with schizophrenia. J Psychiatr Res 2012;46:128–34.

[37] de la Fuente-Sandoval C, Favila R, Gómez-Martin D, Pellicer F, Graff-Guerrero A. Functional magnetic resonance imaging response to experimental pain in drug-free patients with schizophrenia. Psychiatry Res 2010;183:99–104.

[38] De Tommaso M, Serpino C, Difruscolo O, Cormio C, Sciruicchio V, Franco G, Farella I, Livrea P. Nociceptive inputs transmission in Huntington's disease: a study by laser evoked potentials. Acta Neurol Belg 2011;111:33–40.

[39] Defrin R, Pick CG, Peretz C, Carmeli E. A quantitative somatosensory testing of pain threshold in individuals with mental retardation. Pain 2004;108:58–66.

[40] Djaldetti R, Shifrin A, Rogowski Z, Sprecher E, Melamed E, Yarnitsky D. Quantitative measurement of pain sensation in patients with Parkinson disease. Neurology 2004;62:2171–5.

[41] Drewes AM, Gregersen H, Arendt-Nielsen L. Experimental pain in gastroenterology: a reappraisal of human studies. Scand J Gastroenterol 2003;38:1115–30.

[42] Drewes AM, Petersen P, Qvist P, Nielsen J, Arendt-Nielsen L. An experimental pain model based on electric stimulations of the colon mucosa. Scand J Gastroenterol 1999;34:765–71.

[43] Drewes AM, Reddy H, Pedersen J, Funch-Jensen P, Gregersen H, Arendt-Nielsen L. Multimodal pain stimulations in patients with grade B oesophagitis. Gut 2006;55:926–32.

[44] Drewes AM, Schipper KP, Dimcevski G, Petersen P, Andersen OK, Gregersen H, Arendt-Nielsen L. Multimodal assessment of pain in the esophagus: a new experimental model. Am J Physiol Gastrointest Liver Physiol 2002;283:G95–103.

[45] Dunphy RC, Bridgewater L, Price DD, Robinson ME, Zeilman CJ 3rd, Verne GN. Visceral and cutaneous hypersensitivity in Persian Gulf war veterans with chronic gastrointestinal symptoms. Pain 2003;102:79–85.

[46] Dworkin RH, Clark WC, Lipsitz JD, Amador XF, Kaufmann CA, Opler LA, White SR, Gorman JM. Affective deficits and pain insensitivity in schizophrenia. Motiv Emotion 1993;17:245–76.

[47] Dworkin RH. Pain insensitivity in schizophrenia: a neglected phenomenon and some implications. Schizophr Bull 1994;20:235–48.

[48] Edwards RR, Fillingim RB, Ness TJ. Age-related differences in endogenous pain modulation: a comparison of diffuse noxious inhibitory controls in healthy older and younger adults. Pain 2003;101:155–65.

[49] Edwards RR, Fillingim RB. Age-associated differences in responses to noxious stimuli. J Gerontol A Biol Sci Med Sci 2001;56:180–5.

[50] Farrell MJ, Katz B, Helme RD. The impact of dementia on the pain experience. Pain 1996;67:7–15.

[51] Fass R, Naliboff B, Higa L, Johnson C, Kodner A, Munakata J, Ngo J, Mayer EA. Differential effect of long-term esophageal acid exposure on mechanosensitivity and chemosensitivity in humans. Gastroenterology 1998;115:1363–73.

[52] Faure C, Wieckowska A. Somatic referral of visceral sensations and rectal sensory threshold for pain in children with functional gastrointestinal disorders. J Pediatr 2007;150:66–71.

[53] Ford B. Pain in Parkinson's disease. Clin Neurosci 1998;5:63–72.

[54] Ford B. Pain in Parkinson's disease. Mov Disord 2010;25:S98–103.

[55] Frobert O, Arendt-Nielsen L, Bak P, Andersen OK, Funch-Jensen P, Bagger JP. Electric stimulation of the esophageal mucosa. Perception and brain-evoked potentials. Scand J Gastroenterol 1994;29:776–81.
[56] Gagliese L and Melzack R. Pain in the elderly. In: McMahon SB, Koltzenburg M, editors. Wall and Melzack's textbook of pain, 5th ed. Philadelphia: Elsevier Churchill Livingstone; 2006. p. 1169–79.
[57] Gagliese L. Assessment of pain in elderly people. In: Turk DC, Melzack R, editors. Handbook of pain assessment. New York: Guilford Press; 2001. p. 119–33.
[58] Geisser ME, Gracely RH, Giesecke T, Petzke FW, Williams DA, Clauw DJ. The association between experimental and clinical pain measures among persons with fibromyalgia and chronic fatigue syndrome. Eur J Pain 2007;11:202–7.
[59] Gerdelat-Mas A, Simonetta-Moreau M, Thalamas C, Ory-Magne F, Slaoui T, Rascol O, Brefel-Courbon C. Levodopa raises objective pain threshold in Parkinson's disease: a RIII reflex study. J Neurol Neurosurg Psychiatry 2007;78:1140–2.
[60] Gescheider GA. Psychophysics, method, theory and application. Hillsdale, NJ: Lawrence Erlbaum; 1985.
[61] Geuze E, Westenberg HG, Jochims A, de Kloet CS, Bohus M, Vermetten E, Schmahl C. Altered pain processing in veterans with posttraumatic stress disorder. Arch Gen Psychiatry 2007;64:76–85.
[62] Giamberardino MA, Affaitati G, Lerza R, Lapenna D, Costantini R, Vecchiet L. Relationship between pain symptoms and referred sensory and trophic changes in patients with gallbladder pathology. Pain 2005;114:239–49.
[63] Giamberardino MA, De Laurentis S, Affaitati G, Lerza R, Lapenna D, Vecchiet L. Modulation of pain and hyperalgesia from the urinary tract by algogenic conditions of the reproductive organs in women. Neurosci Lett 2001;304:61–4.
[64] Gibson SJ, Farrell M. A review of age differences in the neurophysiology of nociception and the perceptual experience of pain. Clin J Pain 2004;4:227–39.
[65] Gibson SJ, Helme RD. Age-related differences in pain perception and report. Clin Geriatr Med 2001;17:433–56.
[66] Gibson SJ, Voukelatos X, Ames D, Flicker L, Helme RD. An examination of pain perception and cerebral event-related potentials following carbon dioxide laser stimulation in patients with Alzheimer's disease and age-matched control volunteers. Pain Res Manag 2001:6:126–32.
[67] Gierthmühlen J, Arning P, Binder A, Herzog J, Deuschl G, Wasner G, Baron R. Influence of deep brain stimulation and levodopa on sensory signs in Parkinson's disease. Mov Disord 2010;25:1195–202.
[68] Goetz CG, Tanner CM, Levy M, Wilson RS, Garron DC. Pain in Parkinson's disease. Mov Disord 1986;1:45–9.
[69] Goodin BR, McGuire L, Allshouse M, Stapleton L, Haythornthwaite JA, Burns N, Mayes LA, Edwards RR. Associations between catastrophizing and endogenous pain-inhibitory processes: sex differences. J Pain 2009;10:180–90.
[70] Gracely RH. Pain psychophysics. In: Chapman CR, Loeser JD, editors. Issues in pain measurements. Advances in pain research and therapy, vol. 12. New York: Raven Press; 1989. p. 211–30.
[71] Graven-Nielsen T, Arendt-Nielsen L, Mense S. Thermosensitivity of muscle: high-intensity thermal stimulation of muscle tissue induces muscle pain in humans. J Physiol 2002;540:647–56.
[72] Guieu R, Samuelian JC, Coulovrat H. Objective evaluation of pain perception in patients with schizophrenia. Br J Psychiatry 1994;164:253–5.
[73] Haack M, Scott-Sutherland J, Santangelo G, Simpson NS, Sethna N, Mullington JM. Pain sensitivity and modulation in primary insomnia. Eur J Pain 2011; Epub Aug 23.
[74] Hennequin M, Morin C, Feine JS. Pain expression and stimulates localization in individuals with Down's syndrome. Lancet 2000;356:1882–7.
[75] Hickey OT, Burke SM, Hafeez P, Mudrakouski AL, Hayes ID, Keohane C, Butler MA, Shorten GD. Determinants of outcome for patients undergoing lumbar discectomy: a pilot study. Eur J Anaesthesiol 2010;27:696–701.
[76] Holst H, Arendt-Nielsen L, Mosbech H, Elberling J. Increased capsaicin-induced secondary hyperalgesia in patients with multiple chemical sensitivity. Clin J Pain 2011;27:156–62.
[77] Hsu YW, Somma J, Hung YC, Tsai PS, Yang CH, Chen CC. Predicting postoperative pain by preoperative pressure pain assessment. Anesthesiology 2005;103:613–8.
[78] Inui K, Tran TD, Hoshiyama M, Kakigi R. Preferential stimulation of A-delta-fibers by intra-epidermal needle electrode in humans. Pain 2002;96:247–52.

[79] Jardin KG, Gregersen LS, Røsland T, Uggerhøj KH, Arendt-Nielsen L, Gazerani P. Validation of a novel fully-automated brushing device for the assessment of dynamic mechanical allodynia. Pain in Europe VII, 7th Congress of the European Federation of IASP Chapters (EFIC); 2011:S120.

[80] Jepsen JR, Laursen LH, Hagert CG, Kreiner S, Larsen AI. Diagnostic accuracy of the neurological upper limb examination II: relation to symptoms of patterns of findings. BMC Neurol 2006;6:10.

[81] Jespersen A, Dreyer L, Kendall Graven-Nielsen T, Arendt-Nielsen L, Bliddal H, Danneskiold-Samsoe B. Computerized cuff pressure algometry: a new method to assess deep-tissue hyper-sensitivity in fibromyalgia. Pain 2007;131:57–62.

[82] Jones A, Zachariae R, Arendt-Nielsen L. Dispositional anxiety and the experience of pain: gen-der-specific effects. Eur J Pain 2003;7:387–95.

[83] Kemperman I, Russ M, Clark WC, Kakuma T, Zanine E, Harrison K Pain assessments in self-injurious patients with borderline personality disorder using signal detection theory. Psychiatry Res 1997;70:175–83.

[84] Klauenberg S, Maier C, Assion HJ, Hoffmann A, Krumova EK, Magerl W, Scherens A, Treede R-D, Juckel G. Depression and changed pain perception: hints for a central disinhibition mecha-nism. Pain 2008;140:332–43.

[85] Klement W, Arndt JO. The role of nociceptors of cutaneous veins in the mediation of cold pain in man. J Physiol 1992;449:73–83.

[86] Krarup AL, Olesen SS, Funch-Jensen P, Gregersen H, Drewes AM. Proximal and distal esoph-ageal sensitivity is decreased in patients with Barrett's esophagus. World J Gastroenterol 2011;17:514–21.

[87] Kunz M, Mylius V, Scharmann S, Schepelmann K, Lautenbacher S. Influence of dementia on multiple components of pain. Eur J Pain 2009;13:317–25.

[88] Laursen RJ, Graven-Nielsen T, Jensen TS, Arendt-Nielsen L. Quantification of local and referred pain in humans induced by intramuscular electrical stimulation. Eur J Pain 1997;1:105–13.

[89] Lautenbacher S, Krieg J Pain perception in psychiatric disorders: a review of the literature. J Psychiatr Res 1994;28:109–22.

[90] Lautenbacher S, Kunz M, Strate P, Nielsen J, Arendt-Nielsen L. Age effects on pain thresholds, temporal summation and spatial summation of heat and pressure pain. Pain 2005;115:410–8.

[91] Lautenbacher S, Spernal J, Schreiber W, Krieg JC. Relationship between clinical pain com-plaints and pain sensitivity in patients with depression and panic disorder. Psychosom Med 1999;61:822–7.

[92] Lim SY, Farrell MJ, Gibson SJ, Helme RD, Lang AE, Evans AH. Do dyskinesia and pain share common pathophysiological mechanisms in Parkinson's disease? Mov Disord 2008;23:1689–95.

[93] Lind J, Vuorenkoski V, Rosberg G, Paratanen TJ, Wasz-Hockert O. Spectrographic analysis of vocal response to pain stimuli in infants with Down's syndrome. Dev Med Child Neurol 1970;12:478–86.

[94] Liu S, Kopacz DJ, Carpenter RL. Quantitative assessment of differential sensory nerve block after lidocaine spinal anesthesia. Anesthesiology 1995;82:60–3.

[95] Loening-Baucke V, Read NW, Yamada T. Further evaluation of the afferent nervous pathways from the rectum. Am J Physiol 1992;262:927–33.

[96] Lundblad H, Kreicbergs A, Jansson KA. Prediction of persistent pain after total knee replace-ment for osteoarthritis. J Bone Joint Surg Br 2008;90:166–71.

[97] Marini I, Bortolotti F, Bartolucci ML, Inelmen EM, Gatto MR, Alessandri Bonetti G. Aging effect on pressure pain thresholds of head and neck muscles. Aging Clin Exp Res 2011; Epub Oct 3.

[98] Miller LR, Cano A. Comorbid chronic pain and depression: who is at risk? J Pain 2009;10:619–27.

[99] Modir JG, Wallace MS. Human experimental pain models. 2: The cold pressor model. Methods Mol Biol 2010;617:165–8.

[100] Mouraux A, Iannetti GD, Plaghki L. Low intensity intra-epidermal electrical stimulation can activate Aδ-nociceptors selectively. Pain 2010;150:199–207.

[101] Nahman-Averbuch H, Yarnitsky D, Granovsky Y, Sprecher E, Steiner M, Tzuk-Shina T, Pud D. Pronociceptive pain modulation in patients with painful chemotherapy-induced polyneuropa-thy. J Pain Symptom Manage 2011;42:229–3.

[102] Neziri AY, Curatolo M, Nüesch E, Scaramozzino P, Andersen OK, Arendt-Nielsen L, Jüni P. Factor analysis of responses to thermal, electrical, and mechanical painful stimuli supports the importance of multi-modal pain assessment. Pain 2011;152:1146–55.

[103] Nie H, Arendt-Nielsen L, Andersen H, Graven-Nielsen T. Temporal summation of pain evoked by mechanical stimulation in deep and superficial tissue. J Pain 2005;6:348–55.

[104] Nie H, Graven-Nielsen T, Arendt-Nielsen L. Spatial and temporal summation of pain evoked by mechanical pressure stimulation. Eur J Pain 2009;13:592–9.

[105] Nielsen J, Arendt-Nielsen L. The importance of stimulus configuration for temporal summation of first and second pain to repeated painful conducted and radiant heat stimuli. Eur J Pain 1998;2:329–41.

[106] Nielsen PR, Nørgaard L, Rasmussen LS, Kehlet H. Prediction of post-operative pain by an electrical pain stimulus. Acta Anaesthesiol Scand 2007;51:582–6.

[107] Nilsson T, Burström L, Hagberg M, Lundström R. Thermal perception thresholds among young adults exposed to hand-transmitted vibration. Int Arch Occup Environ Health 2008;81:519–33.

[108] Nozu T, Okumura T. Visceral sensation and irritable bowel syndrome; with special reference to comparison with functional abdominal pain syndrome. J Gastroenterol Hepatol 2011;26:122–7.

[109] Osterberg A, Boivie J, Thuomas KA. Central pain in multiple sclerosis: prevalence and clinical characteristics. Eur J Pain 2005;9:531–42.

[110] Otto MW, Dougher MJ, Yeo RA. Depression, pain, and hemispheric activation, J Nerv Mental Dis 1989;177:210–18.

[111] Pavlaković G, Klinke I, Pavlaković H, Züchner K, Zapf A, Bachmann CG, Graf BM, Crozier TA. Effect of thermode application pressure on thermal threshold detection. Muscle Nerve 2008;38:1498–505.

[112] Pazzaglia C, Vollono C, Ferraro D, Virdis D, Lupi V, Le Pera D, Tonali P, Padua L, Valeriani M. Mechanisms of neuropathic pain in patients with Charcot-Marie-Tooth 1 A: a laser-evoked potential study. Pain 2010;149:379–8.

[113] Pedersen J, Gao C, Egekvist H, Bjerring P, Arendt-Nielsen L, Gregersen H, Drewes AM. Pain and biomechanical responses to distention of the duodenum in patients with systemic sclerosis. Gastroenterology 2003;124:1230–9.

[114] Perrotta A, Sandrini G, Serrao M, Buscone S, Tassorelli C, Tinazzi M, Zangaglia R, Pacchetti C, Bartolo M, Pierelli F, Martignoni E. Facilitated temporal summation of pain at spinal level in Parkinson's disease. Mov Disord 2011;26:442–8.

[115] Piché M, Arsenault M, Poitras P, Rainville P, Bouin M. Widespread hypersensitivity is related to altered pain inhibition processes in irritable bowel syndrome. Pain 2010;148:49–58.

[116] Pickering G, Jourdan D, Eschalier A, Dubray C. Impact of age, gender and cognitive functioning on pain perception. Gerontology 2002;48:112–8.

[117] Pinerua-Shuhaibar L, Prieto-Rincon D, Ferrer A, Bonilla E, Maixner W, Suarez-Roca H, Reduced tolerance and cardiovascular response to ischemic pain in minor depression. J Affect Disord 1999;56:119–26.

[118] Polianskis R, Graven-Nielsen T, Arendt-Nielsen L. Computer-controlled pneumatic pressure algometry: a new technique for quantitative sensory testing. Eur J Pain 2001;5:267–77.

[119] Potvin S, Marchand S. Hypoalgesia in schizophrenia is independent of antipsychotic drugs: a systematic quantitative review of experimental studies. Pain 2008;138:70–8.

[120] Potvin S, Stip E, Tempier A, Pampoulova T, Bentaleb LA, Lalonde P, Lipp O, Goffaux P, Marchand S. Pain perception in schizophrenia: no changes in diffuse noxious inhibitory controls (DNIC) but a lack of pain sensitization. J Psychiatr Res 2008;42:1010–6.

[121] Ragé M, Van Acker N, Knaapen MW, Timmers M, Streffer J, Hermans MP, Sindic C, Meert T, Plaghki L. Asymptomatic small fiber neuropathy in diabetes mellitus: investigations with intraepidermal nerve fiber density, quantitative sensory testing and laser-evoked potentials. J Neurol 2011;258:1852–64.

[122] Rago R, Forfori F, Materazzi G, Abramo A, Collareta M, Miccoli P, Giunta F. Evaluation of a preoperative pain score in response to pressure as a marker of postoperative pain and drugs consumption in surgical thyroidectomy. Clin J Pain 2011; Epub Oct 13.

[123] Rainero I, Vighetti S, Bergamasco B, Pinessi L, Benedetti F. Autonomic responses and pain perception in Alzheimer's disease. Eur J Pain 2000;4:267:74.

[124] Rocco AG, Raymond SA, Murray E, Dhingra U, Freiberger D. Differential spread of blockade of touch, cold and pinprick during spinal anesthesia. Anesth Analg 1985;64:917–23.

[125] Rodriguez-Stanley S, Robinson M, Earnest DL, Greenwood-Van Meerveld B, Miner PB Jr. Esophageal hypersensitivity may be a major cause of heartburn. Am J Gastroenterol 1999;94:628–31.

[126] Russ M, Clark WC, Cross L, Kemperman I, Kakuma T, Harrison K. Pain and self-injury in borderline patients: sensory decision theory, coping strategies, and locus of control. Psychiatry Res 1996;63:57–65.

[127] Schattschneider J, Bode A, Wasner G, Binder A, Deuschl G, Baron R. Idiopathic restless legs syndrome: abnormalities in central somatosensory processing. J Neurol 2004;251:977–82.

[128] Scherder E, Oosterman J, Swaab D, Herr K, Ooms M, Ribbe M, Sergeant J, Pickering G, Benedetti F. Recent developments in pain in dementia. BMJ 2005;330:461–4.

[129] Scherder EJ, Bouma A. Is decreased use of analgesics in Alzheimer disease due to change in the affective component of pain? Alzheimer Dis Assoc Disord 1997;11:171–4.

[130] Scherder EJ. Low use of analgesics in Alzheimer's disease: possible mechanism. Psychiatry 2000;63:1–12.

[131] Scherder EJA, Bouma A, Borkent M, Rahman O. Alzheimer patients report less pain intensity and pain affect than non-demented elderly. Psychiatry 1999;62:265–72.

[132] Scherder EJA, Herr K, Pickering G, Gibson S, Benedetti F. Pain in dementia. Pain 2009;145:276–8.

[133] Scherder EJA, Sergeant J, Swaab DF. Pain processing in dementia and its relation to neuropathology. Lancet Neurol 2003;2:677–86.

[134] Schmelz M, Schmid R, Handwerker HO, Torebjörk HE. Encoding of burning pain from capsaicin-treated human skin in two categories of unmyelinated nerve fibers. Brain 2000;123:560–71.

[135] Sharief MK, Priddin J, Delamont RS, Unwin C, Rose MR, David A, Wessely S. Neurophysiologic analysis of neuromuscular symptoms in UK Gulf War veterans: a controlled study. Neurology 2002;59:1518–25.

[136] Sindrup SH, Jensen TS. Efficacy of pharmacological treatments of neuropathic pain: an update and effect related to mechanism of drug action, Pain 1999;83:389–400.

[137] Singh MK, Giles LL, Nasrallah HA. Pain insensitivity in schizophrenia: trait or state marker? J Psychiatr Pract 2006;12:90–102.

[138] Sterling M, Hendrikz J, Kenardy J. Similar factors predict disability and posttraumatic stress disorder trajectories after whiplash injury. Pain 2011;152:1272–8.

[139] Stiasny-Kolster K, Magerl W, Oertel WH, Möller JC, Treede RD. Static mechanical hyperalgesia without tactile allodynia in patients with restless legs syndrome. Brain 2004;127:773–82.

[140] Strigo IA, Simmons AN, Matthews SC, Craig AD, Paulus MP. Increased affective bias revealed using experimental graded heat stimuli in young depressed adults: evidence of "emotional allodynia." Psychosom Med 2008;70:338–44.

[141] Svendsen KB, Jensen TS, Hansen HJ, Bach FW. Sensory function and quality of life in patients with multiple sclerosis and pain. Pain 2005;114:473–81.

[142] Svendsen KB, Sørensen L, Jensen TS, Hansen HJ, Bach FW. MRI of the central nervous system in MS patients with and without pain. Eur J Pain 2011;15:395–401.

[143] Tanaka T, Satoh T, Tanaka A, Yokozeki H. Congenital insensitivity to pain with anhidrosis: a case with preserved itch sensation to histamine and partial pain sensation. Br J Dermatol 2011; Epub Oct 27.

[144] Terhaar J, Viola FC, Franz M, Berger S, Bär K-J, Weiss T. Differential processing of laser stimuli by Aδ and C fibres in major depression. Pain 2011;152:1796–802.

[145] Treister R, Pud D, Ebstein RP, Laiba E, Raz Y, Gershon E, Haddad M, Eisenberg E. Association between polymorphisms in serotonin and dopamine-related genes and endogenous pain modulation. J Pain 2011;12:875–83.

[146] Trimble KC, Pryde A, Heading RC. Lowered oesophageal sensory thresholds in patients with symptomatic but not excess gastro-oesophageal reflux: evidence for a spectrum of visceral sensitivity in GORD. Gut 1995;37:7–12.

[147] Truini A, Padua L, Biasiotta A, Caliandro P, Pazzaglia C, Galeotti F, Inghilleri M, Cruccu G. Differential involvement of A-delta and A-beta fibers in neuropathic pain related to carpal tunnel syndrome. Pain 2009;145:105–9.

[148] Vandenberghe J, Vos R, Persoons P, Demyttenaere K, Janssens J, Tack J. Dyspeptic patients with visceral hypersensitivity: sensitization of pain specific or multimodal pathways? Gut 2005;54:914–9.

[149] Vase L, Nikolajsen L, Christensen B, Egsgaard LL, Arendt-Nielsen L, Svensson P, Staehelin Jensen T. Cognitive-emotional sensitization contributes to wind-up-like pain in phantom limb pain patients. Pain 2011;152:157–62.

[150] Vecchiet L, Montanari G, Pizzigallo E, Iezzi S, de Bigontina P, Dragani L, Vecchiet J, Giamberardino MA. Sensory characterization of somatic parietal tissues in humans with chronic fatigue syndrome. Neurosci Lett 1996;208:117–20.

[151] Vilholm OJ, Cold S, Rasmussen L, Sindrup SH. Sensory function and pain in a population of patients treated for breast cancer. Acta Anaesthesiol Scand 2009;53:800–6.

[152] Waldinger MD, Venema PL, van Gils AP, Schutter EM, Schweitzer DH. Restless genital syndrome before and after clitoridectomy for spontaneous orgasms: a case report. J Sex Med 2010;7:1029–34.

[153] Waldinger MD, Venema PL, van Gils AP, Schweitzer DH. New insights into restless genital syndrome: static mechanical hyperesthesia and neuropathy of the nervus dorsalis clitoridis. J Sex Med 2009;6:2778–87.

[154] Washington LL, Gibson SJ, Helme RD. Age-related differences in the endogenous analgesic response to repeated cold water immersion in human volunteers. Pain 2000;89:89–96.

[155] Weiss T, Giersch DA, Sauer H, Miltner WHR, Bär K-J. Perception to laser heat stimuli in depressed patients is reduced to Aδ- and selective C-fiber stimulation. Neurosci Lett 2011;498:89–92.

[156] Weissman-Fogel I, Granovsky Y, Crispel Y, Ben-Nun A, Best LA, Yarnitsky D, Granot M. Enhanced presurgical pain temporal summation response predicts post-thoracotomy pain intensity during the acute postoperative phase. J Pain 2009;10:628–36.

[157] Werner MU, Duun P, Kehlet H. Prediction of postoperative pain by preoperative nociceptive responses to heat stimulation. Anesthesiology 2004;100:115–9.

[158] Wilder-Smith OH, Schreyer T, Scheffer GJ, Arendt-Nielsen L. Patients with chronic pain after abdominal surgery show less preoperative endogenous pain inhibition and more postoperative hyperalgesia: a pilot study. J Pain Palliat Care Pharmacother 2010;24:119–28.

[159] Wilder-Smith OH, Tassonyi E, Crul BJ, Arendt-Nielsen L. Quantitative sensory testing and human surgery: Effects of analgesic management on postoperative neuroplasticity. Anesthesiology 2003;98:1214–22.

[160] Woodrow KM, Friedmann GD, Siegelaub AB. Pain tolerance: differences according to age, sex and race. Psychosom Med 1972;34:548–56.

[161] Xu YS, Zhang J, Zheng JY, Zhang S, Kang DX, Fan DS. Fully intact contact heat evoked potentials in patients with amyotrophic lateral sclerosis. Muscle Nerve 2009;39:735–8.

[162] Yarnitsky D, Arendt-Nielsen L, Bouhassira D, Edwards RR, Fillingim RB, Granot M, Hansson P, Lautenbacher S, Marchand S, Wilder-Smith O. Recommendations on terminology and practice of psychophysical DNIC testing. Eur J Pain 2010;14:339.

[163] Yarnitsky D, Crispel Y, Eisenberg E, Granovsky Y, Ben-Nun A, Sprecher E, Best LA, Granot M. Prediction of chronic post-operative pain: pre-operative DNIC testing identifies patients at risk. Pain 2008;138:22–8.

[164] Yarnitsky D, Ochoa JL. Warm and cold specific somatosensory systems. Psychophysical thresholds, reaction times and peripheral conduction velocities. Brain 1991;114:1819–26.

[165] Yashiro E, Nozaki-Taguchi N, Isono S, Nishino T. Effects of different forms of dyspnoea on pain perception induced by cold-pressor test. Respir Physiol Neurobiol 2011;177:320–6.

[166] Yeomans DC, Proudfit HK. Nociceptive responses to high and low rates of noxious cutaneous heating are mediated by different nociceptors in the rat: electrophysiological evidence. Pain 1996;68:141–50.

[167] Yoon MS, Obermann M, Dockweiler C, Assert R, Canbay A, Haag S, Gerken G, Diener HC, Katsarava Z. Sensory neuropathy in patients with cryoglobulin negative hepatitis-C infection. J Neurol 2011;258:80–8.

[168] Zambito Marsala S, Tinazzi M, Vitaliani R, Recchia S, Fabris F, Marchini C, Fiaschi A, Moretto G, Giometto B, Macerollo A, Defazio G. Spontaneous pain, pain threshold, and pain tolerance in Parkinson's disease. J Neurol 2011;258:627–33.

[169] Zhou Q, Fillingim RB, Riley JL 3rd, Malarkey WB, Verne GN. Central and peripheral hypersensitivity in the irritable bowel syndrome. Pain 2010;148:454–61.

Correspondence to: Lars Arendt-Nielsen, DMSc, PhD, Center for Sensory-Motor Interaction, Department of Health Science and Technology, Faculty of Medicine, Aalborg University, Fredrik Bajers Vej 7D-3, DK-9220 Aalborg E, Denmark. Email: lan@hst.aau.dk.

A Neurobiological Approach to Chronic Pain and Comorbidities: Evidence from Animal Models

Gordon Munro

Neurodegeneration 2, H. Lundbeck A/S, Valby, Denmark

Over the past two decades information gained from mutant animals with targeted disruption of molecules involved in nociceptive signaling has helped unravel numerous underlying mechanisms (e.g., nociceptor sensitization, local inflammation, loss of spinal inhibitory controls, and central sensitization) that contribute to the pathology of chronic pain [46,55]. In parallel, the development of preclinical pain models with enhanced face (phenomenologically similar) and construct (mechanistically similar) criteria have improved the translational relevance of comparative pharmacology studies [55,87]. Together, these approaches have often yielded impressive preclinical validation packages for novel pain-related targets, and yet for neuropathic pain at least, no specifically developed, bench to bedside orally bioavailable pain therapeutics have entered into clinical practice during this time.

For the sake of argument, if we agree to forego the minefield that encompasses the development of new clinical pain candidates, the ball invariably ends up back in the court of the animal models, some of the shortcomings of which have recently been discussed elsewhere [55]. Moreover,

Pain Comorbidities: Understanding and Treating the Complex Patient
edited by Maria Adele Giamberardino and Troels Staehelin Jensen
IASP Press, Seattle, © 2012

calls have been made for animal pain studies to mirror the design and implementation of their clinical counterparts, as much as possible. Undoubtedly, information pertaining to randomization, blinding, appropriate powering, positive/negative comparator compounds, inclusion of enrichment (responders/nonresponders to standard-of-care medications), more extensive reporting of adverse effects, consideration of pharmacokinetic issues, and repeating dosing regimens are just some of the factors that will benefit this process enormously [5,55,69]. Accordingly, the reporting of non-evoked or spontaneous nociceptive behaviors has recently taken a place in the translational center stage. The use of conditioned place preference or aversion tasks in which a rat with either inflammatory or neuropathic injury learns to pair a specific environment with either a rewarding (e.g., analgesic) or an aversive experience (e.g., suprathreshold sensory stimulation) have proved particularly fruitful. While the former paradigm provides an insight into mechanisms contributing to spontaneous ongoing pain [38], as we shall see shortly, the latter appears to encapsulate aspects of affective pain-like behaviors residing outside of the sensory domain [45] (Table I).Theoretically, we should be able to expand upon these contextual paradigms to include any change in the behavioral repertoire of the animal that is modulated by injury, with the caveat that it has a corresponding clinical correlate in human pain patients.

We know that chronic pain affects the health-related quality of life experienced by the individual. As discussed throughout this book, chronic pain is often associated with a significant comorbid burden, which can consist of changes in affective state (principally depression or anxiety), cognitive impairment (including attentional deficits), and sleep disruption, among a myriad of other behavioral disturbances. Although we can readily assume that pain is the causal factor underpinning the development of such comorbidities, the high prevalence of pain in patients with depressive disorder suggests that the pathological activation of shared brain structures (especially the brainstem monoaminergic nuclei, which lie outside the scope of this discussion, but see [27]) and cellular substrates might be unifying commonalities [18]. This notion is further encapsulated in the concept of the "body-self neuromatrix," which proposes that the multidimensional experience of chronic pain involves a diversity of parallel processing within somatosensory, limbic, and thalamocortical circuitries (Fig. 1) that subserve the *sensory-discriminative* (location, intensity, modality), *affective-motivational* (unpleasantness, fear, emotion), and *cognitive-evaluative* (coping, planning) components of pain [51]. Notably, human imaging studies have implicated many of these same circuits in the pathology of anxiety, depression, and diseases associated with impaired cognitive functioning.

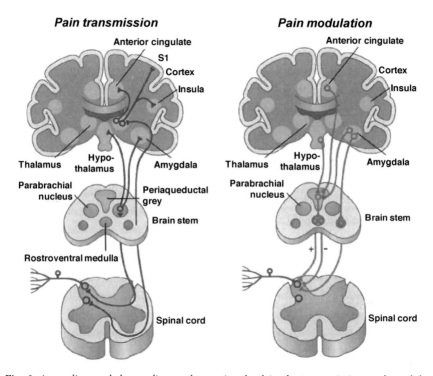

Fig. 1. Ascending and descending pathways involved in the transmission and modulation of pain. *Pain transmission:* Sensory neurons synapse onto second-order neurons in the spinal cord or dorsal column nuclei, which in turn ascend to higher centers of the brain such as the thalamus, hypothalamus, or amygdala. The thalamus, in turn, projects to areas such as the primary somatosensory (S1), anterior cingulate, and insular cortices that are required for the conscious perception of pain. *Pain modulation:* In addition to their contributions to perceiving pain, higher structures such as the hypothalamus and amygdala can in parallel modulate the experience of pain. Neurons in these regions project to regions in the hindbrain such as the periaqueductal gray, which in turn projects to the rostral ventromedial medulla in the brainstem. Descending projections from neurons in the rostral ventromedial medulla modulate neuronal activity in the dorsal spinal cord, and through this process, neurons from higher regions of the brain can inhibit (-) or facilitate (+) nociceptive transmission at the spinal level. Many of these same structures are involved in the neuroplasticity of comorbid burden that includes stress-related illnesses, anxiety, and depression [66]. Figure adapted with permission from Finnerup et al. [19].

Table I
Studies measuring sensory reflex and affective behaviors in animals after injury

Animal*	Pain Model; Behavior	Experimental Design	Main Findings	Ref.
Rat, SD, male, 180–200 g	Formalin-induced CPA; electric foot-shock CPA	Bilateral lesion of ACC or amygdala with quinolinic acid	Formalin-induced CPA reduced by ACC or amygdala lesion. Electric footshock CPA reduced by amygdala lesion. Formalin-induced acute nocifensive behaviors unaffected by either lesion.	[22]
Rat, SD, male, 180–200 g (14 d)	CCI; MA (VFf), MH, PEAP	Systemic injection of morphine, gabapentin, duloxetine, 8-OH-DPAT, WIN 55-212,2 gaboxadol	MA and PEAP reversed by morphine, gabapentin, and 8-OH-DPAT. PEAP reversed by morphine, gabapentin, 8-OH-DPAT, *and* duloxetine.	[64]
Rat, SD, male, 3–4 mo old (3 d)	SNL; MH, PEAP	Muscimol or baclofen injection in rostral ACC	No effect of GABA$_A$-receptor agonist muscimol or GABA$_B$-receptor agonist baclofen on MH. PEAP reversed only by muscimol.	[47]
Rat, SD, male, 180–200 g (14 d)	CCI; MA (VFf), MH, PEAP	Muscimol injection in CeA	MA, MH, and PEAP reversed by muscimol. Muscimol reversal blocked by bicuculline.	[65]
Rat, SD, female, 200 g (12–14 wk)	SCI; mechanical sensitivity (VFf), PEAP	Systemic injection of pregabalin	Mechanical hypersensitivity and increased PEAP in SCI rats vs. sham. PEAP attenuated by pregabalin in SCI vs. sham rats.	[2]
Rat, HW, male, 180–190 g (1–8 wk)	SNI; MA (VFf), PEAP	Glutamate receptor antagonist injection in CeA	MA and PEAP blocked by CPCCOEt (mGluR$_1$ antagonist) and MK-801 (NMDA-receptor antagonist). PEAP blocked by MPEP (mGluR$_5$ antagonist)	[1]

Table I
Continued

Animal*	Pain Model; Behavior	Experimental Design	Main Findings	Ref.
Rat; HW, male, 180–206 g (7–21 d)	SNI; MA (VFf), PEAP	CRF_{6-33} (inhibitor of CRF-binding protein) injection in CeA	CRF_{6-33} differentially increased MA and decreased PEAP; CRF_{6-33} effects blocked by CRF-receptor antagonist, CRF_{9-41}.	[12]

Abbreviations: ACC, anterior cingulate cortex; CCI, chronic constriction injury; CeA, central nucleus of the amygdala; CPA, conditioned place avoidance; CRF, corticotropin-releasing factor; HW, Hannover-Wistar; MA, mechanical allodynia; mGluR, metabotropic glutamate receptors; MH, mechanical hyperalgesia; MPEP, 2-methyl-6-(phenylethynyl)pyridine hydrochloride; NMDA, *N*-methyl-D-aspartate; 8-OH-DPAT, 8-hydroxy-dipropylaminotetralin hydrobromide; PEAP, place escape avoidance behavior; SCI, spinal cord injury; SD, Sprague-Dawley; SNI, spared nerve injury; SNL, spinal nerve ligation; VFf, von Frey filaments.

* Species, strain, sex, age. Typically, the age of animals either at the time of injury or when comorbid behaviors are assessed is not published. Therefore, the body weight of the animal when the study was initiated and the time point thereafter when further behavioral testing occurs (indicated in parentheses in days or weeks in column 1) is provided in the absence of this information. In all studies indicated, rats or mice developed appropriate injury-induced mechanical hypersensitivity.

In this chapter, I will expand on some aspects of these templates to evaluate whether evidence from animal pain models can help to formulate a neurobiological approach to aid our understanding of chronic pain and associated comorbidities. Particular emphasis will be paid to affective behavior comorbidity, which has been the focus of the majority of experimental efforts to date.

Affective Behaviors in Animal Models of Chronic Pain

Behavioral correlates of anxiety and depression have been extensively documented in animal pain models (Table II). The vast majority of these studies have used benzodiazepine-sensitive tests, such as exploration of a novel open-field environment or the elevated plus maze to assess anxiety-like behaviors in models of neuropathic pain. Notably, although simple to perform—and in contrast to other behavioral assays that rely upon the presentation of putative noxious stimuli (e.g., electric footshock) to produce a conditioned behavioral anxiogenic response—these tests rely upon a rodent's preference toward dark, enclosed spaces and an unconditioned

Table II
Studies measuring nociceptive hypersensitivity and comorbidity behaviors in animals

Animal*	Pain Model; Behavior	Behavior/ Endpoint (Test)	Main Findings	Ref.
Rat, SD, male, 150–175 g (14 d)	SNL; MA (VFf), cold (acetone)	Anxiety (OF, EPM), depression (FST), motor (LA)	No change in ALB or DLB vs. sham.	[42]
Rat, W, male, 240–350 g, adult (56 d)	VZV, PNL, SNT; MA (VFe)	Anxiety (OF)	MA in VZV rats reversed by gabapentin. ALB; SNT vs. sham and naive, VZV vs. control and naive. ALB in SNT but not VZV rats attenuated by gabapentin.	[30]
Rat, W, male, 200–250 g (60 d)	HIV-gp120; MA (VFe, VFf)	Anxiety (OF)	ALB vs. sham (14 d). MA reversed by morphine, gabapentin, and WIN 55-212,2; effects on ALB not tested.	[81]
Rat, W, male, 200–250 g (5–50 d)	HIV-gp120, HIV anti-retroviral (ddC); MA (VFe, VFf)	Anxiety (OF)	ALB in gp120 + ddC vs. sham (14d). ALB in ddC rats vs. vehicle (21d).	[82]
Rat, W, male, 200–250 g (19–21 d)	HIV anti-retroviral (ddC); MA (VFe)	Anxiety (OF)	ALB vs. sham, baseline. ALB reversed by morphine, gabapentin, and diazepam vs. sham.	[80]
Rat, WH, male, 230–330 g, 500–600 g, 650–850 g (8 wk, young; 9 mo, mid-age; 21 mo, old), (1 month)	SNI; MA (VFf)	Anxiety (EPM), depression (FST), motor (OF)	Motor deficit in old > mid-age > young SNI rats vs. sham. ALB in young and old SNI rats vs. sham. DLB in mid-age SNI rats vs. sham.	[48]
Rat, W, male, 240–280 g (21–28 d)	CCI, PNL; MA (VFe)	Anxiety (EPM), motor (LA)	ALB; CCI vs. sham. MA, ALB reversed by morphine and gabapentin.	[70]
Rat, SD, female, 200 g (12–14 wk)	SCI; mechanical sensitivity (VFf), PEAP	Anxiety (EPM)	Mechanical hypersensitivity and increased PEAP in SCI rats vs. sham. ALB in SCI and sham rats. PEAP attenuated by pregabalin in SCI vs. sham rats.	[2]

Table II
Continued

Animal*	Pain Model; Behavior	Behavior/ Endpoint (Test)	Main Findings	Ref.
Rat, LE, male, 150–180 g (25 wk)	SNI, MA (VFf), TH, cold (acetone)	Anxiety (EPM), motor (LA), magnetic resonance imaging	MA and cold hyper-sensitivity from 2–24 wk vs. sham. MA correlated with decreased volume in S1 hindlimb cortex, anterior cingulate cortex. ALB from 20–24 wk and decreased frontal cortex volume vs. sham.	[74]
Rat, W, male, 210–230 g (21–28 d)	CCI; MA (VFe)	Depression (FST), motor (LA)	DLB vs. sham. DLB reversed by desipramine. DLB and MA reversed by GW405833 (CB2 agonist).	[34]
Rat, WH, male, 200–250 g (49 d)	SNI; MA (VFf), MH (pinprick)	Anxiety (EPM, OF), depression (FST)	DLB vs. sham. Amygdala volume and cell number increased.	[24]
Rat, SD, male, 160–180 g (29 d)	SNL; MA (VFf)	Depression (FST)	DLB in SNL vs. sham (29d) reversed by amitriptyline and lornoxicam.	[33]
Mouse, C57Bl/6J, male, 25.6 g (6–28 d)	SNL; MA (VFf), cold (acetone)	Anxiety (OF, EPM), depression (FST)	No change in ALB or DLB vs. sham.	[31]
Mouse, C57BL/6, male, 24–28 g; 8 wk old (8 wk)	SNL; MA (VFf), TH	Anxiety (OF, EPM, light/ dark test), depression (FST), motor (Rotarod)	ALB vs. sham. DLB vs. sham. Diurnal activity and circadian rhythms unchanged at 6–7 wk.	[75]
Mouse, C57BL/6J, male, 18–23 g (4 wk)	CFA, PNL; MA (VFf), TH	Anxiety (EPM, light/dark test), $[^{35}S]$GTP-S binding to amygdala membranes	MA and TH in CFA and PNL mice (1, 2, 3, 4 wk) vs. saline, sham. ALB (EPM, light/dark test) in CFA vs. saline. ALB (EPM, light/dark test) in PNL vs. sham. Amygdala opioid receptor binding reduced by CFA and PNL vs. saline, sham.	[56]

Table continues on next page

Table II
Continued

Animal*	Pain Model; Behavior	Behavior/ Endpoint (Test)	Main Findings	Ref.
Mouse, C57Bl/6J, male, adult (35 d)	Sciatic nerve cuff; MA (VFf), TH	Anxiety (EPM, marble burying), depression (tail suspension)	ALB vs. sham (EPM 30d, marble burying 41d). No DLB vs. sham (23d, 35d).	[3]
Mouse, C57Bl/6J, male, 18–23 g (28 d)	PNL; MA (VFf), TH	Anxiety (light/dark test, EPM)	MA, TH, and ALB in PNL mice vs. sham (28d) MA and TH partially reversed by repeated imipramine > milnacipran > paroxetine. ALB in PNL mice reversed by repeated imipramine = milnacipran = paroxetine.	[49]
Mouse, Swiss, male, 25–35 g (14 d)	CCI; (MA (VFf)	Depression (FST), motor (OF)	DLB in CCI vs. sham. MA reversed by bis-selenide > amitriptyline > bupropion = fluoxetine. DLB reversed by bis-selenide > amitriptyline.	[35]
Mouse, C57/BL6, male, 23–30 g (7 d)	SNI; MA (VFf)	Depression (FST), motor (OF), social isolation compared with pair housing	DLB in SNI mice (isolated) vs. sham. Increased IL-1β in prefrontal cortex of SNI mice (isolated) vs. sham. DLB in SNI mice (isolated) reversed by i.c.v. oxytocin.	[59]
Mouse, C57/BL6, male, 23–30 g (7 d)	SNI; MA (VFf)	Depression (FST), motor (OF), 14 days chronic stress prior to SNI	MA and DLB in nonstressed SNI mice vs. sham. DLB potentiated by chronic stress in SNI mice. Increased pre-frontal cortex IL-1β and plasma corticosterone in nonstressed SNI mice vs. sham, potentiated by chronic stress. DLB in nonstressed SNI mice reversed by IL-1 receptor antagonist.	[60]
Mouse, Balb/c and C57Bl/6, male, adult (5 wk)	CFA, SNI, CCI; MA (VFf)	Anxiety (OF, EZM, marble burying), motor (OF)	ALB in Balb/c CFA vs. saline, SNI vs. sham. ALB in C57Bl/6 CCI vs. naive. No ALB in marble-burying test for any groups.	[79]

Table II
Continued

Animal*	Pain Model; Behavior	Behavior/ Endpoint (Test)	Main Findings	Ref.
Rat, SD, male, 180–200 g (7 d)	Colitis (2,4,6-trinitro-benzene-sulfonic acid); tactile cutaneous threshold of low back region (VFf)	Nonselective, nonsustained attention	Referred tactile hyper-sensitivity vs. naive. Attention reduced in colitis rats vs. naive; normal motor and exploratory behavior. Attentional deficit reversed by morphine and acetaminophen.	[53]
Rat, SD, male, adult (60 min)	Formalin-induced nocifensive behaviors	Motor (OF), cognition (5CSRRT)	Cognition/attentional deficit impaired vs. saline control. Pain and attentional deficit attenuated by morphine.	[11]
Rat, SD, male, adult (60 min)	Taxol-induced neuropathy; MA (VFf)	Cognition (5CSRRT)	MA from 1–19 d in Taxol rats vs. vehicle. No change in cognitive function in Taxol rats vs. vehicle.	[10]
Rat, WH, male, 230–330 g, 500–600 g, 650–850 g (8 wk, young; 9 mo, mid-age; 21 mo, old)	SNI; MA (VFf)	Cognition (working memory; MWM: spatial memory; rever-sal: behavioral flexibility)	No change in working memory or spatial reference memory in young, middle-aged, old SNI rats vs. sham. Impaired behavioral flexibility in mid-age SNI rats vs. sham.	[48]
Rat, SD, male, 300–320 g (5 d, 21 d, 56 d)	CFA (tibiotarsal joint); MA (VFf)	Anxiety (EPM), decision making (Rodent Gambling Task)	No ALB in CFA rats vs. shams. Impaired decision making (favoring larger but infrequent rewards) in CFA vs. shams. Reduced dopamine levels in orbital frontal cortex in CFA rats (21d) vs. control.	[62]
Rat, 20–21 d, (6–8 d)	SNI; MA (VFf)	Medial prefron-tal cortex elec-trophysiology and morphology	Increased NMDA-associated synaptic currents in medial prefrontal cortex layer 2/3 pyramidal cells in SNI vs. sham. Basal dendrite length and spine density increased in SNI vs. sham.	[52]

Table continues on next page

Table II
Continued

Animal*	Pain Model; Behavior	Behavior/ Endpoint (Test)	Main Findings	Ref.
Rat, SD, male, 160–180 g (30–34 d)	SNL; MA (VFf)	Spatial learning (MWM), BDNF mRNA/ protein expression	Spatial learning/probing deficits in SNL vs. sham (30–34d) reversed by amitriptyline. Hippocampal BDNF expression decreased in SNI vs. sham; reversed by amitriptyline.	[33]
Rat, SD, male, 220–260 g (10–20 d, 30–40 d); mouse, C57, male, 22–27 g	SNI; MA (VFf)	Cognition (eight-arm radial maze)	Short-term but not long-term memory impaired vs. sham. TNF-α increased in CSF and hippocampus vs. baseline, sham.	[68]
Mouse, ddY strain, male, (4–5 wk)	PNL; MA (VFf)	Motor (OF), cognition (novel-object recognition), hippocampal slice and electrophysiology	CI vs. sham. MA (but not CI) reversed by i.t. glycine transporter-1 inhibitor. NMDAR-dependent hippocampal synaptic plasticity reversed by glycine transporter-1 inhibitor.	[39]

Abbreviations: ALB, anxiety-like behavior; BDNF, brain-derived neurotrophic factor; CB2, cannabinoid receptor 2; CI, cognitive impairment; CCI, chronic constriction injury; CFA, complete Freund's adjuvant; CSF, cerebrospinal fluid; 5CSRRT, five-choice serial reaction time task; ddC, zalcitabine (anti-retroviral); DLB, depressive-like behavior; EPM, elevated plus maze; EZM, elevated zero maze; FST, forced swim test; gp120, glycoprotein I20; i.c.v., intracerebroventricular; IL-1, interleukin-1; i.t., intrathecal; LA, locomotor activity; LE, Long Evans; MA, mechanical allodynia; MWM, Morris water maze; NMDAR, N-methyl-D-aspartate receptor; OF, open field; PEAP, place escape avoidance behavior; PNL, partial nerve ligation; SCI, spinal cord injury; SD, Sprague-Dawley; SNI, spared nerve injury; SNL, spinal nerve ligation; SNT, spinal nerve transection; TH, thermal hyperalgesia; TNF-α, tumor necrosis factor α; VFe, von Frey electronic; VFf, von Frey filaments; VZV, varicella zoster virus; W, Wistar; WH, Wistar-Han.

* Species, strain, sex, age. Typically, the age of animals either at the time of injury or when comorbid behaviors are assessed is not published. Therefore, the body weight of the animal when the study was initiated and the time point thereafter when further behavioral testing occurs (indicated in parentheses in days or weeks in column 1) is provided in the absence of this information. In all indicated studies, rats or mice developed appropriate injury-induced mechanical hypersensitivity.

fear of heights and open spaces [16]. Similarly, the forced swim test can be used to detect a broad spectrum of antidepressant agents in rodents [15,17]. It is relatively simple to use, relying upon a rodent's propensity to develop an immobile posture (a putative state of behavioral despair) following initial escape-oriented movements when placed in an inescapable cylinder of water.

As highlighted in Table II, changes in affective behaviors are frequently observed within 3–4 weeks after neuropathic pain-like behaviors are established in these rodent models. These observations suggest that underlying anatomical changes and accompanying cellular mechanisms must also occur within this timeframe. However, whereas tactile hypersensitivity peaks early in rats with chronic constriction injury (CCI) and is closely correlated to regional cerebral blood flow changes within the ventrolateral thalamic nuclei [63], thermal hypersensitivity is delayed in onset and time-matched to blood flow changes within other distinct structures, principally the hypothalamic paraventricular nucleus (PVN) and the amygdala [63]. As we shall see shortly, these two brain areas are interconnected structures with well-defined roles in stress-related and emotional behaviors [67,76]. Correspondingly, in rats with spared nerve injury (SNI), magnetic resonance imaging showed that the early and sustained changes that occur in neuropathic hypersensitivity are associated with decreased volumes in the bilateral hindlimb area of the primary somatosensory cortex (S1), the anterior cingulate cortex (ACC), and the insula [74]. In contrast, anxiety-like behaviors in SNI rats might not occur until several months after injury; in one study at least, these behaviors have been time-matched to decreased volume within the frontal cortex [74]. Although this structure is more typically implicated in guiding behavior and thought processing using working memory, atrophy within the prefrontal cortex of patients with chronic complex regional pain syndrome has been linked to levels of anxiety [23]. Thus, despite a lack of gross change in amygdala volume being noted in the study in SNI rats [74], the demonstration that increased amygdala neuronal activity is accompanied by decreased prefrontal cortical activation and impaired decision-making in arthritic rats [37] nevertheless suggests that the amygdala is a key structure involved in pain and affective comorbidity.

Shared Structures and Substrates in Pain and Affective Comorbidity

The PVN is an integral component of the hypothalamo-pituitary-adrenal (HPA) axis, which is involved in mediating the neuroendocrine response to stress. Essentially, activation of the HPA axis helps to fuel the rapid sympathetic "flight or fight" response and to enhance arousal, situational appraisal, and cognitive performance. These latter actions are achieved via corticotropin-releasing factor (CRF), which is synthesized within the PVN and acts to induce release of adrenocorticotropic hormone (ACTH) from the pituitary, which in turn promotes release of the glucocorticoid hormone cortisol/corticosterone from the adrenal glands. Negative feedback actions of glucocorticoids ensure that levels are maintained within the physiological range. Abnormal functioning of the HPA axis has been reported in patients with chronic widespread pain, low back pain, and fibromyalgia [14,26,32]. Typically characterized by hypocortisolism, when this state is experimentally induced in human volunteers it is associated with a significant reduction in pain detection thresholds and augmented temporal summation [44]. Although the precise basis for HPA axis dysfunction in these conditions is largely unknown, severe stress (endured either early in life or as part of the pain condition per se) may be a factor [6,86]. Inevitably, variation in stress response genes might also enhance susceptibility to pain [32].

When viewed as a chronic inescapable stressor, chronic pain might modulate HPA axis function in preclinical pain models in a manner similar to that already described for animal models of chronic stress. It has been suggested that such changes might include enhanced basal ACTH/corticosterone levels in plasma, increased CRF expression in the PVN, and reduced glucocorticoid receptor mRNA expression in the hippocampus [7]. However, a pivotal experiment performed in CCI rats failed to show any effect of established neuropathic hypersensitivity on basal or stress-induced plasma ACTH or corticosterone levels, or on basal expression of the peptide hormones arginine vasopressin and CRF within the PVN [8]. Crucially, subsequent studies replicated a number of these unexpected observations but also went on to reveal that neuropathic hypersensitivity did variously modulate extrahypothalamic expression of CRF and glucocorticoid receptor mRNA within the amygdala and the hippocampus [72,78].

In addition to the broader role of the amygdala in emotionality and fear conditioning, neurons within the central nucleus of the amygdala (CeA) can also be activated by noxious stimulation, both directly via the spinoparabrachial pathway and indirectly via thalamic and cingulate cortex projections [9,57,83] (Fig. 1). As already suggested from regional cerebral blood flow changes after nerve injury, this neuronal activation might be maintained indefinitely [63] and is likely to be a precursor to the increased cell proliferation and volume reported within the CeA of neuropathic rats 2 months after injury [24]. These morphological changes, together with reported increases in amygdala volume in depressed patients [20], reinforce the concept that injury-induced neuroplasticity within the amygdala might be a prerequisite to pain and affective comorbidity. At the cellular level, pain-related sensitization of amygdala neurons has been shown to be dependent upon a variety of substrates involving peptidergic (calcitonin gene-related peptide and CRF) receptors, glutamatergic (N-methyl D-aspartate [NMDA] and metabotropic glutamate [mGluR]) receptors, and GABAergic (GABA$_A$) receptors [4,21,28,29,41,58,65]. In the context of pain and anxiety, the involvement of CRF is particularly striking. Electrophysiological recordings made from CeA neurons in arthritic rats have shown that administration of the selective CRF1-receptor antagonist NBI27914 attenuates facilitated synaptic transmission in this structure [21]. Subsequently, when administered locally into the CeA of arthritic rats, NBI27914 reverses spinally mediated withdrawal reflexes and supraspinally mediated audible vocalizations and ultrasonic vocalizations (representative of nocifensive and affective responses, respectively) induced by mechanical stimulation of the inflamed knee joint [21,36]. Importantly, the ability of intra-CeA NBI27914 administration to reduce a recognized measure of pain affect complements its ability to reduce comorbid anxiety-like behaviors in arthritic rats [21].

If a shared neurobiological mechanism exists within the PVN or the amygdala that contributes to chronic pain and affective comorbidity, then it might reasonably be assumed that animal models of depression or anxiety, known to be variously associated with altered HPA axis and amygdala functioning, are associated with heightened pain sensitivity. In this regard, olfactory bulbectomy, prenatal stress, maternal separation, early life stress, and genetically stress-sensitive rat strains [13,25,71,73,77,84,85] have all been shown to modulate nociceptive hypersensitivity, either in the affected adult or in the affected offspring, dependent upon the context of the model. Although these studies have largely focused upon the effects of trait depression or anxiety upon baseline nociceptive thresholds, progress is being made toward understanding the consequences for injury-induced pain pathology and sensitivity to differing analgesic mechanisms. Visceral hypersensitivity provoked by colorectal distension can be reversed by gabapentin in both maternally separated and stress-sensitive Wistar Kyoto rats [61], but a novel stress measure is only attenuated by gabapentin in maternally separated rats. Thus, despite several neurochemical and behavioral similarities in the brain-gut axis [13,50], the origin of stress-related anxiety may be different between these models and may not be related to pain hypersensitivity per se.

Cognitive Impairments in Animal Pain Models

Decline in cognitive ability is usually associated with advancing age and neurodegenerative conditions such as Alzheimer's disease, yet impairments in cognitive function have also been described in chronic pain patients. Typically, these problems affect short-term memory retrieval as well as attentional processing mechanisms (which are not discussed here, but see Table II for more details from preclinical pain models) and involve frontal cortical structures that contribute to the *cognitive-evaluative* component of pain (Fig. 1). Surprisingly (maybe not so much if you are at all acquainted with preclinical cognition models), only a small number of studies have attempted to describe whether similar changes occur in rodent models of chronic pain, with varying levels of success (Table II). In the only study to directly consider the impact of age (young, middle-aged, and old) on cognitive function, neuropathic injury impaired spatial memory performance only in mid-age rats, whereas both young and old rats with neuropathic pain were unaffected [48]. Confusingly, depression-like behaviors were only reported in the mid-age rats, whereas anxiety-like behaviors were only observed in young and old neuropathic rats. If nothing else, this finding serves to highlight the difficulty faced by researchers when trying to determine the translational relevance of such animal pain models. Indeed, although working memory deficits have been described in an alternative rat model of neuropathic pain (SNI) [68], they do not even necessarily correlate to tactile hypersensitivity per se.

These observations aside, the normal induction of hippocampal long-term potentiation—which is generally regarded as a candidate for the cellular basis of learning and memory formation—is blocked in neuropathic rats and mice [40,68]. This finding has been structurally linked to a reduction in presynaptic bouton number within the CA1 region [68], and as we shall see shortly, it also helps provide a foundation for studies to focus upon mechanisms that might contribute in turn to comorbidity in pain and depression. Various lines of evidence have shown that the proinflammatory cytokine tumor necrosis factor-α (TNF-α) participates in the development and maintenance of neuropathic hypersensitivity. Notably, nerve injury also increases levels of TNF-α in hippocampal tissue, suggesting that it contributes to synaptic plasticity in this structure [68]. Indeed, the prevention of memory deficits and rescue of hippocampal LTP induced by nerve injury upon administration of thalidomide (a TNF-α synthesis inhibitor) or genetic deletion of the TNF-α receptor provides compelling evidence to suggest that this cytokine is a key mediator of neuropathy-induced cognitive impairments [68].

Such studies may provide an insight into possible mechanisms that contribute to putative cognitive disturbances associated with chronic pain, but they are less than compelling in pointing toward possible shared neurobiological substrates that contribute to comorbidity across multiple behavioral domains in chronic pain. In this regard, recent studies have reported that neuropathic rats with established mechanical hypersensitivity and comorbid depression-like behaviors also show spatial memory impairments [33]. While administration of either the nonsteroidal anti-inflammatory drug lornoxicam or the antidepressant drug amitriptyline was shown to reverse mechanical hypersensitivity, only amitriptyline reversed depression-like behaviors and cognitive impairments. Furthermore, amitriptyline also increased mRNA expression of brain-derived neurotrophic factor (BDNF) within the hippocampus of SNL rats. Although more traditionally accepted for promoting neuronal differentiation and survival

during development, BDNF has also been shown to modulate glutama-
tergic-mediated synaptic transmission and to contribute to long-term
potentiation within the hippocampus [54]. Moreover, the "neurotrophic
hypothesis" of depression has evolved from studies linking impaired hippocampal BDNF signaling with depression-like behaviors in animals to
those showing reduced hippocampal BDNF levels in postmortem samples
from depressed humans [43].

Conclusions

Overall, the available evidence from animal pain models indicates that
injury-induced sensitization within nociceptive pathways is a prerequisite
to the neuroplasticity that occurs within supraspinal structures mediating
changes in affective state and cognitive function. Simplistically, this line of
reasoning infers that targeting of spinal pain mechanisms should resolve
both pain and comorbidity impairments after injury. Yet it is now apparent
that animal models of chronic stress intimately associated with primary
affective dysfunction are also closely correlated with secondary changes
in nociceptive hypersensitivity. Accordingly, pain-induced neuroplasticity changes within neural structures such as the hypothalamus, amygdala,
and hippocampus underpinning changes in affective state and cognitive
function might persist in the absence of ongoing nociceptive input. Given
that the majority of chronic pain patients never achieve full pain relief or
resolution of quality of life measurements, the realistic scenario is that
distinct disease mechanisms will need to be targeted in parallel for optimal
treatment of pain and comorbidity.

References

[1]   Ansah OB, Bourbia N, Gonçalves L, Almeida A, Pertovaara A. Influence of amygdaloid glutama-
      tergic receptors on sensory and emotional pain-related behavior in the neuropathic rat. Behav
      Brain Res 2010;209:174–8.
[2]   Baastrup C, Jensen TS, Finnerup NB. Pregabalin attenuates place escape/avoidance behavior in
      a rat model of spinal cord injury. Brain Res 2011;1370:129–35.
[3]   Benbouzid M, Pallage V, Rajalu M, Waltisperger E, Doridot S, Poisbeau P, Freund-Mercier
      MJ, Barrot M. Sciatic nerve cuffing in mice: a model of sustained neuropathic pain. Eur J Pain
      2008;12:591–9.
[4]   Bird GC, Lash LL, Han JS, Zou X, Willis WD, Neugebauer V. Protein kinase A-dependent en-
      hanced NMDA receptor function in pain-related synaptic plasticity in rat amygdala neurones. J
      Physiol 2005;564:907–21.

[5] Blackburn-Munro G. Pain-like behaviours in animals: how human are they? Trends Pharmacol Sci 2004;25:299–305.

[6] Blackburn-Munro G, Blackburn-Munro R. Chronic pain, chronic stress and depression: coincidence or consequence? J Neuroendocrinol 2001;13:1009–23.

[7] Bomholt SF, Harbuz MS, Blackburn-Munro G, Blackburn-Munro RE. Involvement and role of the hypothalamo-pituitary-adrenal (HPA) stress axis in animal models of chronic pain and inflammation. Stress 2004;7:1–14.

[8] Bomholt SF, Mikkelsen JD, Blackburn-Munro G. Normal hypothalamo-pituitary-adrenal axis function in a rat model of peripheral neuropathic pain. Brain Res 2005;1044:216–26.

[9] Bourgeais L, Gauriau C, Bernard J-F. Projections from the nociceptive area of the central nucleus of the amygdala to the forebrain: a PHA-L study in the rat. Eur J Neurosci 2001;14:229–55.

[10] Boyette-Davis JA, Fuchs PN. Differential effects of paclitaxel treatment on cognitive functioning and mechanical sensitivity. Neurosci Lett 2009;453:170–4.

[11] Boyette-Davis JA, Thompson CD, Fuchs PN. Alterations in attentional mechanisms in response to acute inflammatory pain and morphine administration. Neuroscience 2008;151:558–63.

[12] Bourbia N, Ansah OB, Pertovaara A. Corticotropin-releasing factor in the rat amygdala differentially influences sensory-discriminative and emotional-like pain response in peripheral neuropathy. J Pain 2010;11:1461–71.

[13] Bravo JA, Dinan TG, Cryan JF. Alterations in the central CRF system of two different rat models of comorbid depression and functional gastrointestinal disorders. Int J Neuropsychopharmacol 2011;14:666–83.

14] Crofford LJ, Pillemer SR, Kalogeras KT, Cash JM, Michelson D, Kling MA, Sternberg EM, Gold PW, Chrousos GP, Wilder RL. Hypothalamic-pituitary-adrenal axis perturbations in patients with fibromyalgia. Arthritis Rheum 1994;37:1583–92.

[15] Cryan JF, Markou A, Lucki I. Assessing antidepressant activity in rodents: recent developments and future needs. Trends Pharmacol Sci 2002;23:238–45.

[16] Cryan JF, Sweeney FF. The age of anxiety: role of animal models of anxiolytic action in drug discovery. Br J Pharmacol 2011;164:1129–61.

[17] Cryan JF, Valentino RJ, Lucki I. Assessing substrates underlying the behavioral effects of antidepressants using the modified rat forced swimming test. Neurosci Biobehav Rev 2005;29:547–69.

[18] Fields H. Depression and pain a neurobiological model. In: Neuropsychiatry, neuropsychology, and behavioral neurology. New York: Raven Press; 1991. p. 83–92.

[19] Finnerup NB, Sindrup SH, Jensen TS. Chronic neuropathic pain: mechanisms, drug targets and measurement. Fundam Clin Pharmacol 2007;21:129–36.

[20] Frodl T, Meisenzahl E, Zetzsche T, Bottlender R, Born C, Groll C, Jäger M, Leinsinger G, Hahn K, Möller HJ. Enlargement of the amygdala in patients with a first episode of major depression. Biol Psychiatry 2002;51:708–14.

[21] Fu Y, Neugebauer V. Differential mechanisms of CRF1 and CRF2 receptor functions in the amygdala in pain-related synaptic facilitation and behavior. J Neurosci 2008;28:3861–76.

[22] Gao YJ, Ren WH, Zhang YQ, Zhao ZQ. Contributions of the anterior cingulated cortex and amygdala to pain- and fear-conditioned place avoidance in rats. Pain 2004;110:343–53.

[23] Geha PY, Baliki MN, Harden RN, Bauer WR, Parrish TB, Apkarian AV. The brain in chronic CRPS pain: abnormal gray-white matter interactions in emotional and autonomic regions. Neuron 2008;60:570–81.

[24] Gonçalves L, Silva R, Pinto-Ribeiro F, Pêgo JM, Bessa JM, Pertovaara A, Sousa N, Almeida A. Neuropathic pain is associated with depressive behaviour and induces neuroplasticity in the amygdala of the rat. Exp Neurol 2008;213:48–56.

[25] Green PG, Chen X, Alvarez P, Ferrari LF, Levine JD. Early-life stress produces muscle hyperalgesia and nociceptor sensitization in the adult rat. Pain 2011;152:2549–56.

[26] Griep EN, Boersma JW, Lentjes EG, Prins AP, van der Korst JK, de Kloet ER. Function of the hypothalamic-pituitary-adrenal axis in patients with fibromyalgia and low back pain. J Rheumatol 1998;25:1374–81.

[27] Hache G, Coudore F, Gardier AM, Guiard BP. Monoaminergic antidepressants in the relief of pain: potential therapeutic utility of triple reuptake inhibitors (TRIs). Pharmaceuticals 2011;4:285–342.

[28] Han JS, Li W, Neugebauer V. Critical role of calcitonin gene-related peptide 1 receptors in the amygdala in synaptic plasticity and pain behavior. J Neurosci 2005;25:10717–28.

[29] Han JS, Adwanikar H, Li Z, Ji G, Neugebauer V. Facilitation of synaptic transmission and pain responses by CGRP in the amygdala of normal rats. Mol Pain 2010;6:10.

[30] Hasnie FS, Breuer J, Parker S, Wallace V, Blackbeard J, Lever I, Kinchington PR, Dickenson AH, Pheby T, Rice AS. Further characterization of a rat model of varicella zoster virus-associated pain: relationship between mechanical hypersensitivity and anxiety-related behavior, and the influence of analgesic drugs. Neuroscience 2007;144:1495–508.

[31] Hasnie FS, Wallace VC, Hefner K, Holmes A, Rice AS. Mechanical and cold hypersensitivity in nerve-injured C57BL/6J mice is not associated with fear-avoidance- and depression-related behaviour. Br J Anaesth 2007;98:816–22.

[32] Holliday KL, Nicholl BI, Macfarlane GJ, Thomson W, Davies KA, McBeth J. Genetic variation in the hypothalamic-pituitary-adrenal stress axis influences susceptibility to musculoskeletal pain: results from the EPIFUND study. Ann Rheum Dis 2010;69:556–60.

[33] Hu Y, Yang J, Hu Y, Wang Y, Li W. Amitriptyline rather than lornoxicam ameliorates neuropathic pain-induced deficits in abilities of spatial learning and memory. Eur J Anaesthesiol 2010;27:162–8.

[34] Hu B, Doods H, Treede RD, Ceci A. Depression-like behaviour in rats with mononeuropathy is reduced by the CB2-selective agonist GW405833. Pain 2009;143:206–12.

[35] Jesse CR, Wilhelm EA, Nogueira CW. Depression-like behavior and mechanical allodynia are reduced by bis selenide treatment in mice with chronic constriction injury: a comparison with fluoxetine, amitriptyline, and bupropion. Psychopharmacology 2010;212:513–22.

[36] Ji G, Fu Y, Ruppert KA, Neugebauer V. Pain-related anxiety-like behaviour requires CRF1 receptors in the amygdala. Mol Pain 20075;3:13.

[37] Ji G, Sun H, Fu Y, Li Z, Pais-Vieira M, Galhardo V, Neugebauer V. Cognitive impairment in pain through amygdala-driven prefrontal cortical deactivation. J Neurosci 2010;30:5451–64.

[38] King T, Qu C, Okun A, Mercado R, Ren J, Brion T, Lai J, Porreca F. Contribution of afferent pathways to nerve injury-induced spontaneous pain and evoked hypersensitivity. Pain 2011;152:1997–2005.

[39] Kodama D, Ono H, Tanabe M. Increased hippocampal glycine uptake and cognitive dysfunction after peripheral nerve injury. Pain 2011;152:809–17.

[40] Kodama D, Ono H, Tanabe M. Altered hippocampal long-term potentiation after peripheral nerve injury in mice. Eur J Pharmacol 2007;574:127–32.

[41] Kolber BJ, Montana MC, Carrasquillo Y, Xu J, Heinemann SF, Muglia LJ, Gereau RW. Activation of metabotropic glutamate receptor 5 in the amygdala modulates pain-like behavior. J Neurosci 2010;30:8203–13.

[42] Kontinen VK, Kauppila T, Paananen S, Pertovaara A, Kalso E. Behavioural measures of depression and anxiety in rats with spinal nerve ligation-induced neuropathy. Pain 1999;80:341–6.

[43] Krishnan V, Nestler EJ. Linking molecules to mood: new insight into the biology of depression. Am J Psychiatry 2010;167:1305–20.

[44] Kuehl LK, Michaux GP, Richter S, Schächinger H, Anton F. Increased basal mechanical pain sensitivity but decreased perceptual wind-up in a human model of relative hypocortisolism. Pain 2010;149:539–46.

[45] LaBuda CJ, Fuchs PN. A behavioral test paradigm to measure the aversive quality of inflammatory and neuropathic pain in rats. Exp Neurol 2000;163:490–4.

[46] Lacroix-Fralish ML, Ledoux JB, Mogil JS. The Pain Genes Database: an interactive web browser of pain-related transgenic knockout studies. Pain 2007;131:3.e1–4.

[47] LaGraize SC, Fuchs PN. GABAA but not GABAB receptors in the rostral anterior cingulate cortex selectively modulate pain-induced escape/avoidance behavior. Exp Neurol 2007;204:182–94.

[48] Leite-Almeida H, Almeida-Torres L, Mesquita AR, Pertovaara A, Sousa N, Cerqueira JJ, Almeida A. The impact of age on emotional and cognitive behaviours triggered by experimental neuropathy in rats. Pain 2009;144:57–65.

[49] Matsuzawa-Yanagida K, Narita M, Nakajima M, Kuzumaki N, Niikura K, Nozaki H, Takagi T, Tamai E, Hareyama N, Terada M, Yamazaki M, Suzuki T. Usefulness of antidepressants for improving the neuropathic pain-like state and pain-induced anxiety through actions at different brain sites. Neuropsychopharmacology 2008;33:1952–65.

[50] McKernan DP, Nolan A, Brint EK, O'Mahony SM, Hyland NP, Cryan JF, Dinan TG, Timmer A. Toll-like receptor mRNA expression is selectively increased in the colonic mucosa of two animal models relevant to irritable bowel syndrome. PloS One 2009;4:e8226.

[51] Melzack R. From the gate to the neuromatrix. Pain 1999;Suppl 6:S121–6.
[52] Metz AE, Yau HJ, Centeno MV, Apkarian AV, Martina M. Morphological and functional reorganization of rat medial prefrontal cortex in neuropathic pain. Proc Natl Acad Sci USA 2009;106:2423–8.
[53] Millecamps M, Etienne M, Jourdan D, Eschalier A, Ardid D. Decrease in non-selective, non-sustained attention induced by a chronic visceral inflammatory state as a new pain evaluation in rats. Pain 2004;109:214–24.
[54] Minichiello L. TrkB signalling pathways in LTP and learning. Nat Rev Neurosci 2009;10:850–60.
[55] Mogil JS. Animal models of pain: progress and challenges. Nat Rev Neurosci 2009;10:283–94.
[56] Narita M, Kaneko C, Miyoshi K, Nagumo Y, Kuzumaki N, Nakajima M, Nanjo K, Matsuzawa K, Yamazaki M, Suzuki T. Chronic pain induces anxiety with concomitant changes in opioidergic function in the amygdala. Neuropsychopharmacology 2006;31:739–50.
[57] Neugebauer V, Li W, Bird GC, Han JS. The amygdala and persistent pain. Neuroscientist 2004;10:221–34.
[58] Neugebauer V, Li W, Bird GC, Bhave G, Gereau RW. Synaptic plasticity in the amygdala in a model of arthritic pain: differential roles of metabotropic glutamate receptors 1 and 5. J Neurosci 2003;23:52–63.
[59] Norman GJ, Karelina K, Morris JS, Zhang N, Cochran M, Courtney DeVries A. Social interaction prevents the development of depressive-like behavior post nerve injury in mice: a potential role for oxytocin. Psychosom Med 2010;72:519–26.
[60] Norman GJ, Karelina K, Zhang N, Walton JC, Morris JS, Devries AC. Stress and IL-1beta contribute to the development of depressive-like behavior following peripheral nerve injury. Mol Psychiatry 2010;15:404–14.
[61] O'Mahony SM, Coelho AM, Fitzgerald P, Lee K, Winchester W, Dinan TG, Cryan JF. The effects of gabapentin in two animal models of co-morbid anxiety and visceral hypersensitivity. Eur J Pharmacol 2011;667:169–74.
[62] Pais-Vieira M, Mendes-Pinto MM, Lima D, Galhardo V. Cognitive impairment of prefrontal-dependent decision-making in rats after the onset of chronic pain. Neuroscience 2009;161:671–9.
[63] Paulson P, Casey K, Morrow T. Long-term changes in behavior and regional cerebral blood flow associated with painful peripheral mononeuropathy in the rat. Pain 2002;95:31–40.
[64] Pedersen LH, Blackburn-Munro G. Pharmacological characterisation of place escape/avoidance behaviour in the rat chronic constriction injury model of neuropathic pain. Psychopharmacology 2006;185:208–17.
[65] Pedersen LH, Scheel-Krüger J, Blackburn-Munro G. Amygdala GABA-A receptor involvement in mediating sensory-discriminative and affective-motivational pain responses in a rat model of peripheral nerve injury. Pain 2007;127:17–26.
[66] Pittenger C, Duman RS. Stress, depression, and neuroplasticity: a convergence of mechanisms. Neuropsychopharmacology 2008;33:88–109.
[67] Prewitt CM, Herman JP. Anatomical interactions between the central amygdaloid nucleus and the hypothalamic paraventricular nucleus of the rat: a dualtract-tracing analysis. J Chem Neuroanat 1998;15:173–85.
[68] Ren WJ, Liu Y, Zhou LJ, Li W, Zhong Y, Pang RP, Xin WJ, Wei XH, Wang J, Zhu HQ, Wu CY, Qin ZH, Liu G, Liu XG. Peripheral nerve injury leads to working memory deficits and dysfunction of the hippocampus by upregulation of TNF-α in rodents. Neuropsychopharmacology 2011;36:979–92.
[69] Rice AS, Cimino-Brown D, Eisenach JC, Kontinen VK, Lacroix-Fralish ML, Machin I; Preclinical Pain Consortium, Mogil JS, Stöhr T. Animal models and the prediction of efficacy in clinical trials of analgesic drugs: a critical appraisal and call for uniform reporting standards. Pain 2008;139:243–7.
[70] Roeska K, Doods H, Arndt K, Treede RD, Ceci A. Anxiety-like behaviour in rats with mononeuropathy is reduced by the analgesic drugs morphine and gabapentin. Pain 2008;139:349–57.
[71] Roeska K, Ceci A, Treede RD, Doods H. Effect of high trait anxiety on mechanical hypersensitivity in male rats. Neurosci Lett 2009;464:160–4.
[72] Rouwette T, Vanelderen P, Reus MD, Loohuis NO, Giele J, Egmond JV, Scheenen W, Scheffer GJ, Roubos E, Vissers K, Kozicz T. Experimental neuropathy increases limbic forebrain CRF. Eur J Pain 2011; Epub Jun 17.

[73] Schwetz I, McRoberts JA, Coutinho SV, Bradesi S, Gale G, Fanselow M, Million M, Ohning G, Taché Y, Plotsky PM, Mayer EA. Corticotropin-releasing factor receptor 1 mediates acute and delayed stress-induced visceral hyperalgesia in maternally separated Long-Evans rats. Am J Physiol Gastrointest Liver Physiol 2005;289:G704–12.

[74] Seminowicz DA, Laferriere AL, Millecamps M, Yu JS, Coderre TJ, Bushnell MC. MRI structural brain changes associated with sensory and emotional function in a rat model of long-term neuropathic pain. Neuroimage 2009;47:1007–14.

[75] Suzuki T, Amata M, Sakaue G, Nishimura S, Inoue T, Shibata M, Mashimo T. Experimental neuropathy in mice is associated with delayed behavioral changes related to anxiety and depression. Anesth Analg 2007;104:1570–7.

[76] Tsubouchi K, Tsumori T, Yokota S, Okunishi H, Yasui Y. A disynaptic pathway from the central amygdaloid nucleus to the paraventricular hypothalamic nucleus via the parastrial nucleus in the rat. Neurosci Res 2007;59:390–8.

[77] Uhelski ML, Fuchs PN. Maternal separation stress leads to enhanced emotional responses to noxious stimuli in adult rats. Behav Brain Res 2010;212:208–12.

[78] Ulrich-Lai YM, Xie W, Meij JT, Dolgas CM, Yu L, Herman JP. Limbic and HPA axis function in an animal model of chronic neuropathic pain. Physiol Behav 2006;88:67–76.

[79] Urban R, Scherrer G, Goulding EH, Tecott LH, Basbaum AI. Behavioral indices of ongoing pain are largely unchanged in male mice with tissue or nerve injury-induced mechanical hypersensitivity. Pain 2011;152:990–1000.

[80] Wallace VC, Segerdahl AR, Blackbeard J, Pheby T, Rice AS. Anxiety-like behaviour is attenuated by gabapentin, morphine and diazepam in a rodent model of HIV anti-retroviral-associated neuropathic pain. Neurosci Lett 2008;448:153–6.

[81] Wallace VC, Blackbeard J, Pheby T, Segerdahl AR, Davies M, Hasnie F, Hall S, McMahon SB, Rice AS. Pharmacological, behavioural and mechanistic analysis of HIV-1 gp120 induced painful neuropathy. Pain 2007;133:47–63.

[82] Wallace VC, Blackbeard J, Segerdahl AR, Hasnie F, Pheby T, McMahon SB, Rice AS. Characterization of rodent models of HIV-gp120 and anti-retroviral-associated neuropathic pain. Brain 2007;130:2688–702.

[83] Wang CC, Willis WD, Westlund KN. Ascending projections from the area around the spinal cord central canal: a Phaseolus vulgaris leucoagglutinin study in rats. J Comp Neurol 1999;415:341–67.

[84] Wang W, Qi WJ, Xu Y, Wang JY, Luo F. The differential effects of depression on evoked and spontaneous pain behaviors in olfactory bulbectomized rats. Neurosci Lett 2010;472:143–7.

[85] Weaver SA, Diorio J, Meaney MJ. Maternal separation leads to persistent reductions in pain sensitivity in female rats. J Pain 2007;8:962–9.

[86] Weissbecker I, Floyd A, Dedert E, Salmon P, Sephton S. Childhood trauma and diurnal cortisol disruption in fibromyalgia syndrome. Psychoneuroendocrinology 2006;31:312–24.

[87] Whiteside GT, Adedoyin A, Leventhal L. Predictive validity of animal pain models? A comparison of the pharmacokinetic-pharmacodynamic relationship for pain drugs in rats and humans. Neuropharmacology 2008;54:767–75.

Correspondence to: Gordon Munro, PhD, Neurodegeneration 2, H. Lundbeck A/S, Ottiliavej 9, DK-2500, Valby, Denmark. Email: gmun@lundbeck.com.

Genetic Factors in Comorbid Pain Disorders

Dan Buskila[a,b] and Antonio Collado Cruz[c]

[a]Department of Medicine, Soroka Medical Center, Beer Sheva, Israel;
[b]Faculty of Health Sciences, Ben Gurion University in the Negev, Beer Sheva, Israel;
[c]Fibromyalgia Unit, Rheumatology Service, Hospital Clinic of Barcelona,
University of Barcelona, Barcelona, Spain

Comorbid pain disorders are common in the general population, and clearly they adversely affect quality of life and physical functioning [8]. Pain perception is a complex process that may be influenced by a variety of environmental and genetic factors [52]. Fibromyalgia syndrome (FMS) is a disorder characterized by chronic widespread musculoskeletal pain and related symptoms (fatigue, disturbed sleep, and cognitive problems). The current concept views FMS as the result of a central nervous system malfunction that amplifies pain transmission and interpretation [9]. Recent evidence suggests that FMS and related syndromes share inheritable pathophysiological features [13–15]. Certain environmental factors may trigger the development of FMS and related conditions in genetically predisposed individuals [17].

Evidence for the role of genetics in the development of FMS and comorbid conditions comes from studies demonstrating familial aggregation in those conditions, which have led to the recognition that specific genes might confer an increased risk of developing FMS. This chapter reviews the current evidence showing that genetic and familial factors may play a role in the development of comorbid pain disorders.

Pain Comorbidities: Understanding and Treating the Complex Patient
edited by Maria Adele Giamberardino and Troels Staehelin Jensen
IASP Press, Seattle, © 2012

Family Studies

Buskila et al. studied the familial occurrence of FMS to try to determine a possible role for genetic and familial factors in this syndrome [10]. Fifty-eight individuals aged 5–46 years (35 males and 23 females) whose mothers had FMS were recruited from 20 complete nuclear families and were clinically evaluated for FMS. Sixteen of these individuals (28%) were found to have FMS. The male/female ratio among those affected was 0.8, compared with 1.5 in the whole study group. Participants with and without FMS did not differ in anxiety, depression, global well-being, quality of life, and physical functioning. In this study, a high prevalence of FMS was observed among offspring of mothers with FMS. Because psychological and familial factors did not differ in offspring with and without FMS, we suggested that the high familial occurrence of this syndrome may be attributable to genetic factors.

We expanded our observations on the prevalence of FMS in relatives of FMS patients in a study of 30 female FMS patients and 117 of their close relatives (parents, brothers, sisters, children, and husbands) [12]. The prevalence of FMS was 26% among blood relatives of patients with FMS and 19% among patients' husbands. FMS prevalence was 14% in male relatives and 41% in female relatives. The mean tender point counts of young male and female relatives was significantly higher than those of controls: 6.1 versus 0.2 for boys ($P < 0.01$), and 4.4 versus 0.4 for girls ($P < 0.01$). Similarly, adult relatives had considerably higher mean tender point counts than controls: 4.0 versus 0.04 for men ($P < 0.01$) and 10.3 versus 0.28 for women ($P < 0.01$).

We concluded that relatives of patients with FMS have a higher prevalence of FMS and are more tender than the general population, based on findings from a study where relatives of FMS patients were compared to a healthy control group. We suggested that these findings can be attributed to genetic and environmental factors. Quality of life was reduced and physical functioning was impaired in relatives of patients with FMS, especially in female relatives and in those who themselves had undiagnosed FMS [54].

Arnold et al. [3] conducted a family study of fibromyalgia, with the aim of assessing familial aggregation of FMS and measures of tenderness and pain, as well as familial coaggregation of FMS and major mood disorder [3]. The investigators collected information regarding 533 relatives of 78 probands with FMS and 272 relatives of 40 probands with rheumatoid arthritis (RA). FMS aggregated strongly in families: the odds ratio (OR) measuring the odds of FMS in a relative of a proband with FMS versus the odds of FMS in a relative of a proband with RA was 8.5. The number of tender points was significantly higher, and the total myalgic score was significantly lower, in the relatives of probands with FMS compared with the relatives of probands with RA. FMS coaggregated significantly with major mood disorder: the OR measuring the odds of major mood disorder in a relative of a proband with FMS versus the odds of major mood disorder in a relative of a proband with RA was 1.8. The authors concluded that FMS coaggregates in families both with reduced pressure pain thresholds and with major mood disorder [3]. Arnold et al. suggested that these findings have important clinical and theoretical implications, including the possibility that genetic factors are involved in the etiology of FMS and in pain sensitivity. In addition, mood disorders and FMS may share some of these inherited factors [3].

Walsh et al. assessed 25 individuals with chronic fatigue syndrome (CFS) and 36 medical control subjects for lifetime psychiatric symptoms [77]. A family history was obtained regarding first-degree relatives. There were significantly higher rates of CFS in the relatives of individuals with CFS compared with the relatives of control subjects. Walsh et al. suggested that familial factors are important in the etiology of CFS. Another study assessed the role of genetic and environmental factors in unexplained chronic fatigue [7]. This classic twin study was conducted using 146 pairs of female twins, in which at least one twin reported at least 6 months of fatigue. The concordance rate was higher in monozygotic than dizygotic twins for each definition of chronic pain. This study provides evidence supporting the familial aggregation of fatigue and suggests that genes may play a role in the etiology of CFS [7].

Irritable bowel syndrome (IBS) was found in 17% of IBS patients' relatives but in only 7% of their spouses' relatives [40]. The authors of this study concluded that familial aggregation of IBS occurs, supporting a genetic or intrafamilial environmental component, but that it may be explained in part by familial aggregation of somatization.

Central sensitization and allodynia, as described in FMS and overlapping conditions [79], have also been reported in migraine [45]. We have reported a high incidence of FMS among female migraine patients, but not in male patients [38]. It has been shown that migraine, along with other comorbid conditions, aggregates in families [38]. Previous studies have demonstrated an association between post-traumatic stress disorder (PTSD) and FMS [2,20].

A twin study of Vietnam veterans has shown a significant genetic contribution to PTSD [41]. In this study, which assessed genetic and environmental influences on trauma exposure and PTSD symptoms, Stein et al. concluded that genetic factors can influence the risk of exposure to some forms of trauma, perhaps through individual differences in personality that influence environmental choices [65].

Genetic Markers in Chronic Pain Disorders

The compelling evidence regarding a genetic basis for FMS and comorbid pain disorders has led researchers to attempt to identify specific target genes involved in the pathogenesis of these disorders. Research performed in recent years has demonstrated a role for polymorphisms of genes in the serotoninergic, dopaminergic, and catecholaminergic systems in the etiology of these chronic pain conditions [8,9,13,15].

Catechol-O-Methyltransferase Polymorphisms

Catechol-O-methyltransferase (COMT) is one of the enzymes that metabolize catecholamines, thereby acting as a key modulator of dopaminergic neurotransmission. There is a common functional polymorphism of the *COMT* gene that encodes the substitution of valine (val) by methionine (met) at codon 158 (val$_{158}$met) [44].

Zubieta and colleagues examined the influence of this common functional genetic polymorphism, which affects the metabolism of catecholamines, on the modulation of responses to sustained pain in humans [80]. Individuals homozygous for val$_{158}$met show diminished regional μ-opioid system responses to pain compared with heterozygotes. These effects were accompanied by higher sensory and affective ratings of pain and a more negative internal affective state. The authors concluded that the COMT val$_{158}$met polymorphism influences the human experience of pain and may underlie interindividual differences in adaptation and responses to pain and other stimuli [80].

Diatchenko et al. identified three genetic variants (haplotypes) of the gene encoding COMT, which they designated as low pain sensitivity (LPS), average pain sensitivity (APS), and high pain sensitivity (HPS) [24]. They showed that these haplotypes encompass 96% of the human population. Five combinations of these haplotypes are strongly associated with variation in the sensitivity to experimental pain. The presence of even a single LPS haplotype diminished the risk of developing myogenous temporomandibular joint disorder (TMD). The LPS haplotype produces much higher levels of COMT enzymatic activity when compared with the APS or HPS haplotypes. Inhibition of COMT activity in the rat results in a profound increase in pain sensitivity. Diatchenko et al. concluded that COMT activity substantially influences pain sensitivity, and that in humans the three major haplotypes determine COMT activity, along with the risk for development of TMD [24].

Gursoy and colleagues [33] have reported on the involvement of a COMT gene polymorphism in patients with FMS. They concluded that a COMT polymorphism is of potential pharmacological importance regarding individual differences in the metabolism of catecholaminergic drugs and may also be involved in the pathogenesis and treatment of FMS through adrenergic mechanisms. A COMT polymorphism may also play a role in genetic predisposition to FMS [33].

The result of a study conducted in Mexican and Spanish patients with FMS showed an association between FMS and two single-nucleotide polymorphisms (SNPs) of the COMT gene that have previously been reported to be related to pain sensitivity, but only in Spaniards [73]. By contrast, the Mexican population displayed only a weak association between the two SNPs and isolated FMS symptoms [73].

Cohen et al. [19] observed an association between FMS and the COMT val$_{158}$met polymorphism and concluded that carriers of the COMT met/met genotype had increased sensitivity to pain. The results of a Brazilian study suggest that SNPs rs4680 and rs4818 of the COMT gene may be associated with FMS and pain sensitivity in Brazilian patients with FMS [4].

Park et al. [58] reported that although the *COMT* polymorphism does not appear to be involved in the predisposition to develop migraine without aura, this genetic factor could be involved in the phenotypic expression of this condition. A gene/environment interaction was indicated between the human *COMT* val$_{158}$met polymorphism and the number of traumatic event types experienced in the risk of developing PTSD [43].

An interesting study provided by McLean et al. [49] demonstrated that *COMT* haplotype predicts immediate musculoskeletal neck pain and psychological symptoms after motor vehicle collision. George et al. [29] provided evidence that the presence of elevated pain catastrophizing and *COMT* diplotype indicative of low COMT enzyme activity may potentially increase the risk of developing chronic pain syndromes. Dai et al. [23] reported on the association of *COMT* genetic variants with the outcome of surgical treatment for lumbar degenerative disk disease. *COMT* haplotypes have been suggested to serve as generic predictors of propranolol treatment outcome, indentifying a subgroup of TMD patients who will benefit from propranolol therapy [67].

Mobascher et al. [51], in a functional MRI study, found that subjects homozygous for the met$_{158}$ allele exhibit a higher blood-oxygen-level-dependent response in the anterior cingulate cortex, particularly in the midcingulate cortex, than do carriers of the val$_{158}$ allele. Lee et al. [47] reported that *COMT* polymorphisms are associated with postoperative pain intensity. Two studies found no evidence for a role of *COMT* haplotypes in chronic musculoskeletal pain [34,55].

Serotonin Transporter Gene Polymorphisms

Research conducted in recent years has demonstrated a role for polymorphisms of genes in the serotoninergic system in the pathogenesis of FMS. Offenbaecher et al. analyzed the genotypes of the promoter region of the serotonin transporter (5-HTT) gene in patients in FMS [56]. A higher frequency of the S/S genotype of 5-HTT was found in FMS patients compared to controls. The S/S subgroup exhibited higher mean levels of depression and psychological distress. The authors suggested that these results support the notion of altered serotonin metabolism in at least a subgroup of patients with FMS.

Bondy et al. investigated a silent polymorphism (T102C) in the 5-HT_{2A}-receptor gene, located on the long arm of chromosome 13, in 168 FMS patients and 115 healthy controls [6]. Their results showed a significantly different genotype distribution in FMS patients, with a decrease in T/T and an increase in both T/C and C/C genotypes as compared to the control population. However, the increase in allele C102 frequency fell short of significance. The pain score was significantly higher in patients of the T/T genotype. The authors suggested that the T102 allele might be involved in the complex circuits of nociception [6].

We performed genotyping in a group of 99 female FMS patients from two Israeli ethnic groups [18]. Additionally, we assessed each patient with the Tridimensional Personality Questionnaire (TPQ), a self-report instrument consisting of 100 yes/no questions. In this study, we confirmed the observation by the German group [56] that the *5-HTTLPR* polymorphism is associated with FMS. There was also a significant association between *5-HTTLPR* genotype and the TPQ harm avoidance trait, which is consistent with the initial report by Lesch et al. that the short allele of this polymorphism is associated with anxiety-related traits [48]. My colleagues and I suggested that the relationship between FMS and the serotonin transporter may be indirect and mediated by anxiety-related traits [18]. Most important, our findings support the idea that a genetic approach to a complex trait such as FMS will help elucidate the biological underpinnings of this disease and allow a more rational approach to drug development and treatment paradigms.

Both serotonin receptor subunit genes, *HTR3A* and *HTR3B*, have been investigated for sequence variations in FMS patients [26]. *HTR3A* mutational analysis revealed one novel as well as five known sequence variations. *HTR3B* mutational analysis revealed seven formerly described mutations and one novel sequence. The authors of that study suggested that these mutations represent the basis for future studies on their pharmacogenetic relevance [26].

The results of a study by Pata et al. [59] suggest that patients with the homozygote C allele of the 102 T/C polymorphism or the homozygote A allele of the 1438 G/A polymorphism of the 5-HT_{2A}-receptor gene have a high risk of IBS. Pata et al. also found that the T/T genotype of the 102T/C polymorphism may be associated with more severe pain in patients with IBS. A significant association was observed between diarrhea-predominant IBS and the *SERT-P* (serotonin reuptake transporter) deletion/deletion genotype, suggesting that the serotonin transporter is a potential candidate gene for diarrhea-predominant IBS in women [78].

Fukudo et al. [27] found that individuals with a weak function of the serotonin transporter have stronger responses to gut signals in emotion-regulating brain regions. The G allele of the rs25531 polymorphism of *SERT* was found to be associated with IBS [42]. The *SERT-P* polymorphism was associated with constipation-predominant IBS in the Indian population [63]. Possible associations of TPH (tryptophan hydroxylase) gene variants with IBS and IBS-related gastrointestinal symptoms have been demonstrated in unrelated Caucasian women [39].

Narita et al. examined a serotonin transporter (5-HTT) gene promoter polymorphism that affects the transcriptional efficiency of 5-HTT, in a study of 78 CFS patients [53]. A significant increase of longer (L and XL) allelic variants was found in the CFS patients compared to the controls, by both genotype-wise and allele-wise analyses. The authors suggested that attenuated concentration of extracellular serotonin due to longer variants may cause higher susceptibility to CFS. A study provided by Smith et al. [64] identified an association of the A allele of the 1438G/A polymorphism of *HTR2A* with CFS and with measures of disability and fatigue.

Corominas et al. [21] suggested a differential involvement of serotonin-related genes in the genetic background of migraine with and without aura. A serotonin transporter gene polymorphism was found to confer an increased risk of inconsistent response to triptans in migraine patients [68].

The association between *5-HTTLPR* polymorphism and the development of acute and persistence of chronic PTSD was investigated [69]. A significant association was found for chronic PTSD, with an increased risk of 4.8 in the group with the S allele compared to the group without it [69].

Grabe et al. [32] studied serotonin transporter gene (*SLC6A4*) promoter polymorphisms and the susceptibility to PTSD in the general population. The results of this study demonstrated a clear gene main effect, with an additive relationship between the number of LA alleles and the diagnosis of PTSD in community residents exposed to at least one traumatic event [32].

Dopaminergic System Polymorphisms

Recent research indicates that the dopaminergic system plays a role in pain perception. Treister et al. [71] have recently suggested that low dopaminergic activity may be associated with high pain sensitivity, and vice versa.

Potvin et al. [60] conducted an experimental study relating DNIC (diffuse noxious inhibitory controls) and thermal pain thresholds to a functional polymorphism of limbic dopamine D_3 receptors. The authors suggested that these results may help identify a subgroup of FMS patients who require closer medical attention [60].

Segman et al. [61] have suggested that genetically determined changes in dopaminergic reactivity may contribute to the occurrence of PTSD among trauma survivors. The results of another study [75] demonstrated an association between a polymorphism in the dopamine D_2 receptor (*DRD2*) gene and PTSD.

Todt et al. [70] have provided evidence for an involvement of components of the dopaminergic system, in particular the dopamine beta-hydroxylase and dopamine transporter genes, to the pathogenesis of migraine with aura. Another study suggests a role of specific dopaminergic gene polymorphisms in migraine susceptibility in the North Indian population [30]. García-Martín et al. [28] found, however, that *DRD3* genotype and allelic variants were not related to the risk of migraine in Caucasian Spanish people.

Adrenergic Receptor Gene Polymorphisms

Adrenergic receptor gene polymorphisms were found to be related to the risk of developing FMS and were also linked to different domains of FMS [74]. Results from the 1958 British Birth Cohort study showed that genetic variation in the β_2-adrenergic receptor gene, but not in *COMT*, predisposes to chronic pain [35]. A significant association was observed between the α_{2A}-adrenergic receptor gene (alpha 2A-1291 C>G) polymorphism and diarrhea-predominant IBS [62].

Other Genetic Polymorphisms in Pain Conditions

The results of a recent study suggest that chronic experience of pain enhances genetic sensitivity to experimentally induced mildly painful stimuli, possibly through a process of epigenetic modification [76].

Feng et al. [25] provided evidence for the association between the *MEFV* structural gene variants (a gene in which various compound heterozygous mutations lead to familial Mediterranean fever) and FMS in a subset of FMS patients. This observation is interesting because we have previously reported on FMS in familial Mediterranean fever patients [46].

The presence of the E*2 allele (an apolipoprotein E allele) was suggested to have a protective action regarding the association between FMS and stress [5]. Su et al. [66] reported on the association between FMS and polymorphisms of monoamine oxidase A and interleukin-4. Holliday et al. [36] reported that genetic variation in the primary stress response system influences susceptibility to musculoskeletal pain in a general population sample (the EPIFUND study). The authors stress, however, that since the associations are modest, replication of these findings is required. Another study investigating cytokine genomic polymorphisms revealed a highly significant increase in tumor necrosis factor (TNF)-857 TT and CT genotypes and a significant decrease in interferon (IFN)-gamma low producers (A/A) among CFS patients compared to controls [16].

A Korean study provided evidence to suggest that the presence of IBS is related to genetic polymorphisms of the cannabinoid receptor [57].

Genetic Factors and the Pathogenesis of Comorbid Pain Disorders

Fibromyalgia and related comorbid pain disorders are syndromes characterized by generalized pain sensitivity as well as a constellation of other symptoms. Our understanding of FMS has made significant advances over the past decade. Research conducted over the past few years has demonstrated a role for polymorphisms of genes in the serotoninergic, dopaminergic, and catecholaminergic systems in the pathogenesis of FMS. Those polymorphisms are not specific to FMS and are found in FMS-related conditions and comorbid pain syndromes.

It remains very probable that no single gene will be identified as the sole cause of these FMS-related conditions. Much more likely, a combination of genetic traits (polygenic inheritance coupled with a chain of environmental events, such as trauma, stress, or infection) will gradually emerge as the explanation [1]. More insight into the genetics involved in

FMS and related conditions may eventually improve our understanding of their pathophysiology and ultimately lead to novel therapeutic strategies.

Clinical Implications of Genetics Findings in Comorbid Pain Conditions

The gene polymorphisms reported in the serotoninergic, dopaminergic, and catecholaminergic systems may help to better understand the pathogenesis of these "central" pain syndromes. Notably, these polymorphisms all affect the metabolism or transport of monoamine compounds that have a critical role in both sensory processing and the human stress response [22].

Knowledge of a patient's genotype may help us to improve the subclassification of FMS patients, since we realize now that FMS is a heterogeneous, rather than homogeneous, disorder. Turk et al. classified FMS patients into three subgroups based on psychosocial and behavioral characteristics [72]. These subgroups showed substantial differences in clinical presentation of their symptoms. Giesecke et al. also reported on distinct subgroups of patients with FMS [31]. There was a group of FMS patients who exhibited extreme tenderness but lacked any associated psychological cognitive factors, an intermediate group who displayed moderate tenderness and had normal mood, and a group in which mood and cognitive factors could have been significantly influencing the report of symptoms [31].

Summary

Recent studies suggest that genetic factors can play a significant role in the perception of pain and in the development of comorbid pain conditions. A strong familial aggregation is reported in FMS and related conditions (central sensitivity syndromes). Polymorphisms of genes in the serotoninergic, dopaminergic, and catecholaminergic systems have been reported in these chronic pain states and may play a role in their pathogenesis. The mode of inheritance of FMS is unknown, but it is most probably polygenic. Environmental factors including trauma and stress may trigger the development of FMS in genetically predisposed individuals. Recognition of these gene polymorphisms may help to better subgroup FMS patients and to treat them in a more targeted pharmacological approach.

References

[1]   Ablin JN, Buskila D. The genetics of fibromyalgia: closing Osler's backdoor. Isr Med Assoc J 2006;8:428–9.

[2]   Amir M, Kaplan Z, Neumann L, Sharabani R, Shani N, Buskila D. Posttraumatic stress disorder, tenderness and fibromyalgia. J Psychosom Res 1997;42:607–13.

[3]   Arnold LM, Hudson JI, Hess EV, Ware AE, Fritz DA, Auchenbach MB, Starck LO, Nech PE Jr. Family study of fibromyalgia. Arthritis Rheum 2004;50:944–52.

[4]   Barbosa RF, Matsuda JB, Mazucato M, de Castro França S, Zingaretti SM, da Silva LM, Martinez-Rossi NM, Júnior MF, Marins M, Fachin AL. Influence of catechol-O-methyltransferase (COMT) gene polymorphisms in pain sensibility of Brazilian fibromyalgia patients. Rheumatol Int 2012;32:427–30.

[5]   Becker RM, da Silva VK, Machado FS, dos Santos AF, Meireles DC, Mergener M, dos Santos GA, de Andrade FM. Association between environmental quality, stress and APOE gene variation in fibromyalgia susceptibility determination. Bras J Rheumatol 2010;50:617–30.

[6]   Bondy B, Spaeth M, Offenbaecher M. Glatzeder K, Startz T, Schwarz M, de Jonge S, Kruger M, Engel RR, Farber L, Pondgratz DE, Ackenheil M. The T102C polymorphism of the 5-HT2A receptor gene in fibromyalgia. Neurobiol Dis 1999;6:433–9.

[7]   Buchwald D, Herreti R, Ashton S, Belcourt M, Schmaling K, Sullivan P, Neale M, Goldberg J. A twin study of chronic fatigue. Psychosom Med 2001;63:936–43.

[8]   Buskila D. Genetics of chronic pain states. Best Pract Res Clin Rheumatol 2007;21:535–47.

[9]   Buskila D. Developments in the scientific and clinical understanding of fibromyalgia. Arthritis Res Ther 2009;11:242.

[10] Buskila D, Neumann L, Hazanov I, Carmi R. Familial aggregation in the fibromyalgia syndrome. Semin Arthritis Rheum 1996;26:605–11.

[11] Buskila D, Cohen H, Neumann L, Ebstein RP. An association between fibromyalgia and the dopamine D4 receptor exon III repeat polymorphism and relationship to novelty seeking personality traits. Mol Psychiatry 2004;9:730–3.

[12] Buskila D, Neumann L. Fibromyalgia syndrome (FM) and nonarticular tenderness in relatives of patients with FM. J Rheumatol 1997;24:941–4.

[13] Buskila D, Neumann L. Genetics of fibromyalgia. Curr Pain Headache Rep 2005;9:313–5.

[14] Buskila D, Neumann L, Press J. Genetic factors in neuromuscular pain. CNS Spectr 2005;10:281–4.

[15] Buskila D, Sarzi Puttini P. Biology and therapy of fibromyalgia. Genetic aspects of fibromyalgia syndrome. Arthritis Res Ther 2006;8:218.

[16] Carlo-Stella N, Badulli C, De Silvestri A, Bazzichi L, Martinetti M, Lorusso L, Bombardieri S, Salvaneschi L, Cuccia M. A first study of cytokine genomic polymorphisms in CFS: positive association of TNF-857 and IFN gamma 874 rare alleles. Clin Exp Rheumatol 2006;24:179–82.

[17] Clauw DJ, Crofford LJ. Chronic widespread pain and fibromyalgia. What we know and what we need to know. Best Pract Res Clin Rheumatol 2003;17:685–701.

[18] Cohen H, Buskila D, Neumann L, Ebstein RP. Confirmation of an association between fibromyalgia and serotonin transporter promoter region (5-HTTLPR) polymorphism, and relationship to anxiety-related personality traits. Arthritis Rheum 2002;46:845–7.

[19] Cohen H, Neumann L, Glazer Y, Ebstein RP, Buskila D. The relationship between a common catechol-0- methyltransferase (COMT) polymorphism val(158)met and fibromyalgia. Clin Exp Rheumatol 2009;27(5 Suppl 56):S51–6.

[20] Cohen H, Neumann L, Haiman Y, Matar MA, Press J, Buskila D. Prevalence of post traumatic stress disorder in fibromyalgia patients: Overlapping syndromes or post traumatic fibromyalgia syndrome? Semin Arthritis Rheum 2002;32:38–50.

[21] Corominas R, Sobrido MJ, Ribases M, Cuenca Leon E, Blanco-Arias P, Narberhaus B, Roig M, Leira R, Lopez-Gonzalez J, Macaya A, Cormand B. Association study of the serotoninergic system in migraine in the Spanish population. Am J Med Genet B Neuropsychiatr Genet 2010;153B:177–84.

[22] Dadabhoy D, Clauw D. Therapy insight: fibromyalgia—a different type of pain needing a different type of treatment. Nat Clin Pract Rheumatol 2006;2:364–72.

[23] Dai F, Belfer I, Schwartz CE, Banco R, Martha JF, Tighioughart H, Tromanhauser SG, Jenis LG, Kim DH. Association of Catechol-O-methyltransferase genetic variants with outcome in patients undergoing surgical treatment for lumbar degenerative disc disease. Spine J 2010;10:949–57.

[24] Diatchenko L, Slade GD, Nackley AG, Bhalang K, Sigurdsson A, Blefer I, Goldman D, Xu K, Shabalina SA, Shagin D, Max MB, Makarov SS, Maixner W. Genetic basis for individual variations in pain perception and the development of a chronic pain condition. Hum Mol Genet 2005;14:135–43.

[25] Feng J, Zhang Z, Li W, Shen X, Song W, Yang C, Chang F, Longmate J, Marek C, St. Amand RP, Krontiris TG, Shively JE, Sommer SS. Missense mutations in the MEFV gene are associated with fibromyalgia syndrome and correlate with elevated IL-1 beta plasma levels. PLOS One 2009;4:e8480.

[26] Frank B, Niesler B, Bondy B, Spathe M, Pongratz DE, Achenheil M, Fischer C, Rappoid G. Mutational analysis of serotonin receptor genes HTR3A and HTR3B in fibromyalgia patients. Clin Rheumatol 2004;23:338–44.

[27] Fukudo S, Kanazawa M, Mizuno T, Hamaguchi T, Kano M, Watanabe S, Sagami Y, Shoj T, Endo M, Hongo M, Itoyama Y, Yanai K, Tashiro M, Aoki M. Impact of serotonin transporter gene polymorphism on brain activation by colorectal distention. Neuroimage 2009;47: 946–51.

[28] García-Martín E, Martínez C, Serrador M, Alonso-Navarro H, Navacerrada F, Agúndez JA, Jiménez-Jiménez FJ. Dopamine receptor 3 (DRD3) polymorphism and risk for migraine. Eur J Neurol 2010;17:1220–3.

[29] George SZ, Dover GC, Wallace MR, Sack BK. Herbstman DM, Aydong E, Fillingim RB. Biopsychosocial influence on exercise-induced delayed onset muscle soreness at the shoulder: pain catastrophizing and catechol-O-methyltransferase (COMT) diplotype predict pain ratings. Clin J Pain 2008;24:793–801.

[30] Ghosh J, Pradhan S, Mittal B. Role of dopaminergic gene polymorphisms (DBH 19 bp Indel and DRD2 NCOI) in genetic susceptibility to migraine in North Indian population. Pain Med 2011;12:1109–11.

[31] Giesecke T, Williams DA, Harris RF, Cupps TR, Tian X, Tian TX, Gracely RH, Clauw DJ. Subgrouping of fibromyalgia patients on the basis of pressure pain thresholds and psychological factors. Arthritis Rheum 2003;48:2916–22.

[32] Grabe HJ, Spitzer C, Schwahn C, Marcinek A, Frahnow A, Barnow S, Lucht M, Freyberger HJ, John U. Serotonin transporter gene (SLC6A4) promoter polymorphisms and the susceptibility to posttraumatic stress disorder in the general population. Am J Psychiatry 2009;166:926–33.

[33] Gursoy S, Erdal E, Herken H, Madenci E, Alasehirli B, Erdal N. Significance of catechol-O-methyltransferase gene polymorphism in fibromyalgia syndrome. Rheumatol Int 2003;23:104–7.

[34] Hagen K, Pettersen E, Stovner LJ. Skorpen F, Zwart JA. No association between chronic musculoskeletal complaints and Val158Met polymorphism in the catechol-O-methyltransferase gene. The HUNT study. BMC Musculoskelet Disord 2006;7:40.

[35] Hocking LJ, Smith BH, Jones GT, Reid DM, Strachan DP, Macfarlane GJ. Genetic variation in the beta2-adrenergic receptor but not catecholamine-O-methyltransferase predisposes to chronic pain: results from the 1958 British Cohort Study. Pain 2010;149:143–51.

[36] Holliday KL, Nicholl B, Macfarlane G, Thomson W, Davies KA, McBeth J. Genetic variation in the hypothalamic-pituitary-adrenal stress axis influences susceptibility to musculoskeletal pain: results from the EPIFUND study. Ann Rheum Dis 2010;69:556–60.

[37] Hudson JI, Mangweth B, Pope HG Jr, De Col C, Hausmann A, Gutweniger S, Laird NM, Biebl W, Tsuang MT. Family study of affective spectrum disorder. Arch Gen Psychiatry 2003, 60: 170–7.

[38] Ifergane G, Buskila D, Simiseshvely N, Zeev K, Cohen H. Prevalence of fibromyalgia syndrome in migraine patients. Cephalgia 2006;26:451–6.

[39] Jun S, Kohen R, Cain KC, Jarrett ME, Heitkemper MM. Associations of tryptophan hydroxylase gene polymorphism with irritable bowel syndrome. Neurogastroenterol Motil 2011;23:233–9.

[40] Kalamtar JS, Loccke GR, Zinsmeister AR, Beighley CM, Talley NJ. Familial aggregation of ir-
      ritable bowel syndrome: a prospective study. Gut 2003;52:1703–7.
[41] Koenen KC, Lyons MJ, Goldenberg J, Simpsom J, Williams WM, Toomey R, Eisen SA, True WR,
      Cloitre M, Wolfe J, Tsuang MT. A high risk twin study of combat related PTSD comorbidity.
      Twin Res 2003;6:218–26.
[42] Kohen R, Jarrett ME, Cain KC, Jun SE, Navaja GP, Symonds S, Heitkemper MM. The serotonin
      transporter polymorphism rs 25531 is associated with irritable bowel syndrome. Dig Dis Sci
      2009;54:2663–70.
[43] Kolassa IT, Kolasa S, Ertl V, Papassotiropoulos A, De Quervain DJF. The risk of posttraumatic
      stress disorder after trauma depends on traumatic load and the catechol-O-methyltransferase
      Val158Met polymorphism. Biol Psychiatry 2010;67:304–8.
[44] Lachman HM, Papolos DF, Saito T. Human Catechol-O-methyltransferase pharmacogenetics:
      description of a functional polymorphism and its potential application to neuropsychiatric dis-
      orders. Pharmacogenetics 1996;6:243–50.
[45] Landy S, Ricek L, Lobo B. Central sensitization and cutaneous allodynia in migraine: implica-
      tions for treatment. CNS Drugs 2004;18:337–42.
[46] Langevitz P, Buskila D, Finklestein R, Zaks N, Neumann L, Sukenik S, Smythe HA, Pras M. Fi-
      bromyalgia in familial Mediterranean fever. J Rheumatol 1994;21:1335–7.
[47] Lee PJ, Delaney P, Koigh J, Sleeman D, Shorten GD. Catecholamine-O-methyltransferase poly-
      morphisms are associated with postoperative pain intensity. Clin J Pain 2011;27:93–101.
[48] Lesch KP, Bengel D, Heils A, Sabol SZ, Greenberg BD, Petri S, Benjamin J, Muller CR, Hamer
      DH, Murphy DL. Association of anxiety-related traits with a polymorphism in the serotonin
      transporter gene regulatory region. Science 1996;274:1527–31.
[49] MacLean SA, Diatchenko L, Lee YM, Swornes RA, Domeir RM, Jones CW, Reed C, Harris RE,
      Maixner W, Clauw DG, Liberzon I. Catechol-O-methyltransferase haplotype predicts immedi-
      ate musculoskeletal neck pain and psychological symptoms after motor vehicle collision. J Pain
      2011;12:101–7.
[50] Mellman TA, Alim T, Brown DD, Gorodetsky E, Buzas B, Lawson WB, Goldman D, Charney
      DS. Serotonin polymorphisms and posttraumatic stress disorder in a trauma-exposed African
      American population. Depress Anxiety 2009;26: 993–7.
[51] Mobascher A, Brinkmeyer J, Thiele H, Toliat MR, Steffens M, Warbrick T, Musso F, Wittsack
      HJ, Saleh H, Schnitzler A, Winterer G. The val158met polymorphism of human catechol-O-
      methyltransferase (COMT) affects anterior cingulated cortex activation in response to painful
      laser stimulation. Mol Pain 2010;6:32.
[52] Mogil JS. The genetic mediation of individual differences in sensitivity to pain and its inhibition.
      Proc Natl Acad Sci USA 1999;96:7744–51.
[53] Narita M, Nishigami N, Narita N, Yamaguti K, Okado N, Yamaguti K, Okado N, Watanabe Y,
      Kuratsune H. Association between serotonin transporter gene polymorphism and chronic fa-
      tigue syndrome. Biochem Biophys Res Commun 2003;311:264–6.
[54] Neumann L, Buskila D. Quality of life and physical functioning of relatives of fibromyalgia pa-
      tients. Semin Arthritis Rheum 1997;26:834–9.
[55] Nicholl BI, Holliday KL, Macfarlane GJ, Thomson W, Davies KA, O'Neill TW, Bartfai G, Boonen
      S, Casanueva F, Finn JD, Forti G, Giwercman A, Huhtaniemi IT, Kuta K, Punab M, Silman AJ,
      Vanderschueren D, Wu FC, McBeth J, European Male Ageing Study Group. No evidence for a
      role of the catechol-O-methyltransferase sensitivity haplotypes in chronic widespread pain. Ann
      Rheum Dis 2010;69:2009–12.
[56] Offenbaecher M, Bondy B, de Jonge S, Glatzede K, Kruger M, Schoeps P, Ackenheil M. possible
      association of fibromyalgia with a polymorphism in the serotonin transporter gene regulation
      region. Arthritis Rheum 1999;42:2482–8.
[57] Park JM, Choi MG, Cho YK, Lee IS, Kim SW, Choi KY, Chung IS. Cannabinoid receptor 1 gene
      polymorphism and irritable bowel syndrome in the Korean population: a hypothesis-generating
      study. J Clin Gastroenterol 2011;45:45–9.
[58] Park JW, Lee KS, Kim JS, Kim YI, Shin HE. Genetic contribution of catechol-O-methyltransfer-
      ase polymorphism in patients with migraine without aura. J Clin Neurol 2007;3:24–30.
[59] Pata C, Erdal E, Yazici K, Camdeviren H, Ozkaya M, Ulu O. Association of the 1438-G/A and 102
      T/C polymorphism of the 5-HT2A receptor gene with irritable bowel syndrome. J Clin Gastro-
      enterol 2004;38:561–6.

[60] Potvin S, Larouche A, Normand E, de Souza JB, Gaumond I, Grignon S, Marchand S. DRD3 Ser-9Gly polymorphism is related to thermal pain perception and modulation in chronic widespread pain patients and healthy controls. J Pain 2009;10:969–75.

[61] Segman RH, Cooper-Kazaz R, Macciardi F, Goltser T, Halfon Y, Dobroborski T, Shalev AY. Association between the dopamine transporter gene and posttraumatic stress disorder. Mol Psychiatry 2002;7:903–7.

[62] Sikander A, Rana SV, Sharma SK, Sinha SK, Arora SK, Prasad KK, Singh K. Association of alpha 2A adrenergic receptor gene (ADRAlpha2A) polymorphism with irritable bowel syndrome, microscopic and ulcerative colitis. Clin Chim Acta 2010;411:59–63.

[63] Sikander A, Rana SV, Sinha SK, Prasad KK, Arora SK, Sharma SK, Singh K. Serotonin transporter promoter variant analysis in Indian IBS patients and control population. J Clin Gastroenterol 2009;43:957–61.

[64] Smith AK, Dimulescu I, Falkenberg VR, Narasimhan S, Heim C, Vernon SD, Rajeevan MS. Genetic evaluation of the serotonergic system in chronic fatigue syndrome. Psychoneuroendocrinology 2008;33:188–97.

[65] Stein MB, Jang KL, Taylor S, Vernon PA, Livesley WJ. Genetic and environmental influences on trauma exposure and posttraumatic stress disorder symptoms: a twin study. Am J Psychiatry 2002;159:1675–81.

[66] Su SY, Chen JJ, Lai CC, Chen CM, Tsai FJ. The association between fibromyalgia and polymorphism of monoamine oxidase A and interleukin-4. Clin Rheumatol 2007;26:12–6.

[67] Tchivileva E, Lim PF, Smith SB, Slade GD, Diatchenko L, McLean SA, Maixner W. Effect of catechol-O-methyltransferase polymorphism on response to propranolol therapy in chronic musculoskeletal pain: a randomized double blind, placebo controlled, crossover pilot study. Pharmacogenet Genomics 2010;20:239–48.

[68] Terrazzinno S, Viana M, Floriddia E, Monaco F, Mittino D, Sances G, Tassorelli C, Nappi G, Rinaldi M, Canonico PL, Genazzani AA. The serotonin transporter gene polymorphism STin2 VNTR confers an increased risk of inconsistent response to triptans in migraine patients. Eur J Pharmacol 2010;641:81–7.

[69] Thakur GA, Joober R, Brunet A. Development and persistence of posttraumatic stress disorder and the 5-HTTLPR polymorphism. J Trauma Stress 2009;22:240–3.

[70] Todt U, Netzer C, Toliat M, Heinze A, Goebel I, Nurnberg P, Gobel H, Freudenberg J, Kubisch C. New genetic evidence for involvement of the dopamine system in migraine with aura. Hum Genet 2009;125:265–9.

[71] Treister R, Pud D, Ebstein RP, Laiba E, Gershan E, Haddad M, Eisenberg E. Associations between polymorphisms in dopamine neurotransmitter pathway genes and pain response in health humans. Pain 2009;147:187–93.

[72] Turk DC, Okifuji A, Sinclair JD, Startz TW. Pain, disability and physical functioning in subgroups of patients with fibromyalgia. J Rheumatol 1996;23:1255–62.

[73] Vargas-Alarcon G, Fragoso JM, Cruz-Robles D, Vargas A, Lao-Villadoniga JI, Garcia-Fructuoso F, Ramus-Kuri M, Hernandez F, Springall R, Bojalil R, Vallejo M, Martinez-Lavin M. Catechol-O-methyltransferase gene haplotypes in Mexican and Spanish patients with fibromyalgia. Arthritis Res Ther 2007;9:R110.

[74] Vargas-Alarcon G, Fragoso JM, Cruz-Robles D, Vargas A, Martinez A, Lao-Villadoniga JI, Garcia-Fructuoso F, Vallejo M, Martinez-Lavin M. Association of adrenergic receptor gene polymorphisms with different fibromyalgia syndrome domains. Arthritis Rheum 2009;60:2169–73.

[75] Voisey J, Swagell CD, Hughes IP, Morris CP, van Daal A, Noble EP, Kann B, Heslop KA, Young RM, Lawford BR. The DRD2 gene 957C>T polymorphism is associated with posttraumatic stress disorder in war veterans. Depress Anxiety 2009;26:28–33.

[76] Vossen H, Kenis G, Rutten B, van Os J, Hermens H, Lousberg R. The genetic influence of the cortical processing of experimental pain and the moderating effect of pain status. PLoS One 2010;5:e13641.

[77] Walsh CM, Zainal NZ, Middleton SJ, Paykel ES. A family history study of chronic fatigue syndrome. Psychiatr Genet 2001;11:123–8.

[78] Yeo A, Boyd P, Lumsden S, Saunders T, Handley A, Stubbins M, Knaggs A, Asquith S, Taylor I, Bahari B, Crocker N, Rallan R, Varsani S, Montgomery D, Alpers DH, Dukes GE, Purvis I. Association between a functional polymorphism in the serotonin transporter gene and diarrhea predominant irritable bowel syndrome in women. Gut 2004;53:1452–8.

[79] Yunus MB. Fibromyalgia and overlapping disorders: the unifying concept of central sensitivity syndromes. Semin Arthritis Rheum 2007;36:339–56.

[80] Zubieta JK, Heitzeg MM, Smith YR, Bueller JA, Xu K, Xu Y, Koeppe RA, Stohler CS, Goldman D. COMT val158met genotype affects mu-opioid neurotransmitter responses to a pain stressor. Science 2003;299:1240–3.

Correspondence to: Prof. Dan Buskila, MD, Department of Medicine H, Soroka Medical Center, POB 151, Beer Sheva, Israel 84101. Email: dbuskila@bgu.ac.il.

Hormonal Contributions to Comorbid Pain Conditions

Roger B. Fillingim[a,b] and Margarete Ribeiro-Dasilva[a]

[a]University of Florida College of Dentistry, [b]North Florida/South Georgia Veterans Health System, Gainesville, Florida, USA

Women are more frequently affected by many of the comorbid pain and non-pain conditions (such as affective disorders) discussed throughout this volume (also see [49]). Therefore, pathophysiological explanations for these comorbidities must account for sex differences in their prevalence. Sex hormones represent one potential contributing mechanism that may explain male-female differences in pain comorbidities. Beyond their reproductive role, gonadal hormones produce multiple effects throughout the peripheral and central nervous systems, and mounting evidence implicates these hormones in pain-related sex differences. Estrogens, progesterone, and testosterone differ substantially across sexes, not only in their concentrations, but also in their temporal patterns, including long-term changes across the lifespan. For example, hormone levels vary with the menstrual cycle throughout most of a woman's reproductive lifetime, and hormonal concentrations change dramatically during and after pregnancy and after menopause. In contrast, men experience less robust fluctuations in hormone levels across the lifespan, the most significant being the reduction of testosterone with aging. This

Pain Comorbidities: Understanding and Treating the Complex Patient
edited by Maria Adele Giamberardino and Troels Staehelin Jensen
IASP Press, Seattle, © 2012

chapter will review the evidence that hormonal influences may contribute to pain comorbidities. First, we will provide a brief overview of clinical and epidemiological findings regarding hormonal effects on pain, followed by a review of the literature regarding hormonal effects on experimental pain in humans. Finally, we will discuss several pathways whereby gonadal hormones can influence pain [19].

Epidemiological and Clinical Evidence of Hormonal Influences on Pain

A growing body of evidence supports the notion that gonadal hormones contribute to numerous clinical pain conditions. Epidemiological studies indicate that sex differences in the prevalence of several pain conditions vary across the lifespan, and these patterns may be based on hormonal factors. For example, prepubertal girls and boys have an approximately equal prevalence of migraine; however, the lifetime prevalence of migraine increases to 18% for women and 6% for men after puberty, but then the female : male prevalence ratio decreases later in life (after menopause) [19,56]. Similar prevalence patterns have been reported for temporomandibular disorders [48]. In addition, before puberty, girls and boys are equally likely to report one or more common pain complaints (back pain, headache, chest pain, abdominal pain, and orofacial pain); however, the frequency of these conditions increases more dramatically in girls as puberty progresses [51]. The female predominance of these conditions peaks during the reproductive years (ages 25–44 years), and in one study, no sex differences in prevalence were observed among individuals 65 years of age and older [49]. One interpretation of these epidemiological findings is that sex differences in the prevalence of many pain conditions are primarily observed at times when the influence of gonadal hormones is greatest (estrogens/progesterone in women and testosterone in men).

Additional evidence of hormonal contributions derives from studies examining menstrual cycle effects on clinical pain. The phases of the female menstrual cycle are characterized by varying levels of estradiol and progesterone. During menstruation, both hormones are at low levels, and during the follicular phase, estradiol slowly rises and then peaks in the late follicular phase, plummeting just before ovulation. After ovulation, estradiol rises modestly during the luteal phase, and then declines in the late luteal phase leading back to menses. Progesterone remains low during the follicular phase, peaking in the mid-luteal phase, then declining before menses. Thus, if estradiol and/or progesterone influences pain responses, one would expect variations in pain-related clinical symptoms across the menstrual cycle. Indeed, in the general population, physical symptoms, including pain, and psychological distress vary across the menstrual cycle, with greatest symptomatology in the perimenstrual phases [10]. Further, in clinical populations, the severity of symptoms has been shown to vary across the menstrual cycle for several pain conditions, including irritable bowel syndrome [36], headache [41], temporomandibular disorders (TMD) [50], interstitial cystitis [71], and fibromyalgia [68], with pain severity peaking perimenstrually for most conditions. However, data suggesting no menstrual cycle effect on pain-related symptoms are also available [66]. Further support for hormonal modulation of clinical pain comes from findings that during pregnancy, migraine frequency declines and TMD pain is reduced [19,53]. Interestingly, as estradiol levels decline sharply postpartum, migraine attacks become more frequent [76], and pain severity in TMD increases [53].

Exogenous hormone use has also been associated with clinical pain. Postmenopausal women using hormone replacement therapy have shown increased risk for back pain [12] and TMD [52], and oral contraceptive use has been related to increased risk for TMD [52] and carpal tunnel syndrome [23]. Moreover, Wise and colleagues [95] found that postmenopausal women on hormone replacement seeking treatment for orofacial pain reported significantly more severe pain compared to facial pain patients not using hormones. However, other research suggests no association of exogenous hormone use with clinical pain [57]. Moreover, discontinuation of hormone replacement therapy in postmenopausal women is associated with higher levels of reported pain or stiffness [65], and after prolonged estradiol administration, estradiol withdrawal has been shown to precipitate migraine headaches [54,83]. Other exogenous agents that have an impact on estrogens may also affect pain. For example, aromatase inhibitors, which reduce estrogen levels by blocking the conversion of androgen to estrogen, have been associated with increased joint pain [38]. In contrast, selective estrogen receptor modulators, which possess both agonist and antagonist effects at estrogen receptors, appear to produce analgesia [31,75]. Taken together, these findings suggest that gonadal hormones can significantly affect clinical pain; however, the nature and direction of these influences is quite complex and not yet understood. Moreover, it can be difficult to distinguish hormonal influences on pain processing from effects on disease processes. For example, use of aromatase inhibitors can produce musculoskeletal pain, which recently has been attributed to the increased frequency of osteoporosis and fracture that accompanies use of these medications [62].

Hormonal Influences on Experimental Pain

Studies of laboratory pain provide more direct evidence of hormonal influences on pain responses, independent of the potential confound of hormonal influences on disease activity. A previous meta-analytic review of studies examining pain perception across the menstrual cycle concluded that pain thresholds for mechanical, thermal, and ischemic muscle pain were generally higher during the follicular phase of the menstrual cycle (when levels of estradiol and progesterone are low to moderate) than during perimenstrual phases of the cycle (when levels of estradiol and progesterone are decreasing). Effect sizes for these menstrual cycle differences were generally small to moderate [73]. Since this systematic review, additional studies have yielded conflicting results, as recently summarized (see [25,78] for more detailed reviews). Electrical pain thresholds were lower in the luteal versus the follicular phase in one study, while another study showed the highest electrical pain threshold in the luteal phase [87], and two other studies reported no such menstrual cycle effects on electrical pain thresholds [67,88]. No menstrual cycle effects on heat pain perception emerged in several studies [81,87], and lower heat pain thresholds during the ovulatory phase were observed only on the abdomen in another study [7]. Menstrual cycle effects on pressure pain threshold (PPT) were absent in pain-free women or among those with TMD pain [79,92]. However, other studies reported varying menstrual cycle effects, including the following findings: PPT was lower during the perimenstrual versus luteal and follicular phases [39]; PPT tested on the back was lower during the ovulatory phase [7]; PPT on the temporalis muscle was higher in the menstrual than the follicular phase [22]; PPT on the forearm peaked during the luteal phase [87]; and masseter and temporalis PPTs were lowest during the periovulatory phase [16]. Recently, Kowalczyk et al. [45] used a signal detection approach to examine menstrual cycle effects on measures of discriminability (sensory processing) and response criterion (stoicism) in response to sustained mechanical pain. Women showed the greatest ability to discriminate among painful stimuli during the luteal phase, and they had the highest response criterion values (thus, a lower inclination to report pain) during the follicular and late luteal phases.

Additional studies have examined menstrual cycle effects on experimental pain modalities that are more tonic in nature. Three studies reported no menstrual cycle effects on ischemic pain [72,79,85]. Cold pressor pain threshold showed menstrual cycle effects in two studies, with lower thresholds in perimenstrual [37] and luteal [84] phases, though these studies found no menstrual cycle effects on pain ratings or pain tolerance. In contrast, another study found that cold pain threshold was lower on Day 7, and pain tolerance was lower on days 7 and 14 of the cycle, compared to the first day of menses (Day 1) [46]. Other investigators have shown no menstrual cycle effect on cold pressor pain [44]. Gazerani et al. [32] reported greater capsaicin-induced pain, allodynia, and mechanical hyperalgesia during the menstrual versus the luteal phase. In addition to subjective pain responses, pain-related cerebral activation [15,21], laser evoked potentials [33], and nociceptive muscle reflexes have varied across the menstrual cycle [86]. Using a diffuse noxious inhibitory controls paradigm to assess pain inhibitory function, Tousignant-Laflamme and Marchand showed that endogenous pain inhibition was greatest during the ovulatory versus the follicular and luteal phases [90]. These studies, using experimental methodologies to examine menstrual cycle effects on pain processing, provide a very mixed and inconsistent picture of such effects. While menstrual cycle effects occasionally emerge, their magnitude and direction are quite variable. As previously noted [73,78], these inconsistent menstrual cycle effects can be attributed to the wide variation in timing of cycle phases, along with other methodological inconsistencies, including varying pain modalities and testing sites.

Some investigators have examined the association of circulating levels of hormones with experimental pain responses. For example, in premenopausal women, higher estradiol levels were associated with increased heat pain sensitivity [26]. In contrast, higher progesterone levels were associated with increased cold pressor pain sensitivity, and this association was attenuated in the presence of higher estradiol levels [84]. Kowalczyk and colleagues reported tendencies for estradiol levels to predict both response criterion and discriminability responses to mechanical stimuli [45], although estradiol did not correlate with cold pain responses [44]. We reported that higher levels of estradiol were associated with lower ischemic pain sensitivity [72]. Ring and colleagues reported a positive relationship between estradiol and progesterone levels and ratings of venipuncture pain [74]. Others have shown no association of estradiol with pain responses, but found that testosterone levels were positively associated with electrical and heat pain thresholds [87]. These findings suggest inconsistent associations between circulating hormone levels and pain responses, and it is likely that hormonal influences on pain cannot be reduced to a simple linear relationship between hormone levels and pain sensitivity.

Some evidence also suggests that exogenous hormones may influence experimental pain responses. We reported that postmenopausal women taking hormone replacement therapy displayed lower thermal pain thresholds and tolerances than postmenopausal women not taking hormones [24]. Subsequently, we found that women using oral contraceptives exhibited greater pressure pain sensitivity compared to their normally cycling counterparts [72]. Similarly, women on oral contraceptives showed greater discriminability of mechanical pain than normally menstruating women, suggesting increased sensory pain responses [45]. In contrast, others reported lower pressure pain sensitivity among oral contraceptive users with and without temporomandibular pain [92]. Thus, the limited available evidence suggests that exogenous hormone use among women may be associated with increased pain sensitivity; however, causal interpretations should be withheld, because none of these studies included random assignment of women to hormone use.

Mechanisms Underlying Hormonal Influences on Pain

Gonadal hormones can influence pain responses via multiple pathways, and many of these effects remain incompletely understood. For example, in addition to their potential effects on disease activity, sex hormones can influence nociceptive processing at virtually all levels of the peripheral nervous system (PNS) and central nervous system (CNS). As we have previously noted [25], one challenge in characterizing these effects is that the magnitude and direction of hormonal influences on pain can be affected by multiple factors, including: (1) the dose and timing of hormonal exposure; (2) the type of pain under consideration; (3) the entire hormonal complement (i.e., the influence of multiple hormonal factors); and (4) the target tissues in which hormones are producing their effects (e.g., peripheral vs. spinal vs. supraspinal). Moreover, it is important to distinguish between organizational and activational effects of sex hormones. Organizational effects refer to long-lasting hormonal influences that occur during development, which may include relatively permanent effects on CNS structure and function. On the other hand, activational effects comprise acute and varying influences of gonadal hormones, such as the influence of menstrual cycle fluctuations in hormone levels and the effects of exogenous hormone administration on pain-related biological processes [47].

Estrogen acts by binding to its receptors, estrogen receptor-α (ER-α) and estrogen receptor-β (ER-β), which are found in PNS and CNS structures involved in nociception, including the dorsal root ganglia [69], the dorsal horn of the spinal cord [5], the periaqueductal gray [64], as well as the hypothalamus, limbic system, spinal cord, and several cortical areas [60]. Also, inflammatory cells such as monocytes express both types of estrogen receptor [70]. Consequently, estrogen can modulate pain via effects on the PNS, the CNS, and immune/inflammatory processes.

In the PNS, estrogen can increase the excitability of nociceptive afferents via multiple mechanisms [19]. One study found that estrogen promoted axon outgrowth in nociceptive neurons, which could contribute to estrogen-mediated augmentation of nociceptive responses [8]. In contrast, estradiol reduced activation of transient receptor potential vanilloid receptor 1 (TRPV1) by capsaicin in dorsal root ganglion neurons, suggesting a peripheral mechanism whereby estrogen may attenuate pain responses [96]. Furthermore, the effects of estrogens on peripheral afferent responses may alter the levels of multiple neuromodulators and neurotransmitters involved in spinal nociceptive processing, possibly causing hyperalgesia and allodynia by increasing glutamatergic nociceptive activity [19]. These findings provide several examples of peripheral mechanisms whereby estrogens may alter nociceptive processing via direct effects on nociceptive neurons, but estrogens acting peripherally could also affect clinical pain by altering disease processes (see Craft [19] for further review).

Estrogenic effects in the CNS can also influence nociceptive responses. Abundant preclinical evidence demonstrates sex-related differences in the functioning of the opioid system. Such sex differences in opioid system function may be influenced by gonadal hormones. In fact, women showed greater baseline mu-opioid receptor availability and higher pain-induced receptor binding in a high-estrogen compared to a low-estrogen state, such that responses of women in the high-estrogen state were comparable to those of men [80]. Moreover, estrogen can modulate hippocampal opioid peptides [94], inhibit the analgesic effect of orphanin FQ (an endogenous ligand of the opioid receptor-like 1 receptor), [17] and increase the concentration of glutamate in the nucleus accumbens, which may explain the lower morphine antinociception observed in female rodents [61]. Indirectly, estrogen may also regulate pain in the CNS by modulating anxiety and depression symptoms, both shown to influence pain response. Indeed, cyclic changes in the concentrations of ovarian hormones across the menstrual cycle can be accompanied by symptoms of irritability and depressed mood [13]. Following childbirth, the sudden change in hormone levels, notably estrogen, has been directly implicated in the development of depression [9], and the hormonal decline that occurs after menopause appears to be associated with a higher risk of depressive symptoms [11]. Moreover, estrogen can influence the levels of neurotransmitters that have been directly implicated in anxiety reduction, such as γ-aminobutyric acid (GABA) [27], and serotonin (5-HT) [97]. Therefore, estrogen can modulate pain indirectly by modulating cognitive and affective factors.

Estrogens may also influence pain responses via effects on immune and inflammatory processes. Immune mediators may strongly influence

neuronal function in many persistent or chronic pain states [58], and cytokines may play an important role in many pain conditions [93]. Estrogen
can modulate the immune system, with high levels of estrogen (e.g., during
the ovulatory and luteal phases) producing an anti-inflammatory effects
[91], and low estrogen levels (e.g., during the follicular phase) increasing pro-inflammatory cytokines [2]. Moreover, estrogen deficiency (e.g.,
after menopause) results in overexpression of the pro-inflammatory cytokines TNF-α [1,14,43], interleukin-1-beta (IL-1β) [14,43], and IL-6 [43].
However, the effects of estrogen on inflammatory processes are poorly
understood, because high estrogen levels have also been shown to result in
increased pro-inflammatory cytokine levels following lipopolysaccharide
challenge [98], contradicting the studies cited above.

Thought These findings together reinforce the idea that estrogen may have
varying effects on the inflammatory response. This complex role of estrogen in inflammation and consequently in pain sensitivity may relate to the
interplay of multiple factors. For example, levels of circulating hormones
can affect the inflammatory response, as discussed above. Also, the estrogen receptor (ER) repertoire may be a factor, because different types of ER
expression may have a different impact on the inflammatory response. Of
note, ER-α is more highly expressed after menopause [70], and ER-α, but
not ER-β, enhances pro-inflammatory cytokine expression in response to
low-dose estrogen [59]. Finally, genetic complement may influence the effects of estrogens on immune and inflammatory processes. A recent study
in postmenopausal women demonstrated that polymorphisms in the ER-α
gene were associated with higher inflammatory responses [63]. Therefore,
despite the complexity of its role in inflammation, estrogen can change
the cytokine balance, potentially leading to increased inflammation and
resulting in heightened acute pain or a hyperalgesic state, and prolonged
inflammation could lead to central sensitization [42]. Additional research
is needed regarding the mechanisms by which estrogen influences the
inflammatory response and subsequent effects on pain sensitivity, which
may elucidate the higher prevalence of inflammatory and painful conditions in women.

In addition to estrogen, other gonadal hormones, including
progesterone and testosterone, may also influence pain comorbidities;
however, the role of these hormones in pain processing has received far

less empirical attention. These hormones differ substantially between the sexes at different life stages and may produce diverse effects on the peripheral and central nervous systems that could affect pain response. Preclinical studies consistently demonstrate a protective effect of progesterone against the development of neuropathic pain [20]. Limited clinical evidence also suggests that progesterone may ameliorate pain. For example, in a large trial of postmenopausal hormone interventions, women adhering to progesterone regimens reported significantly fewer musculoskeletal symptoms compared to women randomized to placebo [34]. Also, women with rheumatoid arthritis showed a trend toward increased pain during menstrual cycle phases characterized by decreasing progesterone [18]. The mechanisms whereby progesterone produces these effects are not fully understood. Progesterone receptors are expressed in the nucleus of the solitary tract, the ventrolateral medulla, and the parabrachial nucleus, implicating progesterone in autonomic regulation as well as in pain processing [40]. However, in contrast to the dense expression of estrogen receptors seen in the superficial dorsal horn [6], progesterone receptors have not been found in that area [40]. Further, expression of progesterone receptors in other parts of the spinal gray matter appears to be inconsistent or absent, suggesting that the effect of progesterone on pain processing may be exerted through descending projections from supraspinal regions, or through intracellular pathways not involving nuclear progesterone receptors [40]. Additional studies are needed to explore the mechanisms whereby progesterone may modulate pain responses.

Preclinical findings suggest that testosterone also has antinociceptive effects on a variety of assays, including attenuation of temporomandibular joint pain or damage in male rats [28,29]. Testosterone replacement reduced nociceptive behaviors after sciatic nerve injury in castrated male rats [55]. Likewise, in male rats, testosterone administration decreased nociceptive responses following inflammatory manipulations, such as administration of formalin or complete Freund's adjuvant [35,89]. Some clinical evidence also supports a protective effect of testosterone. Testosterone supplementation for sex reassignment positively modulated chronic pain [3]. Also, testosterone levels were marginally higher among pain-free workers compared to those with neck, back, or shoulder pain [77]. In addition, testosterone replacement among male chronic pain patients with opioid-induced hypogonadism was associated with reduced scores on the McGill Pain Questionnaire, although visual analogue pain scores failed to improve and opioid doses increased in some patients in this uncontrolled study [4].

In conclusion, despite strong evidence that sex hormones are very important determinants in pain comorbidities, little is known about the mechanism by which these hormones modulate pain. Therefore, more studies must be done to try to reveal the reasons for the conflicting findings and to enable us to tailor better treatments in the future.

Conclusions

The greater prevalence of many pain comorbidities among women, especially during the reproductive years, implicates sex hormones as a potential contributing factor. The literature reviewed above suggests that sex hormones can substantially influence nociceptive responses, but the patterns of association are complex and poorly understood. The magnitude and direction of hormonal effects on pain responses are influenced by the levels or doses of hormones under consideration. Also, the varying hormonal effects at different target tissues can produce conflicting outcomes. For example, estrogen may be protective against bone loss, which could reduce pain due to fractures, while concurrently enhancing nociceptive sensitivity at PNS or CNS sites. Moreover, because hormones may have interactive effects, it is important to consider the total hormonal complement rather than simply levels of a single hormone. The temporal patterns of hormones represent another important issue. For example, the estrogen withdrawal that occurs at certain phases of the menstrual cycle and after pregnancy appears to increase experimental pain sensitivity as well as clinical pain. Investigators must incorporate these factors into future studies in order to advance our understanding of hormonal effects on pain comorbidities. In addition, the overwhelming majority of research in this area has focused on estrogens, and greater empirical attention to other sex-related hormones is warranted. Indeed, a recent large-scale epidemiological study found no associations of gonadal hormones (estradiol, testosterone) with musculoskeletal pain in middle-aged and older men; however, higher levels of gonadotrophins (follicle-stimulating hormone,

luteinizing hormone) were associated with greater odds of musculoskeletal pain. Overall, few studies have examined hormonal influences on
pain among men, which represents another important topic for future research. There is also a need to better understand the mechanisms whereby
sex hormones influence pain-related responses. In addition to the direct
effects discussed above, indirect effects of hormones on pain could occur
via their influence on cognitive and affective processes, which have been
well documented [30,82]. In summary, sex-related hormones can produce
substantial, yet complex, influences on pain responses, and they are likely
to contribute to the increased prevalence of pain comorbidities among
women. Additional research is needed to further characterize these hormonal effects and to elucidate their mechanisms.

References

[1]   Afzal S, Khanam A. Serum estrogen and interleukin-6 levels in postmenopausal female osteoar-
      thritis patients. Pak J Pharm Sci 2011;24:217–9.
[2]   Al-Harthi L, Wright DJ, Anderson D, Cohen M, Matity AD, Cohn J, Cu-Unvin S, Burns D,
      Reichelderfer P, Lewis S, Beckner S, Kovacs A, Landay A. The impact of the ovulatory cycle on
      cytokine production: evaluation of systemic, cervicovaginal, and salivary compartments. J Inter-
      feron Cytokine Res 2000;20:719–24.
[3]   Aloisi AM, Bachiocco V, Costantino A, Stefani R, Ceccarelli I, Bertaccini A, Meriggiola
      MC. Cross-sex hormone administration changes pain in transsexual women and men. Pain
      2007;132(Suppl 1):S60–S67.
[4]   Aloisi AM, Ceccarelli I, Carlucci M, Suman A, Sindaco G, Mameli S, Paci V, Ravaioli L, Passa-
      vanti G, Bachiocco V, Pari G. Hormone replacement therapy in morphine-induced hypogonadic
      male chronic pain patients. Reprod Biol Endocrinol 2011;9:26.
[5]   Alstergren P, Ernberg M, Kvarnstrom M, Kopp S. Interleukin-1beta in synovial fluid from the
      arthritic temporomandibular joint and its relation to pain, mobility, and anterior open bite. J
      Oral Maxillofac Surg 1998;56:1059–65.
[6]   Amandusson A, Hermanson O, Blomqvist A. Estrogen receptor-like immunoreactivity in the
      medullary and spinal dorsal horn of the female rat. Neurosci Lett 1995;196:25–8.
[7]   Bajaj P, Bajaj P, Madsen H, Arendt-Nielsen L. A comparison of modality-specific somatosen-
      sory changes during menstruation in dysmenorrheic and nondysmenorrheic women. Clin J Pain
      2002;18:180–90.
[8]   Blacklock AD, Johnson MS, Krizsan-Agbas D, Smith PG. Estrogen increases sensory nociceptor
      neuritogenesis in vitro by a direct, nerve growth factor-independent mechanism. Eur J Neurosci
      2005;21:2320–8.
[9]   Bloch M, Schmidt PJ, Danaceau M, Murphy J, Nieman L, Rubinow DR. Effects of gonadal ste-
      roids in women with a history of postpartum depression. Am J Psychiatry 2000;157:924–30.
[10] Boyle CA, Berkowitz GS, Kelsey JL. Epidemiology of premenstrual symptoms. Am J Public
      Health 1987;77:349–50.
[11] Bromberger JT, Matthews KA, Schott LL, Brockwell S, Avis NE, Kravitz HM, Everson-Rose SA,
      Gold EB, Sowers M, Randolph JF Jr. Depressive symptoms during the menopausal transition: the
      Study of Women's Health Across the Nation (SWAN). J Affect Disord 2007;103:267–72.
[12] Brynhildsen JO, Bjors E, Skarsgard C, Hammar ML. Is hormone replacement therapy a risk fac-
      tor for low back pain among postmenopausal women? Spine 1998;23:809–13.
[13] Campagne DM, Campagne G. The premenstrual syndrome revisited. Eur J Obstet Gynecol Re-
      prod Biol 2007;130:4–17.

[14] Cantatore FP, Loverro G, Ingrosso AM, Lacanna R, Sassanelli E, Selvaggi L, Carrozzo M. Effect of oestrogen replacement on bone metabolism and cytokines in surgical menopause. Clin Rheumatol 1995;14:157–60.

[15] Choi JC, Park SK, Kim YH, Shin YW, Kwon JS, Kim JS, Kim JW, Kim SY, Lee SG, Lee MS. Different brain activation patterns to pain and pain-related unpleasantness during the menstrual cycle. Anesthesiology 2006;105:120–7.

[16] Cimino R, Farella M, Michelotti A, Pugliese R, Martina R. Does the ovarian cycle influence the pressure-pain threshold of the masticatory muscles in symptom-free women? J Orofac Pain 2000;14:105–11.

[17] Claiborne JA, Nag S, Mokha SS. Estrogen-dependent, sex-specific modulation of mustard oil-induced secondary thermal hyperalgesia by orphanin FQ in the rat. Neurosci Lett 2009;456:59–63.

[18] Colangelo K, Haig S, Bonner A, Zelenietz C, Pope J. Self-reported flaring varies during the menstrual cycle in systemic lupus erythematosus compared with rheumatoid arthritis and fibromyalgia. Rheumatology (Oxford) 2011;50:703–8.

[19] Craft RM. Modulation of pain by estrogens. Pain 2007;132:S3–S12.

[20] Dableh LJ, Henry JL. Progesterone prevents development of neuropathic pain in a rat model: timing and duration of treatment are critical. J Pain Res 2011;4:91–101.

[21] de Leeuw R, Albuquerque RJ, Andersen AH, Carlson CR. Influence of estrogen on brain activation during stimulation with painful heat. J Oral Maxillofac Surg 2006;64:158–66.

[22] Drobek W, Schoenaers J, De Laat A. Hormone-dependent fluctuations of pressure pain threshold and tactile threshold of the temporalis and masseter muscle. J Oral Rehabil 2002;29:1042–51.

[23] Ferry S, Hannaford P, Warskyj M, Lewis M, Croft P. Carpal tunnel syndrome: a nested case-control study of risk factors in women. Am J Epidemiol 2000;151:566–74.

[24] Fillingim RB, Edwards RR. The association of hormone replacement therapy with experimental pain responses in postmenopausal women. Pain 2001;92:229–34.

[25] Fillingim RB, King CD, Ribeiro-Dasilva MC, Rahim-Williams B, Riley JL III. Sex, gender, and pain: a review of recent clinical and experimental findings. J Pain 2009;10:447–85.

[26] Fillingim RB, Maixner W, Girdler SS, Light KC, Harris MB, Sheps DS, Mason GA. Ischemic but not thermal pain sensitivity varies across the menstrual cycle. Psychosom Med 1997;59:512–20.

[27] Finocchi C, Ferrari M. Female reproductive steroids and neuronal excitability. Neurol Sci 2011;32(Suppl 1):S31–5.

[28] Fischer L, Clemente JT, Tambeli CH. The protective role of testosterone in the development of temporomandibular joint pain. J Pain 2007;8:437–42.

[29] Flake NM, Hermanstyne TO, Gold MS. Testosterone and estrogen have opposing actions on inflammation-induced plasma extravasation in the rat temporomandibular joint. Am J Physiol Regul Integr Comp Physiol 2006;291:R343–8.

[30] Foy MR. Ovarian hormones, aging and stress on hippocampal synaptic plasticity. Neurobiol Learn Mem 2011;95:134–44.

[31] Fujita T, Fujii Y, Munezane H, Ohue M, Takagi Y. Analgesic effect of raloxifene on back and knee pain in postmenopausal women with osteoporosis and/or osteoarthritis. J Bone Miner Metab 2010;28:477–84.

[32] Gazerani P, Andersen OK, Arendt-Nielsen L. A human experimental capsaicin model for trigeminal sensitization: gender-specific differences. Pain 2005;118:155–63.

[33] Granot M, Yarnitsky D, Itskovitz-Eldor J, Granovsky Y, Peer E, Zimmer EZ. Pain perception in women with dysmenorrhea. Obstet Gynecol 2001;98:407–11.

[34] Greendale GA, Reboussin BA, Hogan P, Barnabei VM, Shumaker S, Johnson S, Barrett-Connor E. Symptom relief and side effects of postmenopausal hormones: results from the Postmenopausal Estrogen/Progestin Interventions Trial. Obstet Gynecol 1998;92:982–8.

[35] Harbuz MS, Perveen-Gill Z, Lightman SL, Jessop DS. A protective role for testosterone in adjuvant-induced arthritis. Br J Rheumatol 1995;34:1117–22.

[36] Heitkemper MM, Chang L. Do fluctuations in ovarian hormones affect gastrointestinal symptoms in women with irritable bowel syndrome? Gend Med 2009;6(Suppl 2):152–67.

[37] Hellstrom B, Lundberg U. Pain perception to the cold pressor test during the menstrual cycle in relation to estrogen levels and a comparison with men. Integr Physiol Behav Sci 2000;35:132–41.

[38] Henry NL, Giles JT, Stearns V. Aromatase inhibitor-associated musculoskeletal symptoms: etiology and strategies for management. Oncology (Williston Park) 2008;22:1401–8.

[39] Isselee H, De Laat A, Bogaerts K, Lysens R. Long-term fluctuations of pressure pain thresholds in healthy men, normally menstruating women and oral contraceptive users. Eur J Pain 2001;5:27–37.

[40] Kastrup Y, Hallbeck M, Amandusson A, Hirata S, Hermanson O, Blomqvist A. Progesterone receptor expression in the brainstem of the female rat. Neurosci Lett 1999;275:85–8.
[41] Keenan PA, Lindamer LA. Non-migraine headache across the menstrual cycle in women with and without premenstrual syndrome. Cephalalgia 1992;12:356–9.
[42] Kidd BL, Photiou A, Inglis JJ. The role of inflammatory mediators on nociception and pain in arthritis. Novartis Found Symp 2004;260:122–33; discussion 133–8, 277–9.
[43] Kim OY, Chae JS, Paik JK, Seo HS, Jang Y, Cavaillon JM, Lee JH. Effects of aging and menopause on serum interleukin-6 levels and peripheral blood mononuclear cell cytokine production in healthy nonobese women. Age (Dordr) 2011; Epub Apr 13.
[44] Kowalczyk WJ, Evans SM, Bisaga AM, Sullivan MA, Comer SD. Sex differences and hormonal influences on response to cold pressor pain in humans. J Pain 2006;7:151–60.
[45] Kowalczyk WJ, Sullivan MA, Evans SM, Bisaga AM, Vosburg SK, Comer SD. Sex differences and hormonal influences on response to mechanical pressure pain in humans. J Pain 2010;11:330–42.
[46] Kumar M, Narayan J, Verma NS, Saxena I. Variation in response to experimental pain across the menstrual cycle in women compared with one month response in men. Indian J Physiol Pharmacol 2010;54:57–62.
[47] LaCroix-Fralish ML, Tawfik VL, DeLeo JA. The organizational and activational effects of sex hormones on tactile and thermal hypersensitivity following lumbar nerve root injury in male and female rats. Pain 2005;114:71–80.
[48] LeResche L. Epidemiology of temporomandibular disorders: implications for the investigation of etiologic factors. Crit Rev Oral Biol Med 1997;8:291–305.
[49] LeResche L. Epidemiology of pain conditions with higher prevalence in women. In: Chin ML, Ness TJ, Fillingim RB, editors. Pain in women. New York: Oxford University Press; 2011. In press.
[50] LeResche L, Mancl L, Sherman JJ, Gandara B, Dworkin SF. Changes in temporomandibular pain and other symptoms across the menstrual cycle. Pain 2003;106:253–61.
[51] LeResche L, Mancl LA, Drangsholt MT, Saunders K, Korff MV. Relationship of pain and symptoms to pubertal development in adolescents. Pain 2005;118:201–9.
[52] LeResche L, Saunders K, Von Korff MR, Barlow W, Dworkin SF. Use of exogenous hormones and risk of temporomandibular disorder pain. Pain 1997;69:153–60.
[53] LeResche L, Sherman JJ, Huggins K, Saunders K, Mancl LA, Lentz G, Dworkin SF. Musculoskeletal orofacial pain and other signs and symptoms of temporomandibular disorders during pregnancy: a prospective study. J Orofac Pain 2005;19:193–201.
[54] Lichten EM, Lichten JB, Whitty A, Pieper D. The confirmation of a biochemical marker for women's hormonal migraine: the depo-estradiol challenge test. Headache 1996;36:367–71.
[55] Lin SM, Tsao CM, Tsai SK, Mok MS. Influence of testosterone on autotomy in castrated male rats. Life Sci 2002;70:2335–40.
[56] Lipton RB, Stewart WF, Diamond S, Diamond ML, Reed M. Prevalence and burden of migraine in the United States: data from the American Migraine Study II. Headache 2001;41:646–57.
[57] Macfarlane TV, Blinkhorn A, Worthington HV, Davies RM, Macfarlane GJ. Sex hormonal factors and chronic widespread pain: a population study among women. Rheumatology (Oxford) 2002;41:454–7.
[58] Marchand F, Perretti M, McMahon SB. Role of the immune system in chronic pain. Nat Rev Neurosci 2005;6:521–32.
[59] Maret A, Coudert JD, Garidou L, Foucras G, Gourdy P, Krust A, Dupont S, Chambon P, Druet P, Bayard F, Guery JC. Estradiol enhances primary antigen-specific CD4 T cell responses and Th1 development in vivo. Essential role of estrogen receptor alpha expression in hematopoietic cells. Eur J Immunol 2003;33:512–21.
[60] McEwen BS, Alves SE. Estrogen actions in the central nervous system. Endocr Rev 1999;20:279–307.
[61] Mousavi Z, Shafaghi B, Kobarfard F, Jorjani M. Sex differences and role of gonadal hormones on glutamate level in the nucleus accumbens in morphine tolerant rats: a microdialysis study. Eur J Pharmacol 2007;554:145–9.
[62] Muslimani AA, Spiro TP, Chaudhry AA, Taylor HC, Jaiyesimi I, Daw HA. Aromatase inhibitor-related musculoskeletal symptoms: is preventing osteoporosis the key to eliminating these symptoms? Clin Breast Cancer 2009;9:34–8.

[63] Mysliwska J, Rutkowska A, Hak L, Siebert J, Szyndler K, Rachon D. Inflammatory response of coronary artery disease postmenopausal women is associated with the IVS1-397T > C estrogen receptor alpha polymorphism. Clin Immunol 2009;130:355–64.

[64] Nomura M, Akama KT, Alves SE, Korach KS, Gustafsson JA, Pfaff DW, Ogawa S. Differential distribution of estrogen receptor (ER)-alpha and ER-beta in the midbrain raphe nuclei and peri-aqueductal gray in male mouse: predominant role of ER-beta in midbrain serotonergic systems. Neuroscience 2005;130:445–56.

[65] Ockene JK, Barad DH, Cochrane BB, Larson JC, Gass M, Wassertheil-Smoller S, Manson JE, Barnabei VM, Lane DS, Brzyski RG, Rosal MC, Wylie-Rosett J, Hays J. Symptom experience after discontinuing use of estrogen plus progestin. JAMA 2005;294:183–93.

[66] Okifuji A, Turk DC. Sex hormones and pain in regularly menstruating women with fibromyalgia syndrome. J Pain 2006;7:851–9.

[67] Oshima M, Ogawa R, Londyn D. Current perception threshold increases during pregnancy but does not change across menstrual cycle. J Nippon Med Sch 2002;69:19–23.

[68] Pamuk ON, Cakir N. The variation in chronic widespread pain and other symptoms in fibromyalgia patients. The effects of menses and menopause. Clin Exp Rheumatol 2005;23:778–82.

[69] Papka RE, Storey-Workley M, Shughrue PJ, Merchenthaler I, Collins JJ, Usip S, Saunders PT, Shupnik M. Estrogen receptor-alpha and beta- immunoreactivity and mRNA in neurons of sensory and autonomic ganglia and spinal cord. Cell Tissue Res 2001;304:193–214.

[70] Phiel KL, Henderson RA, Adelman SJ, Elloso MM. Differential estrogen receptor gene expression in human peripheral blood mononuclear cell populations. Immunol Lett 2005;97:107–13.

[71] Powell-Boone T, Ness TJ, Cannon R, Lloyd LK, Weigent DA, Fillingim RB. Menstrual cycle affects bladder pain sensation in subjects with interstitial cystitis. J Urol 2005;174:1832–6.

[72] Ribeiro-Dasilva MC, Shinal RM, Glover T, Williams RS, Staud R, Riley JL III, Fillingim RB. Evaluation of menstrual cycle effects on morphine and pentazocine analgesia. Pain 2011;152:614–22.

[73] Riley JL III, Robinson ME, Wise EA, Price DD. A meta-analytic review of pain perception across the menstrual cycle. Pain 1999;81:225–35.

[74] Ring C, Veldhuijzen van Zanten JJ, Kavussanu M. Effects of sex, phase of the menstrual cycle and gonadal hormones on pain in healthy humans. Biol Psychol 2009;81:189–91.

[75] Sadreddini S, Molaeefard M, Noshad H, Ardalan M, Asadi A. Efficacy of Raloxifen in treatment of fibromyalgia in menopausal women. Eur J Intern Med 2008;19:350–5.

[76] Sances G, Granella F, Nappi RE, Fignon A, Ghiotto N, Polatti F, Nappi G. Course of migraine during pregnancy and postpartum: a prospective study. Cephalalgia 2003;23:197–205.

[77] Schell E, Theorell T, Hasson D, Arnetz B, Saraste H. Stress biomarkers' associations to pain in the neck, shoulder and back in healthy media workers: 12-month prospective follow-up. Eur Spine J 2008;17:393–405.

[78] Sherman JJ, LeResche L. Does experimental pain response vary across the menstrual cycle? A methodological review. Am J Physiol Regul Integr Comp Physiol 2006;291:R245–56.

[79] Sherman JJ, LeResche L, Mancl LA, Huggins K, Sage JC, Dworkin SF. Cyclic effects on experimental pain response in women with temporomandibular disorders. J Orofac Pain 2005;19:133–43.

[80] Smith YR, Stohler CS, Nichols TE, Bueller JA, Koeppe RA, Zubieta JK. Pronociceptive and antinociceptive effects of estradiol through endogenous opioid neurotransmission in women. J Neurosci 2006;26:5777–85.

[81] Soderberg K, Sundstrom P, I, Nyberg S, Backstrom T, Nordh E. Psychophysically determined thresholds for thermal perception and pain perception in healthy women across the menstrual cycle. Clin J Pain 2006;22:610–6.

[82] Solomon MB, Herman JP. Sex differences in psychopathology: of gonads, adrenals and mental illness. Physiol Behav 2009;97:250–8.

[83] Somerville BW. The role of estradiol withdrawal in the etiology of menstrual migraine. Neurology 1972;22:355–65.

[84] Stening K, Eriksson O, Wahren L, Berg G, Hammar M, Blomqvist A. Pain sensations to the cold pressor test in normally menstruating women: comparison with men and relation to menstrual phase and serum sex steroid levels. Am J Physiol Regul Integr Comp Physiol 2007;293:R1711–6.

[85] Straneva PA, Maixner W, Light KC, Pedersen CA, Costello NL, Girdler SS. Menstrual cycle, beta-endorphin and pain sensitivity in premenstrual dysphoric disorder. Health Psychol 2002;21:358–67.

[86] Tassorelli C, Sandrini G, Cecchini AP, Nappi RE, Sances G, Martignoni E. Changes in noci-
      ceptive flexion reflex threshold across the menstrual cycle in healthy women. Psychosom Med
      2002;64:621–6.
[87] Teepker M, Peters M, Vedder H, Schepelmann K, Lautenbacher S. Menstrual variation in experi-
      mental pain: correlation with gonadal hormones. Neuropsychobiology 2010;61:131–40.
[88] Tofoli GR, Ramacciato JC, Volpato MC, Meechan JG, Ranali J, Groppo FC. Anesthetic efficacy
      and pain induced by dental anesthesia: the influence of gender and menstrual cycle. Oral Surg
      Oral Med Oral Pathol Oral Radiol Endod 2007;103:e34–8.
[89] Torres-Chavez KE, Sanfins JM, Clemente-Napimoga JT, Pelegrini-Da-Silva A, Parada CA, Fisch-
      er L, Tambeli CH. Effect of gonadal steroid hormones on formalin-induced temporomandibular
      joint inflammation. Eur J Pain 2011; Epub Jul 7.
[90] Tousignant-Laflamme Y, Marchand S. Excitatory and inhibitory pain mechanisms during the
      menstrual cycle in healthy women. Pain 2009;146:47–55.
[91] Trzonkowski P, Mysliwska J, Tukaszuk K, Szmit E, Bryl E, Mysliwski A. Luteal phase of the
      menstrual cycle in young healthy women is associated with decline in interleukin 2 levels. Horm
      Metab Res 2001;33:348–53.
[92] Vignolo V, Vedolin GM, de Araujo CR, Rodrigues Conti PC. Influence of the menstrual cycle on
      the pressure pain threshold of masticatory muscles in patients with masticatory myofascial pain.
      Oral Surg Oral Med Oral Pathol Oral Radiol Endod 2008;105:308–15.
[93] Watkins LR, Maier SF. Implications of immune-to-brain communication for sickness and pain.
      Proc Natl Acad Sci USA 1999;96:7710–3.
[94] Williams TJ, Mitterling KL, Thompson LI, Torres-Reveron A, Waters EM, McEwen BS, Gore
      AC, Milner TA. Age- and hormone-regulation of opioid peptides and synaptic proteins in the
      rat dorsal hippocampal formation. Brain Res 2011;1379:71–85.
[95] Wise EA, Riley JLI, Robinson ME. Clinical pain perception and hormone replacement therapy in
      post-menopausal females experiencing orofacial pain. Clin J Pain 2000;16:121–6.
[96] Xu S, Cheng Y, Keast JR, Osborne PB. 17-Beta-estradiol activates estrogen receptor beta-signal-
      ling and inhibits transient receptor potential vanilloid receptor 1 activation by capsaicin in adult
      rat nociceptor neurons. Endocrinology 2008;149:5540–8.
[97] Zinder O, Dar DE. Neuroactive steroids: their mechanism of action and their function in the
      stress response. Acta Physiol Scand 1999;167:181–8.
[98] Zuckerman SH, Ahmari SE, Bryan-Poole N, Evans GF, Short L, Glasebrook AL. Estriol: a po-
      tent regulator of TNF and IL-6 expression in a murine model of endotoxemia. Inflammation
      1996;20:581–97.

Correspondence to: Roger B. Fillingim, PhD, University of Florida College of
Dentistry and North Florida/South Georgia Veterans Health System, 1329 SW
16th Street, Suite 5180, Gainesville, FL 32610-3628, USA. Email: rfillingim@
dental.ufl.edu.

The Role of the Immune System in Chronic Pain Comorbidities

Peter M. Grace,[a,c] Linda R. Watkins,[c] and Mark R. Hutchinson[b,c]

[a]Discipline of Pharmacology and [b]Discipline of Physiology, School of Medical Sciences, University of Adelaide, Adelaide, South Australia, Australia; [c]Department of Psychology and Center for Neuroscience, University of Colorado at Boulder, Boulder, Colorado, USA

Since the seminal work of Garrison and colleagues [22] demonstrating that peripheral nerve damage results in activation of spinal cord glia, a considerable amount of research has shown that glia and peripheral immune cells contribute to nociceptive hypersensitivity [24,48]. Glia are the most abundant cell type in the central nervous system (CNS), outnumbering neurons ten to one. Microglia (~10%) and astrocytes (~50%), the two predominant glial cell types, are immunocompetent—that is, they are capable of recognizing and responding to traditional immune signals. Originally considered merely as structural support to neurons, glia are increasingly being recognized by the scientific and medical communities as more than just mere neuronal "housekeepers." It is now clear that astrocytes play a pivotal role in maintaining CNS homeostasis, with microglia constantly surveying the CNS microenvironment for damage or danger. Microglia respond quickly, producing large quantities of proinflammatory cytokines. The immediate consequences are astrocyte activation and upregulation of cell-specific activation markers. Glia and cytokines are recognized to contribute substantially to a diverse range of CNS pathologies, not least the common comorbidities of chronic pain, depression, anxiety, and drug abuse. Interestingly, sleep disturbances, which are commonly associated with chronic pain, although not linked to an inflammatory etiology at present, can result in increased proinflammatory effects [27], which may exacerbate the symptoms of chronic pain and its comorbidities. Therefore, glia and proinflammatory cytokines are critically involved in both health and disease.

As will be discussed and introduced here, it is now clear that inflammatory mechanisms contribute to the chronic pain comorbidities of depression, anxiety, and opioid abuse. The common mechanistic link between these comorbid diseases suggests that these conditions are co-occurring on "fertile ground," rather than one disease driving the other. Clearly, distinct and separable neuroanatomical features are responsible for each disease, but perhaps the immune mechanisms that are common to conditions affecting the nervous system, owing to the ever-present glia, form common major risk factors for these diseases.

The following discussion of the immune basis for chronic pain comorbidities will comprise two sections. The first will cover the evidence for an immune component to depression and anxiety, followed by a discussion of the mechanisms by which cytokines contribute to these conditions, given their similarities [71]. The second section will discuss the evidence supporting immune mechanisms of drug abuse—opioid reward and dependence in particular—followed by a summary of these mechanisms.

Evidence for an Immune Component to Depression

There is a reciprocal relationship between major depressive disorders and chronic pain. The incidence of pain among depressed patients is greater than 50% [79], whereas the incidence of major depression among chronic pain patients is reported to range between 1.5% and 87% [82]. The direction of causality is not completely clear, and in some instances, it can go either way. Most studies suggest that depressive disorders tend to occur after chronic pain begins [19]. However, many of those affected have a prior history of depression.

It is now clear that the monoamine hypothesis fails to explain all aspects of major depressive disorder, and a number of observations have implicated inflammatory mechanisms in the pathophysiology of depression. In animals, there is a striking similarity between sickness behavior and depression, as both involve withdrawal from the physical and social environment and are accompanied by pain, malaise, and decreased reactivity to reward. In addition, some components of sickness behavior, such as a decreased preference for sweet solutions and reduced social exploration, are improved by antidepressant treatment [83]. In humans, major depressive disorder occurs in approximately one-third of patients who are treated with the recombinant cytokines interleukin (IL)-2 and interferon (IFN)-α [60]. Indeed, immunotherapy has become an experimental model by which to investigate the pathophysiology of cytokine-induced depression. A recent meta-analysis has found that plasma cytokine levels are elevated in patients with major depression [13], and a post mortem study has revealed increased expression of different pro- and anti-inflammatory cytokines in the prefrontal cortices of unmedicated patients with major depression [66]. In support of these findings, major depressive disorders are more prevalent in patients with conditions that lead to chronic inflammation (such as cardiovascular diseases, type 2 diabetes, and rheumatoid arthritis) than in the general population [12].

A number of rodent studies have also been performed to demonstrate a role for cytokines in depression. Despite the behavioral overlap between sickness behavior and depression, a separation of these effects has been cleverly achieved in several key experiments. Twenty-four hours after lipopolysaccharide (LPS) treatment, which is beyond the peak effect for sickness behavior, mice displayed increased immobility in the tail-suspension and forced-swim tests [21]. Furthermore, preference for a sweetened drinking solution was still decreased when food intake and drinking had returned to normal [21], a behavior that was abolished by pretreatment with antidepressants [83]. An antidepressant pretreatment also attenuated the decreased performance of rats given a sucrose solution reward to a task requiring progressively increased effort following IL-1β treatment [47]. Genetic animal models of depression have also been used. For example, fawn-hooded rats are considered to display many of the animal equivalents of depression and are more sensitive to IL-1β-induced immobility in the forced-swim test than normal Sprague Dawley rats [67]. A strong link between depression and pain has been amply demonstrated in a recent study showing that peripheral nerve injury results in increased depressive behaviors and elevated frontal cortex levels of IL-1β [54]. These findings support the clinical observations that immune proinflammatory activation can cause depression.

A role for cytokines in depression was first proposed in the early 1990s [43,69], but this theory was not well accepted by the psychiatric community because depression was thought to be associated with decreased rather than increased immunity, and many key links between inflammation and depression were limited. The ensuing research has filled in many of these gaps, which will be discussed following an examination of the role of the immune system in anxiety disorders.

Evidence for an Immune Component to Anxiety

Anxiety not only occurs in conjunction with chronic pain, but also accompanies many other chronic pain comorbidities, such as major depression. The overall prevalence of anxiety in chronic pain populations is estimated to range from 16.5% to 28.8% [20]. Despite the close relationship between depression and anxiety, little is known about the association between anxiety and inflammation.

Studies in patients have demonstrated elevated IL-6 and lowered cortisol plasma levels, compared to controls [55]. Furthermore, ex vivo stimulation of peripheral blood mononuclear cells isolated from anxious patients resulted in decreased Th1 and Th2 cytokines, but increased Th17 cytokines (tumor necrosis factor-α [TNF-α] and IL-17) [77]. In contrast to cytokine production from control peripheral blood mononuclear cells, this effect is not inhibited by glucocorticoids, indicating glucocorticoid resistance [3].

The P2X7 purinergic receptor, activated by ATP and other related nucleotides, is considered to be exclusively expressed by microglia in the CNS. Activation of this receptor results in the rapid release of IL-1β, and has been implicated in the induction of chronic pain in rodent models. In a recent study, P2X7 knockout mice displayed attenuated anxiety-like behaviors in the forced-swim test and elevated plus maze [4]. IL-1β-treated mice lacking IL-1 receptor type I also exhibited decreased anxiety-like behaviors in the elevated plus maze and light-dark box, compared to wild-type controls [40], thereby implicating these cytokines in anxiety behaviors in addition to their established roles in chronic pain. Furthermore, mice with experimental autoimmune encephalomyelitis (a model of multiple sclerosis) display anxiety-like behaviors in the light-dark box as well as increased startle responses, correlating with increased TNF-α in the hippocampus [59].

Pathophysiological Mechanisms by Which Cytokines Affect the Brain in Depression and Anxiety

Cytokines are relatively large molecules that do not freely pass through the blood-brain barrier. However, a number of mechanisms have been described to show how cytokine signals are able to reach the brain, including: (1) passage of cytokines through leaky regions of the blood-brain barrier, including the choroid plexus and circumventricular organs; (2) active transport via saturable cytokine-specific transport molecules on brain endothelium; (3) activation of blood-brain barrier endothelial cells, responsible for the subsequent release of second messengers (e.g., prostaglandins and nitric oxide) within the brain parenchyma; (4) transmission of cytokine signals via afferent nerve fibers, such as the vagus nerve; and (5) entry into the brain parenchyma via peripherally activated monocytes [7].

In the CNS, cytokines function as part of an integrated network of cells, including neurons, microglia, and astrocytes, which are able to produce cytokines and amplify cytokine signals. These signals have a range of consequences for depression and anxiety due to their effect on the hypothalamus-pituitary-adrenal (HPA) axis and changes in the metabolism of key monoamines. They also affect neuroendocrine activity, neural plasticity, and brain circuitry.

Effects of Cytokines on Neurotransmitters

Serotonin

Serotonin is the most widely studied of all neurotransmitters in regards to the effects of cytokines on brain and behavior. Studies in rodents have shown that acute administration of cytokines or LPS can alter serotonin metabolism in multiple brain regions [2,15,16]. Clinically, the serotonin reuptake inhibitor paroxetine can significantly reduce depressive symptoms associated with IFN-α therapy [62]. In addition, chronic IFN-α treatment leads to a downregulation of serotonin receptor 1A [6]. The effects of cytokines on the enzyme indoleamine 2,3 dioxygenase (IDO) and the signaling molecule p38 mitogen-activated protein kinase (MAPK) suggest that cytokines may affect both synthesis and reuptake of monoamines, thus contributing to reduced serotonin availability.

Indoleamine 2,3 dioxygenase. Proinflammatory cytokines, including IL-2, IFN-γ, and TNF-α, activate the enzyme IDO [52], which catabolizes tryptophan into kynurenine. The breakdown of tryptophan is believed to contribute to reduced serotonin availability, which may alter CNS serotonin synthesis [12]. Consistent with the role of IDO in cytokine-induced depression, decreased tryptophan and increased kynurenine plasma concentrations have been associated with the development of depression in IFN-α-treated patients [10].

Kynurenine is also metabolized to quinolinic acid and kynurenic acid, two potentially neurotoxic metabolites [51,56]. Kynurenic acid has been shown to inhibit the release of glutamate, which may inhibit the release of dopamine, the release of which is regulated in part by glutamatergic activity. In contrast, quinolinic acid promotes glutamate release through activation of *N*-methyl-D-aspartate (NMDA) receptors. Quinolinic acid also induces oxidative stress, which in combination with glutamate release may contribute to CNS excitotoxicity [52], and perhaps to additional feed-forward glial activation. IFN-α treatment increases the activity of IDO and the plasma concentration of its metabolites [81]. IFN-α treatment has also been associated with increased levels of kynurenine and quinolinic acid in cerebrospinal fluid that correlated with clinical symptoms of depression [61].

p38 Mitogen-activated protein kinase. Recent in vitro studies using direct activators of p38 MAPK, or using IL-1β and TNF-α to indirectly stimulate p38, have shown that activation of p38 signaling pathways can upregulate both the expression and activity of the membrane transporters for serotonin and norepinephrine in cell lines and rat brain synaptosome preparations [84,85]. These findings have recently been extended in vivo to show that LPS-induced activation of p38 MAPK can upregulate serotonin transporter expression and activity in the hippocampus in association with increased extracellular clearance of serotonin [86].

Dopamine

As with serotonin, cytokines influence both the synthesis and reuptake of dopamine (as well as its release, as discussed above in relation to kynurenic acid). For example, administration of IFN-α to rats has been shown to decrease CNS concentrations of tetrahydrobiopterin and dopamine and to stimulate release of nitric oxide (NO) [38]. These effects are reversed by administration of a nitric oxide synthase inhibitor [38]. Tetrahydrobiopterin is an important cofactor for the conversion of tyrosine to L-DOPA and is required for NO synthesis. Activation of microglia is associated with increased NO production, suggesting that cytokine influences on tetrahydrobiopterin via NO may be a common mechanism by which cytokines reduce dopamine availability in relevant brain regions. As with the serotonin transporter, cytokine-induced activation of MAPK pathways has also been shown to upregulate the activity of the dopamine transporter [50].

Glutamate

Cytokines and associated inflammatory mediators have been shown to stimulate the release of glutamate from glia within the brain, as well as decreasing glutamate reuptake, in part through downregulation of astrocyte glutamate transporters [75,78]. Excessive release of glutamate by astrocytes can access extrasynaptic NMDA receptors, which mediate excitotoxicity and decreased production of trophic factors such as brain-derived neurotrophic factor (BDNF) [26]. These potential excitotoxic effects may in turn contribute to glial loss in multiple mood-relevant brain regions, including the subgenual prefrontal cortex and amygdala, which has been associated with major depression [63].

Effects of Cytokines on Neuroendocrine Function

A hyperactive HPA axis is often associated with clinical depression, which is acutely and potently activated by proinflammatory cytokines. Such HPA axis activity leads to the increased production of corticotropin-releasing hormone (CRH) and vasopressin, neuropeptides that have long been considered candidates for causing symptoms of depression [29,74]. Under chronic inflammation, proinflammatory cytokines can cause glucocorticoid resistance in immune cells via induction of the MAP kinases c-jun N-terminal kinase (JNK) and p38 [37], as well as promoting expression of the inactive glucocorticoid receptor isoform [57]. Glucocorticoid resistance is well described in patients with major depression [58]. Cytokine-dependent glucocorticoid receptor resistance explains the reduced ability of glucocorticoids to downregulate the production of CRH in the hypothalamus. It also explains how the normal inhibitory effect of glucocorticoids on cytokine production by immune cells is absent, leading to a positive feedback loop that would result in cumulative production of proinflammatory cytokines.

Effects of Cytokines on Neural Plasticity

Although cytokines provide trophic support to neurons and enhance neuronal integrity under physiological conditions, in the context of chronic stress, excessive cytokine production has been shown to lead to depressive-like behavior, in part through the disruption of growth factor production and neurogenesis. Neurogenesis is believed to play a fundamental role in the maintenance of neural integrity, and reduced neurogenesis, especially in the hippocampus, is a hallmark of chronic exposure to stress in laboratory animals [14]. Not only does chronic stress activate the expression of cytokines, in particular that of IL-1β in the hippocampus, but several studies have shown that blockade of IL-1β (through the administration of IL-1 receptor antagonist (IL-1ra), the transplantation of IL-1ra-secreting neural precursor cells, or the use of IL-1β knockout mice) reverses the reduced production of BDNF and decreased neurogenesis that are associated with chronic stress (while also reversing stress-induced behavioral changes) [5,23,39]. In vitro studies have suggested that the effects of IL-1β on neurogenesis appear to occur through activation of nuclear factor (NF)-κB signaling pathways [39], while in vivo studies indicate that endogenous glucocorticoids are also involved [23].

Effects of Cytokines on Neurocircuitry

Neuroimaging studies have begun to reveal the neurocircuits that appear to be targeted by cytokines. Neurocircuits in both cortical and subcortical brain regions are involved, including the basal ganglia and the subgenual and dorsal aspects of the anterior cingulate cortex (ACC).

The basal ganglia play an important role in motor activity and motivation, whereas the ACC regions are implicated in depression (the subgenual ACC) and in anxiety, arousal, and alarm (the dorsal ACC) [1,17,42]. Supporting the role for cytokines in targeting dopamine neurotransmission, IFN-α induces motor slowing, which is correlated with the development of both depression and fatigue [45]. In addition, neuroimaging studies have found that IFN-α induces altered metabolic activity (as revealed by positron emission tomography) and blood flow (as measured by functional magnetic resonance imaging) in relevant basal ganglia nuclei, including the nucleus accumbens, putamen, and substantia nigra [9].

Activation of the dorsal ACC has also been described in patients receiving IFN-α [8]. Increased activity in the dorsal ACC has been associated with high-trait anxiety, neuroticism, obsessive-compulsive disorder, and bipolar disorder [17], all of which are associated with increased anxiety and arousal. Interestingly, in a recent study, stress-induced inflammatory responses were associated with increased activity in the dorsal ACC, which supports a role for cytokines in targeting dorsal ACC circuits to increase arousal and alarm [68].

Evidence for an Immune Component to Opioid Abuse

Owing to the prominent role opioids play in pain management, many chronic pain patients have significant exposure to opioids and as such, a proportion of these patients may be at risk of elevated opioid abuse liability. Classically, opioids are thought to induce their rewarding effects via activation of the mesolimbic dopamine reward pathway via classical opioid receptors. Despite several decades of research, the non-neuronal CNS effects of opioids have only come to light in at most the past two decades. In addition, it has only recently been acknowledged that these non-neuronal actions of opioids at CNS immunocompetent cells and central immune-signaling pathways may play a significant role in contributing to the behavioral outcomes following drug exposure [32,53,80]. While the immune system has been implicated in the rewarding aspects of many drugs of abuse, opioids remain the most commonly abused drugs among chronic pain patients (with estimates ranging from 2.8% to 50% [46]).

While a recent post mortem study of the brains of opioid abusers supports a role for proinflammatory immune signaling [64], the bulk of evidence comes from animal studies. Fairbanks and Wilcox [18] first implicated spinal proinflammatory immune signaling in opioid tolerance. Soon afterward, Song and Zhao [70] implicated opioid-induced glial reactivity as critical to morphine tolerance. These studies triggered a profound shift in opioid research to include a central immune-signaling hypothesis as part of the several systems involved in the effects of opioids. The first crucial evidence of a link between central immune signaling and reward and development of dependence to opioids has arisen from preclinical animal behavioral models. Numerous in vivo animal behavioral studies have demonstrated that central immune changes affect morphine responses, manifested as behavioral reward (conditionéd place preference [CPP]), naloxone-precipitated withdrawal, and levels of opioid self-administration.

Central immune-signaling modulation of morphine behavior was first implicated by studies showing that direct injection of astrocyte-conditioned medium into the nucleus accumbens heightened morphine CCP [53]. This study, and others to follow, further highlighted the role of central immune signaling following observations that proinflammatory glial activation attenuators could block morphine CPP [33,34,53], block spontaneous and precipitated withdrawal from morphine and oxycodone, and simultaneously prevent increases or caused decreases of cytokines and chemokines in various brain regions shown to mediate withdrawal (e.g., the ventral tegmental area and nucleus accumbens [33]). Further studies have shown that other immune mediators also play a role via alteration in downstream events to initial glial activation. For example, toll-like receptor 4 (TLR4) involvement (discussed in more detail below) is implicated because (+)-naloxone, a TLR4 antagonist with no opioid receptor activity, significantly attenuated morphine withdrawal [36].

Consequences of Opioid-Induced Glial Activation

Upon in vivo or in vitro opioid exposure, several aspects of central immune signaling are altered in a way that can modify neuronal homeostasis and in turn lead to changes in behavioral responses. These effects have been summarized into five principal aspects: cell proliferation/death/survival; cell marker/phenotype (receptor expression); cell function; intracellular signaling; and extracellular signaling. Interestingly, aside from cell proliferation/death/survival, all of the opioid effects on central immune signaling have also been implicated in nerve injury and nociceptive hypersensitivity.

Changes in Cell Proliferation and Survival in the Central Nervous System

The earliest opioid-induced adaptations of non-neuronal cells observed in the CNS were alterations in cellular proliferation and survival. Studies have demonstrated morphine-induced decreases in astrocyte cell proliferation [25]; this effect was found to be naloxone-sensitive [72] and generalizable to astrocytes across multiple brain regions (the striatum, hippocampus, and cerebral cortex) [73]. The inhibitory effect of opioid receptors on epidermal growth factor-induced astrocyte proliferation has been further examined in vitro and demonstrated to be linked to upregulation of extracellular signal-regulated kinase (ERK) phosphorylation. Protein kinase C, arrestin, and calmodulin pathways seem to be involved in the antiproliferative effects of opioids on astrocytes [35].

Morphine has also been shown to induce microglial apoptosis, although astrocytes were resistant to such effects. The role of morphine-induced caspase-3 has been implicated in the apoptotic death of microglia via glycogen synthase kinase-3 and p38 MAPK signaling pathways; morphine also interacts with HIV Tat protein-induced death [35].

Adaptations in Cell Marker and Reactivity Phenotype in the Central Nervous System

Early studies have also demonstrated profound opioid-induced changes in cellular morphology [28] and phenotypic receptor/immunohistological marker expression. After long-term systemic morphine administration, a significant increase in glial fibrillary acidic protein (GFAP) expression, an astrocyte activation marker, was observed in the ventral tegmental area but not in the substantia nigra, locus ceruleus, cerebral cortex, or spinal cord, thereby displaying significant regional heterogeneity [35]. Increased astrocyte expression of cell surface receptors, such as the chemokine receptors CCR2, CCR3, CCR5, and CXCR2 [44] and classical opioid receptors [76], have also been reported after in vitro exposure to morphine. The mechanisms of morphine-induced elevations in GFAP expression have also been examined, implicating NMDA-receptor signaling, CCL5, CCR2, protein kinase C, ceramide synthase, sphingosine kinase, matrix metalloproteinase-9, P2X4, α_2-adrenergic receptors, and alterations in glutamate homeostasis [35]. Several general proinflammatory attenuators have been shown to block opioid-induced GFAP upregulation [35].

Opioid-induced elevations in microglial reactive phenotype cell surface marker expression have also been observed using immunohistochemistry [35]. Again, significant regional heterogeneity was observed; morphine-induced decreases in CD11b expression were reported in the cornu ammonis of the hippocampus, the nucleus accumbens, and the substantia nigra, and no change was reported in the dorsal raphe nucleus and medial prefrontal cortex [35]. Increased microglial expression of other cell surface receptors such as CCR5, TLR2, TLR4, P2X4, and P2X7 have also been reported after opioid exposure [35]. The mechanisms by which these opioid-induced microglial phenotypic changes occur have been characterized pharmacologically and were found to involve ceramide synthase, sphingosine kinase, P2X4, and P2X7 [35]. The microglial responses were also sensitive to general anti-inflammatory treatments [35].

Alterations in Cell Function in the Central Nervous System

Adaptations in other microglial and astrocyte functions have also been observed after opioid exposure, such as chemotaxis. Early studies demonstrated that morphine was able to decrease microglial chemotaxis toward complement protein 5a [11] and CCL5 [31]. Such inhibitory responses by at least CCL5 could be explained by heterologous desensitization of chemokine receptors by opioid receptors [65]. In contrast, microglial chemotaxis toward ATP was potentiated by morphine in a P2X4-dependent fashion [30]. These chemotactic responses were concluded to be induced by classical opioid receptors and Akt/inositol triphosphate (IP3) pathways.

Initiation of Intracellular Signaling in the Central Nervous System

One of the most prominently reported cascades influenced by opioid exposure is the MAPK pathway. The MAPK pathway comprises a collection of serine/threonine-specific protein kinases that are recruited by cell surface receptors and respond to extracellular stimuli and communicate this to elicit various cellular responses, such as gene expression. Three key kinases of this response system are p38, ERK, and JNK (although the effects on JNK are not clear). The phosphorylation of these kinases results in an active functional signaling complex. Morphine causes phosphorylation of p38 within microglia, in a manner dependent on P2X7, calcitonin gene-regulated peptide (CGRP), and neuronal nitric oxide; this effect could be blocked by naloxone and minocycline [35]. Likewise, morphine induces ERK activation in both microglia and astrocytes in a manner dependent on MEK, CGRP, matrix metalloproteinase 9, pertussis toxin, calmodulin, and IP3/Akt kinase [35].

Opioid-Induced Glial Activation and the Extracellular Environment of the Central Nervous System

The intracellular events reviewed above result in the release of a myriad of factors into the extracellular space in the CNS that can act on both neuronal and non-neuronal cells. The proinflammatory cytokines IL-1β, IL-6, and TNF-α, among other factors, show an upregulation of transcription, translation, and release after morphine administration. Importantly, such cytokine release is attenuated by ibudilast, propentofylline, amitriptyline, and etanercept [35].

Morphine also modulates the chemokines CCL2, CCL3, CCL5, CCL20, and CXCL1, as well as complement component C3, 27-kDa heat shock protein, prostaglandin E, and prostaglandin E synthase-1 [35]. It is noteworthy that each of these opioid-induced events directs the CNS toward a proinflammatory reactive phenotype.

Finally, opioid exposure causes alterations in non-neuronal cell control over glutamate homeostasis. It is noteworthy that altered glutamate homeostasis due to decreased glial glutamate transporter expression has been demonstrated in several CNS disturbances in which glia assume a reactive phenotype [75]. Long-term morphine administration results in an elevation of cerebrospinal fluid levels of aspartate and glutamate, most likely resulting from downregulation of glial GLT-1 and GLAST glutamate transporters [75,78]. This elevation of aspartate and glutamate seems to involve aquaporin 4 and is sensitive to coadministration of morphine with dexamethasone, ceftriaxone, naloxone, and amitriptyline [35]. Such changes in glutamate expression have profound implications for neuroexcitability, including increased NMDA receptor signaling, as demonstrated by increased phosphorylation of the NR1 subunit [41].

Conclusions

It is now clear that inflammatory mechanisms contribute to chronic pain comorbidities of depression, anxiety, and opioid abuse. Some of the outstanding questions surrounding this field include the source of the proinflammatory cytokines and the mechanistic explanation for their elevated expression in these patients. The realization of a common immunological link between several of these comorbidities provides an exciting avenue for future research. Moreover, the common link of TLR4 as a possible proinflammatory glial trigger in several of these comorbidities, by either exogenous or endogenous substances, also provides a tantalizing novel avenue for treatment. A great deal of research has investigated these questions with respect to elevated spinal cord cytokines following nerve injury in animal models. However, the relationship between nerve injury and glial activation/cytokine expression in the brain regions associated with depression, anxiety, and drug abuse is not clear. Perhaps further examination and identification of common exogenous or endogenous TLR4 triggers may provide answers to some of these regional heterogeneity questions. More sophisticated use of animal models such as those developed by the Keay group [49] may assist in answering these important questions.

Given the common underlying mechanisms of cytokines on neuronal networks in the brain and spinal cord in chronic pain and its comorbidities, as well as the increased prevalence of other inflammatory disorders with major depressive disorders [12], perhaps these conditions should be understood as occurring on "fertile ground" rather than one disease driving the other. Each disease is multifactorial, but perhaps the central immune mechanisms represent maladaptive versions of the healthy central immune response, forming major risk factors for these diseases. Perhaps these responses occur when activation of the innate immune response is exacerbated in intensity or duration, when taking place in the context of other vulnerabilities. Hence, patients may check the risk factor boxes for multiple diseases. Ultimately, appreciation of the common central immune mechanisms between chronic pain and its comorbidities may lead to more complete treatment approaches and better treatment outcomes for people with chronic pain worldwide.

References

[1]   Alexander GE, Crutcher MD, DeLong MR. Basal ganglia-thalamocortical circuits: parallel substrates for motor, oculomotor, "prefrontal" and "limbic" functions. Prog Brain Res 1990;85:119–46.
[2]   Anisman H, Merali Z, Poulter MO, Hayley S. Cytokines as a precipitant of depressive illness: animal and human studies. Curr Pharm Des 2005;11:963–72.
[3]   Barros PO, Ferreira TB, Vieira MM, Almeida CR, Araujo-Lima CF, Silva-Filho RG, Hygino J, Andrade RM, Andrade AF, Bento CA. Substance P enhances Th17 phenotype in individuals with generalized anxiety disorder: an event resistant to glucocorticoid inhibition. J Clin Immunol 2011;31:51–9.
[4]   Basso AM, Bratcher NA, Harris RR, Jarvis MF, Decker MW, Rueter LE. Behavioral profile of P2X7 receptor knockout mice in animal models of depression and anxiety: relevance for neuropsychiatric disorders. Behav Brain Res 2009;198:83–90.
[5]   Ben Menachem-Zidon O, Goshen I, Kreisel T, Ben Menahem Y, Reinhartz E, Ben Hur T, Yirmiya R. Intrahippocampal transplantation of transgenic neural precursor cells overexpressing interleukin-1 receptor antagonist blocks chronic isolation-induced impairment in memory and neurogenesis. Neuropsychopharmacology 2008;33:2251–62.
[6]   Cai W, Khaoustov VI, Xie Q, Pan T, Le W, Yoffe B. Interferon-alpha-induced modulation of glucocorticoid and serotonin receptors as a mechanism of depression. J Hepatol 2005;42:880–7.
[7]   Capuron L, Miller AH. Immune system to brain signaling: neuropsychopharmacological implications. Pharmacol Ther 2011;130:226–38.
[8]   Capuron L, Pagnoni G, Demetrashvili M, Woolwine BJ, Nemeroff CB, Berns GS, Miller AH. Anterior cingulate activation and error processing during interferon-alpha treatment. Biol Psychiatry 2005;58:190–6.
[9]   Capuron L, Pagnoni G, Demetrashvili MF, Lawson DH, Fornwalt FB, Woolwine B, Berns GS, Nemeroff CB, Miller AH. Basal ganglia hypermetabolism and symptoms of fatigue during interferon-alpha therapy. Neuropsychopharmacology 2007;32:2384–92.
[10] Capuron L, Ravaud A, Neveu PJ, Miller AH, Maes M, Dantzer R. Association between decreased serum tryptophan concentrations and depressive symptoms in cancer patients undergoing cytokine therapy. Mol Psychiatry 2002;7:468–73.
[11] Chao CC, Hu S, Shark KB, Sheng WS, Gekker G, Peterson PK. Activation of mu opioid receptors inhibits microglial cell chemotaxis. J Pharmacol Exp Ther 1997;281:998–1004.
[12] Dantzer R, O'Connor JC, Freund GG, Johnson RW, Kelley KW. From inflammation to sickness and depression: when the immune system subjugates the brain. Nat Rev Neurosci 2008;9:46–56.
[13] Dowlati Y, Herrmann N, Swardfager W, Liu H, Sham L, Reim EK, Lanctot KL. A meta-analysis of cytokines in major depression. Biol Psychiatry 2010;67:446–57.
[14] Duman RS, Monteggia LM. A neurotrophic model for stress-related mood disorders. Biol Psychiatry 2006;59:1116–27.
[15] Dunn AJ, Wang J. Cytokine effects on CNS biogenic amines. Neuroimmunomodulation 1995;2:319–28.
[16] Dunn AJ, Wang J, Ando T. Effects of cytokines on cerebral neurotransmission. Comparison with the effects of stress. Adv Exp Med Biol 1999;461:117–27.
[17] Eisenberger NI, Lieberman MD. Why rejection hurts: a common neural alarm system for physical and social pain. Trends Cogn Sci 2004;8:294–300.
[18] Fairbanks CA, Wilcox GL. Spinal plasticity of acute opioid tolerance. J Biomed Sci 2000;7:200–12.

[19] Fishbain DA, Cutler R, Rosomoff HL, Rosomoff RS. Chronic pain-associated depression: antecedent or consequence of chronic pain? A review. Clin J Pain 1997;13:116–37.

[20] Fishbain DA, Cutler RB, Rosomoff HL, Rosomoff RS. Validity of self-reported drug use in chronic pain patients. Clin J Pain 1999;15:184–91.

[21] Frenois F, Moreau M, O'Connor J, Lawson M, Micon C, Lestage J, Kelley KW, Dantzer R, Castanon N. Lipopolysaccharide induces delayed FosB/DeltaFosB immunostaining within the mouse extended amygdala, hippocampus and hypothalamus, that parallel the expression of depressive-like behavior. Psychoneuroendocrinology 2007;32:516–31.

[22] Garrison CJ, Dougherty PM, Kajander KC, Carlton SM. Staining of glial fibrillary acidic protein (GFAP) in lumbar spinal cord increases following a sciatic nerve constriction injury. Brain Res 1991;565:1–7.

[23] Goshen I, Kreisel T, Ben-Menachem-Zidon O, Licht T, Weidenfeld J, Ben-Hur T, Yirmiya R. Brain interleukin-1 mediates chronic stress-induced depression in mice via adrenocortical activation and hippocampal neurogenesis suppression. Mol Psychiatry 2008;13:717–28.

[24] Grace PM, Rolan PE, Hutchinson MR. Peripheral immune contributions to the maintenance of central glial activation underlying neuropathic pain. Brain Behav Immun 2011;25:1322–32.

[25] Hauser KF, Stiene-Martin A, Mattson MP, Elde RP, Ryan SE, Godleske CC. mu-Opioid receptor-induced Ca^{2+} mobilization and astroglial development: morphine inhibits DNA synthesis and stimulates cellular hypertrophy through a Ca^{2+}-dependent mechanism. Brain Res 1996;720:191–203.

[26] Haydon PG, Carmignoto G. Astrocyte control of synaptic transmission and neurovascular coupling. Physiol Rev 2006;86:1009–31.

[27] Heffner KL, France CR, Trost Z, Ng HM, Pigeon WR. Chronic low back pain, sleep disturbance, and interleukin-6. Clin J Pain 2011;27:35–41.

[28] Holdridge SV, Armstrong SA, Taylor AM, Cahill CM. Behavioural and morphological evidence for the involvement of glial cell activation in delta opioid receptor function: implications for the development of opioid tolerance. Mol Pain 2007;3:7.

[29] Holsboer F. Corticotropin-releasing hormone modulators and depression. Curr Opin Investig Drugs 2003;4:46–50.

[30] Horvath RJ, DeLeo JA. Morphine enhances microglial migration through modulation of P2X4 receptor signaling. J Neurosci 2009;29:998–1005.

[31] Hu S, Chao CC, Hegg CC, Thayer S, Peterson PK. Morphine inhibits human microglial cell production of, and migration towards, RANTES. J Psychopharmacol 2000;14:238–43.

[32] Hutchinson MR, Bland ST, Johnson KW, Rice KC, Maier SF, Watkins LR. Opioid-induced glial activation: mechanisms of activation and implications for opioid analgesia, dependence, and reward. ScientificWorldJournal 2007;7:98–111.

[33] Hutchinson MR, Lewis SS, Coats BD, Skyba DA, Crysdale NY, Berkelhammer DL, Brzeski A, Northcutt A, Vietz CM, Judd CM, Maier SF, Watkins LR, Johnson KW. Reduction of opioid withdrawal and potentiation of acute opioid analgesia by systemic AV411 (ibudilast). Brain Behav Immun 2009;23:240–50.

[34] Hutchinson MR, Northcutt AL, Chao LW, Kearney JJ, Zhang Y, Berkelhammer DL, Loram LC, Rozeske RR, Bland ST, Maier SF, Gleeson TT, Watkins LR. Minocycline suppresses morphine-induced respiratory depression, suppresses morphine-induced reward, and enhances systemic morphine-induced analgesia. Brain Behav Immun 2008;22:1248–56.

[35] Hutchinson MR, Shavit Y, Grace PM, Rice KC, Maier SF, Watkins LR. Exploring the neuroimmunopharmacology of opioids: an integrative review of mechanisms of central immune signaling and their implications for opioid analgesia. Pharmacol Rev 2011;63:772–810.

[36] Hutchinson MR, Zhang Y, Shridhar M, Evans JH, Buchanan MM, Zhao TX, Slivka PF, Coats BD, Rezvani N, Wieseler J, Hughes TS, Landgraf KE, Chan S, Fong S, Phipps S, Falke JJ, Leinwand LA, Maier SF, Yin H, Rice KC, Watkins LR. Evidence that opioids may have toll like receptor 4 and MD-2 effects. Brain Behav Immun 2010;24:83–95.

[37] Irwin MR, Miller AH. Depressive disorders and immunity: 20 years of progress and discovery. Brain Behav Immun 2007;21:374–83.

[38] Kitagami T, Yamada K, Miura H, Hashimoto R, Nabeshima T, Ohta T. Mechanism of systemically injected interferon-alpha impeding monoamine biosynthesis in rats: role of nitric oxide as a signal crossing the blood-brain barrier. Brain Res 2003;978:104–14.

[39] Koo JW, Duman RS. IL-1beta is an essential mediator of the antineurogenic and anhedonic effects of stress. Proc Natl Acad Sci USA 2008;105:751–6.

[40] Koo JW, Duman RS. Interleukin-1 receptor null mutant mice show decreased anxiety-like behavior and enhanced fear memory. Neurosci Lett 2009;456:39–43.

[41] Lin SL, Tsai RY, Shen CH, Lin FH, Wang JJ, Hsin ST, Wong CS. Co-administration of ultra-low dose naloxone attenuates morphine tolerance in rats via attenuation of NMDA receptor neurotransmission and suppression of neuroinflammation in the spinal cords. Pharmacol Biochem Behav 2010;96:236–45.

[42] Lozano AM, Mayberg HS, Giacobbe P, Hamani C, Craddock RC, Kennedy SH. Subcallosal cingulate gyrus deep brain stimulation for treatment-resistant depression. Biol Psychiatry 2008;64:461–7.

[43] Maes M, Smith R, Scharpe S. The monocyte-T-lymphocyte hypothesis of major depression. Psychoneuroendocrinology 1995;20:111–6.

[44] Mahajan SD, Schwartz SA, Shanahan TC, Chawda RP, Nair MP. Morphine regulates gene expression of alpha- and beta-chemokines and their receptors on astroglial cells via the opioid mu receptor. J Immunol 2002;169:3589–99.

[45] Majer M, Welberg LA, Capuron L, Pagnoni G, Raison CL, Miller AH. IFN-alpha-induced motor slowing is associated with increased depression and fatigue in patients with chronic hepatitis C. Brain Behav Immun 2008;22:870–80.

[46] Martell BA, O'Connor PG, Kerns RD, Becker WC, Morales KH, Kosten TR, Fiellin DA. Systematic review: opioid treatment for chronic back pain: prevalence, efficacy, and association with addiction. Ann Intern Med 2007;146:116–27.

[47] Merali Z, Brennan K, Brau P, Anisman H. Dissociating anorexia and anhedonia elicited by interleukin-1beta: antidepressant and gender effects on responding for "free chow" and "earned" sucrose intake. Psychopharmacology (Berl) 2003;165:413–8.

[48] Milligan ED, Watkins LR. Pathological and protective roles of glia in chronic pain. Nat Rev Neurosci 2009;10:23–36.

[49] Mor D, Bembrick AL, Austin PJ, Wyllie PM, Creber NJ, Denyer GS, Keay KA. Anatomically specific patterns of glial activation in the periaqueductal gray of the sub-population of rats showing pain and disability following chronic constriction injury of the sciatic nerve. Neuroscience 2010;166:1167–84.

[50] Moron JA, Zakharova I, Ferrer JV, Merrill GA, Hope B, Lafer EM, Lin ZC, Wang JB, Javitch JA, Galli A, Shippenberg TS. Mitogen-activated protein kinase regulates dopamine transporter surface expression and dopamine transport capacity. J Neurosci 2003;23:8480–8.

[51] Muller N, Myint AM, Schwarz MJ. Inflammatory biomarkers and depression. Neurotox Res 2011;19:308–18.

[52] Muller N, Schwarz MJ. The immune-mediated alteration of serotonin and glutamate: towards an integrated view of depression. Mol Psychiatry 2007;12:988–1000.

[53] Narita M, Miyatake M, Narita M, Shibasaki M, Shindo K, Nakamura A, Kuzumaki N, Nagumo Y, Suzuki T. Direct evidence of astrocytic modulation in the development of rewarding effects induced by drugs of abuse. Neuropsychopharmacology 2006;31:2476–88.

[54] Norman GJ, Karelina K, Zhang N, Walton JC, Morris JS, Devries AC. Stress and IL-1beta contribute to the development of depressive-like behavior following peripheral nerve injury. Mol Psychiatry 2010;15:404–14.

[55] O'Donovan A, Hughes BM, Slavich GM, Lynch L, Cronin MT, O'Farrelly C, Malone KM. Clinical anxiety, cortisol and interleukin-6: evidence for specificity in emotion-biology relationships. Brain Behav Immun 2010;24–:1074–7.

[56] Oxenkrug GF. Tryptophan kynurenine metabolism as a common mediator of genetic and environmental impacts in major depressive disorder: the serotonin hypothesis revisited 40 years later. Isr J Psychiatry Relat Sci 2010;47:56–63.

[57] Pace TW, Hu F, Miller AH. Cytokine-effects on glucocorticoid receptor function: relevance to glucocorticoid resistance and the pathophysiology and treatment of major depression. Brain Behav Immun 2007;21:9–19.

[58] Pariante CM, Miller AH. Glucocorticoid receptors in major depression: relevance to pathophysiology and treatment. Biol Psychiatry 2001;49:391–404.

[59] Peruga I, Hartwig S, Thone J, Hovemann B, Gold R, Juckel G, Linker RA. Inflammation modulates anxiety in an animal model of multiple sclerosis. Behav Brain Res 2011;220:20–9.

[60] Raison CL, Capuron L, Miller AH. Cytokines sing the blues: inflammation and the pathogenesis of depression. Trends Immunol 2006;27:24–31.

[61] Raison CL, Dantzer R, Kelley KW, Lawson MA, Woolwine BJ, Vogt G, Spivey JR, Saito K, Miller AH. CSF concentrations of brain tryptophan and kynurenines during immune stimulation with IFN-alpha: relationship to CNS immune responses and depression. Mol Psychiatry 2010;15:393–403.

[62] Raison CL, Woolwine BJ, Demetrashvili MF, Borisov AS, Weinreib R, Staab JP, Zajecka JM, Bruno CJ, Henderson MA, Reinus JF, Evans DL, Asnis GM, Miller AH. Paroxetine for prevention of depressive symptoms induced by interferon-alpha and ribavirin for hepatitis C. Aliment Pharmacol Ther 2007;25:1163–74.

[63] Rajkowska G, Miguel-Hidalgo JJ. Gliogenesis and glial pathology in depression. CNS Neurol Disord Drug Targets 2007;6:219–33.

[64] Ramos-Miguel A, García-Fuster MJ, Callado LF, La Harpe R, Meana JJ, García-Sevilla JA. Phosphorylation of FADD (Fas-associated death domain protein) at serine 194 is increased in the prefrontal cortex of opiate abusers: relation to mitogen activated protein kinase, phosphoprotein enriched in astrocytes of 15 kDa, and Akt signaling pathways involved in neuroplasticity. Neuroscience 2009;161:23–38.

[65] Rogers TJ, Steele AD, Howard OM, Oppenheim JJ. Bidirectional heterologous desensitization of opioid and chemokine receptors. Ann N Y Acad Sci 2000;917:19–28.

[66] Shelton RC, Claiborne J, Sidoryk-Wegrzynowicz M, Reddy R, Aschner M, Lewis DA, Mirnics K. Altered expression of genes involved in inflammation and apoptosis in frontal cortex in major depression. Mol Psychiatry 2011;16:751–62.

[67] Simmons DA, Broderick PA. Cytokines, stressors, and clinical depression: augmented adaptation responses underlie depression pathogenesis. Prog Neuropsychopharmacol Biol Psychiatry 2005;29:793–807.

[68] Slavich GM, Way BM, Eisenberger NI, Taylor SE. Neural sensitivity to social rejection is associated with inflammatory responses to social stress. Proc Natl Acad Sci USA 2010;107:14817–22.

[69] Smith RS. The macrophage theory of depression. Med Hypotheses 1991;35:298–306.

[70] Song P, Zhao ZQ. The involvement of glial cells in the development of morphine tolerance. Neurosci Res 2001;39:281–6.

[71] Stein MB. Neurobiology of generalized anxiety disorder. J Clin Psychiatry 2009;70:15–9.

[72] Stiene-Martin A, Gurwell JA, Hauser KF. Morphine alters astrocyte growth in primary cultures of mouse glial cells: evidence for a direct effect of opiates on neural maturation. Brain Res Dev Brain Res 1991;60:1–7.

[73] Stiene-Martin A, Hauser KF. Morphine suppresses DNA synthesis in cultured murine astrocytes from cortex, hippocampus and striatum. Neurosci Lett 1993;157:1–3.

[74] Swaab DF, Bao AM, Lucassen PJ. The stress system in the human brain in depression and neurodegeneration. Ageing Res Rev 2005;4:141–94.

[75] Tilleux S, Hermans E. Neuroinflammation and regulation of glial glutamate uptake in neurological disorders. J Neurosci Res 2007;85:2059–70.

[76] Turchan-Cholewo J, Dimayuga FO, Ding Q, Keller JN, Hauser KF, Knapp PE, Bruce-Keller AJ. Cell-specific actions of HIV-Tat and morphine on opioid receptor expression in glia. J Neurosci Res 2008;86:2100–10.

[77] Vieira MM, Ferreira TB, Pacheco PA, Barros PO, Almeida CR, Araujo-Lima CF, Silva-Filho RG, Hygino J, Andrade RM, Linhares UC, Andrade AF, Bento CA. Enhanced Th17 phenotype in individuals with generalized anxiety disorder. J Neuroimmunol 2010;229:212–8.

[78] Viviani B, Bartesaghi S, Gardoni F, Vezzani A, Behrens MM, Bartfai T, Binaglia M, Corsini E, Di Luca M, Galli CL, Marinovich M. Interleukin-1beta enhances NMDA receptor-mediated intracellular calcium increase through activation of the Src family of kinases. J Neurosci 2003;23:8692–700.

[79] von Knorring L, Perris C, Eisemann M, Eriksson U, Perris H. Pain as a symptom in depressive disorders. I. Relationship to diagnostic subgroup and depressive symptomatology. Pain 1983;15:19–26.

[80] Watkins LR, Hutchinson MR, Rice KC, Maier SF. The "toll" of opioid-induced glial activation: improving the clinical efficacy of opioids by targeting glia. Trends Pharmacol Sci 2009;30:581–91.

[81] Wichers MC, Koek GH, Robaeys G, Verkerk R, Scharpe S, Maes M. IDO and interferon-alpha-induced depressive symptoms: a shift in hypothesis from tryptophan depletion to neurotoxicity. Mol Psychiatry 2005;10:538–44.

[82] Worz R. Pain in depression-depression in pain. Pain Clin Updates 2003;XI(5).

[83] Yirmiya R, Weidenfeld J, Pollak Y, Morag M, Morag A, Avitsur R, Barak O, Reichenberg A, Cohen E, Shavit Y, Ovadia H. Cytokines, "depression due to a general medical condition," and antidepressant drugs. Adv Exp Med Biol 1999;461:283–316.

[84] Zhu CB, Blakely RD, Hewlett WA. The proinflammatory cytokines interleukin-1beta and tumor necrosis factor-alpha activate serotonin transporters. Neuropsychopharmacology 2006;31:2121–31.

[85] Zhu CB, Carneiro AM, Dostmann WR, Hewlett WA, Blakely RD. p38 MAPK activation elevates serotonin transport activity via a trafficking-independent, protein phosphatase 2A-dependent process. J Biol Chem 2005;280:15649–58.

[86] Zhu CB, Lindler KM, Owens AW, Daws LC, Blakely RD, Hewlett WA. Interleukin-1 receptor activation by systemic lipopolysaccharide induces behavioral despair linked to MAPK regulation of CNS serotonin transporters. Neuropsychopharmacology 2010;35:2510–20.

Correspondence to: Peter M. Grace, PhD, Department of Psychology and the Center for Neuroscience, University of Colorado at Boulder, Boulder, CO 80309, USA. Email: peter.grace@colorado.edu.

The Influence of Psychosocial Environment in Pain Comorbidities

Akiko Okifuji[a] and Dennis C. Turk[b]

[a]Department of Anesthesiology, University of Utah, Salt Lake City, Utah, USA;
[b]Department of Anesthesiology and Pain Medicine, University of Washington,
Seattle, Washington, USA

Pain is a complex perceptual experience, defined as an "unpleasant sensory and emotional experience associated with actual or potential tissue damage, or described in terms of such damage" [41]. The experience of pain is ubiquitous; the majority of pain is time-limited and heals spontaneously or with a minor intervention. However, some pain persists over and beyond the expected healing time. As pain persists, it may lead to adverse consequences in people's lives and in their ability to function. Chronic pain is a pervasive problem throughout the world, affecting up to a quarter of the population [39]. It is one of the leading conditions for disability in the United States [77]. Problems related to chronic pain are expected to increase as society ages [32].

One of the most critical developments in the past several decades in pain research is progress in our understanding of the multifactorial biobehavioral mechanisms involved in chronic pain [31]. Research has also consistently shown the importance of using multimodal approaches to treat patients with chronic pain [58], given that monotherapies appear to provide less than optimal relief [87]. These developments have suggested that various psychological factors—cognitive, emotional, and behavioral—significantly contribute to pain modulation and pain-related disability [32]. The objective of this chapter is to review psychological factors relevant to pain comorbidities. We will first review several prominent psychological variables that are known to influence pain experience in general. Then we will discuss ways to integrate these psychological variables so as to understand their contributions to pain comorbidities.

Failure of the Somatic Model of Pain

The historically dominant view of pain reflected the persistent assumption that an isomorphic relationship must exist between subjective reports of pain and observable pathology. Even today, this somatic view of pain is popular among many people, including a large number of clinicians. As a consequence, chronic noncancer pain conditions that often do not have observable pathology are considered a medical mystery at best, or else symptom magnification, malingering, or a manifestation of psychopathology, at worst. However, scientific evidence suggests that pain is not linearly related to pathology, even when clear pathological conditions are considered to underline pain complaints.

In knee osteoarthritis, for example, physical findings such as cartilage loss and bone marrow edema are considered to reflect the clinical progression of the disease. However, when the grading of pathology was evaluated by magnetic resonance imaging (MRI), neither bone marrow edema nor cartilage abnormality was linearly related to pain severity [53]. The results of a longitudinal study following groups of elite male athletes and nonathletes for 15 years indicated that the evolution of persistent back pain was not related to the number of problematic disks or changes in MRI findings [8]. The authors found not only that the presence of pain did not predict pathology, but also that the presence of pathology did not predict pain. An MRI study of a total of 256 hips found that the majority of hips that were causing no pain showed various degrees of peritrochanteric abnormalities, comparable to hips that were causing pain [11]. Furthermore, people's expectations about the impact of their pain and the likelihood of recovery from a painful injury have been shown to be more predictive of long-term disability than objective levels of physical pathology [19].

The failure to explain the presence and extent of pain based solely on pathological findings has led the field to widen its view on pain to integrate other factors that may contribute to the pain experience. According to the biopsychosocial view of pain, the pain experience results from a complex web of interaction among nervous and physiological systems (both central and peripheral), psychological factors, and social variables [31].

Psychological Factors Contributing to Pain

Cognitions

Beliefs and Appraisals

People are active processors of their experience, which is always mediated by what we believe and how we interpret a given situation. The influence of beliefs on pain is profound. In acute pain situations, pain is a direct result of tissue damage. In the short term, protecting the area of pain by refraining from activity may be adaptive. However, when the same belief is extended to chronic pain, it often contributes to complications. Such beliefs are unfortunately all too common in chronic pain, and they often lead to activity avoidance and deactivation in general and are significantly related to greater pain and disability [88]. Cancer patients who believed that their pain was related to cancer reported greater pain in response to physical therapy than those who believed that their pain came from other sources [72]. Even for healthy individuals, the belief that the pain is threatening reduces their pain tolerance [42]. On the other hand, modification of maladaptive beliefs about pain seems to predict changes in pain and disability [60].

Catastrophizing

Catastrophizing is a cognitive process where one assumes the worst possible outcomes and interprets even minor problems as major calamities. A large volume of evidence suggests that catastrophizing about pain plays a significant role in defining the actual experience [78]. Catastrophizing is related to higher sensitivity to experimentally induced pain in healthy children [54] and adults [30], as well as in people with acute and chronic pain [33,34,73,75]. For people undergoing surgery, catastrophizing predicts

lengthier time to hospital discharge [64], greater postoperative pain severity, and poor quality of life, as well as the later development of chronic
pain [48]. It is also a significant predictor of pain-related disability [2] in
individuals with chronic pain. The degree to which catastrophizing exerts
its influence may depend on personality factors; catastrophizing seems to
influence pain experience among individuals with a higher degree of anxiety sensitivity in response to physical exertion [36]. Evidence also suggests
that catastrophizing seems to worsen the pain experience by attenuating
diffuse noxious inhibitory controls [92].

Recent imaging studies may offer additional explanations as to
how catastrophizing may influence pain perception. Seminowicz and
Davis [69] examined functional MRI (fMRI) images while their healthy
subjects underwent laboratory pain testing. They found that the effect of
catastrophizing on the neural response to painful stimulation may depend
on stimulus intensity. With mild pain stimulation, there was a positive
relationship between catastrophizing and the neural response in regions
representing attention, vigilance, and emotion, whereas the relationship
was negative with moderate pain, suggesting that catastrophizing attenuates the descending inhibitory system's response to more intense stimuli,
making it more difficult to disengage from pain. Similar results have been
reported in an imaging study of fibromyalgia patients in which catastrophizing, independent of depression, was related to activation in the brain
areas reflecting attentional, anticipatory, and emotional activities in response to pain [37]. These studies suggest that catastrophizing adversely
affects pain experience through increased attention and negative anticipation of pain.

Sense of Control/Helplessness

A sense of control represents the perceived controllability of pain or pain-
related matters. How patients conceptualize their ability to control pain
and associated stress seems to be an important determinant for how they
cope with pain. Indeed, increased sense of control is linearly related to
greater functionality in chronic pain patients [88]. Furthermore, improvement in control beliefs following treatment has typically been shown to
reduce pain and disability [44]. The opposite end of the control spectrum
is a sense of helplessness. The literature generally supports the association

of helplessness with greater pain and poorer physical and psychological adjustment in people with chronic pain [47].

The effects of perceived control are not limited to chronic pain but significantly influence how people experience acute pain. During mammography, for example, when women were allowed to control compression to one breast while a technician controlled the pressure for the other, the patients' pain reports were significantly lower for self-controlled compression, with no compromise in the quality of the images [51]. Similarly, perceived controllability of pain during childbirth has been shown to be associated with lower pain report and distress at a 6-month follow-up [81].

Neural mechanisms accounting for how control affects pain may parallel those reviewed above for catastrophizing. Perceived controllability of pain seems to influence neural activation in the anterior cingulate cortex (ACC) and insula (areas representing attentional and emotional responses). One study showed that the responses in these areas were attenuated in individuals who were led to believe that they could control the stimulus level compared to those who were led to believe that there was nothing they could do to change it [66]. A subsequent study [67] showed that responses in these regions lost their predictability when the effects of the prefrontal cortex (PRF) were controlled for, suggesting that modulation of pain by a sense of control depends on the top-down influence of the PFC on the ACC and insula.

Self-Efficacy

Self-efficacy belief is defined as a personal conviction that one can successfully execute a course of action to produce a desired outcome in a given situation. Self-efficacy beliefs are task specific; in the context of the assessment of chronic pain, they typically include beliefs in one's own ability to manage pain, symptoms, and functioning.

Experimental studies have shown that pain-related self-efficacy is associated with reports of pain sensitivity in response to noxious stimulation [6]. An early study with healthy participants showed that a stronger self-efficacy belief about tolerating a cold pressure test was significantly related to pain tolerance [28]. Similarly, patients with osteoarthritis with a high level of self-efficacy for handling pain rated heat stimuli as less painful than those with a low self-efficacy belief [46].

Self-efficacy belief also plays a role in the clinical presentation of chronic pain. Lower self-efficacy is consistently related to greater clinical pain ratings in various chronic pain conditions [16,22,76]. A low level of self-efficacy belief is related to disability [10,68] and mediates the relationship between pain and physical and psychological functioning [3,4]. Furthermore, recent longitudinal studies suggest that poor self-efficacy belief is a risk factor for work absenteeism [17] and for development of disability associated with chronic pain [23]. Functional self-efficacy at the preoperative stage also predicts postoperative symptoms and function after knee surgery [80].

Whereas low self-efficacy beliefs are related to more severe pain and dysfunction, improvement in self-efficacy is one of the best predictors for successful rehabilitation for pain patients. An elevated level of self-efficacy beliefs before treatment tends to predict better outcomes [15,50]. However, even when the initial level of self-efficacy belief is low, evidence suggests that improved self-efficacy facilitates healthy practices in chronic pain patients [9].

Improvement of self-efficacy following treatment may improve pain by activating the endogenous opioid system. Chronic pain patients who successfully completed cognitive-behavioral therapy and gained increased self-efficacy by the completion of treatment showed significantly increased pain tolerance compared to study participants who did not receive treatment or who just took placebo pills; however, the effect was attenuated by naloxone injection [7].

We have reviewed several cognitive variables that have been implicated in the experience of pain and related disability. Each of these variables has a potent association with pain, disability, and psychological functioning in chronic pain patients. Thus, it makes sense that treatment approaches that target modification of maladaptive cognitions (e.g., cognitive-behavioral therapy) should lead to better outcomes. We would like to offer a word of caution here, however. These cognitive variables do not occur in isolation and are thus likely to be interrelated. Whether these variables represent some aspects of a larger construct or are independent processes associated with pain and stress is not clearly delineated. This dilemma poses a problem in interpreting results from studies that involve several of these factors treated independently. Further investigation on this issue seems warranted.

Mood and Behaviors

Depression

The prevalence of depression as a comorbid psychological condition in chronic pain varies greatly from 5% to 100%, depending on how and where patients were assessed and on the criteria used for depression. However, depression is quite common in specialized pain clinic patients, with more than 50% experiencing significant emotional distress [5]. Depression adds a significant burden to chronic pain patients. It is one of the most significant determinants of pain-related disability [82]. Depression in chronic pain also increases the costs associated with disability and health care utilization [45].

Historically, there has been much debate as to which comes first: depression or pain. The psychogenic tradition of pain asserts that chronic pain is a form of "masked depression" [12]. That is, patients' reports of pain hide underlying depression because it may be more acceptable to complain of pain than to acknowledge that one is depressed, although this acknowledgment does not necessarily occur at a conscious level. Despite the lack of any scientific evidence to substantiate this scenario, it remains a popular notion among the public and, very unfortunately, even among clinicians. Many patients experience undue distress upon facing the assumption that their chronic pain is "all in their head."

The literature typically supports the notion that depression follows the development of chronic pain [14]. Some studies also suggest that the pain-depression relationship is not linear but rather is mediated by how patients view their plight. Turk et al. [83] have demonstrated that the relationship is mediated by a sense of control and by patients' appraisal of interference of chronic pain with their lives. The interaction between cognition and mood in chronic pain makes sense, given the presence of individual differences in depression among patients with the same diagnoses when pain and physical findings are comparable [62].

This is not to say that depression does not make any contributions to pain. It is well established that depressed people tend to have an elevated degree of pain complaints [74]. Longitudinal studies [29,43] suggest that depression is a risk factor for developing chronic pain. However, these results do not necessarily indicate that depression is the sole cause of pain. Regardless of the causal priority, both pain and depression require treatment in chronic pain patients.

Depression in chronic pain presents a particularly difficult concern for clinicians, given the recent increase in the misuse of potent opioid analgesics and unintentional as well as intentional poisoning. Fatalistic thoughts and wishes are common in chronic pain patients. Almost a quarter of treatment-seeking chronic pain patients admit a history of suicidal ideation [71]. Thus, the assessment of depression in chronic pain should also be linked to the screening of medication misuse or abuse as well as suicidal or overdosing history, and a proper referral should be made to address potentially dangerous conditions [21].

Fear and Anxiety

Anxiety and fear-related problems are more prevalent in chronic pain patients than in the general public. The prevalence of any anxiety disorder may be twice as high (35% vs. 18%); both panic disorder and post-traumatic stress disorder (PTSD) are three times more common in chronic pain patients [59]. Although fear and anxiety are often treated as a single mood condition, they are likely to be distinct entities with different types of physiological and emotional experiences. Anxiety is a future-oriented emotion; it is experienced as worry and nervousness related to some often vague future issues, whereas fear is a present-oriented mood state about something specific that one wants to escape from or avoid. The blurred distinction between fear and anxiety may partially come from the fact that psychological problems associated with these states were both included under one category of anxiety disorder as a diagnostic entity. When the patterns of symptom clustering are considered, however, two distinct types seem to emerge: (1) an anxiety-oriented cluster, which includes generalized anxiety disorder and PTSD, which are associated more with depression; and (2) a fear-oriented cluster, where phobia and panic disorder symptoms form an entity [91]. In relation to pain experience, these states may also lead to differential results. When fear and anxiety states were experimentally induced (fear with exposure to shock, and anxiety with the threat of shock), people experiencing anxiety had greater pain reactivity than those who were in the fear group [65].

Fear and anxiety are known to have behavioral consequences, expressed as escape and avoidance behaviors. Escape behaviors are intended to terminate a noxious experience. Some examples that may apply to chronic pain patients include taking medication in response to a pain flare-up, as well as stopping activity and resting. In short, escape behaviors are a reaction to the noxious cues, and they are often negatively reinforced; the probability of the behavior recurring is increased by the positive consequence of removing the aversive experience. Avoidance, on the other hand, is intended to prevent the noxious experience from occurring. People and animals typically respond to cues associated (or possibly associated) with pain by attempting to terminate the cues. For example, chronic pain patients may not walk more than 15 meters (about 50 feet) because they believe that walking any further may worsen their pain. As a response to fear, escape behaviors reduce fear, whereas successful avoidance may cover up fear totally, so that people may not be aware that they are engaging in avoidance behaviors, yet the behaviors are self-reinforced by the termination of the threatening cues and the absence of fear-loaded noxious events (e.g., worsening of pain).

Pain is a naturally fear-producing state (i.e., an unconditioned stimulus), thus being easily subjected to the behavioral principles by which conditioned responses develop. Pain related avoidance and escape behaviors in pain patients may be conceptualized as a set of "safety-seeking behaviors," loosely defined as "behaviors utilized by patients in an attempt to avoid a feared outcome" (p. 242) [70]. These behaviors are known to be integrated into the dysfunctional circle of pain maintenance. The revolving model of fear-avoidance in chronic pain [90] is depicted in Fig. 1. As the model suggests, pain-related fear and avoidance play a significant role in the interplay between pain, dysfunctional cognitive and affective experience, and disability, resulting in the perpetuation of the chronic pain circle. Indeed, pain-related fear-avoidance is significantly associated with functional limitation in various life domains and with perceived disability in patients with acute and chronic pain [25,35,38,79].

Treatment that incorporates fear-extinction strategies has shown impressive results. A typical approach would start with a thorough assessment of fear and avoidance and develop a hierarchy of feared activities, followed by education and graded in vivo exposure. In the exposure

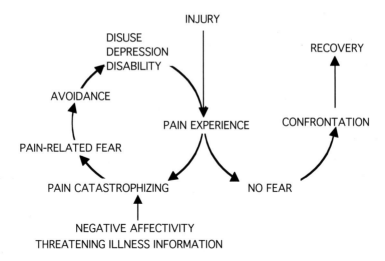

Fig. 1. Fear-avoidance model for chronic pain. Reprinted with permission from Vlaeyen and Linton [90].

series, patients are repeatedly confronted with feared tasks from the low end of the hierarchy, while fear-eliciting beliefs are extinguished. A series of studies evaluating this approach has shown a significant decrease in pain and pain-related fear and an increase in functional ability in various pain conditions, such as chronic back pain [89], complex regional pain syndrome (CRPS) [27], and post-traumatic neck pain [26]. In the study with the CRPS patients, the treatment resulted in elimination or reduction of the cardinal symptoms and signs of CRPS, such as hyperesthesia, edema, and asymmetrical skin color and temperature [27]. Some of the patients in this study first underwent activation therapy, but it was not until they underwent exposure therapy that these changes in symptoms and functions began, suggesting that extinction of patient-specific, maladaptive safety-seeking behaviors is critical in treating chronic pain conditions in general.

Psychological Factors and Pain Comorbidities

An important question is whether there are any specific psychological factors that contribute specifically to the association between various pain conditions. Although the question is intriguing, the current status of pain research does not provide a clear answer. We could speculate, however, about how psychological factors may interact with various pain disorders, leading to high rates of co-occurrence among certain pain disorders.

A number of pain disorders tend to co-occur with no known etiology, often termed "medically unexplained" conditions, such as fibromyalgia, irritable bowel syndrome, headaches, and temporomandibular disorders [55]. One of the common denominators of these conditions is affective distress. Increased prevalence of affective distress in many pain disorders has led to the speculation that perhaps all those medically unexplained, functional pain disorders are actually psychiatrically defined. Pain disorder is an Axis I disorder in the somatoform disorder category that considers pain involving significant life impairment with psychological contribution to be a mental illness [1]. This diagnostic category has been widely criticized for its lack of consideration for the complexity and multifactorial nature of pain. Pain, by definition, has a psychological contribution, and therefore, all chronic pain patients, regardless of the physical findings explaining their pain, would meet the Axis I diagnosis of pain disorder. It has been suggested that it would have more sensible clinical utility to define those pain disorders as the Axis III condition, "physical symptom disorder" [52].

Others have considered that those overlapping pain and distress conditions may represent affective spectrum disorder [40], in which these conditions may share common pathophysiological mechanisms. Abnormalities in serotonin have been suggested as a culprit, as it seems to be dysregulated in both depression and many pain disorders [55]. For example, in fibromyalgia, both pain and depression have a strong family association [13], and some have suggested the involvement of a genetic polymorphism that affects the serotonergic system [18]. However, the actual contribution of impaired serotonergic activities to the experience of depression and chronic pain is still controversial [24]. Thus, it seems reasonable to state that the affective spectrum disorder model is more heuristic at this point than theoretical or empirically guided.

Another common pathway for overlapping pain disorders and psychological factors has been linked to generalized dysregulation of pain and stress modulation. Central sensitization is frequently observed in various pain conditions [49]. Generalized dysfunction in the multiple systems that regulate adaptation to pain and stress may underlie a number of chronic pain conditions [20]. Accordingly, some related concepts have emerged to describe a group of pain and functional disorders as a part of the spectrum syndrome. Dysregulation spectrum syndrome [56] and central sensitization syndrome [49] are two examples attempting to clarify the common characteristics of the dysfunctional central modulatory process involving pain and stress. Although these models are heuristic, there is empirical support for the existence of such dysregulations in diverse pain disorders. However, the state of science is piecemeal, and integration of the evidence into the biopsychosocial framework will be needed to best understand the validity of these syndrome concepts [31].

One comorbid condition that tends to be associated with both psychological distress and pain is sleep disturbance. Sleep disturbance is ubiquitous in chronic pain patients [57]. Epidemiological, experimental, and clinical studies all show a cross-sectional relationship between sleep disturbance and pain as well as adverse effects of sleep deprivation on pain sensitivity [61]. Sleep disturbance is known to adversely affect a range of physical impairments and mental capacities, including alteration in the nervous, metabolic, endocrine, and immune systems, dermal changes, impaired sensory responses, and deterioration in mood and cognition [63]. Many of the psychological factors we have discussed in this chapter are also associated with sleep disturbance. Since maladaptive cognition and avoidance behaviors are likely to lead to deactivation in life functioning, as well as to mood and sleep disturbance, could we consider sleep disturbance to be a potential mediating factor for the contribution of those psychological factors to pain? This is an interesting question that needs empirical testing.

When considering psychosocial factors associated with pain, we have always advocated the importance of not getting trapped into the "patient uniformity myth," where all patients are considered as psychosocially homogeneous within a pain diagnostic group. The review of the effects of various psychosocial and behavioral factors on pain that we have provided should make it clear by now that people vary in their pain-related psychosocial and behavioral presentations. Yet our discussion suggests that the nature of the influence of those factors is consistent across pain conditions.

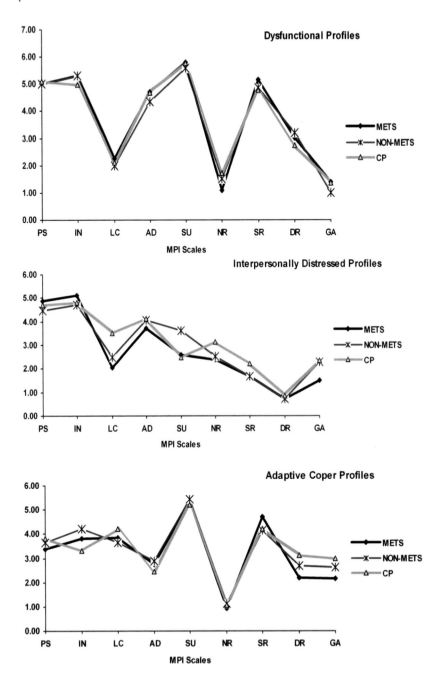

Fig. 2. Psychological adaptation of three types of pain patients (patients with metastatic cancer, regional cancer, or noncancer pain) according to their psychosocial and behavioral profiles. Adapted from Turk et al. [86], with permission.

Past research has demonstrated that patients differ greatly in their pain-related psychosocial and behavioral characteristics, even within the same medical diagnosis [84,85]. Conversely, we have shown that psychosocial and behavioral profiles of pain patients emerge in similar patterns across diagnoses. Fig. 2 shows the within-profile patterns of pain-related psychosocial variables across three types of conditions with diverse pathophysiology (metastatic cancer, regional cancer, and noncancer chronic pain) [86]. Whereas the three groups are quite different in their health status and pain pathophysiology, it is impossible to distinguish them from one another within the psychosocial response profiles. These studies suggest that the influence of the psychological factors on pain is not specific to pain conditions and diagnoses but rather is largely determined by the patterns of psychosocial and behavioral profiles that are specific to individuals.

Summary and Conclusions

Pain is a complex biopsychosocial perceptual phenomenon that cannot be understood solely from the perspective of physiological damage and neural transduction [31]. The literature overwhelmingly supports the contributory impacts of various psychological factors on pain. Recent advancement in imaging technology has also helped us understand that cognitive, behavioral, and affective factors influence the neural activation process of pain experience as well as the endogenous opioid system. Theoretical models delineating how those factors relate to multiple pain comorbidities are in the developmental stages and need additional work. However, research has consistently shown that the impact of psychological factors is not pain condition specific. Individuals greatly vary in their psychosocial profiles, even within a single pain diagnosis, suggesting that we should not assume that we can delineate what their psychological needs are from the pain diagnosis alone. Rather, we must pay attention to the psychological needs of individual pain patients and address them during treatment planning. In considering various pain comorbidities, clinicians and researchers may wish to pay particular attention to psychological factors that are related to functional dysregulations that seem to be common to those pain conditions. Successful treatment of patients with chronic pain will require attention not only to the pathophysiology that may contribute to pain but also to a range of psychosocial and behavioral factors, all of which interact to create the experience of pain; these factors influence the severity, maintenance, and exacerbation of pain, the extent of disability, and response to treatment.

References

[1]   American Psychiatric Association. Diagnostic and statistical manual of mental disorders. Washington, DC: American Psychiatric Press; 1994.
[2]   Arnow BA, Blasey CM, Constantino MJ, Robinson R, Hunkeler E, Lee J, Fireman B, Khaylis A, Feiner L, Hayward C. Catastrophizing, depression and pain-related disability. Gen Hosp Psychiatry 2011;33:150–6.
[3]   Arnstein P. The mediation of disability by self efficacy in different samples of chronic pain patients. Disabil Rehabil 2000;22:794–801.
[4]   Arnstein P, Caudill M, Mandle CL, Norris A, Beasley R. Self efficacy as a mediator of the relationship between pain intensity, disability and depression in chronic pain patients. Pain 1999;80:483–91.
[5]   Bair MJ, Robinson RL, Katon W, Kroenke K. Depression and pain comorbidity: a literature review. Arch Intern Med 2003;163:2433–45.
[6]   Bandura A. Self-efficacy: toward a unifying theory of behavioral change. Psychol Rev 1977;84:191–215.
[7]   Bandura A, O'Leary A, Taylor CB, Gauthier J, Gossard D. Perceived self-efficacy and pain control: opioid and nonopioid mechanisms. J Pers Soc Psychol 1987;53:563–71.
[8]   Baranto A, Hellstrom M, Cederlund CG, Nyman R, Sward L. Back pain and MRI changes in the thoraco-lumbar spine of top athletes in four different sports: a 15-year follow-up study. Knee Surg Sports Traumatol Arthrosc 2009;17:1125–34.
[9]   Beal CC, Stuifbergen AK, Brown A. Predictors of a health promoting lifestyle in women with fibromyalgia syndrome. Psychol Health Med 2009;14:343–53.
[10] Benyon K, Hill S, Zadurian N, Mallen C. Coping strategies and self-efficacy as predictors of outcome in osteoarthritis: a systematic review. Musculoskeletal Care 2010;8:224–36.
[11] Blankenbaker DG, Ullrick SR, Davis KW, De Smet AA, Haaland B, Fine JP. Correlation of MRI findings with clinical findings of trochanteric pain syndrome. Skeletal Radiol 2008;37:903–9.
[12] Blumer D, Heilbronn M. Chronic pain as a variant of depressive disease: the pain-prone disorder. J Nerv Ment Dis 1982;170:381–406.
[13] Bradley LA. Pathophysiologic mechanisms of fibromyalgia and its related disorders. J Clin Psychiatry 2008;69(Suppl 2):6–13.
[14] Brown GK. A causal analysis of chronic pain and depression. J Abnorm Psychol 1990;99:127–37.
[15] Buckelew SP, Huyser B, Hewett JE, Parker JC, Johnson JC, Conway R, Kay DR. Self-efficacy predicting outcome among fibromyalgia subjects. Arthritis Care Res 1996;9:97–104.
[16] Buckelew SP, Murray SE, Hewett JE, Johnson J, Huyser B. Self-efficacy, pain, and physical activity among fibromyalgia subjects. Arthritis Care Res 1995;8:43–50.
[17] Busch H, Goransson S, Melin B. Self-efficacy beliefs predict sustained long-term sick absenteeism in individuals with chronic musculoskeletal pain. Pain Pract 2007;7:234–40.
[18] Buskila D, Sarzi-Puttini P. Biology and therapy of fibromyalgia. Genetic aspects of fibromyalgia syndrome. Arthritis Res Ther 2006;8:218.
[19] Carragee EJ, Alamin TF, Miller JL, Carragee JM. Discographic, MRI and psychosocial determinants of low back pain disability and remission: a prospective study in subjects with benign persistent back pain. Spine J 2005;5:24–35.
[20] Chapman CR, Tuckett RP, Song CW. Pain and stress in a systems perspective: reciprocal neural, endocrine, and immune interactions. J Pain 2008;9:122–45.
[21] Cheatle MD. Depression, chronic pain, and suicide by overdose: on the edge. Pain Med 2011;12(Suppl 2):S43–8.

[22] Chong GS, Cogan D, Randolph P, Racz G. Chronic pain and self-efficacy: the effects of age, sex, and chronicity. Pain Pract 2001;1:338–43.

[23] Costa Lda C, Maher CG, McAuley JH, Hancock MJ, Smeets RJ. Self-efficacy is more important than fear of movement in mediating the relationship between pain and disability in chronic low back pain. Eur J Pain 2011;15:213–9.

[24] Cowen PJ. Serotonin and depression: pathophysiological mechanism or marketing myth? Trends Pharmacol Sci 2008;29:433–6.

[25] Crombez G, Vlaeyen JW, Heuts PH, Lysens R. Pain-related fear is more disabling than pain itself: evidence on the role of pain-related fear in chronic back pain disability. Pain 1999;80:329–39.

[26] de Jong JR, Vangronsveld K, Peters ML, Goossens ME, Onghena P, Bulte I, Vlaeyen JW. Reduction of pain-related fear and disability in post-traumatic neck pain: a replicated single-case experimental study of exposure in vivo. J Pain 2008;9:1123–34.

[27] de Jong JR, Vlaeyen JW, Onghena P, Goossens ME, Geilen M, Mulder H. Fear of movement/(re)injury in chronic low back pain: education or exposure in vivo as mediator to fear reduction? Clin J Pain 2005;21:9–17; discussion 69–72.

[28] Dolce JJ, Doleys DM, Raczynski JM, Lossie J, Poole L, Smith M. The role of self-efficacy expectancies in the prediction of pain tolerance. Pain 1986;27:261–72.

[29] Dworkin RH, Hartstein G, Rosner HL, Walther RR, Sweeney EW, Brand L. A high-risk method for studying psychosocial antecedents of chronic pain: the prospective investigation of herpes zoster. J Abnorm Psychol 1992;101:200–5.

[30] Edwards RR, Smith MT, Stonerock G, Haythornthwaite JA. Pain-related catastrophizing in healthy women is associated with greater temporal summation of and reduced habituation to thermal pain. Clin J Pain 2006;22:730–7.

[31] Flor H, Turk DC. Chronic pain: an integrated biobehavioral approach. Seattle: IASP Press; 2011.

[32] Gatchel RJ, Peng YB, Peters ML, Fuchs PN, Turk DC. The biopsychosocial approach to chronic pain: scientific advances and future directions. Psychol Bull 2007;133:581–624.

[33] Geisser ME, Casey KL, Brucksch CB, Ribbens CM, Appleton BB, Crofford LJ. Perception of noxious and innocuous heat stimulation among healthy women and women with fibromyalgia: association with mood, somatic focus, and catastrophizing. Pain 2003;102:243–50.

[34] George SZ, Wallace MR, Wright TW, Moser MW, Greenfield WH, 3rd, Sack BK, Herbstman DM, Fillingim RB. Evidence for a biopsychosocial influence on shoulder pain: pain catastrophizing and catechol-O-methyltransferase (COMT) diplotype predict clinical pain ratings. Pain 2008;136:53–61.

[35] Gheldof EL, Vinck J, Van den Bussche E, Vlaeyen JW, Hidding A, Crombez G. Pain and pain-related fear are associated with functional and social disability in an occupational setting: evidence of mediation by pain-related fear. Eur J Pain 2006;10:513–25.

[36] Goodin BR, McGuire LM, Stapleton LM, Quinn NB, Fabian LA, Haythornthwaite JA, Edwards RR. Pain catastrophizing mediates the relationship between self-reported strenuous exercise involvement and pain ratings: moderating role of anxiety sensitivity. Psychosom Med 2009;71:1018–25.

[37] Gracely RH, Geisser ME, Giesecke T, Grant MA, Petzke F, Williams DA, Clauw DJ. Pain catastrophizing and neural responses to pain among persons with fibromyalgia. Brain 2004;127:835–43.

[38] Grotle M, Vollestad NK, Veierod MB, Brox JI. Fear-avoidance beliefs and distress in relation to disability in acute and chronic low back pain. Pain 2004;112:343–52.

[39] Gureje O, Von Korff M, Simon GE, Gater R. Persistent pain and well-being: a World Health Organization Study in Primary Care. JAMA 1998;280:147–51.

[40] Hudson JI, Pope HG Jr. Fibromyalgia and psychopathology: is fibromyalgia a form of "affective spectrum disorder"? J Rheumatol Suppl 1989;19:15–22.

[41] International Association for the Study of Pain. Classification of chronic pain. Descriptions of chronic pain syndromes and definitions of pain terms. Pain 1986;3:S1–226.

[42] Jackson T, Pope L, Nagasaka T, Fritch A, Iezzi T, Chen H. The impact of threatening information about pain on coping and pain tolerance. Br J Health Psychol 2005;10:441–51.

[43] Jarvik JG, Hollingworth W, Heagerty PJ, Haynor DR, Boyko EJ, Deyo RA. Three-year incidence of low back pain in an initially asymptomatic cohort: clinical and imaging risk factors. Spine (Phila Pa 1976) 2005;30:1541–8; discussion 1549.

[44] Jensen MP, Turner JA, Romano JM. Changes after multidisciplinary pain treatment in patient pain beliefs and coping are associated with concurrent changes in patient functioning. Pain 2007;131:38–47.

[45] Katon W. The impact of depression on workplace functioning and disability costs. Am J Manag Care 2009;15(11 Suppl):S322–7.

[46] Keefe FJ, Lefebvre JC, Maixner W, Salley AN Jr, Caldwell DS. Self-efficacy for arthritis pain: relationship to perception of thermal laboratory pain stimuli. Arthritis Care Res 1997;10:177–84.

[47] Keefe FJ, Rumble ME, Scipio CD, Giordano LA, Perri LM. Psychological aspects of persistent pain: current state of the science. J Pain 2004;5:195–211.

[48] Khan RS, Ahmed K, Blakeway E, Skapinakis P, Nihoyannopoulos L, Macleod K, Sevdalis N, Ashrafian H, Platt M, Darzi A, Athanasiou T. Catastrophizing: a predictive factor for postoperative pain. Am J Surg 2011;201:122–31.

[49] Kindler LL, Bennett RM, Jones KD. Central sensitivity syndromes: mounting pathophysiologic evidence to link fibromyalgia with other common chronic pain disorders. Pain Manag Nurs 2011;12:15–24.

[50] Kores RC, Murphy WD, Rosenthal TL, Elias DB, North WC. Predicting outcome of chronic pain treatment via a modified self-efficacy scale. Behav Res Ther 1990;28:165–9.

[51] Kornguth PJ, Rimer BK, Conaway MR, Sullivan DC, Catoe KE, Stout AL, Brackett JS. Impact of patient-controlled compression on the mammography experience. Radiology 1993;186:99–102.

[52] Kroenke K. Physical symptom disorder: a simpler diagnostic category for somatization-spectrum conditions. J Psychosom Res 2006;60:335–9.

[53] Link TM, Steinbach LS, Ghosh S, Ries M, Lu Y, Lane N, Majumdar S. Osteoarthritis: MR imaging findings in different stages of disease and correlation with clinical findings. Radiology 2003;226:373–81.

[54] Lu Q, Tsao JC, Myers CD, Kim SC, Zeltzer LK. Coping predictors of children's laboratory-induced pain tolerance, intensity, and unpleasantness. J Pain 2007;8:708–17.

[55] Marcus DA, Deodhar A. Fibromyalgia: a practical clinical guide. New York: Springer; 2011.

[56] Masi AT, Yunus MB. Concepts of illness in populations as applied to fibromyalgia syndromes. Am J Med 1986;81:19–25.

[57] McCracken LM, Iverson GL. Disrupted sleep patterns and daily functioning in patients with chronic pain. Pain Res Manag 2002;7:75–9.

[58] McCracken LM, Turk DC. Behavioral and cognitive-behavioral treatment for chronic pain: outcome, predictors of outcome, and treatment process. Spine (Phila Pa 1976) 2002;27:2564–73.

[59] McWilliams LA, Cox BJ, Enns MW. Mood and anxiety disorders associated with chronic pain: an examination in a nationally representative sample. Pain 2003;106:127–33.

[60] Nieto R, Raichle KA, Jensen MP, Miro J. Changes in pain-related beliefs, coping, and catastrophizing predict changes in pain intensity, pain interference, and psychological functioning in individuals with myotonic muscular dystrophy and facioscapulohumeral dystrophy. Clin J Pain 2012;28:47–54.

[61] Okifuji A, Hare BD. Do sleep disorders contribute to pain sensitivity? Curr Rheumatol Rep 2011;13:528–34.

[62] Okifuji A, Turk DC, Sherman JJ. Evaluation of the relationship between depression and fibromyalgia syndrome: why aren't all patients depressed? J Rheumatol 2000;27:212–9.

[63] Orzel-Gryglewska J. Consequences of sleep deprivation. Int J Occup Med Environ Health 2010;23:95–114.

[64] Pavlin DJ, Rapp SE, Polissar NL, Malmgren JA, Koerschgen M, Keyes H. Factors affecting discharge time in adult outpatients. Anesth Analg 1998;87:816–26.

[65] Rhudy JL, Meagher MW. Fear and anxiety: divergent effects on human pain thresholds. Pain 2000;84:65–75.

[66] Salomons TV, Johnstone T, Backonja MM, Davidson RJ. Perceived controllability modulates the neural response to pain. J Neurosci 2004;24:7199–203.

[67] Salomons TV, Johnstone T, Backonja MM, Shackman AJ, Davidson RJ. Individual differences in the effects of perceived controllability on pain perception: critical role of the prefrontal cortex. J Cogn Neurosci 2007;19:993–1003.

[68] Sarda J Jr, Nicholas MK, Asghari A, Pimenta CA. The contribution of self-efficacy and depression to disability and work status in chronic pain patients: a comparison between Australian and Brazilian samples. Eur J Pain 2009;13:189–95.

[69] Seminowicz DA, Davis KD. Cortical responses to pain in healthy individuals depends on pain catastrophizing. Pain 2006;120:297–306.

[70] Sharp TJ. The "safety seeking behaviours" construct and its application to chronic pain. Behav Cog Psychother 2001;29:241–4.

[71] Smith MT, Perlis ML, Haythornthwaite JA. Suicidal ideation in outpatients with chronic muscu-loskeletal pain: an exploratory study of the role of sleep onset insomnia and pain intensity. Clin J Pain 2004;20:111–8.
[72] Smith WB, Gracely RH, Safer MA. The meaning of pain: cancer patients' rating and recall of pain intensity and affect. Pain 1998;78:123–9.
[73] Somers TJ, Keefe FJ, Carson JW, Pells JJ, Lacaille L. Pain catastrophizing in borderline mor-bidly obese and morbidly obese individuals with osteoarthritic knee pain. Pain Res Manag 2008;13:401–6.
[74] Stahl SM. Does depression hurt? J Clin Psychiatry 2002;63:273–4.
[75] Sterling M, Hodkinson E, Pettiford C, Souvlis T, Curatolo M. Psychologic factors are related to some sensory pain thresholds but not nociceptive flexion reflex threshold in chronic whiplash. Clin J Pain 2008;24:124–30.
[76] Stewart MW, Knight RG. Coping strategies and affect in rheumatoid and psoriatic arthritis. Re-lationship to pain and disability. Arthritis Care Res 1991;4:116–22.
[77] Stewart WF, Ricci JA, Chee E, Morganstein D, Lipton R. Lost productive time and cost due to common pain conditions in the US workforce. JAMA 2003;290:2443–54.
[78] Sullivan MJ, Thorn B, Haythornthwaite JA, Keefe F, Martin M, Bradley LA, Lefebvre JC. Theo-retical perspectives on the relation between catastrophizing and pain. Clin J Pain 2001;17:52–64.
[79] Swinkels-Meewisse EJ, Swinkels RA, Verbeek AL, Vlaeyen JW, Oostendorp RA. Psychometric properties of the Tampa Scale for kinesiophobia and the fear-avoidance beliefs questionnaire in acute low back pain. Man Ther 2003;8:29–36.
[80] Thomee P, Wahrborg P, Borjesson M, Thomee R, Eriksson BI, Karlsson J. Self-efficacy of knee function as a pre-operative predictor of outcome 1 year after anterior cruciate ligament recon-struction. Knee Surg Sports Traumatol Arthrosc 2008;16:118–27.
[81] Tinti C, Schmidt S, Businaro N. Pain and emotions reported after childbirth and recalled 6 months later: the role of controllability. J Psychosom Obstet Gynaecol 2011;32:98–103.
[82] Tripp DA, VanDenKerkhof EG, McAlister M. Prevalence and determinants of pain and pain-re-lated disability in urban and rural settings in southeastern Ontario. Pain Res Manag 2006;11:225–33.
[83] Turk DC, Okifuji A, Scharff L. Chronic pain and depression: role of perceived impact and per-ceived control in different age cohorts. Pain 1995;61:93–101.
[84] Turk DC, Okifuji A, Sinclair JD, Starz TW. Pain, disability, and physical functioning in subgroups of patients with fibromyalgia. J Rheumatol 1996;23:1255–62.
[85] Turk DC, Rudy TE. The robustness of an empirically derived taxonomy of chronic pain patients. Pain 1990;43:27–35.
[86] Turk DC, Sist TC, Okifuji A, Miner MF, Florio G, Harrison P, Massey J, Lema ML, Zevon MA. Adaptation to metastatic cancer pain, regional/local cancer pain and non-cancer pain: role of psychological and behavioral factors. Pain 1998;74:247–56.
[87] Turk DC, Wilson HD, Cahana A. Treatment of chronic non-cancer pain. Lancet 2011;377:2226–35.
[88] Turner JA, Jensen MP, Romano JM. Do beliefs, coping, and catastrophizing independently pre-dict functioning in patients with chronic pain? Pain 2000;85:115–25.
[89] Vlaeyen JW, de Jong J, Geilen M, Heuts PH, van Breukelen G. The treatment of fear of move-ment/(re)injury in chronic low back pain: further evidence on the effectiveness of exposure in vivo. Clin J Pain 2002;18:251–61.
[90] Vlaeyen JW, Linton SJ. Fear-avoidance and its consequences in chronic musculoskeletal pain: a state of the art. Pain 2000;85:317–32.
[91] Watson D. Rethinking the mood and anxiety disorders: a quantitative hierarchical model for DSM-V. J Abnorm Psychol 2005;114:522–36.
[92] Weissman-Fogel I, Sprecher E, Pud D. Effects of catastrophizing on pain perception and pain modulation. Exp Brain Res 2008;186:79–85.

Correspondence to: Akiko Okifuji, PhD, Pain Research and Management Center, Department of Anesthesiology, University of Utah, 615 Arapeen Drive, Suite 200, Salt Lake City, UT 84108, USA. Email: akiko.okifuji@hsc.utah.edu.

Part II

Concurrent Pain and Non-Pain Conditions

Pain and Hypertension

Stephen Bruehl

Department of Anesthesiology, Vanderbilt University School of Medicine, Nashville, Tennessee, USA

Approximately one-quarter of the U.S. population has hypertension (HTN) [21], a condition that is a significant contributor to cardiovascular-related morbidity (stroke, myocardial infarction) and mortality [39,50]. Until relatively recently, the co-occurrence of HTN with chronic pain was not widely recognized. The ubiquity of this association is underscored by findings, for example, that 10.5 million individuals in the United States alone have both chronic back pain and HTN [85].

Although whether chronic pain is causally linked to HTN remains to be proven, even a small influence on HTN development could have a significant public health impact. Chronic pain affects up to 30% of the adult population [7,61,84,85], and once established, it tends to persist. Prospective data indicate that three-quarters of patients reporting chronic pain at baseline were still experiencing ongoing pain at follow-up 4 years later [30]. To the extent that chronic pain does contribute to onset and maintenance of HTN, the persistent nature of chronic pain highlights its potential importance as a public health issue and as a treatment target for reducing cardiovascular morbidity and mortality. An association between pain and HTN in the opposite direction of causality is also well documented. That is, not only might chronic pain affect HTN development, but among individuals free of chronic pain, HTN itself influences *acute* pain responsiveness, with potentially important clinical implications.

This chapter will first provide an overview of the literature regarding the influence of HTN on acute pain. Work suggesting that chronic pain alters associations between elevated blood pressure (BP) and pain responsiveness will then be summarized. Next, epidemiological and clinical data addressing associations between chronic pain and HTN will be examined. Potential mechanisms that might contribute to links between chronic pain and HTN will be described, and implications and future research directions will be discussed.

Hypertension and Diminished Acute Pain Responsiveness

Animal studies conducted more than 30 years ago were the first to document that HTN is associated with reduced acute pain responsiveness [29,88]. These findings were replicated in human studies in hypertensives [42,76], with other work demonstrating links between familial risk for HTN and diminished pain responsiveness, even in the absence of significantly elevated BP [1,37]. However, a number of reports revealed significant linear associations between elevated resting BP level and lower acute pain sensitivity that extended well into the normotensive BP range [12,27,32,33,64,74]. In light of these latter findings, it became clear that the diminished pain responsiveness reported in hypertensive individuals was not a unique feature of HTN per se, but rather, was more accurately referred to as BP-related hypoalgesia.

Hypoalgesia related to BP is not just a phenomenon relevant in the laboratory. For example, elevated ambulatory 24-hour BP is associated with reduced experimental acute pain sensitivity [43], and elevated presurgical resting BP is associated with lower postsurgical pain levels [38]. Of potentially greater clinical importance is the effect of BP-related hypoalgesia on cardiac-related pain. Several studies indicate that the absence of cardiac pain in silent cardiac ischemia is due in part to the influence of hypoalgesia deriving from elevated BP [25,26,31]. Absence of pain-related symptoms among individuals with elevated BP could potentially delay interventions for acute myocardial infarction and chronic cardiovascular disease [47,51].

It is believed that BP-related hypoalgesia is part of a functional inhibitory feedback loop serving to maintain cardiovascular homeostasis in the presence of acutely painful stimuli [41]. Acute pain triggers a somatosensory reflex that increases sympathetic nervous system (SNS) arousal, thereby leading to elevated BP [71,82]. BP elevations, in turn, stimulate baroreceptors in the carotid artery and aorta that send afferent signals to the brain through vagal pathways that traverse the nucleus of the solitary tract. Activation of baroreflex circuits in the nucleus of the solitary tract, via interconnections between that region and brain regions involved in descending pain inhibitory pathways [13], then produces analgesia, which helps restore arousal levels to a state of homeostasis.

The phenomenon of BP-related hypoalgesia might be expected to result in an association between elevated BP and both reduced risk for chronic pain and lower chronic pain intensity. Consistent with this notion, one epidemiological dataset [45] and one laboratory study (in fibromyalgia patients) [72] suggest that elevated resting BP might indeed be linked to reduced risk for chronic pain and to a lesser bodily extent of chronic pain, respectively. Nonetheless, a much larger literature suggests *positive* associations between BP levels and chronic pain, with potential implications for HTN risk.

Effects of Chronic Pain on Blood Pressure-Related Hypoalgesia: A Theoretical Model

The homeostatic model described by Ghione [41] refers to functional interactions between BP and pain-modulatory systems in individuals free of chronic pain. Various experts have proposed [13,20,62,63] that chronic pain alters these functional associations by impairing inhibitory neurotransmitter systems that contribute to BP-related hypoalgesia or otherwise altering the baroreflex systems (feedback systems linking BP changes to modulation of SNS and vagal outflow via baroreceptors) underlying these links between BP and pain modulation. The chronic pain-related dysfunction model (summarized in Fig. 1) proposes that if

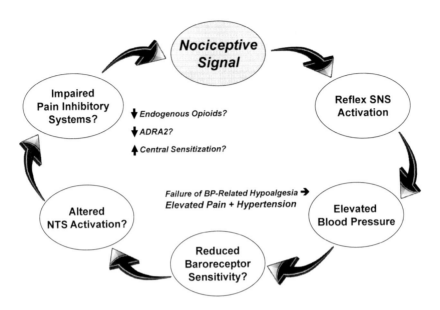

Fig. 1. Model of chronic pain-related alterations in homeostatic cardiovascular/pain-modulatory interactions. ADRA2, α_2-adrenoceptors; BP, blood pressure; NTS, nucleus of the solitary tract; SNS, sympathetic nervous system.

persistent nociceptive input leads to exhaustion or failure of descending pain inhibitory systems that contribute to BP-related hypoalgesia (e.g., those mediated by endogenous opioid or α_2-adrenergic neurotransmitter systems), direct sympathetically mediated increases in BP may predominate in chronic pain. When pain-inhibitory mechanisms fail, resting BP would be expected to increase as clinical pain intensity and related SNS arousal increase. Thus, chronic pain would result simultaneously in failure of descending pain-inhibitory systems and direct SNS-mediated BP increases. This pattern might produce positive associations between resting BP and both acute pain sensitivity and chronic pain intensity in chronic pain patients. The chronic pain dysfunction model postulates that baroreflex impairments also contribute to the absence of BP-related hypoalgesia in chronic pain. To the extent that the proposed chronic pain dysfunction model is valid, absence of BP-related hypoalgesia in chronic pain might serve as a marker of underlying changes in baroreflex function and inhibitory neurotransmitter function that could increase risk for HTN development in chronic pain patients [13,20].

Blood Pressure-Related Hypoalgesia Is Altered in Chronic Pain

Several studies suggest that chronic pain conditions are associated with changes in BP-related hypoalgesia, as proposed in the chronic pain dysfunction model above. BP-related hypoalgesia in response to acute noxious stimuli noted in pain-free controls is not observed in patients with chronic orofacial pain [8,62]. Studies examining patients with chronic back pain in two separate samples reveal similar findings as well, indicating that BP-related hypoalgesia is absent in individuals with chronic back pain, despite only mild to moderate pain intensity and no analgesic medication use in both samples [16,18].

Disruption of normal BP-related hypoalgesic mechanisms in chronic pain is also suggested by results of a study examining wind-up, a phenomenon believed to reflect degree of central sensitization to pain [48]. Elevated BP was found in healthy individuals to be associated with lower wind-up [22], indicating less central sensitization and paralleling findings for more traditional acute pain sensitivity outcomes. Yet, in patients with chronic low back pain, elevated BP was associated with significantly *greater* wind-up [22]. These results hint that alterations in BP-related hypoalgesia among individuals with chronic pain may reflect not only impaired descending inhibitory systems, but also upregulation of ascending pain facilitatory systems.

Recent work has extended findings like those above to more episodic chronic pain conditions and a younger population. Young adults with a documented history of childhood functional abdominal pain (FAP) were compared to matched young adults with no childhood FAP history at an average of 8 years after initial specialty FAP diagnosis [19]. BP-related hypoalgesia to heat pain was observed in those without a history of FAP as expected, but was absent in those who had experienced FAP in childhood [19]. Interestingly, this effect was restricted to females and was evident regardless of whether or not the FAP complaints had resolved in the intervening years. This latter finding raises the possibility that an extended period of chronic pain, even if it resolves, could potentially produce lasting changes in important cardiovascular-pain-modulatory interactions that might have a bearing on future HTN risk.

The results above reflect studies focusing on BP as the independent variable, with resting BP being the end result of the baroreflex mechanisms described previously in the homeostatic model. Functional efficiency of baroreflex BP modulation is a related issue that is also important, and it can be indexed by a spontaneous baroreceptor sensitivity (BRS) measure linking beat-to-beat changes in BP with subsequent alterations in beat-to-beat interval [23]. Among individuals free of chronic pain, elevated BRS was associated with reduced acute pain responsiveness in a pattern similar to that observed in BP-related hypoalgesia, that is, reduced pain ratings and lower wind-up [22,23]. Consistent with the chronic pain dysfunction model, hypoalgesia related specifically to resting BRS was absent in individuals with chronic pain (see Fig. 2) [22,23].

In summary, the studies above indicate that in several very different chronic pain conditions, there are substantial alterations in normally adaptive functional interactions between cardiovascular and pain-modulatory systems. These changes have implications for clinical pain as well. Some evidence suggests that in individuals with chronic pain, elevated BP is associated with significantly *greater* clinical pain intensity [11,17,18], rather than reduced pain intensity, as might be expected. Moreover, at least two studies indicate that elevated BP in chronic pain patients may also be linked to significantly *higher* acute pain sensitivity [16,18]. The similar pattern of associations between elevated BP and both acute and chronic pain responses among individuals with chronic pain is consistent with the influence of impaired central pain-modulatory systems, as in the chronic pain dysfunction model.

While not definitive, one cross-sectional study in 121 chronic pain patients suggests that BP-related hypoalgesia may become progressively dysfunctional in chronically painful states [11]. In patients with chronic pain of 6–14 months' duration, correlations between resting BP and chronic pain intensity were inverse, suggesting some degree of BP-related hypoalgesia like that observed in pain-free individuals, although more modest in magnitude ($r = -0.18$). In contrast, among patients with chronic pain of more than 28 months' duration, the comparable association was strongly positive ($r = 0.50$).

Also consistent with progressive effects of chronic pain on resting BP regulation are findings from a prospective single case study of chronic

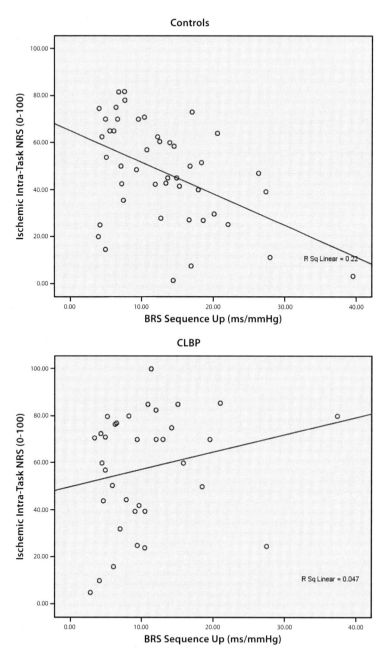

Fig. 2. Scatterplot of association between resting spontaneous baroreceptor sensitivity (BRS), measured in milliseconds per millimeter of mercury, and acute pain, measured on a numeric rating scale (NRS), for the ischemic pain task in healthy pain-free controls and individuals with chronic low back pain (CLBP).

pain development (see Fig. 3) [15]. One otherwise healthy female was followed from the pain-free state to a state of chronic low back pain of increasing duration following an injury. Over a 13-month period, increases
of 11% and 20%, respectively, in resting systolic and diastolic BP were observed following onset of daily low back pain, despite the relatively low
intensity of that pain and the absence of any daily medication use [15].
Interestingly, BP continued to increase substantially from 4 to 13 months
after onset of back pain, despite the daily intensity of that pain remaining
unchanged at each assessment period.

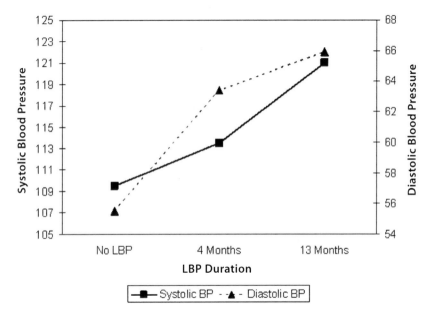

Fig. 3. Prospective changes in resting blood pressure (mm Hg) within one female patient from the healthy pain-free state to mild chronic low back pain (LBP) of 4 and 13
months' duration.

Prevalence of Hypertension in Chronic Pain Samples

A number of large well-designed epidemiological studies have reported
on HTN prevalence as it relates to chronic pain. In one such study, von
Korff et al. [85] reported on prevalence of chronic back pain and comorbid disorders in a large U.S. general population sample (n = 5,692).

A diagnosis of HTN was significantly more likely among individuals experiencing chronic back pain in the past 12 months than in comparable individuals without chronic pain, even when the investigators adjusted for potential demographic confounds. Similar analyses of this epidemiological dataset also indicated a significantly increased risk of HTN in individuals with chronic arthritic pain [81].

Two related studies conducted in the developing world using identical methodology revealed similar findings. In a Nigerian epidemiological sample, the risk for HTN was three times higher in individuals reporting chronic back pain in the past year than in those who were free of chronic pain [44]. This notably increased risk was observed despite the relatively young age of the sample (approximately three-quarters of the participants were below the age of 45). Similar work in a Chinese epidemiological sample revealed that individuals with chronic arthritic pain were at least twice as likely to have HTN compared to individuals without chronic pain [56].

The results of a population study in more than 12,000 elderly Mexican individuals may also be relevant, although the authors did not address chronic pain specifically. Individuals who reported "often" experiencing physical pain (42% of the sample) more often had a diagnosis of HTN (45% prevalence) than did age-matched individuals not experiencing frequent pain (31% prevalence of HTN) [5]. Similar links between clinical pain and HTN are suggested by findings in a large cohort of elderly Danish individuals. Occurrence of back and neck pain in the month prior to the survey was significantly associated with physician-diagnosed HTN, beyond effects of age and gender [46].

Possible dose-response effects of chronic pain on HTN are also suggested. HTN was significantly more common and clinical pain intensity was higher in rheumatoid arthritis (RA) patients with comorbid fibromyalgia than in RA patients without fibromyalgia [86]. Results from the Framingham dataset also support a dose-response effect for chronic pain on HTN, with a greater number of musculoskeletal pain locations being associated in a linear fashion with higher resting BP [58]. Interestingly, links between persistent musculoskeletal pain and BP levels in this latter study were restricted to women [58]. Potential gender specificity of these effects is also suggested by results of a Swedish population study [6]. HTN was the number one ranked comorbidity of back and extremity pain in women, exceeding anxiety and depression, headache, and sleep problems in prevalence. Although pain was also associated with increased prevalence of HTN in men in this study, this association was less prominent than in women.

While the issue of increased prevalence of HTN in the chronic pain population is not the same as the prevalence of chronic pain in the HTN population, work addressing this latter issue might nonetheless be considered additional supporting data. In a sample of 675 rural Canadians [83], those with diagnosed HTN were significantly more likely than patients without HTN to be diagnosed with chronic back/neck pain (15% versus 10%) or osteoarthritis (21% versus 6%). Even after controlling for age, sex, and race, the investigators were able to show that HTN was significantly associated with reports of greater bodily pain. This latter effect has been replicated in large Chinese [60] and Swedish [4] epidemiological datasets.

Beyond epidemiological studies, the best evidence for a link between chronic pain and HTN comes from work examining a pain clinic population. A retrospective review was conducted on the records of 300 chronic pain patients evaluated at a tertiary care pain management center and 300 general internal medicine patients without chronic pain seen at the same institution [17]. Results revealed that over 39% of the chronic pain group was diagnosed with HTN, compared to only 21% of the general medicine group ($P < 0.001$). Analyses by gender (see Fig. 4) revealed significant group differences in both males and females. While HTN prevalence in the general medicine group was comparable to national population values, prevalence in the chronic pain group was significantly higher for both genders ($P < 0.005$). Similar findings were obtained for analyses with antihypertensive medication use as the outcome. One notable finding in this study was that despite females having a lower prevalence of HTN than males in the general medicine sample (and in the general population), female chronic pain patients appeared to be disproportionately affected by HTN (Fig. 4). Stepwise logistic regression within the chronic pain sample in this study revealed that chronic pain intensity was a significant predictor of hypertensive status independent of the effects of traditional risk factors including age, race/ethnicity, and parental history of HTN [17].

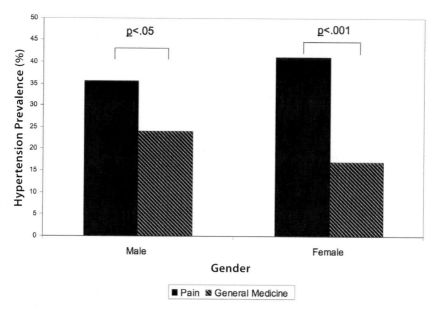

Fig. 4. Prevalence of hypertension by gender in a chronic pain patient sample (n = 300) compared to a non-pain general internal medicine sample (n = 300).

Mechanisms Potentially Linking Chronic Pain and Hypertension

Chronic pain appears to be associated with alterations in BP-related hypoalgesia, consistent with the chronic pain dysfunction model. Evidence supporting specific mechanistic pathways underlying this dysfunction may help strengthen conclusions regarding potential causal links between chronic pain and increased HTN prevalence. Chronic pain-related changes in baroreflex function may be involved. Patients with chronic low back pain [23], fibromyalgia [40,72], or irritable bowel syndrome [80] exhibit significantly lower resting spontaneous BRS levels than healthy pain-free controls. Spectral analysis findings from the Chung et al. [23] dataset indicated that, compared to pain-free controls, patients with chronic back pain had significantly lower heart rate variability (HRV) in the high-frequency domain, both at rest and during orthostatic stress [Diedrich et al., unpublished manuscript]. Simultaneous reductions in high-frequency HRV and spontaneous resting BRS have also been reported in fibromyalgia patients relative to pain-free controls [72]. Given that the high-frequency component of HRV corresponds well with vagal activity, which in turn is the primary mechanism of baroreflex control of beat-to-beat heart rate changes [54], the observations above suggest that vagal withdrawal might contribute to impaired baroreflex function in chronic pain patients.

Other work addressing links between cardiovascular regulation and clinical pain, albeit not necessarily chronic pain per se, is also relevant. Higher ambulatory BP levels were found to be associated with both greater recent bodily pain and an HRV pattern suggesting vagal withdrawal [70]. These findings of reduced vagal inhibitory tone in individuals with greater daily pain are consistent with findings in chronic pain patients [23,40; Diedrich et al., unpublished manuscript].

The reductions in BRS and vagal tone that have been observed in chronic pain patients can impair the ability to regulate BP and could thereby increase HTN risk. This possibility is supported by prospective findings in the general population that lower BRS at baseline predicts greater increases in resting BP 5 years later [28]. Diminished baroreflex function has been associated with increased cardiovascular morbidity [52,53,79], including pathogenesis of HTN [28,54]. While there is as yet no direct evidence that baroreflex alterations in chronic pain patients contribute to HTN development, it is nonetheless notable that correlations between reduced BRS and higher resting BP levels were significantly stronger in patients with chronic pain than in pain-free controls in one study [22].

Inhibitory neurotransmitters, including norepinephrine (acting at α_2-adrenergic receptors) and endogenous opioids, may both play a role in BP-related hypoalgesia, given that they can modulate both pain sensitivity [67] and cardiovascular function [65,66]. Therefore, chronic pain-related dysfunction in either neurotransmitter system might contribute to absence of BP-related hypoalgesia and impaired BP modulation [13]. Experimental human work using placebo-controlled α_2-adrenergic receptor blockade with yohimbine has confirmed that α_2-adrenergic mechanisms contribute to the baroreflex-mediated component of BP-related hypoalgesia. Moreover, this work suggests that changes in α_2-adrenergic receptor systems contribute to the absence of BRS-related hypoalgesia in patients with chronic low back pain [23]. In pain-free healthy controls, spontaneous BRS had a significant hypoalgesic effect on acute pain responses ($r = -0.57$, $P < 0.01$) that was substantially attenuated under α_2-adrenergic receptor blockade ($r = -0.21$, $P > 0.10$). In contrast, individuals with chronic back pain displayed a nonsignificant positive association between BRS and acute pain responses under placebo ($r = 0.18$, $P > 0.10$), but α_2-adrenergic receptor blockade appeared to restore BRS-related hypoalgesia to the levels observed in healthy individuals ($r = -0.40$, $P < 0.10$).

Animal studies also clearly suggest a role for endogenous opioids in BP-related hypoalgesia [77,78]. The role of opioids in human BP-related hypoalgesia has been less clear [2,18,36,64,73]. However, several studies do suggest endogenous opioid involvement in human BP-related hypoalgesia. Enhanced endogenous opioid analgesia has been observed in normotensive individuals at increased risk for HTN [65], and opioid blockade has been shown to eliminate BP-related hypoalgesia on experimental acute pain responses in healthy individuals free of chronic pain [19,59]. The issue of opioid involvement in BP-related hypoalgesia is important in light of evidence that impaired opioid function might increase BP stress reactivity and HTN risk [66]. Data regarding endogenous opioid levels (in plasma and cerebrospinal fluid) suggest that endogenous opioid systems may become dysfunctional in long-term chronic pain [20]. Such changes could result in impaired ability to modulate both pain and BP and potentially contribute to absence of BP-related hypoalgesia in chronic pain [20].

While no studies to date directly indicate that opioid dysfunction contributes to altered BP-related hypoalgesia in chronic pain, other work suggests that this is plausible. Opioid blockade with naloxone was found to impair return to baseline of BP following exposure to acute pain in healthy pain-free controls, but not in individuals with chronic back pain [14]. This finding is consistent with opioid modulation of BP in pain-free controls but not in chronic pain patients.

Other Possible Contributors to Links Between Chronic Pain and Hypertension

In populations not necessarily experiencing chronic pain, use of common nonsteroidal anti-inflammatory drugs (NSAIDs) and analgesic medications such as acetaminophen (paracetamol) has been linked to increased

HTN risk [24,34,35]. Although more frequent use of such medications in chronic pain populations could potentially contribute to HTN, it is important to note that studies of the HTN-pain medication link do not address the potential effects that chronic pain itself and variability in chronic pain intensity may exert on HTN [9]. It is unknown whether analgesic use might to some extent be a surrogate measure for the influence of chronic pain intensity on the HTN-pain medication link. Data from one clinical study in chronic pain patients may be relevant to this issue [17]. The same percentage of chronic pain patients were found to use NSAIDs regularly, regardless of whether or not a comorbid HTN diagnosis was present (44% for each group). In addition, acetaminophen use was nonsignificantly *lower* in chronic pain patients with HTN compared to those without HTN. These findings suggest that among individuals with significant clinical chronic pain, NSAID and analgesic use is unlikely to exert any significant impact on HTN risk beyond that conferred by chronic pain itself.

Another alterative explanation for links between chronic pain and HTN is the role of body mass index (BMI) and metabolic factors. Chronic pain and BMI display at least modest positive associations [49,55,75], with one recent study linking greater intensity of chronic pain with greater BMI [87]. One small study found that patients with widespread chronic pain had significantly higher resting BP, higher BMI, and higher fasting glucose and cholesterol levels than did pain-free controls, with patients who were experiencing more spatially restricted chronic pain showing intermediate levels on these measures [69]. This latter study is consistent with dose-response effects of more extensive chronic pain on potential metabolic mediators of HTN risk. Given the associations between obesity and HTN [3,10], even in relatively young populations [68], there may be a potential pathway linking chronic pain to increased BMI and metabolic abnormalities, and eventually to HTN. There is currently no evidence available to determine whether this hypothesized causal chain is supported. At present, there is no reason to expect that metabolic pathways potentially contributing to the chronic pain-HTN association would necessarily exclude a simultaneous contributory role for chronic pain-related alterations in overlapping BP and pain-modulatory systems.

Conclusions and Directions for Future Work

Elevated BP and HTN are both reliably associated with reduced pain sensitivity in individuals free of chronic pain. This BP-related hypoalgesia is absent or even reversed (i.e., hyperalgesia is present) in individuals experiencing chronic pain. Alterations in baroreflex function, endogenous opioids, and α_2-adrenergic receptors systems may all be contributing factors. Chronic pain-related dysfunction in homeostatic cardiovascular-pain-modulatory interactions may increase the risk for future HTN in the chronic pain population. This possibility is supported by both clinical and epidemiological studies.

From the clinical standpoint, improved recognition of the role that chronic pain plays in the development and maintenance of HTN is important because this issue crosses traditional boundaries of medical specialization. On the one hand, physicians specializing in pain management understandably tend to focus on addressing patients' pain and functional complaints. As a silent disease not traditionally connected with pain, HTN is unlikely to be a treatment target in the pain clinic setting. On the other hand, cardiology or internal medicine physicians, for example, would clearly recognize and treat HTN, yet would be unlikely to appreciate the role that chronic pain could be playing in that condition. Improved recognition of connections between chronic pain and HTN could facilitate more timely HTN diagnosis, improve its treatment in the millions of individuals suffering from both conditions simultaneously, and ultimately contribute to reduced cardiovascular-related morbidity and mortality.

This chapter has detailed a directional hypothesis in which chronic pain is a risk factor for future development of HTN. Although available data addressing issues of causation are extremely limited, one prospective study suggests the possibility of an alternative direction of causation. Higher resting systolic BP and triglyceride levels at baseline were found to predict the occurrence of frequent low back pain 27 years later, even when the investigators controlled for effects of differing BMI [57]. These results raise the possibility that elevated normotensive resting BP and triglyceride levels, both known risk factors for future cardiovascular disease, might also increase the risk of developing chronic pain. In that case, cross-sectional associations between HTN and chronic pain might reflect an underlying and overlapping susceptibility to both conditions. Well-designed prospective studies addressing potential mechanisms are required to clarify whether chronic pain contributes to future HTN development via a dysfunction in overlapping systems that modulate both pain and BP, or rather, whether chronic pain-HTN links are the result of a shared biological vulnerability simultaneously enhancing risks for both conditions.

Acknowledgments

The work described in this chapter was supported in part by National Institutes of Health Grants NS038145, NS050578, and NS046694, and Vanderbilt CTSA grant 1 UL1 RR024975 from the National Center for Research Resources, NIH. The author would like to acknowledge the contribution of Dr. Laura Diedrich to the unpublished spectral analysis data reported.

References

[1]   al'Absi M, Buchanan T, Lovallo WR. Pain perception and cardiovascular responses in men with positive parental history for hypertension. Psychophysiology 1996;33:655–61.

[2]   al'Absi M, France C, Harju A, France J, Wittmers L. Adrenocortical and nociceptive responses to opioid blockade in hypertension-prone men and women. Psychosom Med 2006;68:292–8.

[3]   Al Harakeh AB, Burkhamer KJ, Kallies KJ, Mathiason MA, Kothari SN. Natural history and metabolic consequences of morbid obesity for patients denied coverage for bariatric surgery. Surg Obes Relat Dis 2010;6:591–6.

[4]   Bardage C, Isacson DG. Hypertension and health-related quality of life: an epidemiological study in Sweden. J Clin Epidemiol 2001;54:172–81.

[5]   Barragán-Berlanga AJ, Mejía-Arango S, Gutiérrez-Robledo LM. Pain in the elderly: prevalence and associated factors [Article in Spanish]. Salud Publica Mex 2007;49(Suppl 4):S488–94.

[6]   Bingefors K, Isacson D. Epidemiology, co-morbidity, and impact on health-related quality of life of self-reported headache and musculoskeletal pain: a gender perspective. Eur J Pain 2004;8:435–50.

[7]   Bouhassira D, Lantéri-Minet M, Attal N, Laurent B, Touboul C. Prevalence of chronic pain with neuropathic characteristics in the general population. Pain 2008;136:380–7.

[8]   Bragdon EE, Light KC, Costello NL, Sigurdsson A, Bunting S, Bhalang K, Maixner W. Group differences in pain modulation: pain-free women compared to pain-free men and to women with TMD. Pain 2002;96:227–37.

[9]   Brotman DJ. Acetaminophen and hypertension: a causal association or pain mediated? Arch Intern Med 2003;163:1113–4; author reply 1115–6.

[10] Bruce SG, Riediger ND, Zacharias JM, Young TK. Obesity and obesity-related comorbidities in a Canadian First Nation population. Prev Chronic Dis 2011;8:1–8.

[11] Bruehl S, Burns JW, McCubbin JA. Altered cardiovascular/pain regulatory relationships in chronic pain. Int J Behav Med 1998;5:63–75.

[12] Bruehl S, Carlson CR, McCubbin JA. The relationship between pain sensitivity and blood pressure in normotensives. Pain 1992;48:463–7.

[13] Bruehl S, Chung OY. Interactions between the cardiovascular and pain regulatory systems: an updated review of mechanisms and possible alterations in chronic pain. Neurosci Biobehav Rev 2004;28:395–414.

[14] Bruehl S, Chung OY, Burns JW. Trait anger and blood pressure recovery following acute pain: evidence for opioid-mediated effects. Int J Behav Med 2006;13:138–46.

[15] Bruehl S, Chung OY, Chont M. Chronic pain-related changes in endogenous opioid analgesia: a case report. Pain 2010;148:167–71.

[16] Bruehl S, Chung OY, Diedrich L, Diedrich A, Robertson D. The relationship between resting blood pressure and acute pain sensitivity: effects of chronic pain and alpha-2 adrenergic blockade. J Behav Med 2008;31:71–80.

[17] Bruehl S, Chung OY, Jirjis JN, Biridepalli S. Prevalence of clinical hypertension in chronic pain patients compared to non-pain general medical patients. Clin J Pain 2005;21:147–53.

[18] Bruehl S, Chung OY, Ward P, Johnson B, McCubbin JA. The relationship between resting blood pressure and acute pain sensitivity in healthy normotensives and chronic back pain sufferers: the effects of opioid blockade. Pain 2002;100:191–201.

[19] Bruehl S, Dengler-Crish CM, Smith CA, Walker LS. Hypoalgesia related to elevated resting blood pressure is absent in adolescents and young adults with a history of functional abdominal pain. Pain 2010;149:57–63.

[20] Bruehl S, McCubbin JA, Harden RN. Theoretical review: altered pain regulatory systems in chronic pain. Neurosci Biobehav Rev 1999;23:877–90.

[21] Burt VL, Whelton P, Roccella EJ, Brown C, Cutler JA, Higgins M, Horan MJ, Labarthe D. Prevalence of hypertension in the US adult population. Results from the Third National Health and Nutrition Examination Survey, 1988–1991. Hypertension 1995;25:305–13.

[22] Chung OY, Bruehl S, Diedrich L, Diedrich A. The impact of blood pressure and baroreflex sensitivity on wind-up. Anesth Analg 2008;107:1018–25.

[23] Chung OY, Bruehl S, Diedrich L, Diedrich A, Chont M, Robertson D. Baroreflex sensitivity associated hypoalgesia in healthy states is altered by chronic pain. Pain 2008;138:87–97.

[24] Curhan GC, Willett WC, Rosner B, Stampfer MJ. Frequency of analgesic use and risk of hypertension in younger women. Arch Intern Med 2002;162:2204–8.

[25] Ditto B, D'Antono B, Dupuis G, Burelle D. Chest pain is inversely associated with blood pressure during exercise among individuals being assessed for coronary heart disease. Psychophysiology 2007;44:183–8.

[26] Ditto B, Lavoie KL, Campbell TS, Gordon J, Arsenault A, Bacon SL. Negative association between resting blood pressure and chest pain in people undergoing exercise stress testing for coronary artery disease. Pain 2010;149:501–5.

[27] Ditto B, Séguin JR, Boulerice B, Pihl RO, Tremblay RE. Risk for hypertension and pain sensitivity in adolescent boys. Health Psychol 1998;17:249–54.

[28] Ducher M, Fauvel JP, Cerutti C. Risk profile in hypertension genesis: a five-year follow-up study. Am J Hyper 2006;19:775–80.

[29] Dworkin B, Filewich R, Miller N, Craigmyle N, Pickering T. Baroreceptor activation reduces reactivity to noxious stimulation: Implications in hypertension. Science 1979;205:1299–301.

[30] Elliott AM, Smith BH, Hannaford PC, Smith WC, Chambers WA. The course of chronic pain in the community: results of a 4-year follow-up study. Pain 2002;99:299–307.

[31] Falcone C, Nespoli L, Geroldi D, Gazzaruso C, Buzzi MP, Auguadro C, Tavazzi L, Schwartz PJ. Silent myocardial ischemia in diabetic and nondiabetic patients with coronary artery disease. Int J Cardiol 2003;90:219–27.

[32] Fillingim RB, Maixner W. The influence of resting blood pressure and gender on pain responses. Psychosom Med 1996;58:326–32.

[33] Fillingim RB, Maixner W, Bunting S, Silva S. Resting blood pressure and thermal pain responses among females: Effects on pain unpleasantness but not pain intensity. Int J Psychophys 1998;30:313–8.

[34] Forman JP, Rimm EB, Curhan GC. Frequency of analgesic use and risk of hypertension among men. Arch Intern Med 2007;167:394–9.

[35] Forman JP, Stampfer MJ, Curhan GC. Non-narcotic analgesic dose and risk of incident hypertension in US women. Hypertension 2005;46:500–7.

[36] France CR, al'Absi M, Ring C, France JL, Brose J, Spaeth D, Harju A, Nordehn G, Wittmers LE. Assessment of opiate modulation of pain and nociceptive responding in young adults with a parental history of hypertension. Biol Psychol 2005;70:168–74.

[37] France, CR, Ditto, B, Adler, P. Pain sensitivity in offspring of hypertensives at rest and during baroreflex stimulation. J Behav Med 1991;14:513–25.

[38] France CR, Katz J. Postsurgical pain is attenuated in men with elevated presurgical systolic blood pressure. Pain Res Manage 1999;4:100–3.

[39] Franklin SS, Larson MG, Khan SA, Wong ND, Leip EP, Kannel WB, Levy D. Does the relation of blood pressure to coronary heart disease risk change with aging? The Framingham Heart Study. Circulation 2001;103:1245–9.

[40] Furlan R, Colombo S, Perego F, Atzeni F, Diana A, Barbic F, Porta A, Pace F, Malliani A, Sarzi-Puttini P. Abnormalities of cardiovascular neural control and reduced orthostatic tolerance in patients with primary fibromyalgia. J Rheumatol 2005;32:1787–93.

[41] Ghione S. Hypertension-associated hypalgesia: Evidence in experimental animals and humans, pathophysiological mechanisms, and potential clinical consequences. Hypertension 1996;28:494–504.

[42] Ghione S, Rosa C, Mazzasalma L, Panattoni E. Arterial hypertension is associated with hypalgesia in humans. Hypertension 1988;12:491–7.

[43] Guasti L, Zanotta D, Mainardi LT, Petrozzino MR, Grimoldi P, Garganico D, Diolisi A, Gaudio G, Klersy C, Grandi AM, Simoni C, Cerutti S. Hypertension-related hypoalgesia, autonomic function and spontaneous baroreflex sensitivity. Auton Neurosci 2002;99:127–33.

[44] Gureje O, Akinpelu AO, Uwakwe R, Udofia O, Wakil A. Comorbidity and impact of chronic spinal pain in Nigeria. Spine 2007;32:E495–500.

[45] Hagen K, Zwart JA, Holmen J, Svebak S, Bovim G, Stovner LJ. Nord-Trøndelag Health Study. Does hypertension protect against chronic musculoskeletal complaints? The Nord-Trøndelag Health Study. Arch Intern Med 2005;165:916–22.

[46] Hartvigsen J, Christensen K, Frederiksen H. Back and neck pain exhibit many common features in old age: a population-based study of 4,486 Danish twins 70–102 years of age. Spine 2004;29:576–80.

[47] Hedblad B, Janzon L. Hypertension and silent myocardial ischemia: their influence on cardiovascular mortality and morbidity. Cardiology 1994;85(Suppl 2):16–23.

[48] Herrero JF, Laird JM, López-García JA. Wind-up of spinal cord neurones and pain sensation: much ado about something? Prog Neurobiol 2000;61:169–203.

[49] Heuch I, Hagen K, Heuch I, Nygaard Ø, Zwart JA. The impact of body mass index on the prevalence of low back pain: the HUNT study. Spine 2010;35:764–8.

[50] Ingelsson E, Gona P, Larson MG, Lloyd-Jones DM, Kannel WB, Vasan RS, Levy D. Altered blood pressure progression in the community and its relation to clinical events. Arch Intern Med 2008;168:1450–7.

[51] Kannel WB, Dannenberg AL, Abbott RD. Unrecognized myocardial infarction and hypertension: the Framingham Study. Am Heart J 1985;109:581–5.

[52] La Rovere MT, Bigger JT Jr, Marcus FI, Mortara A, Schwartz PJ. Baroreflex sensitivity and heart-rate variability in prediction of total cardiac mortality after myocardial infarction. ATRAMI (Autonomic Tone and Reflexes After Myocardial Infarction) Investigators. Lancet 1998;351:478–84.

[53] La Rovere MT, Pinna GD, Hohnloser SH, Marcus FI, Mortara A, Nohara R, Bigger JT Jr, Camm AJ, Schwartz PJ; ATRAMI Investigators; Autonomic Tone and Reflexes After Myocardial Infarction. Baroreflex sensitivity and heart rate variability in the identification of patients at risk for life-threatening arrhythmias: implications for clinical trials. Circulation 2001;103:2072–7.

[54] La Rovere MT, Pinna GD, Raczak G. Baroreflex sensitivity: measurement and clinical implications. Ann Noninvasive Electrocardiol 2008;13:191–207.

[55] Leboeuf-Yde C, Kyvik KO, Bruun NH. Low back pain and lifestyle. Part II: Obesity. Information from a population-based sample of 29,424 twin subjects. Spine 1999;24:779–83.

[56] Lee S, Tsang A, Huang YQ, Zhang MY, Liu ZR, He YL, Von Korff M, Kessler RC. Arthritis and physical-mental comorbidity in metropolitan China. J Psychosom Res 2007;63:1–7.

[57] Leino-Arjas P, Solovieva S, Kirjonen J, Reunanen A, Riihimäki H. Cardiovascular risk factors and low back pain in a long-term follow-up of industrial employees. Scand J Work Environ Health 2006;32:12–9.

[58] Leveille SG, Zhang Y, McMullen W, Kelly-Hayes M, Felson DT. Sex differences in musculoskeletal pain in older adults. Pain 2005;116:332–8.

[59] Lewkowski MD, Young SN, Ghosh S, Ditto B. Effects of opioid blockade on the modulation of pain and mood by sweet taste and blood pressure in young adults. Pain 2008;135:75–81.

[60] Li W, Liu L, Puente JG, Li Y, Jiang X, Jin S, Ma H, Kong L, Ma L, He X, Ma S, Chen C. Hypertension and health-related quality of life: an epidemiological study in patients attending hospital clinics in China. J Hypertens 2005;23:1667–76.

[61] Magni G, Caldieron C, Rigatti-Luchini S, Merskey H. Chronic musculoskeletal pain and depressive symptoms in the general population. An analysis of the 1st National Health and Nutrition Examination Survey data. Pain 1990;43:299–307.

[62] Maixner W, Fillingim R, Kincaid S, Sigurdsson A, Harris MB. Relationship between pain sensitivity and resting arterial blood pressure in patients with painful temporomandibular disorders. Psychosom Med 1997;59:503–11.

[63] Maixner W, Sigurdsson A, Fillingim RB, Lundeen T, Booker DK. Regulation of acute and chronic orofacial pain. In: Fricton JR, Dubner R, editors. Orofacial pain and temporomandibular disorders. New York: Raven Press; 1995.

[64] McCubbin JA, Bruehl S. Do endogenous opioids mediate the relationship between blood pressure and pain sensitivity in normotensives? Pain 1994;57:63–7.

[65] McCubbin JA, Helfer SG, Switzer FS 3rd, Galloway C, Griffith WV. Opioid analgesia in persons at risk for hypertension. Psychosom Med 2006;68:116–20.

[66] McCubbin JA, Surwit RS, Williams RB Jr. Endogenous opiate peptides, stress reactivity, and risk for hypertension. Hypertension 1985;7:808–11.

[67] Millan MJ. Descending control of pain. Prog Neurobiol 2002;66:355–474.

[68] Movahed MR, Bates S, Strootman D, Sattur S. Obesity in adolescence is associated with left ventricular hypertrophy and hypertension. Echocardiography 2011;28:150–3.

[69] Nilsson PM, Kandell-Collen A, Andersson HI. Blood pressure and metabolic factors in relation to chronic pain. Blood Press 1997;6:294–8.

[70] Okano Y, Tochikubo O, Umemura S. Relationship between base blood pressure during sleep and health-related quality of life in healthy adults. J Hum Hypertens 2007;21:135–40.

[71] Reis DJ, Ruggiero DA, Morrison SF. The C1 area of the rostral ventrolateral medulla oblongata. Am J Hypertens 1989;2:363–74S.

[72] Reyes Del Paso GA, Garrido S, Pulgar A, Martín-Vázquez M, Duschek S. Aberrances in autonomic cardiovascular regulation in fibromyalgia syndrome and their relevance for clinical pain reports. Psychosom Med 2010;72:462–70.

[73] Ring C, France CR, al'Absi M, Edwards L, McIntyre D, Carroll D, Martin U. Effects of naltrexone on electrocutaneous pain in patients with hypertension compared to normotensive individuals. Biol Psychol 2008;77:191–6.

[74] Rosa C, Ghione S, Mezzasalma L, Pellegrini M, Fasolo B, Giaconi S, Gazzetti P, Ferdeghini M. Relationship between pain sensitivity, cardiovascular reactivity to cold pressor test, and indexes of activity of the adrenergic and opioid system. Clin Exp Hypertens A 1988;10(Suppl 1):383–90.

[75] Rosmond R, Björntorp P. Quality of life, overweight, and body fat distribution in middle-aged men. Behav Med 2000;26:90–4.

[76] Sheps DS, Bragdon EE, Gray TF, Ballenger M, Usedom JE, Maixner W. Relationship between systemic hypertension and pain perception. Am J Cardiol 1992;70:3F–5F.

[77] Sitsen JM, DeJong W. Hypoalgesia in genetically hypertensive rats (SHR) is absent in rats with experimental hypertension. Hypertension 1983;5:185–90.

[78] Sitsen JM, De Jong W. Observations on pain perception and hypertension in spontaneously hypertensive rats. Clin Exp Hypertens A 1984;6:1345–56.

[79] Sleight P. The importance of the autonomic nervous system in health and disease. Aust N Z J Med 1997;27:467–73.

[80] Spaziani R, Bayati A, Redmond K, Bajaj H, Bienenstock J, Collins SM, Kamath MV. Vagal dysfunction in irritable bowel syndrome assessed by rectal distension and baroreceptor sensitivity. Neurogastroenterol Motil 2008;20:336–42.

[81] Stang PE, Brandenburg NA, Lane MC, Merikangas KR, Von Korff MR, Kessler RC. Mental and physical comorbid conditions and days in role among persons with arthritis. Psychosom Med 2006;68:152–8.

[82] Stornetta RL, Morrison SF, Ruggiero DA, Reis DJ. Neurons of the rostral ventrolateral medulla mediate the somatic pressor reflex. Am J Physiol 1989;256:R448–62.

[83] Thommasen HV, Zhang W. Impact of chronic disease on quality of life in the Bella Coola Valley. Rural Remote Health 2006;6:528.

[84] Tsang A, Korff MV, Lee S, Alonso J, Karam E, Angermeyer MC, Borges GL, Bromet EJ, de Girolamo G, de Graaf R, Gureje O, Lepine JP, Haro JM, Levinson D, Browne MA, Posada-Villa J, Seedat S, Watanabe M. Common chronic pain conditions in developed and developing countries: gender and age differences and comorbidity with depression-anxiety disorders. J Pain 2008;9:883–91.

[85] Von Korff M, Crane P, Lane M, Miglioretti DL, Simon G, Saunders K, Stang P, Brandenburg N, Kessler R. Chronic spinal pain and physical-mental comorbidity in the United States: results from the national comorbidity survey replication. Pain 2005;113:331–9.

[86] Wolfe F, Michaud K. Severe rheumatoid arthritis (RA), worse outcomes, comorbid illness, and sociodemographic disadvantage characterize RA patients with fibromyalgia. J Rheumatol 2004;31:695–700.

[87] Wood D, Goodnight S, Haig AJ, Nasari T. Body mass index, but not blood pressure is related to the level of pain in persons with chronic pain. J Back Musculoskelet Rehabil 2011;24:111–5.

[88] Zamir N, Segal M. Hypertension-induced analgesia: changes in pain sensitivity in experimental hypertensive rats. Brain Res 1979;160:170–3.

Correspondence to: Stephen Bruehl, PhD, Vanderbilt University Medical Center, 701 Medical Arts Building, 1211 Twenty-First Avenue South, Nashville, TN 37212, USA. Email: stephen.bruehl@vanderbilt.edu.

Neuropathic Pain in Diabetes: Diagnosis and Management

Solomon Tesfaye

Consultant Physician and Honorary Professor of Diabetic Medicine at the University of Sheffield, Royal Hallamshire Hospital, Sheffield, United Kingdom

Diabetes mellitus is a metabolic disorder resulting from a dysfunction in the mechanisms that maintain normal blood glucose levels. Over the past decade the prevalence of diabetes has been increasing by epidemic proportions. The International Diabetes Federation recently announced that the global diabetes map is changing rapidly. Currently, an estimated 366 million people have diabetes throughout the world [31]. Unfortunately, this rise is associated with 4.6 million deaths directly attributable to diabetes, and health care spending on diabetes has reached nearly half a trillion U.S. dollars per annum [31]. The chronic complications of diabetes also continue to pose major challenges both to society and to affected patients. Diabetes is now the most common cause of blindness in working-age adults, as well as being the leading cause of end-stage renal disease and nontraumatic lower-limb amputations. Most amputations are performed in cases in which the first presentation was a foot ulcer, and most ulcers occur in a limb affected by diabetic peripheral neuropathy (DPN).

Diabetic neuropathy is a very common feature of both type 1 and type 2 diabetes, occurring in approximately 50% of patients [11]. It has

Pain Comorbidities: Understanding and Treating the Complex Patient
edited by Maria Adele Giamberardino and Troels Staehelin Jensen
IASP Press, Seattle, © 2012

major detrimental effects on patients because it confers high morbidity and is associated with increased mortality [51]. Diabetic neuropathy is not a single entity, but encompasses a number of neuropathic syndromes in which pain is a prominent feature (Table I) [52].

Symmetrical neuropathies can manifest as typical or atypical DPNs. Atypical DPNs present as acute painful neuropathies and are relatively rare. By far the most common presentation of diabetic neuropathy (more than 90% of cases) is typical DPN, also known as chronic distal symmetrical neuropathy. Unless specified otherwise, the term "DPN" is synonymous with "typical DPN" in this chapter. The Toronto Diabetic Neuropathy Expert Group recently defined DPN [52] as a symmetrical, length-dependent sensorimotor neuropathy attributable to metabolic and microvessel alterations as a result of chronic hyperglycemia exposure and cardiovascular risk covariates. An abnormality of nerve conduction tests, which is frequently subclinical, appears to be the first objective quantitative indication of the condition. The occurrence of diabetic retinopathy and nephropathy in a given patient strengthens the case that the neuropathy is attributable to diabetes.

Neuropathic pain can be a feature of DPN. Painful diabetic neuropathy (PDN) is often found in association with autonomic neuropathy and other microvascular complications of diabetes [52]. The other manifestations of diabetic neuropathy (focal/multifocal neuropathies and atypical DPNs) are relatively rare (Table I), and neuropathic pain can also be a feature of these conditions. For example, the third cranial nerve palsy

Table I
Classification of diabetic neuropathy

Focal and Multifocal Neuropathies
    Mononeuropathies (e.g., cranial nerve palsies)
    Multiple focal lesions (mononeuritis multiplex)
    Radiculopathies/plexopathies (e.g., proximal motor neuropathy)
    Entrapment neuropathies (e.g., carpal, ulnar, peroneal)

Symmetrical Neuropathies
    Typical DPN (chronic distal symmetrical neuropathy)
    Atypical DPN (acute painful neuropathies)
    Autonomic neuropathy

Source: Adapted from Tesfaye et al. [52].
Abbreviation: DPN, diabetic peripheral neuropathy.

associated with diabetes can lead to pain around the orbit. Proximal motor neuropathy can present with pain in the affected focal area of muscle weakness, such as deep in the thigh. However, these rare focal and multifocal neuropathies will not be discussed further in this chapter.

Clinical Features of Diabetic Peripheral Neuropathy

History

The onset of DPN is indicated by sensory symptoms that start in the toes and then progress proximally to involve the feet and legs in a "stocking" distribution. When the disease is well established in the lower limbs, in more severe cases, there is upper-limb involvement, with a similar progression proximally starting in the fingers. As the disease advances further, motor manifestations, such as wasting of the small muscles of the hands and limb weakness, become apparent. In some cases there may be sensory loss that the patient may not be aware of, and the first presentation may be a foot ulcer. Approximately 50% of neuropathic subjects experience a progressive increase in unpleasant sensory symptoms in the lower limbs, including tingling (paresthesias), pain (burning, shooting or "electric-shock like," lancinating or "knife-like," "crawling," or "aching" in character), evoked pain (allodynia, hyperesthesia), or unusual sensations (such as a feeling of swelling of the feet or severe coldness of the legs when clearly the lower limbs look and feel fine to the clinician, or odd sensations on walking likened to "walking on pebbles" or "walking on hot sand") (Fig. 1). Painful diabetic neuropathy (PDN) is characteristically more severe at night and often interferes with normal sleep [56]. It also has a major impact on the ability to function normally (both mental and physical functioning, such as the ability to work), as well as on mood and quality of life [56].

In a study from the United States, the burden of PDN was found to be considerable, resulting in persistent discomfort despite polypharmacy and high resource use, and leading to limitations in daily activities and poor satisfaction with treatments [29]. Chronic persistent PDN can be extremely distressing and might be associated with profound depression [58,60], together with anxiety [29] and sleep loss [65]. In one study conducted in a tertiary referral multidisciplinary clinic for PDN, in patients with moderate or severe symptoms, over 50% were found to have anxiety and/or depression [45].

The natural history of PDN has not been well studied, but it is generally believed that painful symptoms may wax and wane over the years, and eventually the pain becomes less prominent as the sensory loss worsens. This view is supported by a study that reported improvements in painful symptoms with worsening of quantitative measures of nerve function over 3.5 years [6]. However, 3.5 years later, one-third of the 50 patients from the original cohort had died or were lost to follow-up, which is a major drawback of this study. There was symptomatic improvement in painful DPN in the majority of the remaining patients [6]. Many of the subjects were being treated with pain-relieving drugs, which might also have influenced the findings. Despite symptomatic improvement, small-fiber function deteriorated significantly [6]. Another school of thought is that there is no appreciable occurrence of significant remission [11]. This view is supported by one study that reported that neuropathic symptoms persist or get worse over a 5-year period in patients with DPN [10]. A major drawback of this study was that it involved highly selected patients from a hospital base. There is thus a need for large, population-based, prospective studies of patients with PDN aimed at examining the natural history and potentially modifiable risk factors.

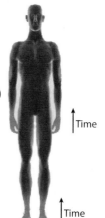

Symptoms of diabetic peripheral neuropathy

Positive Symptoms
— Persistent burning pain
— Paroxysmal, electric-shock-like, or stabbing pain
— Unusual sensations (e.g., crawling or ice-cold sensations)
— Dysesthesias (painful paresthesias)
Evoked pain (hyperalgesia, allodynia)

Negative Symptoms (Deficits)
— Numbness ("dead" feeling)
— Hypoalgesia, analgesia
— Hypoesthesia, anesthesia

Fig. 1. Symptoms of diabetic peripheral neuropathy.

Examination

Diabetic peripheral neuropathy is usually easily detected by simple clinical examination of the peripheral nervous system. Shoes and socks should be removed and the feet examined at least annually, and more often if neuropathy is present. The most common presenting abnormality is a reduction or absence of vibration sense in the toes. As the disease progresses, there is sensory loss in a "stocking" and sometimes in a "glove" distribution involving all sensory modalities. Rarely, when there is severe sensory loss, proprioception may also be impaired, leading to a positive Romberg's sign. Ankle tendon reflexes are lost (although these reflexes may also be lost with old age in nondiabetic people). With more advanced neuropathy, knee reflexes are often reduced or absent.

Muscle strength is usually normal during the early course of the disease, although mild weakness may be found in the toe extensors. However, with progressive disease there is a significant generalized muscular wasting, particularly in the small muscles of the hand and feet. Fine movements of the fingers would then be affected, causing difficulty in handling small objects. This impairment is often considered a major handicap because we use our hands almost all the time. Wasting of dorsal interosseous muscles is, however, usually due to entrapment of the ulnar nerve at the elbow. The clawing of the toes seen in DPN is believed to be due to unopposed pulling of the long extensor and flexor tendons (unopposed because of wasting of the small muscles of the foot). This scenario results in elevated plantar pressure points at the metatarsal heads that are prone to callus formation and foot ulceration. Deformities such as a bunion can form the focus of ulceration, and with more extreme deformities, such as those associated with Charcot arthropathy, the risk is further increased. Given that one of the most common precipitants of foot ulceration is inappropriate footwear, a thorough assessment should also include examination of shoes for poor fit, abnormal wear, and internal pressure areas or foreign bodies.

Autonomic neuropathy affecting the feet can cause a reduction in sweating and consequently dry skin that is likely to crack easily, predisposing the patient to the risk of infection. The "purely" neuropathic foot is also warm due to arteriovenous shunting, as first described by Ward [63]. This situation results in the distension of foot veins that fail to collapse even when the foot is elevated. It is not unusual to observe a gangrenous toe in a foot that has bounding arterial pulses, as there is impairment of the nutritive capillary circulation due to arteriovenous shunting.

Assessing Severity of Diabetic Peripheral Neuropathy

The Toronto Diabetic Neuropathy Consensus Panel suggested that a reliable objective and quantitative measure, nerve conduction abnormality, should be used as the minimal criterion for the diagnosis of DPN [52]. When nerve conduction values have not been assessed, the Consensus Panel recommended that it is not possible to provide a "confirmed" diagnosis of DPN—only a "possible" or "probable" diagnosis. There are several instruments that evaluate combinations of neuropathy symptoms, signs, and neurophysiological test abnormalities to provide scores for severity of DPN [13,17,22,52,64]. For clinical trials where accurate assessment of DPN is necessary, an approach to estimating severity suggested by Dyck et al. can be used [17]. It is important to exclude other causes of sensorimotor neuropathy. For epidemiological surveys or controlled clinical trials of DPN, the Toronto Consensus Panel advocated nerve conduction testing as an early and reliable indicator of the occurrence of neuropathy [52]. The group also emphasized that, to be reliable, the test must be carried out rigorously, using appropriate reference values corrected for applicable variables [52]. Moreover, recent studies emphasize the importance of the proficiency of the clinical neurological assessment [18].

Epidemiology

Although the epidemiology of DPN and the risk factors associated with this condition have been studied extensively [47,53], very few studies have specifically looked at the prevalence of pain. Pain prevalence varies from 10% to 26% of all diabetic people in a number of studies [15,16]. In one population-based study in urban Liverpool, United Kingdom, the prevalence of PDN, as assessed by a structured questionnaire and examination, was estimated at 16% [15]. Sadly, 12.5% of these patients had never reported their symptoms to their doctor, and notably, 39% had never received treatment for their pain [15]. Similarly, because of a lack of studies, it is difficult to confirm specific risk factors for PDN, although the incidence appears to be much higher in females [21].

Atypical Diabetic Peripheral Neuropathy (Acute Painful Neuropathies)

Atypical DPNs or acute painful neuropathies associated with diabetes are well recognized as a rare, yet distinct, variety of the symmetrical neuropathies [52]. They are characterized by severe sensory symptoms similar to those described above, but with a relatively rapid onset (weeks) and very few neurological signs on examination. The overriding symptom reported by all patients is severe pain, and there may be associated weight loss, depression, and, in men, erectile dysfunction [55]. This acute neuropathy typically follows some rapid change in glycemic control. It might occur after a sudden improvement in glycemic control, as in the case of "insulin neuritis" [55] (the term "insulin neuritis" is, strictly speaking, a misnomer because this condition might also be precipitated by sudden improvement of glycemic control with oral hypoglycemic agents). Alternatively, it might occur after an episode of very poor glycemic control, typically in young type 1 patients, such as following diabetic ketoacidosis, with the symptoms coming on after successful treatment of the acute exacerbation [11,55]. Fortunately, the prognosis of acute painful neuropathies is good, with complete resolution of all symptoms usually occurring within a year of onset [55].

Small-Fiber Neuropathy

The existence of a "small-fiber neuropathy" as a distinct entity has been advocated by some authorities [19,35,49], usually within the context of young type 1 patients and prediabetes [50]. A dominant feature of this syndrome is neuropathic pain, which may be very severe, with relative sparing of large-fiber functions (e.g., detection of vibration and proprioception). The pain is described as burning, deep, and aching. A sensation of pins and needles (paresthesias) is often experienced. Hypersensitivity to touch may be present. However, rarely, patients with small-fiber neuropathy may not have neuropathic pain, and some may occasionally have foot ulceration. Autonomic involvement is common, and severely affected patients may be disabled by postural hypotension and/or gastrointestinal symptoms. The syndrome tends to develop within a few years of onset of diabetes (and also in prediabetes) as a relatively early complication, and there is some evidence that lifestyle intervention may improve cutaneous reinnervation and improve pain [50].

On clinical examination there is little evidence of objective signs of nerve damage, apart from a reduction of pinprick and temperature sensations, which are reduced in a "stocking" and "glove" distribution. There is relative sparing of vibration and position sense (due to relative sparing of the large-diameter Aβ fibers). Muscle strength is usually normal, and reflexes are also usually normal. However, autonomic function tests are frequently abnormal, and affected male patients usually have erectile dysfunction. Electrophysiological tests are usually normal. Quantitative sensory testing to assess the psychophysical thresholds for cold and warm sensations and skin biopsy with quantification of somatic intraepidermal nerve fibers may be used to determine the damage to small nerve fibers [54].

Mechanisms of Neuropathic Pain in Diabetes

The exact pathophysiology of neuropathic pain in diabetes remains elusive, although several mechanisms have been postulated, as listed in Table II [54]. Other potential mechanisms include the association of increased blood glucose instability with the genesis of neuropathic pain [18], an increase in peripheral nerve epineurial blood flow [47], altered foot skin microcirculation [53], reduced intraepidermal nerve fiber density in the context of early neuropathy [15], increased thalamic vascularity [16], and autonomic dysfunction [21].

Assessment of Neuropathic Pain Severity

As discussed above, the diagnosis of PDN relies on two determinants: (1) the patient's description of pain in distal extremities initially of the lower limbs, associated with nocturnal exacerbation, and (2) peripheral neuro-

Table II
Mechanisms of neuropathic pain

Peripheral Mechanisms	Central Mechanisms
Changes in sodium channel distribution and expression	Central sensitization
Changes in calcium channel distribution and expression	Aβ-fiber sprouting into lamina II of the dorsal horn
Altered neuropeptide expression	Reduced inhibition of descending pathways
Sympathetic sprouting	
Peripheral sensitization	
Altered peripheral blood flow	
Axonal atrophy, degeneration, or regeneration	
Damage to small fibers	
Increased glycemic flux	

Source: Adapted from Tesfaye and Kempler [54].

logical examination. The clinical diagnosis may be supported by nerve conduction studies and quantitative sensory testing. Predominant small-fiber neuropathy is diagnosed by skin biopsy and by the presence of reduced intraepidermal nerve fiber density [50]. Nerve conduction studies are particularly important to exclude other causes of pain, such as entrapment syndromes. As diabetic neuropathy is a diagnosis of exclusion, a careful clinical history and a peripheral neurological and vascular examination of the lower extremities are essential to exclude other causes of neuropathic pain and leg or foot pain such as peripheral vascular disease, arthritis, malignancy, alcohol abuse, or spinal canal stenosis. Patients with asymmetrical symptoms or signs should be carefully assessed for other etiologies of their symptoms because PDN is invariably symmetrical.

The frequency and severity of painful symptoms can be assessed by a number of simple numeric rating scales [14]. It is important to appreciate the difficulties in the description and assessment of painful symptoms that patients experience. After all, pain is a very individual sensation, and even patients with similar pathological lesions may describe their symptoms in markedly different ways. It must also be emphasized that, since pain is a personal psychological experience, the external observer can play no part in its assessment or interpretation. Hence, the use of simple scales is recommended, such as the simple visual analogue scale (VAS), which is the oldest and best-validated measure, or the numerical rating scale (NRS), such as an 11-point Likert scale (0 = no pain to 10 = worst possible pain). Other validated scales and questionnaires include the Neuropathic Pain Symptom Inventory [9], the modified Brief Pain Inventory [66], the Neuropathic Pain Questionnaire [4], the LANNS pain scale [7], and the McGill Pain Questionnaire, often used in its shortened format [37]. Quality of life might be assessed by generic instruments that may allow cross-comparison with other chronic medical conditions. However, it is also important to use validated, neuropathy-specific measures of quality of life, such as the NeuroQol [59], the Norfolk Quality of Life Scale [62], and the Neuropathic Pain Impact on Quality-of-Life questionnaire (NePIQoL) [41]. The impact of painful symptomatology on mood can be evaluated using scales such as the Hospital Anxiety and Depression Scale (HADS) [69]. Similarly, a number of scales can be used to assess pain behavior and sleep interference and to predict response to therapy [61].

For clinical trials of potential new therapies for PDN, careful patient selection with the use of neuropathic pain scales and outcome measures is indicated. Inclusion criteria for such trials would normally include neuropathic pain associated with diabetes for more than 6 months and a mean weekly pain score of between 4 and 10 on an 11-point graphic rating scale, with exclusion of pain not associated with DPN.

Management of Painful Diabetic Neuropathy

It is not easy to assess and treat PDN. Ideally, a multidisciplinary approach is required because the impact of PDN is varied and multidimensional. A multidisciplinary team might include the involvement of a diabetologist, a neurologist, the pain clinic team, specialist nurses, podiatrists, psychologists, physiotherapists, and others. However, in most clinical settings this level of care is not possible, and management falls mainly on the diabetes physician, the primary care physician, or the neurologist. Whereas strong evidence implicates poor glycemic control as a pathogenetic mechanism in the etiology of DPN, there is no proof from randomized, controlled trials (RCTs) that it is the cause of neuropathic pain. However, there is some evidence that increased blood glucose flux might contribute to neuropathic pain [40]. An RCT in this area is unlikely, and there is therefore general consensus that good blood glucose control should be the first step in the management of any form of diabetic neuropathy. Other risk factors for large-vessel disease (such as hypertension and hyperlipidemia) are also common in DPN, and it is important to address these abnormalities in addition.

Pharmacological Management

A large number of pharmacological treatments with known efficacy in PDN are listed in Table III, although only duloxetine and pregabalin are approved for the treatment of neuropathic pain in diabetes by both the Food and Drug Administration of the United States and the European Medicines Agency.

Tricyclic Antidepressants

Tricyclic antidepressants (TCAs) have been used to treat neuropathic pain for over 25 years. Several RCTs and meta-analyses have confirmed the efficacy of TCAs in PDN [23]. These agents have been shown to promote successful analgesia to thermal, mechanic, and electrical stimuli in

Table III
Pharmacological treatment approaches for
painful diabetic peripheral neuropathy showing
some of the commonly prescribed treatments

Tricyclic antidepressants
Amitriptyline, 25–75 mg/day
Imipramine, 25–75 mg/day
Serotonin norepinephrine reuptake inhibitors
Duloxetine, 60–120 mg/day
Venlafaxine, 150–225 mg/day
Anticonvulsants
Gabapentin, 900–3600 mg/day
Pregabalin, 300–600 mg/day
Carbamazepine, 200–800 mg/day
Opiates
Tramadol, 200–400 mg/day
Oxycodone, SR, 20–80 mg/day
Morphine sulfate, SR, 20–80 mg/day
Capsaicin cream, 0.075%
Applied sparingly 3–4 times per day

Abbreviation: SR, sustained release.

diabetic patients. Putative mechanisms underlying these effects include the inhibition of norepinephrine and/or serotonin reuptake synapses of central descending pain control systems, and more recently, the antagonism of N-methyl-D-aspartate (NMDA) receptors, which mediate hyperalgesia and allodynia [48]. Amitriptyline and imipramine provide balanced inhibition of norepinephrine and serotonin, which may confer an advantage with respect to efficacy over noradrenergic compounds such as nortriptyline and desipramine, which, on the other hand, are better tolerated. In addition, drugs such as nortriptyline have reduced anticholinergic properties and create fewer symptoms caused by cholinergic blockade. As TCAs have predictable and frequent side effects, including drowsiness and anticholinergic effects, it is recommended to start with a small dose, especially in older patients (who are at risk of falls), of 10 mg/day, increasing to 75 mg/day gradually, if required. Data from a large retrospective study of patients on TCA therapy showed an increased risk of sudden cardiac death associated with doses greater than 100 mg/day [43], and additional caution should be taken in any patient with a history of cardiovascular disease. Some authorities recommend that an electrocardiogram (ECG) should be done, and if there is prolongation of the PR or QT interval, these drugs should not be used. However, others feel that this screening is not necessary, and often it is not feasible, particularly in resource-poor countries.

Serotonin and Norepinephrine Reuptake Inhibitors

Serotonin and norepinephrine reuptake inhibitors (SNRIs) have dual antidepressant and pain-relieving characteristics. SNRIs, such as duloxetine, relieve pain by increasing the synaptic availability of serotonin (5-hydroxytryptamine, 5-HT) and norepinephrine in the descending pathways that are inhibitory to pain impulses. The efficacy of duloxetine has been confirmed in PDN in several similarly designed clinical trials at doses of 60 or 120 mg/day [23,32]. The pooled data from three trials confirmed that treatment efficacy started within 1 week and was maintained throughout the treatment period of 12 weeks, and moreover, approximately 50% of patients achieved at least 50% pain reduction [32]. The number needed to treat (NNT) to achieve at least 50% pain reduction (generally accepted to be clinically meaningful) was 4.9 for 120 mg/day and 5.2 for 60 mg/day

[41]. An advantage of this agent is that it is not associated with weight gain; the most frequent adverse effects include nausea, somnolence, dizziness, constipation, dry mouth, and reduced appetite, and these effects tend to be mild to moderate and are transient.

Another SNRI, venlafaxine (at a dose of 150 to 225 mg/day) is also effective in relieving neuropathic pain [23], although clinically significant cardiovascular adverse events were reported. As diabetes is associated with cardiovascular disease, caution should be applied with regard to venlafaxine use in patients with PDN, many of whom will have comorbid cardiovascular disease.

Anticonvulsants

Of the many anticonvulsants that have been employed to treat neuropathic pain, gabapentin and pregabalin are the two most widely used. The evidence for the efficacy of the first-generation agents (such as carbamazepine and phenytoin) is limited and mainly comes from small single-center studies. Furthermore, these agents are associated with a relatively high frequency of adverse events, particularly central effects, such as somnolence and dizziness [23].

Gabapentin and pregabalin bind to the $\alpha_2\delta$ subunit of the calcium channel, reducing calcium influx and thus reducing synaptic neurotransmitter release in the hyperexcited neuron. Gabapentin is well established as a treatment of PDN, although doses typically prescribed in clinical practice are much lower than the doses of up to 3.6 g/day used in the main clinical trial [3]. Pregabalin is also commonly used to treat PDN because it has been shown to be highly effective in several RCTs [23,24]. Based on these and other studies supporting its efficacy and tolerability, doses of 150 to 600 mg/day (in divided doses) are recommended for the treatment of PDN. The pooled analysis of seven RCTs in PDN has confirmed the efficacy and safety of pregabalin [24]. The most frequent side effects for pregabalin are dizziness, somnolence, peripheral edema, headache, and weight gain.

Local Anesthetic/Antiarrhythmic Agents

Intravenous (i.v.) lidocaine (5 mg/kg over 30 minutes) was found to be beneficial in relieving PDN in a randomized, double-blind, placebo-controlled trial [33]. However, oral dosing is unavailable, and ECG monitoring is necessary during administration, thus limiting its use to refractory cases of PDN. Many patients experience pain relief for up to 1 month after i.v. lidocaine treatment. A multicenter randomized, open-label, parallel-group study of lidocaine patch vs. pregabalin, with a drug washout phase of up to 2 weeks and a comparative 4-week treatment period, showed that lidocaine was as effective as pregabalin in reducing pain and had no side effects [23].

Opioids

Opioids are now generally regarded as second-line agents for the treatment of PDN. Many physicians are reluctant to prescribe opioids for neuropathic pain, probably because of fear of addiction. However, there is clinical trial evidence for some opioids, and there is thus a good rationale for their use in appropriate patients after first-line therapy has been tried. Of the orally administered opioids, tramadol is the best studied. It is a centrally acting synthetic opioid with an unusual mode of action, working on both opioid and monoaminergic pathways. It has a lower abuse potential than conventional stronger opioids, and development of tolerance is uncommon. In an RCT, tramadol at doses of up to 200 mg/day was effective in the management of PDN, with a follow-up showing that symptomatic relief could be maintained for at least 6 months [30]. Finally, two randomized trials have confirmed the efficacy of controlled-release oxycodone for neuropathic pain in diabetes [23,57]. All studies of opioids have only assessed relatively short-term use, so the risks of tolerance and dependence over the longer term have yet to be quantified. In recognition of these potential problems, physicians should be alert to signs of abuse and should use opioids only if other therapies have failed to provide sufficient pain relief.

Comparator Trials

A major problem in the area of the treatment of neuropathic pain in diabetes is the relative lack of comparative or combination studies. Most of the studies cited in this chapter tested active agents against placebo. There is a need for more studies that test a new drug against an active comparator or compare two existing drugs with known efficacy.

A recent example of such a trial was published by Bansal et al. [5], who compared amitriptyline with pregabalin in PDN in a small, randomized, double-blind trial. This study found little difference in efficacy, but confirmed that pregabalin was the preferred drug because of a superior adverse-event profile. Another recent study compared duloxetine with amitriptyline [34]. This small crossover study found that both drugs were equally efficacious, although among the reported adverse events, dry mouth was more common with amitriptyline than duloxetine (55% vs. 24%; $P < 0.01$). A greater number of patients preferred duloxetine, although this finding was not statistically significant (48% vs. 36%; $P = 0.18$) [34].

An indirect meta-analysis by Quilici et al. compared the efficacy and tolerability of duloxetine versus pregabalin and gabapentin in participants with PDN, using placebo as a common comparator [42]. The authors conducted a search of regulatory websites, as well as PubMed, EMBASE, and CENTRAL databases, for available data from randomized, double-blind, placebo-controlled clinical trials that had assessed these three drugs in the treatment of PDN [42]. Efficacy criteria were a reduction in 24-hour pain severity score for all three treatments, and treatment response rate (at least 50% pain reduction) and overall health improvement (as measured on the Patient Global Impression of Improvement/Change questionnaire) for duloxetine and pregabalin only [42]. Eleven studies met the inclusion criteria: three of duloxetine, six of pregabalin, and two of gabapentin. Direct comparison found all three drugs to be superior to placebo for all efficacy parameters, although there were some tolerability trade-offs [42]. Indirect analyses were performed between duloxetine and each of pregabalin and gabapentin, using placebo as a common comparator [42]. An indirect comparison between duloxetine and gabapentin found no statistically significant differences [42]. Comparing duloxetine with pregabalin, the authors found significant differences in overall health improvement, favoring pregabalin, and in dizziness, favoring duloxetine. There was no significant difference in the 24-hour pain severity score between duloxetine and gabapentin [42].

The Combo study that has just finished compared the efficacy of a combination treatment of duloxetine and pregabalin with the maximal dose of each drug in monotherapy, in patients with PDN who had not responded to the standard recommended dose of either drug [20]. It is hoped that it will provide an answer to a common clinical question: Is it better to increase the dose of the current monotherapy or to combine both treatments early on, in patients who do not respond to standard doses of duloxetine or pregabalin?

Combination Trials

Gilron et al. studied nortriptyline and gabapentin either in combination or alone in a randomized trial and confirmed that, when given together, the two drugs were more efficacious than either one given alone [27]. In another crossover study, low-dose combination therapy with gabapentin and morphine was significantly more effective than higher doses of either drug alone [26].

Topical Treatments

Topical capsaicin works by depleting substance P from nerve terminals, and there might be worsening of neuropathic symptoms for the first few weeks of application. Topical capsaicin (0.075%) applied sparingly 3–4 times per day to the affected area has been found to relieve neuropathic pain [67] (see the section above on the use of lidocaine in PDN).

Disease-Modifying Treatments

Although several disease-modifying agents are under investigation, only the antioxidant α-lipoic acid, which is available in certain countries, is supported by a meta-analysis [68]. Evidence supports the use of this agent at a dose of 600 mg i.v. per day over a 3-week period in reducing neuropathic pain [2]. The meta-analysis confirmed that the treatment was associated with a significant and clinically meaningful improvement in positive neuropathic symptoms as well as deficits [52]. The results of long-term trials of oral α-lipoic acid for neuropathic symptoms and neuropathic deficits are less convincing, and more data are required.

Previous Guidelines on Treatment of Painful Diabetic Neuropathy

The European Federation of Neurological Societies (EFNS) has published guidelines proposing that first-line treatments might comprise TCAs, SNRIs, or gabapentin or pregabalin [20]. Most recently, the U.K. National Institute for Health and Clinical Excellence (NICE) published guidelines on the management of neuropathic pain in nonspecialist settings, in which the management of PDN featured prominently [38]. NICE ranked the level of evidence for pain outcomes with duloxetine, pregabalin, and gabapentin as similar, yet they propose that oral duloxetine should be the first line of treatment with amitriptyline as an alternative, and pregabalin as a second-line treatment [12]. The proposal that oral duloxetine should be first-line therapy does not appear to be based on efficacy but rather on cost-effectiveness. Yet another consensus statement was given by the American Academy of Neurology that recommended that pregabalin is "established as effective and should be offered for relief of PDN (Level A evidence)" [12]. Venlafaxine, duloxetine, amitriptyline, gabapentin, valproate, opioids (morphine sulfate, tramadol, and controlled-release oxycodone), and capsaicin were considered to be "probably effective and should be considered for treatment of PDN (Level B evidence)" [12].

Recommendations for a Treatment Algorithm

Recently, the International Consensus Panel on Diabetic Neuropathy met in Toronto and recommended a treatment algorithm based on the clinical trial evidence for the various pharmacological agents for PDN [52,56]. The panel compared the relative efficacy and safety of treatments for PDN and recommended that a TCA, SNRI, or $\alpha_2\delta$-receptor agonist should be considered for first-line treatments, provided there are no contraindications. On the basis of trial data, duloxetine would be the preferred SNRI and pregabalin would be the preferred $\alpha_2\delta$-receptor agonist. If pain is inadequately controlled despite a change in monotherapy, depending on contraindications and side effects, the first-line agents could be combined (e.g., pregabalin + duloxetine, or amitriptyline + pregabalin). If pain is inadequately controlled despite a combination of first-line agents, opioids such as tramadol and oxycodone might be added in a combination treatment [52,56].

Initial selection of treatment will be influenced by the assessment of contraindications, and by consideration of comorbidities and cost. For example, in diabetic patients with a history of heart disease, elderly patients who are taking concomitant medications such as diuretics and antihypertensives, and patients with comorbid orthostatic hypotension, TCAs would have greater contraindications. In patients with liver disease, duloxetine should not be prescribed, and in those with edema, pregabalin or gabapentin should be avoided.

Nonpharmacological Treatments

Nonpharmacological approaches have a theoretical advantage of fewer unwanted side effects, but unfortunately there are few well-designed trials in this area. A full review of studies on nonpharmacological treatments for PDN is beyond the remit of this chapter. Briefly, there have been some studies in PDN of interventions such as acupuncture [1], near-infrared phototherapy [36], low-intensity laser therapy [70], transcutaneous electrical nerve stimulation (TENS) [39], frequency-modulated electromagnetic neural stimulation (FREMS) therapy [2,8], high-frequency external muscle stimulation [44], and as a last resort, the implantation of an electrical spinal cord stimulator [57].

Conclusions

Painful diabetic neuropathy affects around 20% of all diabetic people and confers a significant clinical burden to the patient. Nevertheless, it continues to be underdiagnosed and undertreated, and this unsatisfactory scenario must change. The minimum requirements for diagnosis of PDN are assessment of symptoms and neurological examination, with shoes and socks removed. Bilateral sensory impairment is usually present. Other causes of pain should be excluded, and contraindications for the use of individual drugs should be taken into account. Based upon trial evidence, the Toronto Consensus Panel on Diabetic Neuropathy recommends that first-line therapies for PDN should be either a TCA, the SNRI duloxetine, or the anticonvulsants pregabalin or gabapentin. The physician's decision for each patient should take into account comorbidities and costs.

Combination therapy might be useful for those with more severe pain, but there is a paucity of studies, and further research is required. Studies are also required on direct head-to-head comparative trials and long-term efficacy of drugs, as most trials have lasted less than 6 months. Despite many trials looking for effective pathogenetic treatments for painful DPN, only i.v. administration of the antioxidant α-lipoic acid has evidence from a meta-analysis and is in wide clinical use in certain countries. Thus, further research is required to find novel and more effective pathogenetic treatments for PDN.

Finally, key peripheral and central nervous system target areas generating or modulating pain in PDN, including peripheral small fibers with modulation at the level of the spinal cord, the thalamus [46], and the other pain matrix areas in the brain, require further studies in order to lead to development of more effective treatments. The association of PDN with autonomic neuropathy also merits further investigation [25].

References

[1]   Abuaisha BB, Constanzi JB, Boulton AJM. Acupuncture for the treatment of chronic painful diabetic neuropathy: a long-term study. Diabetes Res Clin Pract 1998;39:115–21.

[2]   Attal N, Cruccu G, Baron R, Haanpää M, Hansson P, Jensen TS, Nurmikko T; European Federation of Neurological Societies. EFNS guidelines on the pharmacological treatment of neuropathic pain: 2010 revision. Eur J Neurol 2010;17:1113–e88.

[3]   Backonja M, Beydoun A, Edwards KR, Schwartz SL, Fonseca V, Hes M, LaMoreaux L, Garofalo E. Gabapentin for symptomatic treatment of painful neuropathy in patients with diabetes mellitus. JAMA 1998;280:1831–6.

[4]   Backonja MM, Krause SJ. Neuropathic pain questionnaire: short form. Clin J Pain 2003;19:315.

[5]   Bansal D, Bhansali A, Hota D, Chakrabarti A, Dutta P. Amitriptyline vs pregabalin in painful diabetic neuropathy: a randomised double-blind clinical trial. Diabetic Med 2009;26:1019–26.

[6]   Benbow SJ, Chan AW, Bowsher D, McFarlane IA, Williams G. A prospective study of painful symptoms, small fibre function and peripheral vascular disease in chronic painful diabetic neuropathy. Diabet Med 1994;11:17–21.

[7]   Bennett M.The LANSS Pain Scale: the Leeds assessment of neuropathic symptoms and signs. Pain 2001;92:147–57.

[8]   Bosi E, Conti M, Vermigli C, Cazzetta G, Peretti E, Cordoni MC, Galimberti G, Scionti L. Effectiveness of frequency-modulated electromagnetic neural stimulation in the treatment of diabetic peripheral neuropathy. Diabetologia 2005;48:817–23.

[9]   Bouhassira D, Attal N, Fermanian J, Alchaar H, Gautron M, Masquelier E, Rostaing S, Lanteri-Minet M, Collin E, Grisart J, Boureau F. Development and validation of the Neuropathic Pain Symptom Inventory. Pain 2004;108:248–57.

[10] Boulton AJM, Armstrong WD, Scarpello JHB, Ward JD. The natural history of painful diabetic neuropathy: a 4 year study. Postgrad Med J 1983;59:556–9.

[11] Boulton AJM, Malik RA, Arezzo J, Sosenko JM. Diabetic somatic neuropathies. Diabetes Care 2004;27:1458–86.

[12] Bril V, England J, Franklin GM, Backonja M, Cohen J, Del Toro D, Feldman E, Iverson DJ, Perkins B, Russell JW, Zochodne D; American Academy of Neurology; American Association of Neuromuscular and Electrodiagnostic Medicine; American Academy of Physical Medicine and Rehabilitation. Evidence-based guideline: treatment of painful diabetic neuropathy: report of the American Academy of Neurology, the American Association of Neuromuscular and Electrodiagnostic Medicine, and the American Academy of Physical Medicine and Rehabilitation. Neurology 2011;76:1758–65.

[13] Bril V, Perkins BA. Validation of the Toronto Clinical Scoring System for diabetic polyneuropathy. Diabetes Care 2002;25:2048–52.

[14] Cruccu G, Sommer C, Anand P, Attal N, Baron R, Garcia-Larrea L, Haanpaa M, Jensen TS, Serra J, Treede RD. EFNS guidelines on neuropathic pain assessment: revised 2009. Eur J Neurol 2010;17:1010–8.

[15] Daousi C, McFarlane IA, Woodward A, Nurmikko TJ, Bendred PE, Benbow SJ. Chronic painful peripheral neuropathy in an urban community: a control comparison of people with and without diabetes. Diabet Med 2004;21:976–82.

[16] Davies M, Brophy S, Williams R, Taylor A. The prevalence, severity, and impact of painful diabetic peripheral neuropathy in type 2 diabetes. Diabetes Care 2006;29:1518–22.

[17] Dyck PJ. Detection, characterization, and staging of polyneuropathy: assessed in diabetics. Muscle Nerve 1988;11:21–32.

[18] Dyck PJ, Overland CJ, Low PA, Litchy WJ, Davies JL, Dyck PJB, O'Brien PC, Andersen H, Albers JW, Bolton CF, England J, Klein CJ, Llewelyn G, Mauermann ML, Russell JW, Singer W, Smith G, Tesfaye S, Vella A. Signs and symptoms vs nerve conduction studies to diagnose diabetic sensorimotor polyneuropathy. Muscle Nerve 2010;42:157–64.

[19] Ebenezer GJ, Hauer P, Gibbons C, McArthur JC, Polydefkis M. Assessment of epidermal nerve fibers: a new diagnostic and predictive tool for peripheral neuropathies. J Neuropathol Exp Neurol 2007;66:1059–73.

[20] Eli Lilly and Company. A study in painful diabetic neuropathy (COMBO-DN). Available at: http://clinicaltrials.gov/ct2/show/NCT01089556.

[21] Elliott J, Tesfaye S, Chaturvedi N, Gandhi RA, Stevens LK, Emery C, Fuller JH; EURODIAB Prospective Complications Study Group. Large-fiber dysfunction in diabetic peripheral neuropathy is predicted by cardiovascular risk factors. Diabetes Care 2009;32:1896–900.

[22] Feldman EL, Stevens MJ, Thomas PK, Brown MB, Canal N, Greene DA. A practical two-step quantitative clinical and electrophysiological assessment for the diagnosis and staging of diabetic neuropathy. Diabetes Care 1994;17:1281–9.

[23] Finnerup NB, Sindrup SH, Jensen TS. The evidence for pharmacological treatment of neuropathic pain. Pain 2010;150:573–81.

[24] Freeman R, Durso-Decruz E, Emir B. Efficacy, safety, and tolerability of pregabalin treatment for painful diabetic peripheral neuropathy: findings from seven randomised, controlled trials across a range of doses. Diabetes Care 2008;31:1448–54.

[25] Gandhi R, Marques JLB, Selvarajah D, Emery CJ, Tesfaye S. Painful diabetic neuropathy is associated with greater autonomic dysfunction than painless diabetic neuropathy. Diabetes Care 2010;33:1585–90.

[26] Gilron I, Bailey JM, Tu D, Holden RR, Weaver DF, Houlden RL. Morphine, gabapentin, or their combination for neuropathic pain. N Engl J Med 2005;352:1324–34.

[27] Gilron I, Bailey JM, Tu D, Holden RR, Jackson AC, Houlden RL. Nortriptyline and gabapentin, alone and in combination for neuropathic pain: a double-blind, randomised controlled crossover trial. Lancet 2009;374:1252–61.

[28] Gimbel JS, Richards P, Portenoy RK. Controlled-release oxycodone for pain in diabetic neuropathy: a randomised controlled trial. Neurology 2003;60:927–34.

[29] Gore M, Brandenburg NA, Dukes E, Hoffman DL, Tai KS, Stacey B. Pain severity in diabetic peripheral neuropathy is associated with patient functioning, symptom levels of anxiety and depression, and sleep. J Pain Symptom Manage 2005;30:374–85.

[30] Harati Y, Gooch C, Swenson M, Edelman S, Greene D, Raskin P, Donofrio P, Cornblath D, Sachdeo R, Siu CO, Kamin M. Double-blind randomized trial of tramadol for the treatment of the pain of diabetic neuropathy. Neurology 1998;50:1842–6.

[31] International Diabetes Foundation. New IDF data reveals diabetes epidemic continues to escalate. Available at: http://www.idf.org/new-idf-data-reveals-diabetes-epidemic-continues-escalate.

[32] Kajdasz DK, Iyengar S, Desaiah D, Backonja MM, Farrar JT, Fishbain DA, Jensen TS, Rowbotham MC, Sang CN, Ziegler D, McQuay HJ. Duloxetine for the management of diabetic peripheral neuropathic pain: evidence-based findings from post hoc analysis of three multicentre, randomised, double-blind, placebo-controlled, parallel-group studies. Clin Ther 2007;29:2536–46.

[33] Kastrup J, Petersen P, Dejgard A, Angelo HR, Hilsted J. Intravenous lidocaine infusion: a new treatment of chronic painful diabetic neuropathy. Pain 1987;28:69–75.

[34] Kaur H, Hota D, Bhansali A, Dutta P, Bansal D, Chakrabarti A. Comparative trial to evaluate amitriptyline and duloxetine in painful diabetic neuropathy: a randomized, double-blind, crossover clinical trial. Diabetes Care 2011;34:818–22.

[35] Kennedy WR, Wendelschafer-Crabb G, Johnson T. Quantitation of epidermal nerves in diabetic neuropathy. Neurology 1996;47:1042–8.

[36] Leonard DR, Farooqu MH, Myers S. Restoration of sensation, reduced pain, and improved balance in subjects with diabetic peripheral neuropathy: a double-blind, randomised placebo-controlled study with monochromatic infrared treatment. Diabetes Care 2004;27:168–72.

[37] Melzack R. The short-form McGill Pain Questionnaire. Pain 1987;30:191–7.

[38] National Institute for Health and Clinical Excellence. NICE Clinical Guideline 96: Neuropathic pain. The pharmacological management of neuropathic pain in adults in non-specialist settings. March 2010. Available at: www.nice.org.uk.

[39] Oyibo S, Breislin K, Boulton AJM. Electrical stimulation therapy through stocking elec-
      trodes for painful diabetic neuropathy: a double-blind controlled crossover study. Diabet Med
      2004;21:940–4.
[40] Oyibo SO, Prasad YDM, Jackson NJ Boulton AJM. The relationship between blood glucose ex-
      cursions and painful diabetic peripheral neuropathy: a pilot study. Diabet Med 2002;19:870–3.
[41] Poole HM, Murphy P, Nurmikko TJ. Development and preliminary validation of the NePIQoL:
      a quality-of-life measure for neuropathic pain. J Pain Symptom Manage 2009;37:233–45.
[42] Quilici S, Chancellor J, Löthgren M, Simon D, Said G, Le TK, Garcia-Cebrian A, Monz B. Meta-
      analysis of duloxetine vs. pregabalin and gabapentin in the treatment of diabetic peripheral neu-
      ropathic pain. BMC Neurol 2009;9:6.
[43] Ray WA, Meredith S, Thapa PB, Hall K, Murray KT. Cyclic antidepressants and the risk of sud-
      den cardiac death. Clin Pharmacol Ther 2004;75:234–41.
[44] Reichstein L, Labrenz S, Ziegler D, Martin S. Effective treatment of symptomatic diabetic poly-
      neuropathy by high-frequency external muscle stimulation. Diabetologia 2005;48:824–8.
[45] Sankar A, Selvarajah D, Gandhi R, Oleolo M, Emery C, Tesfaye S. Significant impact of mood
      disturbances of pain perception inpainful DPN: time to re-evaluate current practice? Diabetolo-
      gia 2010;53:S446.
[46] Selvarajah D, Wilkinson ID, Gandhi R, Emery CJ, Griffiths PD, Tesfaye S. Unique thalamic mi-
      crovascular perfusion abnormalities in painful but not painless diabetic polyneuropathy; a clue
      to the pathogenesis of pain in type 1 diabetes mellitus. Diabetes Care 2012; in press.
[47] Shaw JE, Zimmet PZ, Gries FA, Ziegler D: Epidemiology of diabetic neuropathy. In: Gries FA,
      Cameron NE, Low PA, Ziegler D, editors. Textbook of diabetic neuropathy. Stuttgart: Thieme;
      2003. p. 64–82.
[48] Sindrup S, Otto M, Finnerup NB, Jensen TS. Antidepressants in the treatment of neuropathic
      pain. Basic Clin Pharmacol Toxicol 2005;96:399–409.
[49] Singleton JR, Smith AG, Bromberg MB Increased prevalence of impaired glucose tolerance in
      patients with painful sensory neuropathy. Diabetes Care 2001;24:1448–53.
[50] Smith AG, Russell J, Feldman EL, Goldstein J, Peltier A, Smith S, Hamwi J, Pollari D, Bixby
      B, Howard J, Singleton JR. Lifestyle intervention for pre-diabetic neuropathy. Diabetes Care
      2006;29:1294–9.
[51] Soedamah-Muthu SS, Chaturvedi N, Witte DR, Stevens LK, Porta M, Fuller JH; EURODIAB
      Prospective Complications Study Group. Relationship between risk factors and mortality in type
      1 diabetic patients in Europe: the EURODIAB Prospective Complications Study (PCS). Diabetes
      Care 2008;31:1360–6.
[52] Tesfaye S, Boulton AJ, Dyck PJ, Freeman R, Horowitz M, Kempler P, Lauria G, Malik RA, Spal-
      lone V, Vinik A, Bernardi L, Valensi P; Toronto Diabetic Neuropathy Expert Group. Diabetic
      neuropathies: update on definitions, diagnostic criteria, estimation of severity and treatments.
      Diabetes Care 2010;33:2285–93.
[53] Tesfaye S, Chaturvedi N, Eaton SEM, Witte D, Ward JD, Fuller J. Vascular risk factors and dia-
      betic neuropathy. New Engl J Med 2005;352:341–50.
[54] Tesfaye S, Kempler P. Painful diabetic neuropathy. Diabetologia 2005;48:805–7.
[55] Tesfaye S, Malik R, Harris N, Jakubowski JJ, Mody C, Rennie IG, Ward JD. Arterio-venous shunt-
      ing and proliferating new vessels in acute painful neuropathy and rapid glycaemic control (insu-
      lin neuritis). Diabetologia 1996;39:329–35.
[56] Tesfaye S, Vileikyte L, Rayman G, Sindrup S, Perkins B, Baconja M, Vinik A Boulton A; on behalf
      of the Toronto Expert Panel on Diabetic Neuropathy. Painful diabetic peripheral neuropathy:
      consensus recommendations on diagnosis, assessment and management. Diabetes Metab Res
      Rev 2011; Epub Jun 21.
[57] Tesfaye S, Watt J, Benbow SJ, Pang KA, Miles J, Macfarlane IA. Electrical spinal-cord stimulation
      for painful diabetic peripheral neuropathy. Lancet 1996;348:1698–701.
[58] Vileikyte L, Leventhal H, Gonzalez JS, Peyrot M, Rubin RR, Ulbrecht JS, Garrow A, Waterman
      C, Cavanagh PR, Boulton AJ. Diabetic peripheral neuropathy and depressive symptoms: the as-
      sociation revisited. Diabetes Care 2005;28:2378–83.
[59] Vileikyte L, Peyrot M, Bundy C, Rubin RR, Leventhal H, Mora P, Shaw JE, Baker P, Boulton AJ.
      The development and validation of a neuropathy- and foot ulcer-specific quality of life instru-
      ment. Diabetes Care 2003;26:2549–55.

218

S. Tesfaye

[60] Vileikyte L, Peyrot M, Gonzalez JS, Rubin RR, Garrow AP, Stickings D, Waterman C, Ulbrecht JS, Cavanagh PR, Boulton AJ. Predictors of depressive symptoms in persons with diabetic peripheral neuropathy: a longitudinal study. Diabetologia 2009;52:1265–73.
[61] Vinik A. The approach to the management of the patient with neuropathic pain. J Clin Endocrinol Metab 2010;95:4802–11.
[62] Vinik E, Hayes R, Oglesby A, Bastyr E, Barlow P, Ford-Molvik S, Vinik A. The development and validation of the Norfolk QOL-DN, a new measure of patients' perception of the effects of diabetes and diabetic neuropathy. Diabetes Technol Ther 2005;7:497–508.
[63] Ward JD, Simms JM, Knight G, Boulton AJM, Sandler DA. Venous distension in the diabetic neuropathic foot (physical sign of arteriovenous shunting). J R Soc Med 1983;76:1011–14.
[64] Young MJ, Boulton AJ, MacLeod AF, Williams DR, Sonksen PH. A multicentre study of the prevalence of diabetic peripheral neuropathy in the United Kingdom hospital clinic population. Diabetologia 1993;36:150–4.
[65] Zelman DC, Brandenburg NA, Gore M. Sleep impairment in patients with painful diabetic peripheral neuropathy. Clin J Pain 2006;22:681–5.
[66] Zelman DC, Gore M, Dukes E, Tai KS, Brandenburg N. Validation of a modified version of the Brief Pain Inventory for painful diabetic peripheral neuropathy. J Pain Symptom Manage 2005;29:401–10.
[67] Zhang WY, Li Wan Po A. The effectiveness of topically applied capsaicin: a meta-analysis. Eur J Clin Pharm 1994;46:517–22.
[68] Ziegler D, Nowak H, Kempler P, Vargha P, Low PA. Treatment of symptomatic diabetic polyneuropathy with the antioxidant alpha-lipoic acid: a meta-analysis. Diabet Med 2004;21:114–21.
[69] Zigmond AS, Snaith RP. The Hospital Anxiety and Depression Scale. Acta Psychiatr Scand 1983;67:361–70.
[70] Zinman LH, Ngo M, Ng ET, Nwe KT, Gogov S, Bril V. Low-intensity laser therapy for painful symptoms of diabetic sensorimotor polyneuropathy: a controlled trial. Diabetes Care 2004;27:921–4.

Correspondence to: Professor Solomon Tesfaye, MB ChB, MD, FRCP, Consultant Physician and Honorary Professor of Diabetic Medicine at the University of Sheffield, Royal Hallamshire Hospital, Glossop Road, Sheffield S10 2JF, United Kingdom. Email: solomon.tesfaye@sth.nhs.uk.

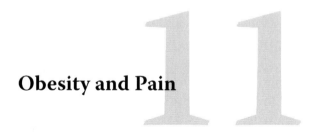

Obesity and Pain

Peggy Mason

Department of Neurobiology, University of Chicago, Chicago, Illinois, USA

The overweight and obesity epidemic is a modern phenomenon that came about when industrialization released us from constraints that have been present throughout evolutionary time. In the past, human adults, like other animals, needed to expend energy to acquire and consume food. Even for clever primates, the "profit" margin associated with feeding in a natural setting is slim, thereby ensuring an upper limit on adiposity. Situations that shift the balance—by decreasing the need for energy expenditure or by increasing the easy availability of energy-dense food, or both—produce net energy gain, with the result that animals gain weight. This scenario has occurred in diverse settings, from squirrels happening upon backyard bird feeders to laboratory rats fed a cafeteria diet [33] to olive baboons exposed to a dump containing discarded food [31].

Today, most Americans are overweight, with a steadily increasing proportion of the population qualifying as obese. Most Americans also experience some form of pain, such as lower back pain or headache, and often the condition is chronic. Thus, it is no surprise that a large number of overweight individuals experience chronic pain. The probability of two

Pain Comorbidities: Understanding and Treating the Complex Patient
edited by Maria Adele Giamberardino and Troels Staehelin Jensen
IASP Press, Seattle, © 2012

very common conditions occurring concurrently is simply the product of their individual probabilities. Clearly, the trick here is to tease apart whether a significant relationship exists between weight and pain and to discern any causal factors involved. It may be, as is often assumed, that extra weight leads to conditions such as lower back pain. It may also be that the pain experience alters neural control of energy balance, resulting in either under- or overweight individuals. Alternatively, there may be a common factor that predisposes individuals to both an abnormal energy balance state, either obesity or an underweight condition, and chronic pain. Finally, there may be different answers for different types of pain and for different energy imbalances.

Overweight or obesity is often defined by body mass index or BMI, a mass (kilograms) to height (square meters) calculation, with BMI values from 25 up to 30 defining overweight and those of 30 and above defining obesity. In particular, excess adipose tissue within the abdominal cavity, known as "central obesity," is thought to be mechanistically linked to adverse health outcomes, and therefore, variables that reflect central girth, such as waist circumference, are preferred over BMI. When central obesity occurs with hyperglycemia, hyperinsulinemia, glucose tolerance, high cholesterol, or related measures, the condition is known as "metabolic syndrome." Metabolic syndrome, more so than overweight or obesity, is the important condition to consider because it is the strongest predictor of cardiovascular disease and diabetes [20].

Does Being Overweight or Obese Lead to Chronic Pain Conditions?

Evidence for a significantly higher co-occurrence than would occur by chance of pain and obesity is underwhelming among the general adult population [16]. Among older adults (>55 years old), the prevalence of pain in men and women in the top quartile of weight (BMI or waist circumference) is about twice that of those in the lowest quartile [14]. In a population of elderly mobile adults (>70 years old), central obesity was associated with a doubling of reported chronic pain [27].

The pain conditions most often postulated to result from excess weight are musculoskeletal ones, including low back pain and osteoarthritis of the knee or hip [16]. Of these three conditions, the strongest association is between overweight and knee osteoarthritis. Even small increases in weight above normal levels are associated with an increase in the risk of knee osteoarthritis [5]. However, even pain conditions other than musculoskeletal pain are more prevalent in the obese, older population.

Mechanisms Supporting the Co-occurrence of Pain and Excess Weight

Even if we accept that there is a significant co-occurrence of at least some forms of chronic pain with being overweight or obese, we are no closer to understanding causality. To achieve any insight into potential underlying mechanisms we need to dissect the differences, and there are many, between overweight individuals and individuals of normal weight. Perhaps most obviously, the overweight person is mechanically carrying more mass than someone of normal weight, and indeed more than humans evolved to carry. Second, there are changes in the metabolic and hormonal internal milieu, including not only changes in directly relevant hormones such as leptin (released by adipocytes and associated with satiation) and ghrelin (opposes leptin-mediated functions by stimulating feeding), but also changes in less obviously related neuroactive substances such as endogenous opioid peptides. Third, there are a number of comorbidities such as diabetes, arteriosclerosis, lung disease and depression in people with pain [14]. Finally, pain may occur secondary to behaviors such as a sedentary lifestyle or smoking, which are more common among overweight and obese individuals than among individuals of normal weight.

Is Extra Mass Responsible for Increased Prevalence of Pain?

Standing humans have a center of mass located within the abdomen in the plane of the ankle joints. The ankle joints stabilize the standing body so that only a minimal contribution of force, mostly from contraction of the soleus muscle, is needed to maintain posture. In the case of overweight individuals, the center of mass is shifted so that it is no longer in the plane of the ankle joints. Thus, in the overweight and obese population, maintaining an upright posture requires steady muscular force to bring the center of body mass back to a point located above the feet. Even sitting may constitute a strenuous activity for an individual with a large waist circumference. More challenging postures associated with walking, running, jumping, and so on require an even greater contribution of muscular force to maintain balance and prevent falling. The steady strain placed on muscles and joints by excess weight and the shift away from the evolved center of mass are widely thought to contribute to painful conditions such as osteoarthritis and low back pain. Yet, as mentioned above, evidence for a significantly higher co-occurrence (than would occur by chance) of lower back pain and obesity is underwhelming.

There are several potential mitigating factors that may protect overweight individuals from musculoskeletal pain. First, the steady exercise required for overweight and obese individuals to maintain posture may lead to stronger postural muscles and hence more stabilized joints. In essence, even the sedentary life of sitting, standing, and walking while obese may involve a comparable amount of muscle strength in postural muscles as is required for an individual of normal weight to lead an active life. Second, the hormonal, neurochemical, and inflammatory milieu in overweight and obese individuals differs from that of normal and underweight individuals; whether these differences exacerbate or protect against pain is poorly understood.

In the natural experiment of pregnancy, a woman transiently carries up to 25–35 or so extra pounds and has a forward-shifted center of mass. The prevalence of lumbar or pelvic girdle pain occurring sometime during pregnancy is >50% [12,13,34,35], evidence that the mechanical impact of carrying extra weight can lead to musculoskeletal pain. The relatively high prevalence in pregnant women compared to overweight women is interesting in light of the different hormonal environments. Although the extra weight carried during pregnancy is not adipose tissue, the end of the second trimester is marked by high levels of leptin and low levels of ghrelin, the same mix that occurs in obese individuals [10, 32]. Accompanying these gut-active peptides is a mix of sex hormones specific to pregnancy. The complement of neuroactive substances present during pregnancy comes as a package deal, and any attempt to tease out the contribution of each substance to modulation of pain is likely to be relatively uninformative. Of greater importance is the effect of the total pregnancy "package." One estimate of this effect comes from a study on pregnant rats that showed analgesia in response to noxious cutaneous and visceral stimuli on the final day of gestation [15].

Most comorbidities that coexist along with pain fail to explain the increased prevalence of pain in obese individuals. For example, the inflammatory marker, C-reactive protein, is elevated in elderly adults with chronic pain, but this factor does not account for the high prevalence of pain in obese individuals [27]. Similarly insulin resistance, depression, and anxiety do not account for the high prevalence of pain in obese individuals. However, smoking may be a common risk factor for both pain and obesity [18].

Can Animal Studies Shed Any Light on Whether Obesity Causes Pain?

Most, but not all, animal studies report an increase in acute nociceptive responsiveness in obese rodents relative to lean controls [1,23,29; cf. 26]. Likely to be of more clinical importance are reports that obese rodents show a longer time course of pain behavior in response to peripheral nerve injury than do lean rats [23]. Yet even these studies do not demonstrate a causal linkage between obesity and pain behavior. The difficulty stems from the multitude of hormonal, physiological, and structural changes that accompany obesity.

Muncey et al. [23] studied rats selectively bred for either long or short exercise endurance. Animals with long endurance had a high aerobic capacity and were lean, and those with short endurance had low aerobic capacity and were more than 100 grams heavier. Thus, the animals with low aerobic capacity had physiological characteristics similar to those of patients with central obesity or metabolic syndrome. Correlating with the different aerobic capacities are differences in sleep, principally a loss of slow-wave sleep and an increase in wakefulness during the light phase of the day (the inactive period). As discussed in several reviews, sleep loss or fragmentation and chronic pain, particularly fibromyalgia, are mutually reinforcing [8,21]. Thus, even Muncey et al.'s finding that rats with low aerobic capacity, the obese ones, exhibit hyperalgesia for a significantly longer period after a chronic constriction injury than do lean rats is difficult to interpret. The prolonged pain response in these obese animals may be secondary to sleep disturbance, or it may indeed be caused by the excess weight, independently of any other factor.

Obesity does not occur in isolation. Obesity is inevitably accompanied by physiological, hormonal, and behavioral changes in rats as well as humans. For example, rats made obese by a high-fat diet show a decreased amount of exploratory behavior and spend more time stationary [1]. Associated with obesity are a number of hormonal and neurochemical changes including high levels of leptin, beta-endorphin, and corticosterone along with low levels of hormones such as ghrelin. Of course, there are critical changes in metabolism that can lead to insulin resistance and ultimately to the development of type 2 diabetes mellitus. The altered glucose and hormonal environment in obese individuals in turn can result in the development of diabetic neuropathy. Since so many bodily processes covary in obese animals, human and otherwise, ascribing causation to one or the other of the covarying measures is difficult or impossible.

Animal studies cannot provide us with information about spontaneous pain. While a human can attest to experiencing pain in one part of the body or another, an animal cannot. A frank decrease in motor activity, which could represent a pain response, is only likely to accompany severe pain. In order to infer mild to moderate nociception in an animal, we need to have a place to look—an injured paw, a flicking tail, and so on. To accomplish this, a stimulus is typically applied to query the animal. For example, heat or mechanical force is applied to the foot or tail, and the withdrawal latency is recorded. Alternatively, an injury to a nerve can produce measurable pain behaviors such as guarding or lifting a limb. However, if obesity causes a variety of aches and pains in the trunk and vertebral column, it is not clear that we would be able to recognize such sensations if they occurred. While it is possible that the obese animal that stays stationary is doing so because movement is painful, it is also possible that the animal is tired from a lack of sleep. In sum, animal studies are inherently limited when it comes to assessing widespread, spontaneous pain.

Does Chronic Pain Lead to Obesity?

Common sense suggests that some painful conditions may lead to a reduction in physical activity expended. In the light of modern society's ready access to energy-dense food, a reduction in energy expended may lead to net weight gain and perhaps eventually to obesity. However, there are hints of the converse relationship: nociception leading to anorexia and weight loss. Anorexia and cachexia are associated with rheumatoid arthritis, cancer (even in the absence of chemotherapy), and fever [4,22]. For example, during a fever, headache and muscle pains are common and are typically accompanied by anorexia [4]. Studies in rodents support a relationship between pain and anorexia. For example, as the tumor load in rats increases to roughly 1% of body weight, cortical, subcortical, and brainstem neurons are engaged, and rats reduce their food intake by 20% [17,30]. As another example, when a mixture of inflammatory agents is placed on the dura, a model of migraine, rats stop eating, just as humans do at the onset of a migraine attack [19]. Finally, migraine attacks affect 75% of those who suffer from anorexia nervosa (compared to 25% of the control population) and typically precede the onset of the eating disorder [25]. Thus, animal studies suggest that either chronic pain leads to anorexia or that a common physiological factor leads to both chronic pain and anorexia.

An Operational View of Feeding and Nociception

The weight of the evidence reviewed above suggests two speculative conclusions. The first conclusion is that individuals with excess weight, ranging from overweight to obese to metabolic syndrome, have a heightened risk of developing certain chronic pain conditions, especially when they are elderly. The second conclusion is that chronic pain may bias an individual toward anorexia and consequent loss of weight. However, both conclusions are only inconsistently supported by evidence, with numerous exceptions threatening to topple each conclusion altogether. Below, I argue that a more mechanistic, "nuts-and-bolts" approach may shed more light than the epidemiological or population-comparison approaches favored by the studies discussed above.

An operational approach differs from an epidemiological approach in several ways. Instead of looking at the relationship between obesity and pain by examining population statistics, emphasis is placed on how the neural systems regulating energy balance and nociception interact. A focus on nociception rather than pain is inclusive of reductions as well as increases in pain sensitivity. It is also inclusive of neuropathic pain, which is pain that occurs independently of a peripheral stimulus. In a parallel fashion, a focus on energy balance rather than on obesity allows for a full consideration of changes in both energy intake and energy expenditure. The relationship between energy balance and nociception is likely to be nuanced and heterogeneous. For example, noxious input from the oral cavity is likely to affect feeding in different ways compared to noxious input from an area uninvolved in the mechanics of eating. Finally, there is behavioral inertia, the principle that a current action is far more likely to be the action in the next moment in time than is any of a myriad of possible other actions. Because of behavioral inertia, the relative timing of nociceptive input, feeding, and energy expenditure will influence the actions that ensue.

From an operational point of view, the fundamental issue comes down to choices between (1) pain reactions or feeding, (2) pain reactions or exercise, and (3) feeding or exercise. The third choice is clearly important, but just as clearly beyond the purview of this chapter. Therefore, I will focus on the first two choices, particularly the choice between pain reactions and feeding. Most evidence supports the idea that animals across a wide phylogenetic range continue to eat and react minimally or not at all to noxious stimulation [2,3,9,11,36]. In other words, for a number of vertebrates and invertebrates, feeding trumps acute nociception, even in the absence of food restriction [9]. While consuming food, rats either do not withdraw or withdraw at long latency from a noxious stimulus [9]. Remarkably, this same selection of feeding occurs even when palatable substances are infused directly into the rat's oral cavity [7], evidence that food consumption rather than appetite or food procurement is the defended action. In other words, the action of consuming food takes precedence over reacting to a noxious stimulus. For animals in natural circumstances where food availability is unpredictable, such a bias toward feeding is likely to be advantageous.

In order to test whether a strong, yet ethical, noxious stimulus disrupts feeding, rats received either a saline or a formalin injection in the paw [6]. In response to formalin, rats show a stereotyped biphasic reaction, indicative of persistent, moderate pain, which includes favoring, lifting, and licking the paw over the course of about 1 hour. Remarkably, the amount of food consumed and the speed of food consumption were the same in rats receiving saline or formalin injections [6]. It is striking that rats almost always ate without exhibiting any pain behaviors. Occasionally they ate while favoring the paw, rarely while lifting the paw, and *never* while licking the paw. The simplest interpretation of the latter result is that licking the paw and eating are simply mutually exclusive actions because they employ common muscles. Favoring or lifting the paw are actions that *can* and do sometimes occur while eating, but eating while not fully balanced on the two hind legs renders the animal prone to falling over, and is therefore not a preferred solution. In short, action selection provides a heuristic framework within which to interpret the conflict between eating and reacting to noxious stimulation [28].

Many factors modulate the outcome of the eating versus pain behavior battle. At rest, eating is of high priority, an evolutionary holdover from the unpredictable and energy-poor food that dominates in the natural world. While ethical considerations preclude scientists from applying intense or enduring noxious stimuli, intensely injurious events as well as neuropathic pain do occur and are predicted to tip the balance away from eating and toward pain behavior. The location of perceived pain is also very important, with a wound on the nondominant hand wielding less influence than a cut on the lip, an attack of trigeminal neuralgia, or even a headache. Food deprivation, strenuous exercise, and energy-depleted states such as pregnancy are likely to tip action selection toward eating. Similarly, we are more apt to ingest highly palatable food than unpalatable food, so that we will more readily eat ice cream than a piece of dry toast when we have a sore throat. Thus whether eating or pain reactions win out depends on the type, intensity, location, and duration of pain on one hand and energy status and food palatability on the other. The bias toward eating observed in laboratory rats in the context of ad libitum chow and brief, mild to moderate noxious stimulation applied to the hindpaw probably reflects only one of many solutions to this conflict.

Because of individual differences, different people will react differently when confronted with the choice between eating and reacting to pain. Among a myriad of potentially important individual differences, two stand out. First, cultural differences heavily influence reactions to pain, biasing people more or less toward stoicism and high pain tolerance [37]. Second, there are huge differences in human eating patterns. For example, overweight individuals eat with little attention to satiety clues, whereas underweight and normal-weight individuals regulate food intake based on such clues [24]. Factoring in individual variability to the already complex relationship between energy balance and pain experience leads to an exponential increase in the possible outcomes to one choice, simple though it may be at its core.

References

[1]   Buchenauer T, Behrendt P, Bode FJ, Horn R, Brabant G, Stephan M, Nave H. Diet-induced obesity alters behavior as well as serum levels of corticosterone in F344 rats. Physiol Behav 2009;98:563–9.
[2]   Casey KL, Morrow TJ. Supraspinal nocifensive responses of cats: spinal cord pathways, monoamines, and modulation. J Comp Neurol 1988;270:591–605.
[3]   Davis WJ, Mpitsos GJ, Pinneo JM. The behavioral hierarchy of the mollusk *Pleurobranchaea*. I. The dominant position of the feeding behavior. J Comp Physiol 1974;90:207–24.
[4]   Eccles R. Understanding the symptoms of the common cold and influenza. Lancet Infect Dis 2005;5:718–25.
[5]   Flugsrud GB, Nordsletten L, Espehaug B, Havelin LI, Engeland A, Meyer HE. The impact of body mass index on later total hip arthroplasty for primary osteoarthritis: a cohort study in 1.2 million persons. Arthritis Rheum 2006;54:802–7.
[6]   Foo H, Crabtree K, Thrasher A, Mason P. Eating is a protected behavior even in the face of persistent pain in male rats. Physiol Behav 2009;97:426–9.
[7]   Foo H, Mason P. Analgesia accompanying food consumption requires ingestion of hedonic foods. J Neurosci 2009;29:13053–62.
[8]   Foo H, Mason P. Brainstem modulation of pain during sleep and waking. Sleep Med Rev 2003;7:145–54.
[9]   Foo H, Mason P. Sensory suppression during feeding. Proc Natl Acad Sci 2005;102:16865–9.
[10]   Fuglsang J, Skjaerbaek C, Espelund U, Frystyk J, Fisker S, Flyvbjerg A, Ovesen P. Ghrelin and its relationship to growth hormones during normal pregnancy. Clin Endocrinol 2005;62:554–9.
[11]   Gillette R, Huang RC, Hatcher N, Moroz LL. Cost-benefit analysis potential in feeding behavior of a predatory snail by integration of hunger, taste, and pain. Proc Natl Acad Sci USA 2000;97:3585–90.
[12]   Gutke A, Ostgaard HC, Oberg B. Pelvic girdle pain and lumbar pain in pregnancy: a cohort study of the consequences in terms of health and functioning. Spine 2006;31:E149–55.
[13]   Han IH. Pregnancy and spinal problems. Curr Opin Obstet Gynecol 2010;22:477–81.
[14]   Heim N, Snijder MB, Deeg DJ, Seidell JC, Visser M. Obesity in older adults is associated with an increased prevalence and incidence of pain. Obesity 2008;16:2510–7.
[15]   Iwasaki H, Collins JG, Saito Y, Kerman-Hinds A. Naloxone-sensitive, pregnancy-induced changes in behavioral responses to colorectal distention: pregnancy-induced analgesia to visceral stimulation. Anesthesiology 1991;74:927–33.

[16] Janke EA, Collins A, Kozak AT. Overview of the relationship between pain and obesity: What do we know? Where do we go next? J Rehabil Res Dev 2007;44:245–62.

[17] Konsman JP, Blomqvist A. Forebrain patterns of c-Fos and FosB induction during cancer-associated anorexia-cachexia in rat. Eur J Neurosci 2005;21:2752–66.

[18] Lake JK, Power C, Cole TJ. Back pain and obesity in the 1958 British birth cohort. cause or effect? J Clin Epidemiol 2000;53:245–50.

[19] Malick A, Jakubowski M, Elmquist JK, Saper CB, Burstein R. A neurohistochemical blueprint for pain-induced loss of appetite. Proc Natl Acad Sci USA 2001;98:9930–5.

[20] McKeigue PM, Shah B, Marmot MG. Relation of central obesity and insulin resistance with high diabetes prevalence and cardiovascular risk in South Asians. Lancet 1991;337:382–6.

[21] Moldofsky H. The significance of the sleeping-waking brain for the understanding of widespread musculoskeletal pain and fatigue in fibromyalgia syndrome and allied syndromes. Joint Bone Spine 2008;75:397–402.

[22] Morley JE. Anorexia in older persons: epidemiology and optimal treatment. Drugs Aging 1996;8:134–55.

[23] Muncey AR, Saulles AR, Koch LG, Britton SL, Baghdoyan HA, Lydic R. Disrupted sleep and delayed recovery from chronic peripheral neuropathy are distinct phenotypes in a rat model of metabolic syndrome. Anesthesiology 2010;113:1176–85.

[24] Nisbett RE. Determinants of food intake in obesity. Science 1968;159:1254–5.

[25] Ostuzzi R, D'Andrea G, Francesconi F, Musco F. Eating disorders and headache: coincidence or consequence? Neurol Sci 2008;29(Suppl 1):S83–7.

[26] Ramzan I, Wong BK, Corcoran GB. Pain sensitivity in dietary-induced obese rats. Physiol Behav 1993;54:433–5.

[27] Ray L, Lipton RB, Zimmerman ME, Katz MJ, Derby CA. Mechanisms of association between obesity and chronic pain in the elderly. Pain 2011;152:53–9.

[28] Redgrave, P, Prescott, TJ, Gurney, K. The basal ganglia: a vertebrate solution to the selection problem? Neuroscience 1999;89:1009–23.

[29] Roane DS, Porter JR. Nociception and opioid-induced analgesia in lean (Fa/-) and obese (fa/fa) Zucker rats. Physiol Behav 1986;38:215–8.

[30] Ruud J, Blomqvist A. Identification of rat brainstem neuronal structures activated during cancer-induced anorexia. J Comp Neurol 2007;504:275–86.

[31] Sapolsky RM. A primate's memoirs: a neuroscientist's unconventional life among the baboons. New York: Scribner; 2001.

[32] Sattar N, Greer IA, Pirwani I, Gibson J, Wallace AM. Leptin levels in pregnancy: marker for fat accumulation and mobilization? Acta Obstet Gynecol Scand 1998;77:278–83.

[33] Sclafani A, Springer D. Dietary obesity in adult rats: similarities to hypothalamic and human obesity syndromes. Physiol Behav 1976;17:461–71.

[34] Smith MW, Marcus PS, Wurtz LD. Orthopedic issues in pregnancy. Obstet Gynecol Surv 2008;63:103–11.

[35] Vermani E, Mittal R, Weeks A. Pelvic girdle pain and low back pain in pregnancy: a review. Pain Pract 2010;10:60–71.

[36] Wylie LM, Gentle MJ. Feeding-induced tonic pain suppression in the chicken: reversal by naloxone. Physiol Behav 1998;64:27–30.

[37] Zatzick DF, Dimsdale JE. Cultural variations in response to painful stimuli. Psychosom Med 1990;52:544–57.

Correspondence to: Peggy Mason, PhD, Department of Neurobiology, University of Chicago, 947 East 58th Street, Chicago, IL 60637, USA. Email: pmason@uchicago.edu

Headache and Cardiovascular Disease

Paolo Martelletti and Andrea Negro

Department of Clinical and Molecular Medicine, Sapienza University of Rome, and Regional Referral Headache Center, Sant'Andrea Hospital, Rome, Italy

Migraine affects 12% of adults in Western countries. Its prevalence is three times higher in women, but it is still the most prevalent neurological disorder in men [10]. The highest prevalence occurs between the ages of 25 and 55 years. Studies have found that migraine patients have a greater incidence of other illnesses than is seen in the general population.

Comorbidity in migraine is important from several perspectives: (1) Co-occurrence of diseases can complicate diagnosis, as in the case of the similar focal signs of migraine and stroke; (2) one disease can remind the clinician to rule out other diseases, as in the case of migraine and coronary disease; (3) one treatment can be used for two diseases, such as angiotensin-converting enzyme (ACE) inhibitors or sartans (angiotensin receptor blockers) for migraine patients with hypertension; and (4) comorbidities can provide clues to the pathophysiology of migraine.

Evidence of a link between headache symptoms and cardiovascular disease (CVD) has grown rapidly in recent years. This chapter provides a brief overview of different cardiovascular diseases that may be related to headache, including stroke, subclinical vascular brain lesions,

Pain Comorbidities: Understanding and Treating the Complex Patient
edited by Maria Adele Giamberardino and Troels Staehelin Jensen
IASP Press, Seattle, © 2012

hypertension, coronary heart disease, patent foramen ovale, atrial septal defects, atrial septal aneurysms, mitral valve prolapse, pulmonary arteriovenous malformations, and congenital heart disease.

Stroke

The association between migraine and ischemic stroke is well known from many case-control and cohort studies. The Atherosclerosis Risk in Communities Study in the United States, recording data from 12,750 African-American and white men and women, evaluated the occurrence of transient ischemic attack (TIA) symptoms and ischemic stroke events among those with a lifetime history of migraine or other headaches with some migrainous features [125]. The results showed that migraine with aura (MA) was associated with stroke symptoms (odds ratio [OR], 5.46), TIA symptoms (OR, 4.28), and verified ischemic stroke events (OR, 2.81). Similarly, other headaches with aura were significantly associated with stroke symptoms (OR, 3.68) and TIA symptoms (OR, 4.53). In contrast, the association for migraine without aura (MO) and other headaches without aura was not consistent. A meta-analysis of data pooled from 11 case-control and 3 cohort studies conducted prior to 2004 suggested a twofold risk of stroke in migraine (relative risk [RR], 2.16), both without aura (RR, 1.83) and with aura (RR, 2.27) [32].

Another important piece of evidence comes from a large prospective cohort analysis on the risk of ischemic stroke in the Women's Health Study (WHS) [70]. Nearly 40,000 U.S. health professionals aged 45 years and older, without a history of stroke, TIA, or an abnormal neurological examination, were followed for a mean of 9 years. In this prospective study, MA, but not MO, was associated with incidents of ischemic stroke (hazard ratio [HR], 1.70), with the risk most evident for those under 55 years of age (HR, 2.25). Data from the WHS have yielded a rich array of information on the risk of CVD in migraineurs. In a subgroup of 27,840 women from the WHS, those with MA were found to have a significantly increased risk of major CVD (multivariable-adjusted HR, 2.15; $P < 0.001$) [65]. After adjustment of the risk factors for major CVD, women with active MA, compared with women without a history of migraine, were shown to have an increased risk of ischemic stroke (HR, 1.9; $P = 0.01$).

Importantly, women who reported active MO did not show a significantly increased risk of any cardiovascular event, having incidence rates similar to women with no migraine history.

Furthermore, a recent report indicates that in the same study population, the association between MA and CVD varies according to vascular risk status. Ischemic stroke was associated with MA in women only in the lowest cardiovascular risk group (those with a low Framingham risk score, whose 10-year risk of coronary heart disease was less than 1%; HR, 3.88) [68]. Analysis of the individual components of the Framingham risk score revealed that this diametric pattern of association was driven by a particularly increased risk of ischemic stroke among women with active MA who were 45–49 years old (HR, 5.35; $P < 0.001$) and had low total cholesterol concentrations (HR, 4.01; $P = 0.03$). Among participants with any level of cardiovascular risk, those with MO were no more likely than nonmigraineurs to experience vascular events.

In the WHS population, the association between migraine and CVD varied by migraine frequency. Significant associations were only found among women with MA. Ischemic stroke was the only outcome associated with a high frequency of MA attacks (HR, 4.25), while a low frequency of attacks was associated with any vascular event (HR, 1.55) [69]. Data from WHS suggest that the association between MA and ischemic stroke is stronger in the absence of nausea and vomiting (HR, 3.27; $P < 0.0001$) than in the presence of these factors (HR, 0.91; $P = 0.80$) [114]. Additional discussions of the WHS data suggest that MA might be a predisposing factor for hemorrhagic stroke (HR, 2.25; $P = 0.024$), but definitive conclusions cannot be drawn because of the low number of events observed [66].

More recently, Becker et al. investigated the risk of stroke and TIA in migraineurs in a large retrospective case-control study using a research database of 3 million patients in the United Kingdom [7]. The study population consisted of 103,376 participants less than 80 years old who were identified within a 7-year study period, of whom 51,688 were classified as migraineurs. The relative risk of stroke of all types (thrombotic, hemorrhagic, and unspecified) was 2.2 among migraineurs compared with nonmigraineurs. Similarly, a history of migraine was associated with an odds ratio of 2.71 for the occurrence of stroke of all types after adjustment for age and cardiovascular risk factors. Other findings of interest from this study are that men with migraine were associated with nearly double (RR, 4.0) the already increased risk of TIA observed in female migraineurs (RR, 2.4).

With regard to the association between migraine and CVD in men, significant prospective data come from the Physicians' Health Study, which enrolled 20,084 apparently healthy U.S. male physicians aged 40–84 without a history of CVD [64]. Within this cohort, 1449 men (7.2%) reported migraine, and they were followed for a mean of 15.7 years. Migraine was not statistically significantly associated with increased risk of ischemic stroke (multivariable-adjusted HR, 1.12; $P = 0.43$). The association between migraine and ischemic stroke, however, was significantly modified by age, indicating an increased risk of ischemic stroke for men with migraine who were younger than 55 years old (RR, 1.84), but not for older age groups. The associations between migraine and major CVD and ischemic stroke are compatible with findings from the WHS.

One recent population-based study, part of the American Migraine Prevalence and Prevention (AMPP) study, with more than 120,000 Americans of both genders participating, found a positive association between MA and stroke in both men and women [9]. The results showed that migraine in general and MA were associated with stroke (OR, 1.61), although MO was not. After adjustment for age, gender, disability, treatment, and CVD risk factors, MA remained significantly associated with stoke (OR, 1.5).

In a population-based cohort study in 18,725 men and women, with a median follow-up of 25.9 years, people with MA were at increased risk of mortality from CVD (sex- and multivariable-adjusted HR, 1.27) and mortality from stroke (HR, 1.40), compared with people with no headache, while those with MO and nonmigraine headache were not at increased risk [48].

A recent systematic review and meta-analysis concluded that MA, as compared to MO, conferred a twofold increase in the risk of ischemic stroke (RR, 2.16 vs. RR, 1.23; meta-regression for aura status, $P = 0.02$). The risk appeared to be magnified in patients less than 45 years of age (RR, 2.65), females (RR, 2.08), smokers (RR, 9.03), and women using oral contraceptives (RR, 7.02) [116]. The risk of TIA among migraineurs was higher than that for ischemic stroke, being increased more than twofold (RR, 2.34).

Why MA might increase the risk of early-onset ischemic stroke is presently unknown. Possible mechanisms include hyperhomocystein-emia, patent foramen ovale, mitral valve prolapse, vasospasm, prothrom-botic factors, and endothelial dysfunction.

Subclinical Vascular Brain Lesions

Migraine has also been linked to silent infarct-like lesions. In a communi-ty-based cohort evaluated as a part of the CAMERA neuroimaging study, even if no significant difference was found between patients with migraine and controls in overall infarct prevalence (8.1% vs. 5.0%), individuals with migraine had a sevenfold increased risk for infarcts in the cerebellar re-gion of the posterior circulation territory (5.4% vs. 0.7%; P = 0.02; adjusted OR, 7.1) [61]. The adjusted OR for posterior infarct varied by migraine subtype and attack frequency, being 13.7 for patients with MA compared with controls, with a lesser risk of 9.3 for migraineurs whose attacks oc-curred less than once per month, and the highest risk of 15.8 in patients with MA with one or more attacks per month. However, it was unclear whether these findings have any clinical significance or whether there is any association with symptomatic stroke or vascular dementia later in life.

The same study group also demonstrated that 88% of infratentorial infarct-like lesions had a vascular border zone location in the cerebellum. They concluded that a combination of hypoperfusion (possibly migraine attack-related) and embolism is the most likely mechanism for posterior circulation infarction in migraine [60].

In the large cohort of Icelandic adults of the AGES-Reykjavik Study (2693 women and 1996 men), 12.2% of the participants (5.7% of men; 17.0% of women) were classified as having migraine. After more than 26 years since their initial headache diagnosis, an MRI scan was per-formed [112]. After adjustments were made for age, sex, and follow-up time in a pooled model for men and women, participants with mid-life MA were at increased risk for total infarcts (adjusted OR, 1.4). In unad-justed comparisons, infarcts overall were more prevalent in women with MA compared with women without headache (31% vs. 25%; P = 0.04), but there was no difference in prevalence for men (41% vs. 39%). This figure mainly reflects the risk associated with lesions located in the cerebellum (adjusted OR, 1.6). Infarcts in the cerebellum, but not in other locations, were more prevalent in women with MA compared with women without headache (23% vs. 15%; $P < 0.001$). The relationship between MA and cerebellar infarcts was significant only in women (men, adjusted OR, 1.0; women, adjusted OR, 1.9; $P = 0.04$ for interaction by sex). The study suggested that women who reported MA in middle age were at increased risk of late-life infarcts relative to those with no migraine symptoms, primarily as a result of cerebellar lesions.

More recently, the Epidemiology of Vascular Ageing study, recording data from 780 participants, confirmed that MA is the only headache type strongly associated with brain infarcts (OR, 3.4) [67]. The location of infarcts was predominantly outside the cerebellum and brainstem. However, there was no evidence that MA by itself or in combination with brain lesions was associated with cognitive impairment.

Hypertension

Although the possibility of a comorbidity between migraine and hypertension has long been suspected, the epidemiological evidence is controversial, with studies demonstrating positive, negative, or no correlation between the two diseases. Repeated migraine attacks over prolonged periods result in endothelial dysfunction and inflammatory arteriopathy of the cranial vessels, which leads to a reduction in the bioavailability of vasodilators and to an increase in endothelium-derived contracting factors [53]. Hypertension probably amplifies the effects of migraine on the vascular wall, further enhancing the endothelial dysfunction in the cerebral vasculature. It is also known that endothelial dysfunction leads to migraine [129]. The renin-angiotensin system, which is certainly involved in hypertension and has activity in the central nervous system, may be relevant in migraine pathogenesis [1].

Insulin resistance underlies the pathogenesis of obesity, diabetes, and hypertension, which are components of metabolic syndrome, and recent studies suggest that insulin resistance is more common in patients with migraine. Migraine prevalence in metabolic syndrome is higher

(11.9% in men and 22.5% in women) than in the general population. Of the various metabolic syndrome components, diabetes, increased waist circumference, and body mass index (BMI) are significantly more frequent in patients with migraine than in those without migraine ($P < 0.05$) [50].

Severe hypertension in the setting of new acute headache may indicate a serious underlying cause and requires urgent investigation. Hypertensive crises represent more than one in four medical emergencies. Hypertensive emergencies frequently involve headache (22%). Severe sustained hypertension, malignant hypertension, and paroxysmal hypertension (a sudden rise in blood pressure) are associated with severe headache. Transient hypertension can occur during an attack of migraine or cluster headache (CH).

A particular form of hypertension, pregnancy-induced hypertension with proteinuria (preeclampsia), is linked to increased vascular reactivity, endothelial damage, and platelet hyperaggregation, which are also typical features seen in migraine patients. In a case-control study, headache was significantly more frequent in women with preeclampsia than in controls (OR, 4.95), and it was more frequent in severe cases than in those with moderate preeclampsia (OR, 5.63). MO was more frequently present in cases than in controls, whereas episodic tension-type headache (TTH) was equally distributed among groups [33]. These findings are confirmed by a prospective cohort study in which a positive personal history of migraine in previously normotensive women was associated with a higher risk of hypertensive disorders compare to nonmigraineurs (9.1% vs. 3.1%; OR, 2.85) [34].

The prevalence of hypertension-migraine comorbidity was investigated in the MIRACLES study, a multicenter, cross-sectional survey including 2973 participants with a known diagnosis of hypertension or migraine [84]. The investigators reported that 17% of participants had hypertension-migraine comorbidity, whereas 43% had hypertension only, and 40% had migraine only. In the comorbidity group, the onset of comorbidity occurred at about 45 years of age, with migraine starting significantly later than in the migraine-only group, and hypertension occurring significantly earlier than in the hypertension-only group. Compared to participants with only hypertension (3.1%) or migraine (0.7%), the comorbidity group had a higher prevalence (4.4%) of history of cerebrovascular events, with an odds ratio of a predicted history of stroke/TIA of 1.76 compared to the hypertension group. Within the age range of 40–49 years, the prevalence of history of stroke/TIA was five times as great in the co-morbidity group (4.8% in the comorbidity group vs. 0.9% in the hypertension group).

Similar findings come from a study on the prevalence of cardio-vascular risk factors in 1343 patients with severe headache. Compared to controls, headache patients of both sexes had a higher prevalence of hypertension, independent of age (OR, 1.51) [26]. Furthermore, hypertension was the only cardiovascular risk factor that was highly prevalent in both male and female patients with headache, particularly in younger adults.

One indirect indication of a link between migraine and hypertension is also represented by the usefulness of some antihypertensive drugs in migraine preventive therapy. ACE inhibitors and sartans have migraine prophylactic properties similar to those of some currently used migraine-preventive agents. Thus, they may represent reasonable second- or third-line drugs [41]. Furthermore, drugs commonly used in the treatment of headache, such as beta-blockers and calcium channel antagonists, are also powerful antihypertensive drugs.

In patients with migraine and established hypertension, good control of blood pressure may be beneficial in controlling the frequency and severity of headache. However, given that many of the drugs used to treat hypertension may *cause* headache and some agents used to treat migraine can exacerbate hypertension, a careful consideration of the therapeutic options is needed. Moreover, if beta-blockers or calcium channel antagonists are used to treat headache, they could mask the development of hypertension in originally normotensive individuals; in these cases, hypertension could become evident only after withdrawal of the drugs used for headache treatment.

In a study in 1486 headache patients, 28% of the participants had hypertension, which was common in MO (23%) and MA (16.9%), and much more so in medication overuse headache (MOH) (60.6%), chronic TTH (55.3%), CH (35%), and episodic TTH (31.4%) [99]. In all headache groups, the prevalence of hypertension was higher than in the general population, within all age groups. Similar findings come from a study evaluating the distribution of hypertension in a sample of migraineurs in comparison with a group with TTH. Hypertension prevalence was highest in patients with TTH, supporting the hypothesis that this type of headache might have vascular mechanisms [102]. There also appears to be an association between hypertension and the prevalence of MA [26].

Migraine is positively correlated with diastolic blood pressure (DBP), but negatively correlated with systolic blood pressure (SBP) and pulse pressure. In a population-based study, for an increase in DBP of one standard deviation (SD), the probability of having migraine increased by 14% (P = 0.11) for men and 30% (P < 0.0001) for women, whereas for similar increases in SBP and pulse pressure, respectively, the probability of having migraine decreased by 19% (P = 0.007) and 13% (P = 0.005) for men and by 25% (P < 0.0001) and 14% (P < 0.0001) for women [49].

Individuals affected by chronic daily headache (CDH) evolving from initially episodic migraine are more likely to be hypertensive than individuals with episodic headaches [87]. According to the AMPP study, hypertension occurs with greater frequency in chronic migraine than in episodic migraine (33.7 vs. 27.9%, OR, 1.23; P = 0.021) [17]. Hypertension is also more frequent in CDH than in chronic TTH (16.2% vs. 6.6%; P < 0.01) [45]. It is possible to conclude that there is an association between CDH and hypertension, but it is not necessarily a causal relationship. However, hypertension may increase the frequency and severity of migraine in migraineurs and may transform episodic migraine into CDH [88].

A randomized case-control study on chronic migraine and comorbidities related to migraine transformation demonstrated a strong association between chronic migraine and hypertension when compared to both episodic migraine (OR, 6.9; P < 0.0001) and chronic post-traumatic headache (OR, 5.1; P = 0.0003) [11]. Hypertension has also been identified as the second most important factor, after drug overuse, favoring the transformation of episodic to chronic migraine [46].

In age-controlled analyses, the prevalence of cardiovascular risk factors is not significantly different among patients with different forms of headache, except for CH. Compared to patients with other types of headache, men with CH, but not women, had a greater prevalence of cigarette smoking, a lower prevalence of hypercholesterolemia, and a trend toward a low prevalence of hypertension [26]. The prevalence of hypertension in

CH patients is 35% [99]. During a cluster period, but outside an actual attack, DBP is higher than outside a cluster period (80.3 [SD, 12.2] vs. 74.8 [SD, 9.0]; $P = 0.04$) [133].

Cardiac Cephalgia

The 2004 International Classification of Headache Disorders includes cardiac cephalgia in the group of secondary headaches attributed to disorders of homeostasis. This type of headache is associated with an ischemic cardiovascular event and is difficult for the physician to recognize [54]. Patients with ischemic heart disease typically present with chest pain and breathlessness either on exertion or at rest.

Likewise, several population-based studies have found that participants with migraines are more likely to report chest pain, although others have reported no association. Symptoms of atypical presentation of acute coronary syndrome include shortness of breath, dyspnea on exertion, toothache, abdominal pain, back pain, and throat pain.

Cardiac ischemia can also lead to headache, especially exertional headache, that can mimic a form of migraine, sometimes accompanied by autonomic symptoms (such as photophobia, phonophobia, osmophobia, and nausea) in 30% of cases. Sometimes cardiac cephalgia can resemble a form of TTH; on other occasions, it exhibits characteristics that can hardly be interpreted as typical of primary headache. Symptoms related to the underlying disorder—such as chest constriction, pain in the left arm radiating up to the mandible, or epigastric pain—occur in 50% of reported cases [12]. In 27% of the cases described in the literature, however, cardiac cephalgia is the only manifestation of a cardiovascular ischemic event [12].

The explanation as to why a referred headache can appear as one (or the only) manifestation of myocardial ischemia is speculative. Possible mechanisms are (1) the anatomical convergence of cardiac nerve fibers and somatic efferents from the head, (2) increased intracranial pressure secondary to decreased cardiac output during ischemia, and (3) unidentified headache mediators released by cardiac ischemia. The clinician should suspect a myocardial cause if the headache is exercise-induced and is relieved by nitrates [98]. Headache as the only manifestation of an acute coronary event should be suspected in case of (1) older age at onset, (2) no past medical history of headache, (3) risk factors for vascular disorders, and (4) onset of headache under stress [120].

Because it is associated with a cardiovascular event, cardiac cephalgia generally occurs after the fifth decade of life in subjects at risk for CVD who may not have previously suffered from headache [3,14,28,86,56]. The headache may start after physical exertion, even after a mild physical activity such as walking. In the so-called "walk headache" [22,27,63,73], pain appears almost instantly after starting exercise, but will disappear in a few minutes as soon as the patient stops exercising. In 33% of cases, headache appears at rest. The frequency of this type of headache is highly variable; it may appear only in concomitance with an acute cardiovascular event [3,5,15,35,47,58,121], or it may be more frequent, sometimes occurring daily [14,86], for periods lasting from a few weeks [14,22,77,111] to several years [28,38,73,111]. Pain location is highly variable.

Fifty-seven percent of cardiac cephalgia patients show pathological alterations of the baseline ECG trace, such as ST-segment elevations or depressions and T-wave inversions [3,14,15,22,35,38,47,58,103,111,121], as well as elevated cardiac enzymes [3,15,35,38,47,58,73,121]. However, there are cases in which the ECG may look perfectly normal at rest, with pathological alterations only under stress [22,73,77,86,111,135]. Exertional headache may reflect underlying symptomatic coronary artery disease, even when conventional ECG stress testing does not indicate ischemia [28]. Sometimes routine examinations, cardiac enzymes, ECG tests, and even exercise stress tests prove negative. In such cases, only a coronary angiogram can provide sufficient evidence for diagnosis. Cardiac cephalgia may occur again in the event of coronary artery restenosis.

This form of headache does not respond to nonsteroidal anti-inflammatory drugs [103,111], and triptans are contraindicated. In contrast, it responds to therapy with nitrate derivatives, drugs that are used to treat CVD.

Coronary Heart Disease

For decades, the association between migraine and coronary disease has been a topic of great debate. An underlying vascular component suggests the plausibility of an association between migraine and coronary heart disease (CHD). In support of a shared genetic basis, previous studies have reported that migraineurs are more likely than controls to report a family history of early myocardial infarction [113]. However, the literature is inconclusive. Some population-based studies report an increased occurrence of CHD among migraineurs [23,76,90], but others have found no association [27].

Findings from the WHS suggest that women with MA (but not MO) have a twofold increased risk of major cardiovascular events (multivariable-adjusted HR, 2.15; $P < 0.001$), myocardial infarction (HR, 2.08; $P = 0.002$), coronary revascularization (HR, 1.74; $P = 0.002$), angina (HR, 1.71; 95% CI, 1.16–2.53; $P = 0.007$), and death because of ischemic cardiovascular disease (HR, 2.33; $P = 0.01$) compared with those with no migraine history. Conversely, women with continued active MO did not appear to be at greater risk for ischemic vascular events [65]. In contrast to ischemic stroke, the association between myocardial infarction and active MA was demonstrated only in those with a high Framingham risk score (a 10-year risk of coronary heart disease of more than 10%; HR, 3.34), particularly among women with high total cholesterol concentrations [114].

In post hoc subgroup analyses of the WHS, a randomized trial tested 100 mg aspirin on alternate days in primary prevention of CVD among 39,876 women aged 45 years and older. Women with MA who were taking aspirin had an increased risk of myocardial infarction (RR, 3.72) when compared with women with MA assigned to aspirin placebo, but the difference was only apparent among those who had ever smoked or who had a history of hypertension (P for interaction < 0.01) [63].

The Physicians' Health Study yielded data on the association of migraine and CVD in men. Within a cohort of 20,084 apparently healthy U.S. male physicians aged 40–84 without a history of CVD, 1449 individuals (7.2%) had migraine, with a subset of 434 patients (2.2%) having "frequent migraine." During a 15.7-year mean follow-up, men with migraine showed an increased incidence of cardiovascular events, primarily myocardial infarction. After adjusting for cardiovascular risk factors, investigators found that male migraineurs had a hazard ratio of 1.24 ($P = 0.008$) for major CVD, 1.42 ($P < 0.001$) for myocardial infarction, 1.05 ($P = 0.54$) for coronary revascularization, 1.15 ($P = 0.068$) for angina, and 1.07 ($P = 0.65$) for ischemic cardiovascular death. Unfortunately, it is not clear whether these risks were occurring in patients with MA or MO because those data were not available [64].

A systematic meta-analysis of case-control and cohort studies investigated the association between any migraine or specific migraine subtypes and CVD. Although the sensitivity analysis found no significant overall association between any migraine and myocardial infarction (RR, 1.12), sex-stratified analyses revealed that the pooled RR was 1.41 among women and 1.38 among men [116]. The analysis did not suggest an overall association (pooled RR, 1.03), but it did detect an increased risk among women (RR, 1.60).

Recently, the AMPP study in 120,000 adults showed that both MA and MO are associated with CVD and with risk factors for CVD. In multivariate analyses, after adjustment for gender, age, disability, treatment, and CVD risk factors, overall migraine was significantly associated with myocardial infarction (OR, 2.16) and claudication (OR, 2.69). In this study, both MA and MO were associated with myocardial infarction (OR, 2.86 for MA; OR, 1.85 for MO) and claudication (OR, 4.61 for MA; OR, 3.11 for MO) [9].

Conversely, in a population-based cohort study with 18,725 men and women, MA was associated with an increased risk of mortality from CVD (sex- and multivariable-adjusted HR, 1.27) and coronary heart disease (HR, 1.28) compared with no headache [48]. No such association was found for MO and nonmigraine headache.

Angina

In 1971, Sampson reported that in a group of 150 patients with angina pectoris, only 6% complained of headache [110]. Since then, case reports and clinical studies have suggested a positive association between migraine and variant angina [71,75,89]. The high prevalence of migraine and Raynaud's phenomenon in variant angina raises the possibility that a common underlying defect or mechanism may partially account for all three conditions [8,51].

Headache could be the only manifestation of angina pectoris, occurring both at rest and after exertion [24]. The Atherosclerosis Risk in Communities Study found that patients with migraine and other types of headache are more likely to have a history of angina than those without a headache history [107]. After more than 10 years of follow-up, the associations were stronger for migraine and other headaches with aura symptoms (prevalence ratio [PR], 3.0 and PR, 2.0 for women; PR, 2.2 and PR, 2.4 for men) than for migraine and other headaches without aura (PR, 1.5 and PR, 1.3 for women; PR, 1.9 and OR, 1.4 for men). Nevertheless, there was no significant association between migraine and other headaches with CHD, regardless of the presence of aura.

Additional analysis of the WHS data found the strongest association for angina among women with prior migraine (HR, 1.70; $P = 0.001$), but there was also an association for women with active migraine occurring with a frequency of less than once a month (HR, 1.48; $P = 0.01$) [69]. Results of a recent systematic review and meta-analysis on the association between migraine or specific migraine subtypes and CVD indicate that the risk of angina in relation to migraine was slightly, but significantly, increased by about 30% (pooled RR, 1.29), with a higher risk in women than in men [116]. Only one study has presented analyses stratified by migraine aura status, suggesting a significantly increased risk in people who had MA (RR, 1.71; $P = 0.007$) but not in people with MO [65].

Cardiovascular Risk Factors

The mechanisms that link migraine to ischemic vascular disease remain uncertain. Cortical spreading depression, the presumed substrate of aura, may directly predispose the patient to brain lesions, which would explain why MA is consistently demonstrated as a risk factor for cerebral ischemia, while for MO the evidence is less consistent [8]. The precise biological mechanism by which MA may increase the risk of vascular events is currently unknown and is likely to be complex.

An unfavorable cardiovascular risk profile could itself be a predisposing factor for the development of headache. Several important risk factors for long-term vascular morbidity cluster in children and adolescents with severe or recurrent headache or migraine. Mean values for BMI, C-reactive protein, and homocysteine were higher in children with headache than in those without headache, and more children with headache were in the highest quintile of risk for these factors. Serum and red blood cell folate levels were lower in children with headache [95].

Data from the WHS indicate statistically significant odds of higher total cholesterol (OR, 1.09; P = 0.02), non-high-density lipoprotein cholesterol (OR, 1.14; P = 0.002), apolipoprotein B-100 (OR, 1.09; P = 0.03), and C-reactive protein (OR, 1.13; P = 0.002) among women who reported any history of migraine [62].

A study in 620 current migraineurs from the Genetic Epidemiology of Migraine (GEM) study, a population-based study in the Netherlands, showed that compared to controls, migraineurs with aura were more likely to have an unfavorable cholesterol profile, with total cholesterol ≥240 mg/dL) (OR, 1.43), a ratio of total cholesterol to high-density lipoprotein of more than 5.0 (OR, 1.64), and elevated blood pressure (SBP > 140 mm Hg or DBP > 90 mm Hg) (OR, 1.76) [113].

The AMPP study indicated that cardiac risk factors, including hypertension, diabetes, high cholesterol, and obesity, are also significantly more likely to be reported by those with chronic migraine than those with episodic migraine [17]. In another study, compared with control subjects, participants with migraine had elevated SBP, DBP, glucose, insulin, and plasma endothelin, and increased intima-media thickness of the carotid artery. The association with vascular risk factors strongly suggests that migraine could increase the risk for atherosclerosis [52].

Peripheral concentrations of endothelin—a vasoactive peptide produced by vascular smooth muscle cells and a marker for endothelial injury and atherosclerosis—were found to be increased during CH attacks (P < 0.05) [40]. In keeping with data on endothelial dysfunction in migraineurs, a recent study measured levels of circulating endothelial progenitor cells (EPCs) in patients with TTH, MA, and MO and in healthy nonmigraine controls. The study provided evidence of reduced endothelial repair capacity in patients with migraine [74]. Migraineurs, especially those with MA, presented lower levels of EPCs (P < 0.001 in TTH vs. MO; P = 0.001 in MO vs. MA), whereas patients with TTH did not differ in EPC number from the healthy controls. Decreased numbers of EPCs have been independently associated with increased risk of cardiovascular events, and elevated EPCs have been associated with a more favorable prognosis after stroke [55,123].

A possible mechanism linking headache to cardiovascular risk profile is that headache, especially if frequent, may lead to decreased physical activity [134] and an unhealthy lifestyle [105]. Data from the HUNT study, a Norwegian study that examined the relationship between recurrent headache disorders and lifestyle factors, indicate that Framingham risk score is elevated in nonmigraine headache (OR, 1.17) and MO (OR, 1.17) and is most pronounced among individuals with MA (OR, 1.54). In both MO and nonmigrainous headache, increased vascular risk was based on unhealthy lifestyle behaviors (smoking, high BMI, and low physical activity), but such factors did not explain the elevated risk associated with MA [139]. One longitudinal study found that adolescents with frequent headache are twice as likely to be smokers in adulthood [138].

Unique to CH compared with all other primary headache conditions is its association with a personal history of cigarette smoking. Studies have indicated that greater than 80% of CH patients have a prolonged history of tobacco usage prior to CH onset [115]. Furthermore, results from the United States Cluster Headache Survey, the largest survey ever done of CH patients living in the United States, suggest that CH may result from secondhand cigarette smoke exposure during childhood [108]. More than 60% of nonsmoking CH patients have parents who smoke; in comparison, in the U.S. population as a whole, 25% of children aged 3–11 years lives with at least one parent who smokes [132].

Cardiovascular risk factors such as smoking and dyslipidemia are also known to cause endothelial dysfunction, which recent evidence implicates to be part of migraine pathogenesis [52,74,129]. A recent review and meta-analysis of data prior 2009 indicate that MA is associated with a twofold increased risk of ischemic stroke (RR, 2.16 vs. RR, 1.23; meta-regression for aura status, $P = 0.02$). Risk of ischemic stroke proved to be further increased for MA patients who smoke (RR, 9.03) [116].

Another possibility is that there are genetic or environmental causes common to both headache and an unfavorable cardiovascular risk profile. In this line, chronic migraine patients are more likely to have a negative family history of stroke compared to other headache types (OR, 0.11; $P = 0.036$), suggesting that chronic migraine is more likely to be a neuronal disease rather than a vascular one [141].

Cardiovascular risk factors should be addressed and managed when possible, and MA itself should be treated as a modifiable risk factor, especially in the context of data suggesting that more frequent attacks increase the risk for myocardial infarction and stroke [68]. Some risk factors are avoidable, such as smoking and use of oral contraceptives, which have been shown to result in markedly increased risk of a vascular event in the headache patient. In the GEM study, women with MA were more likely to be using oral contraceptives (OR, 2.06) [113].

Findings from Stroke Prevention in Young Women study indicate that women with MA who smoke and are using oral contraceptives are at a 1.5-fold increased risk of stroke, but women with MA who use oral contraceptives but do not smoke are not at increased risk of stroke. The combined effect of MA, smoking, and use of oral contraceptives was surprising, however, carrying a statistically significant odds ratio of 7.0 compared with individuals with MO and similar use of tobacco and oral contraceptives. This increased risk was even more prominent (OR, 10.0) when compared with nonsmoking women without a history of migraine who were not using oral contraceptives [83].

Strong recommendations have been made for women with active MA to avoid oral contraceptives, especially if they smoke or have other risk factors for CVD, or a history of thrombosis. There is some controversy about the absolute versus relative contraindication regarding the use of oral contraceptives. Although the Stroke Prevention in Young Women study [83] suggests no additional risk of ischemic stroke in women with MA who are taking oral contraceptives, many studies and a meta-analysis indicate that MA and oral contraceptive use are associated with an eightfold increase in stroke risk [32].

Structural Cardiac Anomalies

Migraine is more prevalent among people with a right-to-left shunt (caused by atrial septal defects or pulmonary arteriovenous malformations) and among those with altered cardiac anatomy (mitral valve prolapse, atrial septal aneurysm, or congenital heart disease) [118].

Patent Foramen Ovale

Patent foramen ovale (PFO), an abnormality in the atrial septum allowing blood flow between the right and left atrium, is present in around 27% of the normal adult population [51]. Although mean pressure in the left atrium is mostly higher than that at the opposite side, a right-to-left shunt (RLS) may occur in these patients during transient reversals of the pressure gradient, specially during the Valsalva maneuver or with diseases leading to increased pulmonary vascular resistance. PFO has been implicated in various pathological conditions such as paradoxical embolism, platypnea-orthodeoxia syndrome, and diving decompression syndromes, as well as cryptogenic stroke (i.e., stroke of unknown cause) and migraine.

Although the mechanism for a potential causal relationship between PFO and migraine is not clear, recent evidence suggests that microembolization resulting in brief episodes of cerebral hypoxia/ischemia can trigger cortical spreading depression, a phenomena that is felt to be the underlying mechanism of MA [97]. Consistent with the hypothesis of paradoxical embolization, both aspirin and warfarin have reduced the incidence of migraine [16,39].

The RLS of blood in a patient with a PFO, whatever the mechanism, may be the most potent trigger of migraine attacks in both MA and MO and the main determinant of aura in MA, serving as a conduit for chemicals that would exert a trigger effect on hyperexcitable neurons, leading to the development of migraine. Furthermore, MA is more prevalent in clinical entities associated with RLS (e.g., cryptogenic stroke, decompression illness in divers, hereditary hemorrhagic telangiectasia, and pulmonary arteriovenous fistulas).

Two Italian groups were the first to report a higher prevalence of PFO in subjects with MA, but not MO, suggesting that RLS could be associated with an increased risk of stroke and also involved in the mechanism of aura [30]. These preliminary data were later confirmed by a study in a cohort of 581 young ischemic stroke patients [72] that showed a prevalence of migraine in 27% of subjects with PFO and in 14% of patients without PFO. PFO was significantly associated with migraine after adjustment for age and sex (OR, 1.75).

Following initial reports, case-control, meta-analytic, and population-based studies over the past decade have suggested that PFO is more common in MA patients and that MA is more common in patients with PFO than in the general population [29,57,117]. PFO is found in 40–70% of subjects with MA and MO as compared to 25% of people in the general population [21,29,36,51,126]. There is a positive connection between prevalence of migraine and the size of the PFO and RLS activity [4,21,56,119].

The odds of a patient with migraine having a PFO is 2.5 times greater than the odds of PFO in those without migraine [117]. For a person with a PFO, the odds of having migraine is 5.1 times greater and the odds of having MA is 3.21 greater than for a person without a PFO [117]. The combination of MA and RLS has also been shown to be a strong and independent predictor for persistent migraine [57]. Moreover, PFO prevalence in MA patients is associated with the clinical features of their aura, being statistically significantly higher in association with an atypical than with a typical presentation (79.2% vs. 46.3%; $P = 0.009$) [85].

However, conflicting data on the association or independence of these conditions have been reported by various study groups around the world. A large-scale case-control study found no association between migraine and the presence of PFO or the severity of shunt across the PFO, nor did it find a difference in PFO prevalence in those with MA and those without [42]. Even though there were a number of methodological flaws in this study, these findings are consistent with those of a population-based study that evaluated more than 1000 healthy volunteers and found no difference in the prevalence of PFO between subjects with and without self-reported migraine [109].

A recent study observed the occurrence of attacks of MA in close temporal relationship with the injection of microbubbles. The attacks occurred in patients with permanent RLS, while no attacks were reported in patients with latent or no shunt, suggesting that shunting itself may have triggered the attacks [19]. These data suggest RLS may represent the trigger of MA in a subset of migraineurs who have PFO.

The association of PFO with other primary headaches has been investigated less than the association with migraine. PFO does not appear to be significantly associated with TTH [91]. Conversely, a relatively higher PFO rate was found in CH, a distinct primary head pain disorder, suggesting that RLS could facilitate headaches in a nonspecific way [79]. Three Italian studies have reported on RLS in CH. Finocchi et al. demonstrated that RLS was 2.5 times more frequent in 40 CH patients than in 40 controls who were free of headache and cerebrovascular diseases (42.5% vs. 17.5%; $P = 0.029$; OR, 3.48) [37]. Morelli et al. showed that RLS was significantly more frequent in CH than in controls (37% vs. 18.3%; $P < 0.005$) [92]. Dalla Volta et al. found that in a population of 38 patients with CH, 14 subjects (36.8%) were PFO carriers [29]. An interesting, although not statistically significant, finding was that the frequency of RLS was also higher in subjects with hemicrania continua and paroxysmal hemicrania and SUNCT (short-lasting unilateral neuralgiform headache with conjunctival injection and tearing) (60%) as compared to controls (20%). These results indicate that RLS may be nonspecifically linked to distinct primary headaches [2].

Several surgical techniques are available to correct PFO, and the link between PFO closure and resolution of migraine has been investigated in various studies. Multiple open-label, retrospective, and case-controlled studies have noted a link between PFO closure and improvement of migraine headache. Benefits were apparent in patients undergoing PFO closure for secondary prevention of paradoxical embolism [43,81,130,137], in patients with high-risk anatomical and functional characteristics predisposing them to paradoxical embolism without previous cerebral ischemia [81,104], and in patients undergoing PFO closure solely for migraine headaches refractory to medical treatment [118]. The benefit was evident at a mid-term follow-up and also seemed to persist for a longer period (4–5 years) [43,104].

A recent systematic review of 11 studies (1306 patients) evaluating PFO closure found that the procedure resolved or significantly improved migraine in 83% of patients, providing a complete cure in 46%. Forty percent of the participants had migraines, and most had a previous history of TIA/stroke. A greater proportion (84%) of subjects with MA experienced complete resolution or significant improvement compared to those with MO (77%) ($P = 0.03$, with a risk difference between the two forms of migraine of 0.10) [18]. These results suggest that a significant group of subjects with migraine, particularly if treated after a neurological event, may benefit from percutaneous closure of their PFO. The improvement in MA and MO appears to be independent of migraine type, gender, age, cerebrovascular risk factors and cerebrovascular events, type of cardiac defect, and thrombophilic conditions [25].

Because of the clear limitations of the early uncontrolled studies that reported a benefit of PFO closure on migraine outcome, the Migraine Intervention with STARFlex Technology (MIST) trial was undertaken [31].

This was the first, and remains the only completed, randomized, double-blind, sham-controlled trial analyzing the effect of PFO closure on migraine. One hundred forty-seven patients with a history of severe migraine headache and without other indications for PFO closure were randomized to undergo either PFO closure (via implantation of a septal repair device) or a sham procedure. The trial failed to reach its primary endpoint (complete cessation of migraines) or its secondary goal (a 50% reduction in migraine days). However, it did confirm an association between MA and severe PFO shunts (38% of patients had RLS consistent with a moderate or large PFO) and showed a significant reduction of MA after device implantation, compared with the sham procedure. MIST demonstrated much less benefit from PFO closure than the other studies with patients who had experienced neurological events. However, a significant difference between the MIST trial and the other studies must be underlined—the MIST trial treated only patients with MA and no history of previous paradoxical embolization, while in retrospective studies the majority of migraine patients had a history of embolic stroke. It is possible that subjects with MA, but without a history of previous paradoxical embolization, such as those treated in the MIST trial, could represent a subset of patients in whom PFO closure has little impact.

The MIST trial, despite significant limitations, does show that there is little support for advocating PFO closure to prevent migraine attacks. Moreover, clinical experience indicates that closure of a PFO or atrial septal defect can aggravate migraine suddenly. Currently, the labeled indication for PFO device closure is recurrent stroke in patients who have had an event despite treatment, or who are not candidates for anticoagulation. The data we have at present suggest that PFO closure be considered for migraineurs only if there are also risk factors for ischemic stroke, such as atrial septal aneurysm, hypercoagulability disorder, peripheral venous thrombosis, or previous paradoxical embolism [33,122].

Atrial Septal Defects

There is evidence that migraine is associated with atrial septal defects (ASDs). Although ASDs are characterized by a predominant left-to-right shunt (LRS) of blood, RLS may occur during the Valsalva maneuver or other activities increasing pressure in the right atrium [93]. Interatrial communications may play a role in the etiology of migraine attacks, either through paradoxical embolism or via humoral factors that escape degradation in bypassing the pulmonary circulation.

Several studies, most of them primarily examining the relationship between PFO and migraine, also included small numbers of subjects with ASDs. Findings on the effects of ASD repair and the prevalence and outcome of migraine have not constantly shown any significant benefit [6,93], but when there was a benefit, it was greater for MA than for MO [82]. Moreover, as in the case of PFO closure, new-onset migraine may occur following ASD closure. The problem may be due to the formation of thrombi on the occlusion device, an intra-atrial pressure imbalance, or the liberation of vasoactive substances [93,140].

After ASD closure, new-onset MA occurs in 7% of patients and persists in most cases after a mean follow-up of 2 years. ASD closure was the only independent predictor of migraine attack occurrence after the procedure [106]. Patients with ASDs are at increased risk of atrial tachyarrhythmias for a variety of reasons when compared with the general population [80]. Furthermore, iatrogenic ASDs due to atrial septal puncture during catheter ablation for atrial fibrillation rarely (2.3%) cause new-onset migraine, and when they do, it is usually temporary [96].

Atrial Septal Aneurysm

Only one study has investigated the prevalence of atrial septal aneurysm (ASA) in migraineurs. ASA was identified in 13.3% of migraine subjects compared to 1.9% of controls ($P < 0.05$). The increased frequency of ASA among migraineurs was isolated to subjects with aura [20].

Migraine was more common in patients with PFO (27.3%) than in those without PFO (14.0%). PFO (OR, 1.75; 95% CI, 1.08–2.82), particularly when associated with atrial septal aneurysm (OR, 2.71; 95% CI, 1.36–5.41), was significantly associated with migraine after adjustment for age and sex [72]. Although ASA has an association with MA, it does not seem to be significantly associated with TTH [91].

Mitral Valve Prolapse

Results from several observational studies have suggested an association between mitral valve prolapse (MVP) and migraine. In MVP patients, the prevalence of migraine is 27.8%, higher than that in the general population, and the migraine occurs with aura in 30% of cases [78]. The odds ratio of having MVP in the presence of MA is 2.7 [124].

The nature of the association between MVP and migraine is uncertain. Arguments for a causal association are based on reduced platelet survival and platelet aggregation in individuals with MVP. Damaged platelets release serotonin, which has been implicated to play a role in the generation of migraine headache. Furthermore, in patients with migraine, MVP can be associated with abnormalities of hemostasis, such as positive anticardiolipin titers, especially in migraine with aura [127]. There also seems to be an association between irritable bowel syndrome and MVP and autonomic and hemostatic abnormalities in migraineurs of all ages [59].

Pulmonary Arteriovenous Malformations

An increased prevalence of MA was also found in subjects with noncardiac causes of RLS, such as in patients with pulmonary arteriovenous malformations (AVMs). There is evidence that the presence of pulmonary AVMs increases the risk of migraine.

Pulmonary AVMs are found in more than one-third of people with hereditary hemorrhagic telangiectasia (HHT), and HHT is the underlying disorder accounting for pulmonary AVMs in 70% of cases [94]. Since pulmonary AVMs result in RLS of blood, the HHT population is an interesting group within which to examine the association between RLS and migraine. In a cohort of 588 patients with HHT, pulmonary AVMs were found in 208 subjects (38.7%). The occurrence of pulmonary AVMs in patients with migraine was significantly higher than in those without migraine (50% vs. 36.4%; P = 0.02) [100]. Retrospective studies on the effect of AVM embolization and the prevalence and outcome of migraine have shown conflicting results [101,128].

Congenital Heart Disease

A study of adults with congenital heart disease found an increased prevalence of migraine compared to controls with acquired cardiovascular diseases (45.3% vs. 11%; P < 0.001) [131]. Aura was more frequent in those with congenital heart disease than in the control group (80% vs. 36%; P < 0.001). The frequency of migraine was highest among congenital heart disease subjects with RLS (52%), followed by those with LRS (44%). Of note is that the prevalence of migraine was also elevated in congenital heart disease subjects without any atrial shunt as compared to control subjects (38% vs. 11%; not significant). The most frequent underlying condition was tetralogy of Fallot (36.3%) in the case of RLS and ASDs (55.9%) in LRS, while the most frequent condition in the no-shunt group was a defect of the bicuspid aortic valve (38.5%). Furthermore, a relatively high prevalence of migraine (38%) was found in female adult patients with coarctation of the aorta [13].

Summary

Evidence of a link between headache symptoms and cardiovascular disease (CVD) has grown rapidly in recent years. This chapter provides a brief overview of different cardiovascular diseases that may be related to headache, including stroke, subclinical vascular brain lesions, hypertension, coronary heart disease, patent foramen ovale, atrial septal defects, atrial septal aneurysms, mitral valve prolapse, pulmonary arteriovenous malformations, and congenital heart disease. Knowledge of these comorbidities is essential in the correct management of primary headaches.

References

[1]   Agostoni E, Aliprandi A. Migraine and hypertension. Neurol Sci 2008;29:S37–39.
[2]   Amaral V, Freitas GR, Rodrigues BC, Christoph D de H, Pinho CA, Góes C de F, Vincent MB. Patent foramen ovale in trigeminal autonomic cephalalgias and hemicrania continua: a nonspecific pathophysiological occurrence? Arq Neuropsiquiatr 2010;68:627–31.
[3]   Amendo MT, Brown BA, Kossow LB, Weinberg FM. Headache as the sole presentation of acute myocardial infarction in two elderly patients. Am J Geriatr Cardiol 2001;10:100–1.
[4]   Anzola GP, Morandi E, Casilli F, Onorato E. Different degrees of right-to-left shunting predict migraine and stroke: data from 420 patients. Neurology 2006;66:765–7.
[5]   Auer J, Berent R, Lassnig E, Eber B. Headache as a manifestation of fatal myocardial infarction. Neurol Sci 2001;22:395–7.
[6]   Azarbal B, Tobis J, Suh W, Chan V, Dao C, Gaster R. Association of interatrial shunts and migraine headaches: impact of transcatheter closure. J Am Coll Cardiol 2005;45:489–92.
[7]   Becker C, Brobert GP, Almqvist PM, Johansson S, Jick SS, Meier CR. Migraine and the risk of stroke, TIA, or death in the UK (CME). Headache 2007;47:1374–84.
[8]   Bigal ME, Kurth T, Hu H, Santanello N, Lipton RB. Migraine and cardiovascular disease: possible mechanisms of interaction. Neurology 2009;72:1864–71.
[9]   Bigal ME, Kurth T, Santanello N, Buse D, Golden W, Robbins M, Lipton RB. Migraine and cardiovascular disease: a population-based study. Neurology 2010;74:628–35.
[10] Bigal ME, Lipton RB. The epidemiology, burden, and comorbidities of migraine. Neurol Clin 2009;27:321–34.

[11] Bigal ME, Sheftell FD, Rapoport AM, Tepper SJ, Lipton RB. Chronic daily headache: identification of factors associated with induction and transformation. Headache 2002;42:575–81.

[12] Bini A, Evangelista A, Castellini P, Lambru G, Ferrante T, Manzoni GC, Torelli P. Cardiac cephalgia. J Headache Pain 2009;10:3–9.

[13] Borin C, Troost E, Thijs V, Moons P, Budts W. Migraine and coarctation of the aorta: prevalence and risk factors. Acta Cardiol 2008;63:431–5.

[14] Bowen J, Oppenheimer G. Headache as a presentation of angina: reproduction of symptoms during angioplasty. Headache 1993;33:238–9.

[15] Broner S, Lay C, Newman L, Swerdlow M. Thunderclap headache as the presenting symptom of myocardial infarction. Headache 2007;47:724–33.

[16] Buring JE, Peto R, Hennekens CH. Low dose aspirin for migraine prophylaxis. JAMA 1990;264:1711–3.

[17] Buse DC, Manack A, Serrano D, Turkel C, Lipton RB. Sociodemographic and comorbidity profiles of chronic migraine and episodic migraine sufferers. J Neurol Neurosurg Psychiatry 2010;81:428–32.

[18] Butera G, Biondi-Zoccai GGL, Carminati M, Caputi L, Usai S, Bussone G, Meola G, Derlogu AB, Sheiban I, Sangiorgi G. Systematic review and meta-analysis of currently available clinical evidence on migraine and patent foramen ovale percutaneous closure. Much ado about nothing? Catheter Cardiovasc Interv 2010;75:494–504.

[19] Caputi L, Usai S, Carriero MR, Grazzi L, D'Amico D, Falcone C, Anzola GP, Del Sette M, Parati E, Bussone G. Microembolic air load during contrast-transcranial Doppler: a trigger for migraine with aura? Headache 2010;50:1320–7.

[20] Carerj S, Narbone MC, Zito C, Serra S, Coglitore S, Pugliatti P, Luzza F, Arrigo F, Oreto G. Prevalence of atrial septal aneurysm in patients with migraine: an echocardiographic study. Headache 2003;43:725–8.

[21] Carod-Artal FJ, da Silveira Ribeiro L, Braga H, Kummer W, Mesquita HM, Vargas AP. Prevalence of patent foramen ovale in migraine patients with and without aura compared with stroke patients. A transcranial Doppler study. Cephalalgia 2006;26:934–9.

[22] Chen SP, Fuh JL, Yu WC, Wang SJ. Cardiac cephalalgia: case report and review of the literature with new ICHD-II criteria revisited. Eur Neurol 2004;51:221–6.

[23] Chen TC, Leviton A, Edelstein S, Ellenberg JH. Migraine and other diseases in women of reproductive age. The influence of smoking on observed associations. Arch Neurol 1987;44:1024–8.

[24] Cheng PY, Sy HN, Chen WL, Chen YY. Cardiac cephalalgia presented with a thunderclap headache and an isolated exertional headache: report of 2 cases. Acta Neurol Taiwan 2010;19:57–61.

[25] Chessa M, Colombo C, Butera G, Negura D, Piazza L, Varotto L, Bussadori C, Fesslova V, Meola G, Carminati M. Is it too early to recommend patent foramen ovale closure for all patients who suffer from migraine? A single-centre study. J Cardiovasc Med 2009;10:401–5.

[26] Cirillo M, Stellato D, Lombardi C, De Santo NG, Covelli V. Headache and cardiovascular risk factors: positive association with hypertension. Headache 1999;39:409–16.

[27] Cook NR, Benseñor IM, Lotufo PA, Lee IM, Skerrett PJ, Chown MJ, Ajani UA, Manson JE, Buring JE. Migraine and coronary heart disease in women and men. Headache 2002;42:715–27.

[28] Cutrer FM, Huerter K. Exertional headache and coronary ischemia despite normal electrocardiographic stress testing. Headache 2006;46:165–78.

[29] Dalla Volta G, Guindani M, Zavarise P, Griffini S, Pezzini A, Padovani A. Prevalence of patent foramen ovale in a large series of patients with migraine with aura, migraine without aura and cluster headache, and relationship with clinical phenotype. J Headache Pain 2005;6:328–30.

[30] Del Sette M, Angeli S, Leandri M, Ferriero G, Bruzzone GL, Finocchi C, Gandolfo C. Migraine with aura and right-to-left shunt on transcranial Doppler: a case-control study. Cerebrovasc Dis 1998;8:327–30.

[31] Dowson A, Mullen MJ, Peatfield R, Muir K, Khan AA, Wells C, Lipscombe SL, Rees T, De Giovanni JV, Morrison WL, Hildick-Smith D, Elrington G, Hillis WS, Malik IS, Rickards A. Migraine intervention with STARFLEX technology (MIST) trial: a prospective, multicenter, double-blind, sham-controlled trial to evaluate the effectiveness of patent foramen ovale closure with STARFLEX septal repair implant to resolve refractory migraine headache. Circulation 2008;117:1397–404.

[32] Etminan M, Takkouche B, Isorna FC, Samii A. Risk of ischaemic stroke in people with migraine: systematic review and meta-analysis of observational studies. BMJ 2005;330:63–6.

[33] Facchinetti F, Allais G, D'Amico R, Benedetto C, Volpe A. The relationship between headache and preeclampsia: a case-control study. Eur J Obstet Gynecol Reprod Biol 2005;121:143–8.

[34] Facchinetti F, Allais G, Nappi RE, D'Amico R, Marozio L, Bertozzi L, Ornati A, Benedetto C. Migraine is a risk factor for hypertensive disorders in pregnancy: a prospective cohort study. Cephalalgia 2009;29:286–92.

[35] Famularo G, Polchi S, Tarroni P. Headache as a presenting symptom of acute myocardial infarction. Headache 2002;42:1025–8.

[36] Ferrarini G, Malferrari G, Zucco R, Gaddi O, Norina M, Pini LA. High prevalence of patent foramen ovale in migraine with aura. J Headache Pain 2005;6:71–6.

[37] Finocchi C, Del Sette M, Angeli S, Rizzi D, Gandolfo C. Cluster headache and right-to-left shunt on contrast transcranial Doppler: a case-control study. Neurology 2004;63:1309–10.

[38] Fleetcroft R, Maddocks JL. Headache due to ischaemic heart disease. J R Soc Med 1985;78:676.

[39] Fragoso YD. Reduction of migraine attacks during the use of warfarin. Headache 1997;37:667–8.

[40] Franceschini R, Tenconi GL, Leandri M, Zoppoli F, Gonella A, Staltari S, Barreca T. Endothelin-1 plasma levels in cluster headache. Headache 2002;42:120–4.

[41] Gales BJ, Bailey EK, Reed AN, Gales MA. Angiotensin-converting enzyme inhibitors and angiotensin receptor blockers for the prevention of migraines. Ann Pharmacother 2010;44:360–6.

[42] Garg P, Servoss SJ, Wu JC, Bajwa ZH, Selim MH, Dineen A, Kuntz RE, Cook EF, Mauri L. Lack of association between migraine headache and patent foramen ovale: results of a case-control study. Circulation. 2010;121:1406–12.

[43] Giardini A, Donti A, Formigari R, Salomone L, Palareti G, Guidetti D, Picchio FM. Long-term efficacy of transcatheter patent foramen ovale closure on migraine headache with aura and recurrent stroke. Catheter Cardiovasc Interv 2006;67:625–9.

[44] Giardini A, Donti A, Formigari R, Salomone L, Prandstaller D, Bonvicini M, Palareti G, Guidetti D, Gaddi O, Picchio FM. Transcatheter patent foramen ovale closure mitigates aura migraine headaches abolishing spontaneous right-to-left shunting. Am Heart J 2006;151:922:e1–5.

[45] Gipponi S, Venturelli E, Rao R, Liberini P, Padovani A. Hypertension is a factor associated with chronic daily headache. Neurol Sci 2010;31:S171–3.

[46] Granella F, Farina S, Malferrari G, Manzoni GC. Drug abuse in chronic headache: a clinico-epidemiologic study. Cephalalgia 1987;7:15–9.

[47] Greiner F, Rothrock J. Thunderclap headache, cardiopulmonary arrest, and myocardial infarction. Headache 2006;46:512.

[48] Gudmundsson LS, Scher AI, Aspelund T, Eliasson JH, Johannsson M, Thorgeirsson G, Launer L, Gudnason V. Migraine with aura and risk of cardiovascular and all cause mortality in men and women: prospective cohort study. BMJ 2010;341:c3966.

[49] Gudmundsson LS, Thorgeirsson G, Sigfusson N, Sigvaldason H, Johannsson M. Migraine patients have lower systolic but higher diastolic blood pressure compared with controls in a population-based study of 21,537 subjects. The Reykjavik Study. Cephalalgia 2006;26:436–44.

[50] Guldiken B, Guldiken S, Taskiran B, Koc G, Turgut N, Kabayel L, Tugrul A. Migraine in metabolic syndrome. Neurologist 2009;15:55–8.

[51] Hagen PT, Scholz DG, Edwards WD. Incidence and size of patent foramen ovale during the first 10 decades of life: an autopsy study of 965 normal hearts. Mayo Clin Proc 1984;59:17–20.

[52] Hamed SA, Hamed EA, Ezz Eldin AM, Mahmoud NM. Vascular risk factors, endothelial function, and carotid thickness in patients with migraine: relationship to atherosclerosis. J Stroke Cerebrovasc Dis 2010;19:92–103.

[53] Hamed SA. The vascular risk associations with migraine: relation to migraine susceptibility and progression. Atherosclerosis 2008;205:15–22.

[54] Headache Classification Subcommittee of the International Headache Society. The international classification of headache disorders, 2nd edition. Cephalalgia 2004;24(Suppl 1):1–160.

[55] Hill JM, Zalos G, Halcox JP, Schenke WH, Waclawiw MA, Quyyumi AA, Finkel T. Circulating endothelial progenitor cells, vascular function, and cardiovascular risk. N Engl J Med 2003;348:593–600.

[56] Jesurum JT, Fuller CJ, Velez CA, Spencer MP, Krabill KA, Likosky WH, Gray WA, Olsen JV, Reisman M. Migraineurs with patent foramen ovale have larger right-to-left shunt despite similar atrial septal characteristics. J Headache Pain 2007;8:209–16.

[57] Koppen H, Palm-Meinders IH, Mess WH. What makes migraine persist? Results from a population-based 8.5 years follow up study. Cephalalgia 2009; 29:1353.

[58] Korantzopoulos P, Karanikis P, Pappa E, Dimitroula V, Kountouris E, Siogas K. Acute non-St-el-evation myocardial infarction presented as occipital headache with impaired level of conscious-ness. Angiology 2005; 56:627–30.
[59] Kountouras J, Zavos C, Papadopoulos A, Deretzi G, Polyzos S. Irritable bowel syndrome as-sociated with mitral valve prolapse and autonomic and haemostatic abnormalities in children, adolescents and adults with migraine. Acta Neurol Scand 2011;123:366–7.
[60] Kruit MC, Launer LJ, Ferrari MD, van Buchem MA. Infarcts in the posterior circulation territory in migraine. The population-based MRI CAMERA study. Brain 2005;128:2068–77.
[61] Kruit MC, van Buchem MA, Hofman PA, Bakkers JT, Terwindt GM, Ferrari MD, Launer LJ. Migraine as a risk factor for subclinical brain lesions. JAMA 2004;291:427–34.
[62] Kurth K, Ridker PM, Buring JE: Migraine and biomarkers of cardiovascular disease in women. Cephalalgia 2007;28:49–56.
[63] Kurth T, Diener HC, Buring JE. Migraine and cardiovascular disease in women and the role of aspirin: subgroup analyses in the Women's Health Study. Cephalalgia 2011;31:1106–15.
[64] Kurth T, Gaziano JM, Cook N, Bubes V, Logroscino G, Diener HC, Buring JE. Migraine and risk of cardiovascular disease in men. Arch Intern Med 2007;167:795–801.
[65] Kurth T, Gaziano JM, Cook NR, Logroscino G, Diener HC, Buring JE. Migraine and risk of car-diovascular disease in women. JAMA 2006;296:283–91.
[66] Kurth T, Kase CS, Schürks M, Tzourio C, Buring JE. Migraine and risk of haemorrhagic stroke in women: prospective cohort study. BMJ 2010;341:c3659.
[67] Kurth T, Mohamed S, Maillard P, Zhu YC, Chabriat H, Mazoyer B, Bousser MG, Dufouil C, Tzourio C. Headache, migraine, and structural brain lesions and function: population based Epidemiology of Vascular Ageing-MRI study. BMJ 2011;342:c7357.
[68] Kurth T, Schürks M, Logroscino G, Gaziano JM, Buring JE. Migraine, vascular risk, and cardio-vascular events in women: prospective cohort study. BMJ 2008;337:a636.
[69] Kurth T, Schürks M, Logroscino G. Migraine frequency and risk of cardiovascular disease in women. Neurology 2009;73:581–8.
[70] Kurth T, Slomke MA, Kase CS, Cook NR, Lee IM, Gaziano JM, Diener HC, Buring JE. Migraine, headache, and the risk of stroke in women: a prospective study. Neurology 2005;64:1020–6.
[71] Lafitte C, Even C, Henry-Lebras F, de Toffol B, Autret A. Migraine and angina pectoris by coro-nary artery spasm. Headache 1996;36:332–4.
[72] Lamy C, Giannesini C, Zuber M, Arquizan C, Meder JF, Trystram D, Coste J, Mas JL. Clinical and imaging findings in cryptogenic stroke patients with and without patent foramen OVALE: the PFO-ASA Study. Atrial septal aneurysm. Stroke 2002;33:706–11.
[73] Lanza GA, Sciahbasi A, Sestito A, Maseri A. Angina pectoris: a headache. Lancet 2000;356:998.
[74] Lee ST, Chu K, Jung KH, Kim DH, Kim EH, Choe VN, Kim JH, Im WS, Kang L, Park JE, Park HJ, Park HK, Song EC, Lee SK, Kim M, Roh JK. Decreased number and function of endothelial progenitor cells in patients with migraine. Neurology 2008;70:1510–7.
[75] Leon-Sotomayor LA. Cardiac migraine-report of twelve cases. Angiology 1974;25:161–71.
[76] Leviton A, Malvea B, Graham JR. Vascular diseases, mortality, and migraine in the parents of migraine patients. Neurology 1974;24:669–72.
[77] Lipton RB, Lowenkopf T, Bajwa ZH, Leckie RS, Ribeiro S, Newman LC, Greenberg MA. Cardiac cephalgia: a treatable form of exertional headache. Neurology 1997;49:813–6.
[78] Litman GI, Friedman HM. Migraine and the mitral valve prolapse syndrome. Am Heart J 1978;96:610–4.
[79] Loder E. Cluster headache and the heart. Curr Pain Headache Rep 2006;10:142–6.
[80] Loomba RS, Chandrasekar S, Sanan P, Shah PH, Arora RR. Association of atrial tachyarrhyth-mias with atrial septal defect, Ebstein's anomaly and Fontan patients. Expert Rev Cardiovasc Ther 2011;9:887–93.
[81] Luermans JG, Post MC, Temmerman F, Thijs V, Schonewille WJ, Plokker HW, Suttorp MJ, Budts WI. Closure of a patent foramen ovale is associated with a decrease in prevalence of migraine: a prospective observational study. Acta Cardiol 2008;63:571–7.
[82] Luermans JG, Post MC, Temmerman F, Thijs V, Schonewille WJ, Plokker HW, Ten Berg JM, Sut-torp MJ, Budts WI. Is a predominant left-to-right shunt associated with migraine? A prospective atrial septal defect closure study. Catheter Cardiovasc Interv 2009;74:1078–84.
[83] MacClellan LR, Giles W, Cole J, Wozniak M, Stern B, Mitchell BD, Kittner SJ. Probable migraine with visual aura and risk of ischemic stroke: the Stroke Prevention in Young Women study. Stroke 2007;38:2438–45.

[84] Mancia G, Rosei EA, Ambrosioni E, Avino F, Carolei A, Daccò M, Di Giacomo G, Ferri C, Grazioli I, Melzi G, Nappi G, Pinessi L, Sandrini G, Trimarco B, Zanchin G; MIRACLES Study Group. Hypertension and migraine comorbidity: prevalence and risk of cerebrovascular events: evidence from a large, multicenter, cross-sectional survey in Italy (MIRACLES study). J Hypertens 2011;29:309–18.

[85] Marchione P, Ghiotto N, Sances G, Guaschino E, Bosone D, Nappi G, Giacomini P. Clinical implications of patent foramen ovale in migraine with aura. Funct Neurol 2008;23:201–5.

[86] Martínez HR, Rangel-Guerra RA, Cantú-Martínez L, Garza-Gómez J, González HC. Cardiac headache: hemicranial cephalalgia as the sole manifestation of coronary ischemia. Headache 2002;42:1029–32.

[87] Mathew NT. Chronic refractory headache. Neurology 1993;43:S26–33.

[88] Mathew NT. Migraine and hypertension. Cephalalgia 1999;19:17–19.

[89] Miller D, Waters DD, Warnica W, Szlachcic J, Kreeft J, Theroux P. Is variant angina the coronary manifestation of a generalized vasospastic disorder? N Engl J Med 1981;304:763–6.

[90] Mitchell P, Wang JJ, Currie J, Cumming RG, Smith W. Prevalence and vascular associations with migraine in older Australians. Aust NZ J Med 1998;28:627–32.

[91] Moaref AR, Petramfar P, Aghasadeghi K, Zamirian M, Sharifkazemi MB, Rezaian S, Afifi S, Zare N, Rezaian GR. Patent foramen ovale in patients with tension headache: is it as common as in migraineurs? An age- and sex-matched comparative study. J Headache Pain 2009;10:431–4.

[92] Morelli N, Gori S, Cafforio G, Gallerini S, Baldacci F, Orlandi G, Murri L. Prevalence of right-to-left shunt in patients with cluster headache. J Headache Pain 2005;6:244–6.

[93] Mortelmans K, Post M, Thijs V, Herroelen L, Budts W. The influence of percutaneous atrial septal defect closure on the occurrence of migraine. Eur Heart J 2005;26:1533–7.

[94] Nanthakumar K, Graham AT, Robinson TI, Grande P, Pugash RA, Clarke JA, Hutchison SJ, Mandzia JL, Hyland RH, Faughnan ME. Contrast echocardiography for detection of pulmonary arteriovenous malformations. Am Heart J 2001;141:243–6.

[95] Nelson KB, Richardson AK, He J, Lateef TM, Khoromi S, Merikangas KR. Headache and biomarkers predictive of vascular disease in a representative sample of US children. Arch Pediatr Adolesc Med 2010;164:358–62.

[96] Noheria A, Roshan J, Kapa S, Srivathsan K, Packer DL, Asirvatham SJ. Migraine headaches following catheter ablation for atrial fibrillation. J Interv Card Electrophysiol 2011;30:227–32.

[97] Nozari A, Dilekoz E, Sukhotinsky I, Stein T, Eikermann-Haerter K, Liu C, Wang Y, Frosch MP, Waeber C, Ayata C, Moskowitz MA. Microemboli may link spreading depression, migraine aura and patent foramen ovale. Ann Neurol 2010;67:221–9.

[98] Petersen JA, Nielsen FE. Headache: a rare manifestation of angina pectoris. Ugeskr Laeger 2002;164:2515–6.

[99] Pietrini U, De Luca M, De Santis G. Hypertension in headache patients? A clinical study. Acta Neurol Scand 2005;112:259–64.

[100] Post MC, Letterboer TGW, Mager JJ, Plokker TH, Kelder JC, Westermann CJJ. A pulmonary right-to-left shunt in patients with hereditary hemorrhagic teleangiectasia is associated with an increased prevalence of migraine. Chest 2005;128:2485–9.

[101] Post MC, Thijs V, Schonewille WJ, Budts W, Snijder RJ, Plokker HW, Westermann CJ. Embolization of pulmonary arteriovenous malformations and decrease in prevalence of migraine. Neurology 2006;66:202–5.

[102] Prudenzano MP, Monetti C, Merico L, Cardinali V, Genco S, Lamberti P, Livrea P. The comorbidity of migraine and hypertension. A study in a tertiary care headache centre. J Headache Pain 2005;6:220–2.

[103] Rambihar VS. Headache angina. Lancet 2001;357:72.

[104] Rigatelli G, Dell'Avvocata F, Ronco F, Cardaioli P, Giordan M, Braggion G, Aggio S, Chinaglia M, Rigatelli G, Chen JP. Primary transcatheter patent foramen ovale closure is effective in improving migraine in patients with high-risk anatomic and functional characteristics for paradoxical embolism. J Am Coll Cardiol Interv 2010;3:282–7.

[105] Robberstad L, Dyb G, Hagen K, Stovner LJ, Holmen TL, Zwart JA. An unfavorable lifestyle and recurrent headaches among adolescents. The HUNT study. Neurology 2010;75:712–7.

[106] Rodés-Cabau J, Mineau S, Marrero A, Houde C, Mackey A, Côté JM, Chetaille P, Delisle G, Bertrand OF, Rivest D. Incidence, timing, and predictive factors of new-onset migraine headache attack after transcatheter closure of atrial septal defect or patent foramen ovale. Am J Cardiol 2008;101:688–92.

[107] Rose KM, Carson AP, Sanford CP, Stang PE, Brown CA, Folsom AR, Szklo M. Migraine and other headaches: associations with Rose angina and coronary heart disease. Neurology 2004;63:2233–9.

[108] Rozen TD. Cluster headache as the result of secondhand cigarette smoke exposure during childhood. Headache 2010;50:130–2.

[109] Rundek T, Elkind MS, Di Tullio MR, Carrera E, Jin Z, Sacco RL, Homma S. Patent foramen ovale and migraine: a cross-sectional study from the Northern Manhattan Study (NOMAS). Circulation 2008;118:1419–24.

[110] Sampson JM. Pathophysiology and differential diagnosis of cardiac pain. Prog Cardiovascular Dis 1971;13:507–31.

[111] Sathirapanya P. Anginal cephalgia: a serious form of exertional headache. Cephalalgia 2004;24:231–4.

[112] Scher AI, Gudmundsson LS, Sigurdsson S, Ghambaryan A, Aspelund T, Eiriksdottir G, van Buchem MA, Gudnason V, Launer LJ. Migraine headache in middle age and late-life brain infarcts. JAMA 2009;301:2563–70.

[113] Scher AI, Terwindt GM, Picavet HS, Verschuren WM, Ferrari MD, Launer LJ. Cardiovascular risk factors and migraine: the GEM population-based study. Neurology 2005;64:614–20.

[114] Schürks M, Buring JE, Kurth T. Migraine, migraine features, and cardiovascular disease. Headache 2010;50:1031–40.

[115] Schürks M, Diener HC. Cluster headache and lifestyle habits. Curr Pain Headache Rep 2008;12:115–21.

[116] Schürks M, Rist PM, Bigal ME, Buring JE, Lipton RB, Kurth T. Migraine and cardiovascular disease: systematic review and meta-analysis. BMJ 2009;339:b3914.

[117] Schwedt TJ, Demaerschalk BM, Dodick DW. Patent foramen ovale and migraine: a quantitative systematic review. Cephalalgia 2008;28:531–40.

[118] Schwedt TJ. The migraine association with cardiac anomalies, cardiovascular disease and stroke. Neurol Clin 2009;27:513–23.

[119] Schwerzmann M, Nedeltchev K, Lagger F, Mattle HP, Windecker S, Meier B, Seiler C. Prevalence and size of directly detected patent foramen ovale in migraine with aura. Neurology 2005;65:1415–18.

[120] Sendovski U, Rabkin Y, Goldshlak L, Rothmann MG. Should acute myocardial infarction be considered in the differential diagnosis of headache? Eur J Emerg Med 2009;16:1–3.

[121] Seow VK, Chong CF, Wang TL, Ong JR. Severe explosive headache: a sole presentation of acute myocardial infarction in a young man. Am J Emerg Med 2007;25:250–1.

[122] Slavin L, Tobis JM, Rangarajan K, Dao C, Krivokapich J, Liebeskind DS. Five-year experience with percutaneous closure of patent foramen ovale. Am J Cardiol 2007;99:1316–20.

[123] Sobrino T, Hurtado O, Moro MA, Rodríguez-Yáñez M, Castellanos M, Brea D, Moldes O, Blanco M, Arenillas JF, Leira R, Dávalos A, Lizasoain I, Castillo J. The increase of circulating endothelial progenitor cells after acute ischemic stroke is associated with good outcome. Stroke 2007;38:2759–64.

[124] Spence JD, Wong DG, Melendez LJ, Nichol PM, Brown JD. Increased prevalence of mitral valve prolapse in patients with migraine. Can Med Assoc J 1984;131:1457–60.

[125] Stang PE, Carson AP, Rose KM, Mo J, Ephross SA, Shahar E, Szklo M. Headache, cerebrovascular symptoms, and stroke: the Atherosclerosis Risk in Communities Study. Neurology 2005;64:1573–7.

[126] Tembl J, Lago A, Sevilla T, Solis P, Vilchez J. Migraine, patent foramen ovale and migraine triggers. J Headache Pain 2007;8:7–12.

[127] Termine C, Trotti R, Ondei P, Gamba G, Montani N, Gamba A, De Simone M, Marni E, Balottin U. Mitral valve prolapse and abnormalities of haemostasis in children and adolescents with migraine with aura and other idiopathic headaches: a pilot study. Acta Neurol Scand 2010;122:91–6.

[128] Thenganatt J, Schneiderman J, Hyland RH, Edmeads J, Mandzia JL, Faughnan ME. Migraines linked to intrapulmonary right-to-left shunt. Headache 2006;46:439–43.

[129] Tietjen GE. Migraine as a systemic vasculopathy. Headache 2009;29:989–96.

[130] Trabattoni D, Fabbiocchi F, Montorsi P, Galli S, Teruzzi G, Grancini L, Gatto P, Bartorelli AL. Sustained long-term benefit of patent foramen ovale closure on migraine. Catheter Cardiovasc Interv 2011;77:570–4.

[131] Truong T, Slavin L, Kashani R, Higgins J, Puri A, Chowdhry M, Cheung P, Tanious A, Child JS, Perloff JK, Tobis JM. Prevalence of migraine headaches in patients with congenital heart disease. Am J Cardiol 2008;101:396–400.
[132] U.S. Department of Health and Human Services. The health consequences of involuntary exposure to tobacco smoke: a report of the Surgeon General. Atlanta: U.S. Department of Health and Human Services, Centers for Disease Control and Prevention, Coordinating Center for Health Promotion, National Center for Chronic Disease Prevention and Health Promotion, Office on Smoking and Health; 2006.
[133] van Vliet JA, Vein AA, Ferrari MD, van Dijk JG. Cardiovascular autonomic function tests in cluster headache. Cephalalgia 2006;26:329–31.
[134] Varkey E, Hagen K, Zwart JA, Linde M. Physical activity and headache: results from the Nord-Trondelag Health Study (HUNT). Cephalalgia 2008;28:1292–7.
[135] Vernay D, Deffond D, Fraysse P, Dordain G. Walking headache: an unusual manifestation of ischemic heart disease. Headache 1989;29:350–1.
[136] Wahl A, Praz F, Findling O, Nedeltchev K, Schwerzmann M, Tai T, Windecker S, Mattle HP, Meier B. Percutaneous closure of patent foramen ovale for migraine headaches refractory to medical treatment. Catheter Cardiovasc Interv 2009;74:124–9.
[137] Wahl A, Praz F, Tai T, Findling O, Walpoth N, Nedeltchev K, Schwerzmann M, Windecker S, Mattle HP, Meier B. Improvement of migraine headaches after percutaneous closure of patent foramen ovale for secondary prevention of paradoxical embolism. Heart 2010;96:967–73.
[138] Waldie KE, McGee R, Reeder AI, Poulton R. Associations between frequent headaches, persistent smoking, and attempts to quit. Headache 2008;48:545–52.
[139] Winsvold BS, Hagen K, Aamodt AH, Stovner LJ, Holmen J, Zwart JA. Headache, migraine, and cardiovascular risk factors. The HUNT study. Eur J Neurol 2011;18:504–11.
[140] Yankovsky AE, Kuritzky A. Transformation into daily migraine with aura following transcutaneous atrial septal defect closure. Headache 2003;43:496–8.
[141] Yoon G, Baggaley S, Bacchetti P, Fu YH, Digre KB, Ptácek LJ. Clinic-based study of family history of vascular risk actors and migraine. J Headache Pain 2005;6:412–6.

Correspondence to: Paolo Martelletti, MD, Department of Clinical and Molecular Medicine, Sapienza University of Rome and Regional Referral Headache Center, Sant'Andrea Hospital, Via di Grottarossa 1035-I, 00161 Rome, Italy. Email: paolo.martelletti@uniroma1.it.

Neuropathic Pain in Metabolic and Inflammatory Diseases

Troels Staehelin Jensen

Department of Neurology and Danish Pain Research Center,
Aarhus University Hospital, Aarhus, Denmark

Neuropathic pain is not a single disease but a syndrome caused by multiple etiologies and with a characteristic core of symptoms and signs. Thus, it is practical and reasonable from a clinical perspective to group these pain conditions under a common label. A key characteristic of these disorders is the presence of pain and sensory abnormalities in body parts that have lost their normal peripheral innervations—or, in the case of central lesions, part of their sensory representation in the brain. Neuropathic pain disorders should be distinguished from other types of pain because their underlying pathophysiology and treatment are different. Neuropathic pain was until recently defined as "Pain initiated or caused by a primary lesion, dysfunction or transitory perturbation in the peripheral or central nervous system" [19]. The word "dysfunction" in the IASP definition of neuropathic pain has been a steady source of confusion because it allowed inclusion of painful conditions for which there are no objective signs of nervous system pathology. IASP has for that reason now strengthened the criteria for neuropathic pain, which is now defined as "Pain caused by a lesion or disease affecting the somatosensory system" (www.iasp-pain.org/painterms).

Pain Comorbidities: Understanding and Treating the Complex Patient
edited by Maria Adele Giamberardino and Troels Staehelin Jensen
IASP Press, Seattle, © 2012

A large number of specific diseases and conditions that differ not only in their underlying etiology but also in their anatomical localization have been associated with neuropathic pain. Inflammatory and metabolic disorders of different etiologies are important examples of conditions giving rise to neuropathic pain. This chapter will briefly outline physiological and clinical types of pain, metabolic and inflammatory causes of neuropathic pain, and the mechanisms and treatment of these conditions.

Physiological and Clinical Types of Pain

Physiological (nociceptive) pain is pain caused by specific activation of high-threshold nociceptors by tissue-damaging noxious mechanical, chemical, or thermal stimuli [4,7,24,27,32]. Nociceptive pain represents an alarm system warning the organism of impending tissue damage. Once pain has been signaled by specialized high-threshold receptors, sensory discrimination is replaced by a less well-defined but emotionally powerful experience driving the individual to stop the pain or escape from the stimulus that is causing it. Nociceptive neurons express a series of transducer receptors and ion channels that respond to a broad range of different noxious stimuli. Acute nociceptive pain occurs only in the presence of noxious stimuli and diminishes shortly after the damaging stimulus is removed. In rare cases where nociception is lacking, such as congenital insensitivity to pain, severe tissue damage may occur. Thus, the nociceptive system is a powerful warning system of tissue damage and is probably necessary for survival.

Clinical pain can be divided into three major classes: inflammatory pain, neuropathic pain, and pain of unknown origin [2,3,17]. These phenomena are all characterized by a heightened sensitivity and response to noxious or non-noxious stimuli, resulting in an experience of pain. There are certain differences in the clinical presentation of these types of pain; Table I summarizes their similarities and differences.

Inflammatory Pain

Inflammatory pain occurs in response to tissue injury and is accompanied by neurogenic inflammation. It is usually caused by sensitizing or directly activating inflammatory substances reducing the activation

Table I
Characteristic features of neuropathic, inflammatory, and other pain types

Symptoms and Signs	Neuropathic Pain	Inflammatory Pain	Pain of Unknown Origin
Positive			
Spontaneous pain in damaged area	Yes	Yes	Yes
Heat hyperalgesia	Rarely	Often	Variable
Cold allodynia	Often	Rarely	Rarely
Hyperpathia (increased threshold and explosive suprathreshold pains)	Often	Never	Never
Aftersensations	Often	Rarely	Often
Specific symptoms	Paroxysms and burning pain	Throbbing pain	No
Pain outside damaged area	No	No	Often
Negative			
Sensory loss in damaged nerve territory	Yes	No	No
Motor deficit in damaged nerve territory	Often	No	No

threshold of nociceptors innervating the inflamed tissue. The result is an exaggerated response to external stimuli and to abnormal (usually increased) responses in the central nervous system (CNS). These phenomena, although evoked within minutes, can outlast the tissue injury that caused it for hours or days. In principle, the inflammatory changes are reversible, and the sensitivity of the system will be restored when the inflammation disappears. Signs of inflammation, such as swelling, reddening, and increased temperature, are usually present, and consequently the inflamed area is often protected and immobilized to reduce further damage and pain. The somatosensory system is completely intact in the inflammatory state, which probably explains the return to normal when the inflammation dies down.

Neuropathic Pain

Neuropathic pain is pain that occurs after injury or disease affecting nerves or the central sensory pathways in the spinal cord or brain. It can be classified according to disease and anatomical location of nerve damage (Table II). When lesions occur, they may cause sensory loss in the innervation territory of damaged nerve fibers. Sensory loss may also occur in parts of the body that correspond to a brain territory that has been damaged directly or indirectly by a cerebral lesion or disease. An important distinguishing feature in several neuropathic types of pain is the paradoxical combination of sensory loss and pain with or without sensory hypersensitivity phenomena in the painful area. This feature will be described in more detail below.

Table II
Classification of neuropathic pain according to disease
and anatomical region

Peripheral	Spinal	Brain
Neuropathies	Multiple sclerosis	Stroke
Herpes zoster	Spinal cord injury	Multiple sclerosis
Nerve injuries	Arachnoiditis	Neoplasms
Amputations	Neoplasms	Syringomyelia
Plexopathies	Syringomyelia	Parkinson's disease
Radiculopathies	Spinal stroke	Epilepsy
Avulsions	Chordotomy	Encephalitis
Neoplasms	Inflammatory myelopathy	
Trigeminal neuralgia		

Pain of Unknown Origin

Pain of unknown origin has also been termed "functional pain," "dysfunctional pain," or "idiopathic pain." These types of pain refer to a group of disorders in which there are no signs of inflammation or nerve injury and no major psychiatric illness. Because of a lack of documented pathology, these conditions represent exclusion diagnoses. A characteristic feature of chronic pain of unknown origin is a local or generalized heightened sensitivity to noxious or non-noxious stimuli. Chronic pain conditions of unknown origin are to be clearly separated from malingering, which in the case of pain refers to the conscious simulation of painful symptoms.

Neuropathic Pain Syndrome

An essential part of neuropathic pain is a partial or complete loss of afferent sensory function and the paradoxical presence of hyperalgesia or allodynia in the painful area [2,3,10,16]. The sensory deficit may be marked in some patients, and subtle in others. The distribution of sensory loss represents an important initial step for pain assessment and for identification of which parts of the nervous system have been damaged (nerve roots, nerves, fascicles, dermatomes, or the somatosensory map in lesioned central brain structures). In general, the distribution of spontaneous or evoked positive sensory phenomena may correspond to the innervation territory of the damaged part of the nervous system, but it may also be a fraction of it or may extend beyond it. The discrepancy between areas of negative and positive sensory phenomena has created some confusion in terms of clarifying mechanisms. For example, hypothetically, in some patients an extension of the distribution of positive sensory phenomena may be a consequence of central sensitization in a spinal cord segment due to damage of a peripheral nerve.

Neuropathic Pain Types

There are two types of neuropathic pain: spontaneous and evoked [2,3,10,16,17].

Spontaneous Pain

Spontaneous pain can be shooting, shock-like, aching, cramping, crushing, smarting, or burning. Paroxysmal pain is the prototypical type of neuropathic pain. In its most typical form, paroxysmal pain is seen in tic douloureux and entrapment neuropathies, but it can also occur in metabolic and inflammatory neuropathic pains. The pain is likely to reflect an increased discharge in sensitized C-nociceptors [23].

Stimulus-Dependent Pain

Stimulus-evoked pain is classified according to the type of stimulus that provokes it: mechanical, thermal, or chemical [2,16]. In some patients several of these phenomena may be present, while in others there may be only one type of hyperalgesia. For example, patients with nerve injury pain or amputation may have trigger points to mechanical stimuli, but entirely normal thermal sensation. In others, cold allodynia may be the only abnormality. Therefore, a series of stimuli must be used to document or exclude abnormalities. The evoked pains are usually brief, lasting only for the period of stimulation, but sometimes they can persist even after cessation of stimulation, causing aftersensations (see below) that can last for hours. In such cases, the distinction between evoked and spontaneous types of pain can be difficult.

Sensory Deficit and Pain

As described above, an essential part of neuropathic pain is a partial or complete loss of afferent sensory function, together with the paradoxical presence of certain hyperphenomena in the painful area. In some patients the sensory deficit may be gross, while in others it can be subtle and difficult to detect with bedside methods, but quantitative measures can usually reveal minor changes [10,13]. The sensory loss may involve all sensory abnormalities, but a loss of spinothalamic functions (cold, warmth, and pinprick detection) appears to be crucial. In fact, the possibility has been raised that loss of spinothalamic functions is a requirement for diagnosis of neuropathic pain.

Allodynia and Hyperalgesia

Hyperalgesia (the lowering of pain threshold and an increased response to noxious stimuli), allodynia (pain in response to non-noxious stimuli) are typical elements of neuropathic pain. Three types of mechanical hyperalgesia can be distinguished: (1) static hyperalgesia: gentle pressure on the skin evokes pain; (2) punctate hyperalgesia: punctate stimuli, such as pinprick, evoke pain; and (3) dynamic hyperalgesia: light brushing evokes a sensation of pain.

With regard to thermal stimuli, both cold and heat can evoke abnormal pain: (1) Cold hyperalgesia: cold stimuli evoke a sensation of pain (the underlying mechanism is unclear, but cortical reorganization due to loss of cold-sensitive $A\delta$ fibers is one possibility). (2) Heat hyperalgesia: warm and heat stimuli evoke pain (via sensitization of C-nociceptors and a corresponding sensitization of second-order neurons).

Dynamic mechanical allodynia is mediated by Aβ fibers, whereas the static high-threshold type is evoked by blunt pressure and appears to be a C-nociceptor-mediated response. The static type of hyperalgesia would be expected to be associated with thermal hyperalgesia, but that is not always the case [26]. Punctate hyperalgesia evoked by pinprick, usually a stiff von Frey filament, is mediated by sensitized Aδ nociceptors. While certain types of hyperalgesia reflect sensitization of receptors, allodynia is always a central phenomenon mediated by large myelinated fibers [18].

Specific Inflammatory Neuropathic Pain Conditions

Table III provides a list of inflammatory and metabolic diseases that may be accompanied by pain that is assumed to be neuropathic. These diseases have been summarized in recent textbooks and reviews (for example [9,12,26,28]).

Postherpetic Neuralgia

Postherpetic neuralgia (PHN) is pain along the course of one or a series of nerves following an acute segmental rash of herpes zoster, usually starting

Table III
Inflammatory and metabolic causes of neuropathic pain

Inflammatory Neuropathic Pain	Metabolic Neuropathic Pain
Guillain-Barré syndrome	Diabetes
Neuroborreliosis	Uremic neuropathy
Vasculitic neuropathy	Hypothyroid neuropathy
Sjögren's disease	B_{12} myelopathy
Postherpetic neuralgia	
HIV/HAART	
Leprosy	
Sarcoidosis	

Abbreviations: HIV, human immunodeficiency virus; HAART, highly active antiretroviral therapy.

within 1–3 months and in some cases up to 6 months after healing of the rash. The incidence of PHN varies, with figures ranging from 3% to 14% depending on the definition of time of onset of PHN after the acute rash. There is pathology of spinal ganglion cells, with necrosis of small and large neurons in the dorsal root ganglion (DRG) and a corresponding axonal loss. There may be secondary pathological changes in cells in the dorsal horn of the spinal cord. Patients with PHN, compared to patients without PHN, have more extensive lesions in the DRG and in the affected skin. The risk of pain is more pronounced in older than in younger patients. In herpes zoster patients less than 40 years of age, the risk for PHN is 10% or lower, while in patients more than 70 years old it may be as high as 75%.

Acute Inflammatory Demyelinating Polyneuropathy

Acute inflammatory polyneuropathy (Guillain-Barré syndrome) is an autoimmune disease affecting the peripheral nerves and roots. This condition usually has an acute onset with rapidly progressing sensory and motor symptoms starting peripherally and ascending to include the trunk and all four extremities and even the lower cranial nerves. Pain is a very common and debilitating symptom in patients. Pain in Guillain-Barré syndrome can be severe and is described as pricking, sticking, lancinating, or shooting; it is mostly present in the acute and subacute phases of the disease and then gradually resolves. In other cases the pain is a deep localized sensation along the distribution of major nerves. It is assumed that the pain is due to local inflammation of the nervi nervorum rather than related to direct activity in the nerve roots themselves. In the acute stages there is demyelination, and as such, the condition is considered to mainly affect large fibers. However, in many cases there is also involvement of small fibers. The chronic version of this disease, termed chronic inflammatory demyelinating polyneuropathy, has an insidious onset with development of a sensory-motor neuropathy, which likewise may be associated with pain.

HIV and HAART Neuropathy

Patients with human immunodeficiency virus (HIV) infection and those treated with highly active antiretroviral therapy (HAART) are subject to development of a distal symmetrical polyneuropathy. Up to 30% of patients with HIV develop this type of neuropathy. They often complain of painful numbness in the feet, spreading upwards. It is often a small-fiber neuropathy, mainly associated with thermal and pinprick sensations. Large-fiber function may be less severely affected. Patients with HIV-related neuropathy often have reduced sensitivity to cold and warm stimuli [5], and this hyposensitivity to stimuli associated with small-fiber function correlates with a reduction of intraepidermal nerve fiber density [21]. In addition to the neuropathy that may be seen as a direct consequence of HIV and HAART, HIV patients may develop a Guillain-Barré-like syndrome. This syndrome is associated with an increased cell count in the cerebrospinal fluid (CSF), unlike the usual Guillain-Barré syndrome, where "albuminocytologic dissociation" is the characteristic picture.

Neuroborreliosis

Neuroborreliosis is an inflammation in the nervous system caused by the spirochete *Borrelia burgdorferi* giving rise to a meningo-radiculo-neuropathy affecting a variety of nerve roots and nerves [20]. The North American form of neuroborreliosis is dominated by a meningeal clinical picture, while in the European form the clinical features mainly consist of variable degrees of facial or limb weakness, sensory abnormalities and pain in the same body parts. The pain types in neuroborreliosis are multiple, including radiating, shooting, pricking, and lancinating pains, associated with different degrees of sensory loss. When located in the thoracic region, the pain is often due to a thoracic radiculitis with a band-like distribution, either unilaterally or bilaterally. When pain occurs in the extremities, the disease can be caused by a plexopathy or a neuropathy. A characteristic feature in these patients is nightly worsening of pains with allodynia and hyperalgesia. The triad of radicular pains, peripheral facial palsy, and a lymphocytic pleocytosis in the CSF is known as Bannwarth's syndrome. The diagnosis of neuroborreliosis depends on the demonstration of increased cell counts in the CSF and intrathecal antibodies against the causative agent. The disorder can be causally treated with antibiotics, and pain generally disappears within a period of weeks to months.

Vasculitic Disorders

Vasculitic disorders, as observed in different connective tissue disorders such as systemic lupus, Wegner's granulomatosis, polyarteritis nodosa, and sarcoidosis, may give rise to neuropathies. These disorders usually present as single or multiple mononeuropathies that can be painful or nonpainful. These neuropathies are assumed to be due to a necrotizing vasculitis causing ischemic damage to the axons because of thrombotic occlusion of vasa nervorum. In Sjögren's syndrome, a small-fiber neuropathy is a characteristic feature.

Leprosy

This disorder, also known as Hansen's disease, which is endemic in certain parts of the developing world, was originally characterized as a nonpainful neuropathy with patchy sensory losses mainly related to large fibers. It has now become clear that leprosy can also be painful.

Specific Metabolic Neuropathic Pain Conditions

Endocrinological Diseases

A number of endocrinological diseases may give rise to neuropathic types of pain. Diabetes mellitus, by far the most common endocrine disorder and the prototypic condition causing neuropathic pain, is dealt with elsewhere in this volume (see, for example, the chapters by Tesfaye and Wittink). Thyroid diseases, including both hyperthyroid and hypothyroid conditions, can cause pain. Patients with hepatitis C may develop a painful neuropathy, which may be related to toxic or ischemic nerve damage.

Fabry's Disease

Fabry's disease is an X-linked lipid disorder characterized by the accumulation of glycosphingolipids in different tissues including the heart, kidney, and cornea, and in peripheral and autonomic nerves. The accumulation of glycosphingolipids is due to a deficiency of the enzyme α-galactosidase A. Patients with this disorder present paresthesia and severe burning pain in the toes, feet, and fingers. A particular character-istic feature is the occurrence of crises with severe pain attacks provoked by fever and movements. These patients, not exclusively males but also females with a less prominent form of the condition, display signs of a small-fiber neuropathy.

Vitamin Deficiencies

Vitamin B_1 (thiamine), B_6 (pyridoxine), and B_{12} (cobalamin) and a few other vitamin deficiencies can all give rise to a polyneuropathy, which may or may not be associated with pain. These vitamin deficiencies are often associated with other forms of malnutrition such as reduced food intake, malabsorption syndromes, and alcoholism, factors that may have an additional negative effect and increase the risk of further devel-opment and maintenance of a neuropathy. Lack of vitamin B_{12}, which occurs in older people with a frequency of >1%, gives rise to both a my-elopathy and a neuropathy. Patients characteristically develop a degen-eration of the dorsal columns, with loss of vibration and position sense together with ataxia. In addition, patients may develop a burning pain sensation in the feet and paresthesias or painful pricking dysesthesias in the limbs.

Mechanisms of Neuropathic Pain

An understanding of neuropathic pain requires an understanding of the mechanisms that cause neuronal hyperexcitability despite a reduced or lost input to the nervous system. The reduction of afferent input caused by a nervous system lesion is the starting point for both regeneration and disinhibition, with secondary development of hypersensitivity.

The changes giving rise to this hypersensitivity occur at different levels. At the molecular level, formation of new channels, upregulation of certain receptors and downregulation of others, expression of novel receptors, and induction of new genes are some of the phenomena that contribute to hyperexcitability [4,6–8,14,15,18,22–24,27,30]. At the cel-lular level, the translation of molecular changes takes multiple forms, in-cluding discharges in nociceptors, a reduced threshold to depolarize cell bodies, an increased response to suprathreshold stimulation, recruitment of silent nociceptors, expansion of receptive fields, changes in cell phenotypes, and secondary changes in spinal cord and brain relay stations [4,6,18,27,30]. The clinical expressions of these cellular manifestations include exaggerated and prolonged pains, different types of evoked pains, and an extraterritorial spread of pain to undamaged tissue [2,10,16]. It is now clear that a series of mechanisms are involved in generating neuropathic pain symptoms and signs and that there is no simple translation of each mechanism into specific symptoms and signs [16]. This is generally the case for most neuropathic types of pain, including those resulting from neuropathies.

The possible translation of neuronal hyperexcitability into clinical symptoms is important because it is the key to understanding potential mechanisms of neuropathic pain and how they can be targeted, for example by pharmacological interventions. At present, the relationship between symptoms and signs on the one hand and mechanisms on the other is not clear because of lack of a one-to-one relationship between a symptom or sign and a mechanism.

An important clinical observation in neuropathic pain is the combination of sensory loss due to damage of transmitting pathways and the development of maladaptive neuroplastic changes in the nervous system, resulting in, for example, pain and hypersensitivity in the affected area. Changes can be divided into peripheral and central sensitization phenomena. The following sections will briefly describe some of these sensitization phenomena that play a role in neuropathic pain.

Sensitization of Primary Afferents

Sensitization of nociceptors may result in spontaneous nociceptor activity as well as decreased threshold and increased response to suprathreshold stimuli. Various mechanisms of nociceptor sensitization are possible. After a nerve injury or inflammation of the nerve trunk, proinflammatory cytokines, chemokines, and neurotrophic factors released from immune cells may sensitize nociceptors, which have immune receptors. Changes in gene expression of both injured and uninjured primary afferents, with increased expression of brain-derived neurotrophic factor (BDNF) and transient receptor potential (TRP) channels, have been shown to alter pain behavior in neuropathic pain models. Neurotransmitter release may also be increased by an upregulation of the $\alpha_2\delta$ subunit of voltage-gated calcium channels.

Central Sensitization

Central sensitization refers to increased responsiveness of nociceptive neurons in the CNS to their normal or subthreshold afferent input. Central sensitization may be a result of the increased peripheral neuronal barrage following peripheral sensitization, but it is also believed that central sensitization can become independent of peripheral input in certain chronic pain conditions. This scenario has important treatment perspectives because treating the initiating mechanisms at the peripheral level will then no longer be effective. Central sensitization is also thought to explain how low-threshold Aβ mechanoreceptors gain access to pain-transmitting systems, causing normally nonpainful stimuli to be perceived as painful.

Activation of N-methyl D-aspartate (NMDA) receptors plays a crucial role in central sensitization by increasing influx of calcium ions and initiating a cascade of intracellular events [22]. Peripheral and central nervous system lesions have also been shown to activate spinal cord glial cells. Microglia activation following peripheral nerve injury leading to the release of proinflammatory cytokines acting upon neurons is likely to be an important mechanism of exaggerated pain and of spreading of pain to neighboring healthy tissue outside the area of nerve injury [24]. Spinal inhibition plays a significant role in controlling nociceptive transmission. The ongoing activity from primary afferents may give rise to a degeneration of inhibitory dorsal horn interneurons containing γ-aminobutyric acid (GABA), which may further contribute to disinhibition and increased neuronal sensitivity. Downregulation of GABA and opioid receptors may also contribute to decreased tonic inhibition. Several recent studies have shown that changes in the balance between descending inhibition and facilitation may contribute to the maintenance of neuropathic pain [29].

In addition to increased afferent barrage from primary afferents, loss of primary nociceptors may also be associated with central sensitization, spontaneous pain, and evoked pain. How such loss of neurons and the resulting imbalance of sensory input may cause pain is not clear, but changes in the CNS due to deafferentation, such as decreased inhibition and bursting activity, may play a role.

Treatment of Inflammatory and Metabolic Neuropathic Pain

Causal treatment is the optimal option for all types of neuropathic pain, including those associated with or caused by metabolic or inflammatory conditions. Even if treatment of the underlying cause of neuropathy is possible, the pain may not necessarily disappear, because nerve damage has already occurred. In many instances, symptomatic treatment is therefore the best that can be provided. Pharmacological management is the mainstay in patients with painful inflammatory or metabolic neuropathies. It is also important to remember that symptomatic pain treatment should be offered even if causal treatment is possible. The following paragraphs will concentrate on pharmacological treatment for these disorders.

Before choosing a neuropathic pain treatment, clinicians need to consider the benefits and risks of a specific treatment. There are no exact data that permit the presentation of a treatment algorithm for all types of neuropathic pain. The data are mainly based on results from painful diabetic neuropathy and HIV neuropathy. It is unknown if results from these studies can be extrapolated to other painful neuropathies. In practice, treatments are often combined. In the future we will see more studies of combined treatments, which makes sense, given the multiple mechanisms contributing to neuropathic pain in individual patients. But side effects are a limiting factor for any type of systemic therapy applied [11].

In general, simpler and less harmful treatments should be chosen, and the efficacy of any compound should always be balanced against its adverse effects. It is mandatory that clinicians are familiar with contraindications, particularly when treating the elderly. Cardiac conduction abnormalities (e.g., AV block), congestive heart failure, and convulsive disorders are contraindications for treatment with tricyclic antidepressants. For anticonvulsants the contraindications are fewer, but side effects such as sedation, dizziness, tremor, and skin rashes are not uncommon.

Before prescribing pharmacological treatment, the physician must address the patient's age, concomitant medical conditions, depression, sleep disturbances, and other psychosocial factors. Realistic expectations for the outcome of a given treatment should be discussed with the patient, and it should be explained that sometimes only partial pain relief can be expected.

The treatment effect is not always predictable, and patients with the same disease or symptom may respond differently to treatment. There is little evidence for specific symptoms to be treated with specific drugs

Table IV
Pharmacological treatment of neuropathic pain

Drug	Starting Dose; Maximum Dose	Documented Effect	Side Effects
Gabapentin	Start: 300 mg/day; Max: 3600 mg/day	PHN, PDN, mixed neuropathic pain	Sedation, dizziness, edema
Pregabalin	Start: 25 mg/day; Max: 600 mg/day	PHN, PDN, HIV, mixed neuropathic pain	Sedation, dizziness, edema
Tricyclic antidepressants	Start: 25 mg/day; Max: 75–150 mg/day	PHN, PDN, mixed neuropathic pain	Cardiac conduction disturbances, anticholinergic side effects, sedation
SNRIs	Venlafaxine: Start: 37.5 mg; Max: 225–375 mg/day Duloxetine: Start: 60 mg; Max: 120 mg/day	Painful neuropathy	Sedation
Carbamazepine (oxcarbazepine)	Start: 300 mg/day; Max: 1200–1800 mg (1/3 higher dose for oxcarbazepine)	Trigeminal neuralgia	Sedation, dizziness, ataxia
Tramadol	Start: 50 mg/day; Max: 400 mg/day	Painful neuropathies	Sedation, dizziness, constipation
Opioids	Start: 5–10 mg/day, titrate, substitute long-acting opioids; Max: variable	PHN, PDN, HIV, mixed neuropathic pains	Sedation, dizziness, tolerance, drug abuse
Lidocaine patch	5%	PHN	Allergic reaction
Capsaicin cream	0.075% and 8%	PHN, PDN, HIV	Pain

Abbreviations: HIV, human immunodeficiency virus; PDN, painful diabetic neuropathy; PHN, postherpetic neuralgia; SNRIs, serotonin norepinephrine reuptake inhibitors.

[10,11]. Although sodium channel blockers, such as carbamazepine, are the drug of choice for treating paroxysmal pain in trigeminal neuralgia, there is little evidence for choosing sodium channel blockers for pain dominated by paroxysms or antidepressants for burning, pricking, and ongoing pain. Based on the current evidence, the European Federation of Neurological Societies (EFNS) has provided guidelines for the pharmacological treatment of neuropathic pain [1]. Table IV presents a list of drugs for the treatment of neuropathic pain with recommended doses for different conditions and their major side effects.

Concluding Remarks

Neuropathic pain caused by or associated with inflammatory diseases and metabolic disorders is an important problem that reduces quality of life. Most of these disorders are dominated by a distal sensory neuropathy, but the clinical picture is also heavily influenced by the underlying causative agent. Just as the neuropathic pain phenotype is variable, so are the underlying mechanisms, which include both peripheral and central factors. Treatment is difficult and has previously relied on symptomatic reduction of neuronal hyperexcitability, either in the peripheral nerves or in the CNS. There is now a desire to move from a simple reduction of symptoms to a disease-modifying strategy. It is assumed that a more radical treatment of the underlying pain generator will result in better pain relief. How far this approach will lead us has yet to be seen.

Acknowledgments

This chapter was made possible in part by grants from the Velux Foundation and the Lundbeck Foundation, and by the Innovative Medicines Initiative Joint Undertaking (IMI JU) grant no. 115007 (EUROPAIN).

References

[1]   Attal N, Cruccu G, Baron R, Haanpaa M, Hansson P, Jensen TS, Nurmikko T. EFNS guidelines on the pharmacological treatment of neuropathic pain: 2010 revision. Eur J Neurol 2010;17:1113–e88.
[2]   Baron R. Mechanisms of disease: neuropathic pain – a clinical perspective. Nat Clin Pract Neurol 2006;2:95–106.

[3] Baron R, Binder G, Wasner G. Neuropathic pain: diagnosis, pathophysiological mechanisms, and treatment. Lancet Neurol 2010;9:807–19.

[4] Basbaum AI, Bautista DM, Scherrer G, Julius D. Cellular and molecular mechanisms of pain. Cell 2009;139:267–84.

[5] Bouhassira D, Attal N, Willer JC. Painful and painless peripheral sensory neuropathies due to HIV infection: a comparison using quantitative sensory evaluation. Pain 1999;80:265–72.

[6] Campbell JN, Meyer RA. Mechanisms of neuropathic pain. Neuron 2006;52:77–92.

[7] Costigan M, Scholz J, Woolf CJ. Neuropathic pain: A maladaptive response of the nervous system to damage. Annu Rev Neurosci 2009;32:1–32.

[8] Dib-Hajj SD, Cummins TR, Black JA, Waxman SG. Sodium channels in normal and pathological pain. Annu Rev Neurosci 2010;33:325–47.

[9] Dyck, PJ, Thomas PK, editors. Peripheral neuropathies I, II. Philadelphia: Saunders; 2005.

[10] Finnerup NB, Jensen TS. Mechanism-based classification of neuropathic pain: a critical analysis. Nat Clin Prac Neurol 2006;2:107–15.

[11] Finnerup NB, Sindrup SH, Jensen TS. The evidence of pharmacological treatment of neuropathic pain. Pain 2010;150:573–81.

[12] Ginsberg L. Specific painful neuropathies. In: Cervero F, Jensen TS, editors. Pain. Handbook of clinical neurology, Vol. 81. London: Elsevier; 2006. p. 635–52.

[13] Haanpaa M, Attal N, Backonja M, Baron R, Bennett M, Bouhassira D, Cruccu G, Hansson P, Haythornthwaite J, Iannetti G, Jensen T, Kauppila T, Nurmikko T, Rice A, Rowbotham M, Serra J, Sommer C, Smith B, Treede RD. NeuPSIG guidelines on neuropathic pain assessment. Pain 2011;152:14–27.

[14] Heinzmann S, McMahon SB. New molecules for the treatment of pain. Curr Opin Support Palliat Care 2011;5:111–5.

[15] Hunt SP, Mantyh PW. The molecular dynamics of pain control. Nat Rev Neurosci 2001;2:83–91.

[16] Jensen TS, Baron R. Translation of symptoms and signs into mechanisms in neuropathic pain. Pain 2003;102:1–8.

[17] Kehlet H, Jensen TS, Woolf CJ. Persistent postsurgical pain: risk factors and prevention. Lancet 2006;367:1618–25.

[18] Latremoliere A, Woolf CJ. Central sensitization: a generator of pain hypersensitivity by central neural plasticity. J Pain 2009;10:895–926.

[19] Merskey H, Bogduk N. Classification of chronic pain: descriptions of chronic pain syndromes and definitions of pain terms. In: Merskey H, Bogduk N, editors. Classification of chronic pain. Seattle: IASP Press; 1994.

[20] Pachner AR, Steiner I. Lyme neuroborreliosis: infection, immunity, and inflammation. Lancet Neurol 2007;6:544–52.

[21] Polydefkiss M, Yiannoutsos CT, Cohen BA, Hollander H, Schifitto G, Clifford DB, Simpson DM, Katzenstein D, Shriver S, Hauer P, Brown A, Haidich AB, Moo L, McArthur JC. Reduced intraepidermal nerve fiber density in HIV-associated sensory neuropathy. Neurology 2002;58:115–9.

[22] Ren K, Dubner R. Pain facilitation and activity-dependent plasticity in pain modulatory circuitry: role of BDNF-TrkB signaling and NMDA receptors. Mol Neurobiol 2007;35:224–35.

[23] Reichling DB, Levine JD. Pain and death: neurodegenerative disease mechanisms in the nociceptor. Ann Neurol 2011;69:13–21.

[24] Saab CY, Waxman SG, Hains BC. Alarm or curse? The pain of neuroinflammation. Brain Res Rev 2008;58:226–35.

[25] Saadé NE, Jabbur SJ. Nociceptive behavior in animal models for peripheral neuropathy: spinal and supraspinal mechanisms. Prog Neurobiol 2008;86:22–47.

[26] Scadding JW, Koltzenburg M. Painful peripheral neuropathies. In: McMahon SB, Koltzenburg M, editors. Textbook of pain. London: Churchill Livingstone; 2006. p. 973–99.

[27] Scholz J, Woolf CJ. Can we conquer pain? Nat Neurosci 2002;5(Suppl):1062–7.

[28] Sommer C, Lauria G. Painful small-fiber neuropathies. In: Cervero F, Jensen TS, editors. Pain. Handbook of clinical neurology, Vol. 81. London: Elsevier; 2006. p. 621–33.

[29] Tracey I, Mantyh PW. The cerebral signature for pain perception and its modulation. Neuron 2007;55:377–91.

[30] Zhuo M, Wu G, Wu LJ. Neuronal and microglial mechanisms of neuropathic pain. Mol Brain 2011;4:31:1–12.

[31] Xu Q, Yaksh TL. A brief comparison of the pathophysiology of inflammatory versus neuropathic
      pain. Curr Opin Anaesthesiol 2011;4:400–7.

Correspondence to: Prof. Troels S. Jensen, MD, DMSc, Danish Pain Research
Center, Aarhus University Hospital, Norrebrogade 44, Building 1A, DK 8000 Aarhus C, Denmark. Email: tsjensen@ki.au.dk.

Pain and Affective Disorders: Looking Beyond the "Chicken and Egg" Conundrum

Ephrem Fernandez[a] and Robert D. Kerns[b,c]

[a]Department of Psychology, University of Texas at San Antonio, San Antonio, Texas, USA; [b]Departments of Psychiatry, Neurology, and Psychology, Yale University, New Haven, Connecticut, USA; [c]PRIME Center, VA Connecticut Healthcare System, West Haven, Connecticut, USA

Pain and Affective Quality

Pain, as defined by the International Association for the Study of Pain, is a physical sensation associated with tissue damage; it is also unpleasant, and therefore an affective experience (www.iasp-pain.org/painterms). The affective concomitant of pain can extend well beyond unpleasantness to a host of negatively valenced emotions or moods. Most common among these are fear, sadness, and anger, or their clinical equivalents of anxiety, depression, and anger disorders. These moods and emotions, according to Fernandez and Kerns [30], make up the "core of negative affect" in chronic pain patients and in many other medical populations too.

The Chicken and Egg Conundrum

In its literal sense, the chicken versus egg conundrum has been solved, or so we are told by biologists. The reasoning goes like this: mutation from one form to another can only occur during the embryonic stage of development. Thus, it was not some specimen of fowl that turned into

Pain Comorbidities: Understanding and Treating the Complex Patient
edited by Maria Adele Giamberardino and Troels Staehelin Jensen
IASP Press, Seattle, © 2012

a chicken, but an egg laid by a proto-chicken that mutated into the first chicken egg that hatched into the first chicken. The chicken egg was the point of origin for that species; the rest, as they say, is reproductive history.

As a figure of speech, the chicken versus egg conundrum continues to be applied whenever there is a question about the origination of two interdependent entities. In the current context, there is less preoccupation with a historical starting point for pain or affective disturbance. Rather, the question is typically framed in terms of whether pain causes affective disturbance or affective disturbance causes pain [34,35].

In this chapter, we tackle this question by examining research from several different angles. The first viewpoint comes from epidemiological studies on comorbidity of pain and affective disturbance. This discussion is followed by findings on the correlation between these two constructs. Finally, we propose a broader exploration of the ways in which these two phenomena may dynamically influence each other.

Comorbidity

The co-occurrence of pain and affective disturbance, like any co-occurrence of two or more diagnoses in an individual, is termed "comorbidity." It can be reported as a simple frequency count or a tally of the number of people with pain who also happen to have affective disturbance. Alternatively, a relative frequency can be reported, which is no different from a percentage, proportion, or probability. Another index of comorbidity is the odds ratio, which is an estimate of the relative risk of a disorder (e.g., depression) in a particular group (e.g., those with pain) as compared to another group (e.g., those without pain). The probability of the disorder in the first group (p_1) can be compared to the probability of the same disorder in the second group (p_2). The odds ratio is calculated by $p_1/(1 - p_1)$ divided by $p_2/(1 - p_2)$. A result that exceeds 1 indicates that the disorder is more likely in the p_1 group than the p_2 group.

Recognizing the comorbidity of pain and affective disturbance is important because if chronic pain carries with it the additional likelihood of depression, anxiety, or anger, the burden on the patient is augmented. This consideration may parallel some of the interesting observations of symptom load in comorbid visceral conditions. Giamberardino and colleagues [37] have demonstrated that pathology in two affected organs or districts of the viscera leads to more than an additive outcome in pain; for example, patients with coronary artery disease and gallbladder calculosis have more episodes of angina as well as more episodes of biliary pain plus hyperalgesia in the left chest and cystic point areas as compared to patients who just have coronary artery disease or just have biliary calculosis alone. For a full description, see the chapter in this volume by Giamberardino et al. The authors provide many more clinical examples of the compounding of symptoms in comorbid visceral conditions. Could it be the case that the patient who has chronic low back pain as well as depression may actually have more pain as well as more depression as compared to the patient who has just one of those two conditions? Not only could there be an added burden for the patient but also further responsibilities for health care providers. Yet, as pointed out by Sherbourne et al. [59], the majority of pain patients seen in primary care have distress, and only a minority of them talk to their provider about emotional problems.

Research continues to draw attention to the comorbidity of pain and affective disturbance. Asmundson and Katz [5] have graphed the rapid increase in publications on this issue over the last 15–20 years. We now turn to some of the comorbidity data that have emerged from various studies. Findings are organized according to the particular types of affective disturbance—anxiety, depression, and anger.

Comorbidity of Pain and Anxiety

A classic study by Fishbain et al. [33] reported that in a sample of 283 chronic pain patients, 19.5% had at least one anxiety disorder. Subsequent studies have reported similar figures. However, findings differ as to which particular type of anxiety disorder is most prevalent in persons with pain. Whereas generalized anxiety disorder (GAD) has been identified as by far the most common by some researchers (e.g., [6,33]), others have reported as low as 2% prevalence of GAD in pain patients (e.g., [53]). More recent research lends support to the early findings that the comorbidity of pain and GAD exceeds that between pain and other anxiety disorders (e.g., [9]). Other anxiety disorders found with varying prevalence in the pain population are panic disorder, obsessive-compulsive disorder, and post-traumatic stress disorder (PTSD).

In their recent update of the literature on comorbidity of chronic pain and anxiety disorders, Asmundson and Katz [5] emphasize that anxiety disorders have a much higher prevalence (35%) in community samples of patients with chronic arthritic pain than in the general population (17%). They highlight the findings from the World Mental Health Surveys [22] that in comparison to the general community, those with chronic back or neck pain are two to three times more likely to have panic disorder, agoraphobia, or social anxiety disorder, and nearly three times more likely to have GAD or PTSD.

Anxiety is particularly prevalent in those with chest pain. Since a person experiencing chest pain often views it as a symptom of a life-threatening condition, it is quite understandable that a sense of emergency or even outright panic would arise. Worthington et al. [73] studied a pool of 1254 emergency ward patients who presented with chest pain as the chief complaint and found that a random sample of 44 revealed high rates of panic disorder. Beitman and colleagues [11] found that of 30 atypical or nonanginal chest pain patients, 13 were positive for panic disorder.

Cancer pain often brings on anxiety, especially when the pain is construed as a sign of progression of a life-threatening disease. Such misinterpretation may evolve into symptom preoccupation so that the slightest increase in pain is sensed and interpreted as tumor development [65]. In a sample of 47 ambulatory male outpatients with prostate cancer, those with pain were significantly more anxious (or depressed) than those without pain [40].

While pain is not a criterion for diagnosis of anxiety disorders, it is the case that many patients seeking help for the latter also experience the former. For example, 71% of panic disorder patients reported pain [58]. In their review of military veterans with a primary diagnosis of PTSD, Otis and colleagues [51] reported that (depending on the study in question) anywhere from 25% to 80% of these individuals also had some kind of pain. Of course, this finding does not imply directionality, but it gives an idea of the range of probability of having pain when one has PTSD. The co-occurrence may be coincidental rather than a conversion reaction, especially since many combat soldiers sustain physical injuries in addition to being psychologically traumatized.

In a sample of patients with chronic rhinosinusitis, 48% had low anxiety, 26% had moderate anxiety, and 26% had high anxiety [70]. Beesdo and colleagues [10] extracted data from the German National Health Interview and Examination Survey. In this representative community sample of 4181 individuals, 31.7% of those with a lifetime pain disorder had anxiety disorder in the preceding 12 months. Logistic regression revealed somewhat of a dose-response relationship in which the odds ratio of having affective disorders was significantly greater in unexplained pain (OR, 2.4 to 7.3) than in medically explainable pain (OR, 1.9 to 2.0).

Comorbidity of Pain and Depression

The American Psychiatric Association [2] estimates the point prevalence of major depression in adult community samples at 2% to 3% for men and 5% to 9% for women. The prevalence of dysthymia is about 3%. In medical populations, especially those experiencing chronic pain, these rates are understandably higher [8,30].

For pain and depression, the comorbidity statistics are even more variable than for pain and anxiety. Estimates of this comorbidity vary from 30% to 87% [61]. Some reviewers place it even further apart at 10% to 100% [54]. An extensive review by Fernandez [29] found the range to be even wider, from a minimum of 0% [26] to an absolute maximum of 100% [68]. This review is consistent with findings that have appeared since. For example, in their study across 17 countries, Tsang and colleagues [64] found the comorbidity of pain and affective disturbance to be as low as 2.4%. On the whole, the pronounced variability may be attributed to differences in sample demographics, heterogeneity of pain syndromes, differences in operationalization of measures, and procedural variations in data collection.

In the early study by Fishbain and colleagues [33], pain patients were interviewed for 2 hours by a senior psychiatrist in order to generate applicable DSM-III (*Diagnostic and Statistical Manual of Mental Disorders*) diagnoses. The investigators found that 56.2% of patients had clinically diagnosable depressive disorder. This percentage was disaggregated into 28.3% with adjustment disorder plus depressed mood, 23.3% with dysthymia, and 4.6% with major depression disorder (MDD).

Particularly high rates of depression have appeared in those with head pain. Substantial depressive symptoms occur in 84% of individuals with headaches [23,68]. The rates may be particularly high when migraine and tension-type headache persist in the absence of organic pathology

[57]. Among patients with chronic low back pain, depression prevalence has been reported at 26% in general practice settings [46] and as high as 78% in specialty pain clinics [63]. However, a recent telephone survey of 1179 adults in Michigan revealed no significant differences in depression as a function of the location or type of pain [49]. What it did find was that comorbid pain and depression were more common in those who were older, female, less educated, and employed less than full-time, as compared to their counterparts without pain or depression.

One underlying variable in the comorbidity of pain and depression may be the number of distinct pain sites. With only one chronic pain complaint, the coprevalence of major depression was only 1%, but this figure rose to 9% in persons with two chronic pain complaints, and reached 12% for those with three chronic pain complaints [25]. Findings may also vary according to the setting of the study. Patients referred to pain clinics generally have a greater prevalence of depression than those seen in primary care clinics. It is likely that the apparent presence of psychosocial distress may account for increased referral to specialists.

Different findings also emerge from different parts of the world. In a sample of 400 patients evaluated at a university pain clinic in Brazil, 42% had depressive episodes and 54% had dysthymia [20]. In a sample of 337 patients with chest pain seen at a university hospital in India, 23% had an ICD-10 (*International Classification of Diseases*) diagnosed psychiatric disorder, and anxiety and depression were equally common among these diagnoses [62]. A study in Turkey found that of 77 patients with myofascial pain, 39% were diagnosed with major depression, as contrasted with 4% in the control group of healthy subjects [1].

Tsang and colleagues [64] surveyed more than 85,000 individuals for chronic pain and affective disturbance; this sample was spread out over 17 countries across the Americas, Europe, Asia, the Middle East, and Oceania. While chronic pain was prevalent in varying degrees in both developing and developed countries, the proportion of chronic pain patients with depression or anxiety ranged from as low as 2.4% in Nigeria to a maximum of 24% in the United States. It is important to note that a large majority of the chronic pain patients did not meet all criteria for diagnoses of depressive or anxiety disorders, thus leading the authors to the suggestion that chronic pain is not a mask for affective disturbance.

Recent studies in Europe also point to a trend toward lower rates of pain comorbid with depression. At a university hospital in Denmark, chronic pain patients had only slightly higher rates of depression than healthy controls, but the prevalence of depression was much lower (7.1%) in fibromyalgia patients and even lower in neuropathic pain patients (3.3%) [38]. The report on the German National Health Interview and Examination Survey found that 24.5% of 4181 individuals had a depressive disorder in the preceding 12 months [10]. As reported earlier, logistic regression revealed a dose-response function in which the odds ratio of having affective disorders was significantly greater in lifetime pain disorder (OR, 3.3 to 14.8) than in unexplained pain (OR, 2.4 to 7.3) which was greater than in medically explainable pain (OR, 1.9 to 2.0).

Depressives with Pain?

In addition to the prevalence of depression in pain patients, the converse, pain in depressives, has also attracted research interest. Lindsay and Wyckoff [44] reported 59% of 191 depressed patients as having pain in the 3 months prior to diagnosis. A survey of 11,000 medical patients revealed that 35% of those with depressive symptoms also reported pain [72]. In depressed geriatric inpatients, 62% reported chronic pain [48].

Results are conflicting regarding the intensity of the pain found among persons with depression. Pain reported among 46% of individuals hospitalized for depressive disorder was in most cases low in intensity [69]. Similarly, in 66% of 51 geriatric patients with major depression, pain severity was moderate [47]. Arnow and colleagues [3] surveyed 5808 patients subscribing to a health maintenance organization. They found that 66% of those with depression also reported chronic pain while 41% reported disabling chronic pain, as compared to 43% and 10%, respectively, in a sample of patients without depression.

Comorbidity of Pain and Anger

Relatively few studies have investigated anger in chronic pain patients, partly because the DSM does not provide a diagnostic category for anger, per se. However, intermittent explosive disorder, though lumped with other impulse control diagnoses rather than affective disorders, can be characterized as an anger disorder. It has been found in about 10% of pain patients, according to the early study by Fishbain and colleagues [33], which is much higher than its 12-month prevalence in the community, which is 3.9% according to the National Comorbidity Survey Replication study of U.S. households [42].

Since Fishbain's study, the comorbidity of anger and pain has also been investigated using customized questionnaires. For example, Kristjansdottir [43] administered a 256-item questionnaire pertaining to pain, distress, attitudes, and behaviors to a sample of 2400 schoolchildren in Iceland. Anger emerged as the most common issue in 76.5% of those with weekly back pain, 76.9% of those with weekly headache, and 78.3% of those with weekly stomach pain. This percentage surpassed the corresponding statistics for anxiety and sadness, respectively.

Comorbidity of Anxiety, Depression, and Anger

Not only do anxiety, depression, and anger tend to co-occur with pain, but they also tend to co-occur with one another. In other words, affective disorders may "pair up," as revealed in the co-prevalence and bivariate correlations reported below.

Evidently the strongest "bond" is between depression and anxiety. About one-third of patients diagnosed with anxiety disorder are also diagnosed with a depressive disorder [56]. Dobson's [24] review of measures of anxiety and depression showed that the average correlation between the two is +0.61, with a range of 0.27 to 0.94. Anxiety and depression are also correlated in the pain population. Smith and Zautra [60] reported $r = +0.70$ in a sample of women with pain associated with rheumatoid arthritis or osteoarthritis.

There is insufficient research on the comorbidity of anxiety and anger, but anger and depression have been linked together. Synthesizing the results of various studies, Bruehl and colleagues [15] reported that the correlation between a standardized measure of the outward expression of anger and measures of depressive symptom severity ranges from +0.32 to +0.43. Estlander and colleagues [27] did not replicate this finding, but instead found a correlation of +0.50 between a standardized measure of "anger-in" and the summary score on a measure of depressive symptom severity, the Beck Depression Inventory (BDI).

This comorbidity of affective disorders among themselves is important from both a clinical and a research standpoint. Clinically, each additional affective disturbance adds an increased burden on the mental and physical health of the pain patient. For example, in a sample of patients with musculoskeletal pain, presence of both depression and anxiety was associated with greater severity of pain and pain interference than was observed for those reporting depression or anxiety alone [7]. In fact, those with pain, depression, and anxiety had twice the number of disability days than those with pain with either depression or anxiety. The authors called this phenomenon "added morbidity," which is strikingly similar to the increased pain and hyperalgesia observed in individuals with comorbid visceral conditions [37].

From a research standpoint, however, the question is why affective disorders are interrelated. Fernandez and Kerns [30] offer multiple explanations. The first relates to construct overlap. DSM diagnoses of anxiety and depression tend to have several shared criteria, especially when one compares dysthymia and generalized anxiety disorder. A second argument relates to test-taking style. This hypothesis derives from the classic work of Bentler [12], which showed that when given multiple self-report tests, subjects often have acquiescent response styles that lead to spurious correlations among the test results. In fact, about a dozen studies have been cited by Russell and Carroll [55] as empirical evidence for how acquiescent response sets may influence measures of affect. This tendency may account, at least partially, for the observed correlations between self-report measures of anxiety and depression (and pain).

Fernandez and Kerns [30] also consider the possibility of a phenomenological basis for the co-occurrence of anxiety, depression, and anger. A single event can generate these three affective reactions via different appraisal pathways. For example, failure on a work project can leave an employee feeling sorry or sad for himself/herself, angry at the supervisor negatively evaluating the project, and worried about the ramifications for one's job. "Mixed emotions," as they are popularly called, can also arise in the context of pain. A person with persistent pain may feel sad or depressed about the misfortune of an accidental injury, anxious because of the danger of disability, and angry at the failure of the health care system to provide a cure.

Dynamic Interactions

The preceding part of this chapter has centered around comorbidity statistics as a window into the relationship between pain and affective disturbance. However, whether they are in the form of percentages, proportions, probabilities, or odds ratios, such numbers do not enlighten us about the interaction between the phenomena in question. In that sense, they are static rather than dynamic indices. To say "Where there is chicken, there is egg" or "Where there is chicken, there is sometimes egg" is merely stating something about joint probability, without offering information about covariation, let alone causation. We now turn to some of the dynamic interactions that are important extensions of the comorbidity findings presented earlier.

Covariation

Improving on relative frequency, the bivariate correlation coefficient, r, conveys how two variables *change* in relation to each other, r^2 indicating the degree of variation in one explained by variation in the other. In comparison to comorbidity, the correlation reveals how variables are dynamically related.

The correlations between pain and affective disturbance vary according to type of affect as well as type of pain. Altindag et al. [1] reported a correlation of 0.65 between visual analogue scale (VAS) ratings of pain and BDI scores on depression in myofascial pain patients.

With regard to anger and pain, Kerns and colleagues [41] were among the first to dissect the anger of pain patients into internalized anger ("anger-in") versus anger expression ("anger-out") and relate it to chronic pain and adjustment difficulties. A research review by Bruehl and colleagues [15] concluded that 79% of 14 studies provided some support for a significant positive relationship between pain severity/dysfunction and anger expression. However, the correlation coefficients vary considerably across these studies. For example, in chronic pain patients, Spielberger State-Trait Anxiety Expression Inventory (STAXI) anger-out scores were significantly correlated with McGill Pain Questionnaire (MPQ) affective scores ($r = 0.38$), but not with MPQ sensory scores ($r = 0.24$) [14]. In a subsequent study, this correlation was only

0.16 [17]. In studies of experimental pain, correlations between anger expression and pain were either nonsignificant (e.g., [16]) or negligible [18]. Furthermore, research by another independent team [19] has found very low to zero correlations between each of the four measures of the MPQ versus each of the four measures of the STAXI, with the exception of significant positive correlations between pain severity and state anger. Similarly, Estlander and colleagues [27] found low-to-no correlations between STAXI measures of anger-in or anger-out versus VAS ratings of pain severity in a sample of patients at a pain clinic. Even in a large sample of more than 500 veterans with chronic pain, the correlations between pain versus anger-out and anger-in scores were 0.15 and 0.089, respectively [45].

A limitation of the correlation coefficient is that it does not tell us anything about temporal precedence or temporal succession. Neither r nor r^2 allows inferences of causation. Caution in making causal inferences from simple correlations or indices of shared variance is usually exercised when findings are limited to such cross-sectional designs and methods.

Affective Disturbance as Predisposing Factor

In an editorial, Weisberg and Boatwright [71] agree with the established position that chronic pain precipitates mood disorders. However, they go on to redirect interest to the yet uncertain relation between temperament or character traits and chronic pain.

An early example of this process came from the psychoanalytically oriented formulations of Blumer and Heilbronn [13]. These authors used the term "pain prone patient" to refer to patients who are self-sacrificing and guilt-ridden to such an extent as to complain about pain as a socially acceptable alternative to more direct expressions of guilt or depression. In their recent review, Gatchel and Dersh [35] caution that even though DSM personality disorders are found in over 50% of low back pain patients, there is a lack of specificity as far as what type of personality disorder prevails in this population.

The study by Beesdo and colleagues [10] based on the German National Health Interview and Examination Survey offers some support for affective disturbance predisposing individuals to pain. In their representative community sample of 4181 individuals, 31.7% of those with a lifetime pain disorder had an anxiety disorder in the preceding 12 months, and 24.5% had a depressive disorder in the preceding 12 months. What is interesting is that 92.6% of those with any 12-month anxiety disorder had any significant lifetime pain, and 91.3% of those with any 12-month depressive disorder had any significant lifetime pain.

Recently, Arola and colleagues [4] undertook a longitudinal study of pain interference and affective disturbance in older adults from the community. Data were analyzed by logistic regression and expressed in the form of odds ratios. Pain interference (with work) was rated on a five-point scale, and depression and anxiety were measured so that scores between 8 and 21 indicate increasing levels of symptoms for each affective disturbance. The same measures were readministered at follow-up 3 years later. In this way, the onset of symptoms could be identified in cohorts that were previously symptom-free. The investigators found that probable depression and anxiety at baseline actually predicted the onset of new pain-related interference 3 years later. This suggests that affective disturbance may have been a contributor to pain onset, if not a distinct "cause" of pain.

Affective Disturbance as Precipitant

In contrast to the distal or cumulative cause, a precipitant is a sudden or relatively immediate trigger of pain. One of the strongest bits of evidence for this kind of interaction comes from research on anxiety in relation to pain. As reviewed by Fernandez [29], both experimental designs and prospective studies have produced evidence that preoperative anxiety leads to postoperative pain. In a recent 11-week study of women with rheumatoid arthritis or osteoarthritis [60], multilevel analysis was used to predict weekly changes in pain on the basis of affective disturbance. For every standard deviation increase in anxiety, there was a 10.13-point increase in pain severity, though the effect of depression was about half of this magnitude, with every standard deviation increase producing a 5.41-point increase in pain severity.

Van Middendorp and colleagues [67] instructed 333 women with fibromyalgia to monitor anger and pain as part of a diary study lasting 28 consecutive days. Pain was assessed at the end of each day using a VAS, and any event that triggered irritability or anger was recorded throughout the day. Notwithstanding considerable individual differences, a higher level of anger during the day significantly predicted more severe pain at the end of the day.

Affective Disturbance as Exacerbating Factor

Affective disturbance can have exacerbating or attenuating influences on pain. The disturbance may be a result of pain itself, or else it may originate from extraneous factors (e.g., family discord, job dissatisfaction, or social stress). Either way, this negative affect can modulate pain. In reviewing the available literature, Fernandez [29] found that the direction of modulation of pain depends on the particular affective quality. Clearly, anxiety aggravates pain; however, there is evidence that depression dampens pain. The findings on anger are mixed.

Affective Disturbance as Consequence

Revisiting the definition of pain, we can see that physical sensation and affective quality are both important components of the human experience of pain. As closely coupled as the two components are, the unpleasantness is typically viewed as a reaction to the sensory component of pain, with anxiety, depression, and anger usually emerging later on.

As emphasized by Fernandez and Wasan [32], the affective consequence does not occur in a vacuum. It occurs within a psychosocial context with agents and actions. Attributions to the agents and appraisals of their actions are what fuel the affective distress of pain into full-blown emotional disorders. Arola and colleagues [4] have cited several recent studies in support of the idea that pain leads to the new onset of depression [36,21,52]. In one particularly interesting study, pain patients referred to a multidisciplinary pain center reported varying levels of anger, and anger was commonly directed at specific individuals [50]. About 60% of patients in this study were angry toward health care providers, about 20% toward attorneys, about 30% toward insurance companies, 26% to employers, 39% to significant others, but by far the most pain patients (about 70%) were angry at themselves. The appraisal content is illustrated in these anecdotes from two pain patients who were asked to write about their anger related to pain [39]: "I am in constant pain due to your negligence. I wish

I could make you understand what it feels like. ... I feel so mad. ... I hope you never have another good night's sleep in your life. I know I won't." "I can't believe that after all this I have to listen to a druggist [who] has no idea how I feel. ... You make me feel like a criminal and a drug addict." (p. 201). Similarly, appraisals of misfortune and loss among pain patients lead to depression, and appraisals of danger lead to anxiety.

Affective Disturbance as Perpetuating Factor

Whereas pain exacerbation involves an increase in the intensity of pain, perpetuation of pain refers to an increase in the duration of pain. Affective disturbance may prolong preexisting pain. Much research has shown that there is a significant risk of acute pain turning into chronic pain under certain circumstances. One of these circumstances involves solicitude by significant others in response to depression, anxiety, or anger on the part of pain patients. This particular affective exchange between patient and caregiver or even between patient and health care provider can be instrumental in the reinforcement of pain. While this factor is fairly well documented clinically, and in the interpretation of behavioral studies of pain, there is a need for more prospective research in this area.

Conclusions

"Did the chicken come before the egg, or the egg come before the chicken?" Samuel Butler gave primacy to the egg in his quip that "A hen is only an egg's way of making another egg." As explained earlier, biologists now claim to have solved the chicken versus egg conundrum by delivering a concrete and unambiguous answer: the egg! Ever since the first egg (laid by a proto-chicken) mutated into a chicken egg that hatched the first chicken, both chicken and egg have simply been taking turns in the seat of the chicken's nest. What is more important is to ask how the chicken influences the egg it lays and how the egg influences the chicken that is hatched. In other words, the point of inception is settled, but the interplay between the two is of great interest.

The relationship between pain and affective disturbance has been handled largely by comorbidity statistics. These statistics range widely, especially in the case of pain and depression. How affective disturbance changes with pain is a more challenging question that has been addressed largely with the aid of correlation coefficients. These statistics too fall across a broad range, though there is consensus that the relationship is positive and often statistically significant and clinically meaningful. This, however, does not shed light on whether it is pain that causes the affective disturbance or the latter that causes the former. Some progress in answering this question has been enabled by prospective studies. The weight of evidence favors anxiety as a precipitant of pain and depression as a consequence of pain. The evidence is inconclusive with regard to anger as a precipitant of pain, though anecdotal reports suggest that anger is often a consequence of pain.

Answering the question of cause or consequence is an advancement upon statements of relative frequency, but it is not without its own limitations. The answer is constrained to only two possibilities within a bidirectional context. In reality, there are many ways in which pain exerts influences on affect and vice versa. This interaction can be placed within the broader context of psychosomatics, with its continued interest in how psyche and soma interact. No longer is there a question of bidirectional causation. Five discrete types of interactions prevail in psychosomatics and are particularly relevant to the interplay between pain and affect [28,31,30]. These interactions pertain to affective disturbance as a predisposing factor, precipitant, exacerbating factor, consequence, and perpetuating factor in pain. Through programmatic research on these five dynamic interactions, it is hoped that a more complete picture on the relationship between pain and affect will evolve.

Acknowledgments

Thanks to Alyssa Salazar, Sarah Starkweather, and Stephen Doyle for help with citations and referencing and thanks to Elizabeth Endres, Associate Editor at IASP. Support for this manuscript was provided by a grant from the Department of Veterans Affairs, Veterans Health Administration, Office of Research and Development, Health Services Research and Development Service (REA 08-266). Disclaimer: The views expressed in this article are those of the authors and do not necessarily reflect the position or policy of the Department of Veterans Affairs.

294 E. Fernandez and R.D. Kerns

References

[1] Altindag O, Gur A, Altindag A. The relationship between clinical parameters and depression level in patients with myofascial pain syndrome. Pain Med 2008;9:161–5.
[2] American Psychiatric Association. Diagnostic and statistical manual of mental disorders Fourth edition Text Revision (DSM-IV-TR). Washington, DC: American Psychiatric Association; 2000.
[3] Arnow BA, Hunkeler EM, Blasey CM, Lee J, Constantino MJ, Fireman B, Kraemer HC, Dea R, Robinson R, Hayward C. Comorbid depression, chronic pain, and disability in primary care. Psychosom Med 2006;68:262–8.
[4] Arola H, Nicholls E, Mallen C, Thomas E. Self-reported pain interference and symptoms of anxiety and depression in community-dwelling older adults: can a temporal relationship be determined? Eur J Pain 2010;14:966–71.
[5] Asmundson GJG, Katz J. Understanding the co-occurrence of anxiety disorders and chronic pain: state-of-the-art. Depress Anxiety 2009;26:888–901.
[6] Atkinson JH, Slater MA, Patterson TL, Grant I. Prevalence, onset, and risk of psychiatric disorders in men with chronic low back pain: a controlled study. Pain 1991;45:111–21.
[7] Bair MJ, Wu J, Damush TM, Sutherland JM, Kroenke K. Association of depression and anxiety alone and in combination with chronic musculoskeletal pain in primary care patients. Psychosom Med 2008;70:890–7.
[8] Banks SM, Kerns RD. Explaining high rates of depression in chronic pain: a diathesis-stress framework. Psychol Bull 1996;119:95–110
[9] Beesdo K, Hoyer J, Jacobi F, Low N, Hofler M, Wittchen H. Association between generalized anxiety levels and pain in a community sample: evidence for diagnostic specificity. J Anxiety Disord 2009;24:684–93.
[10] Beesdo K, Hoyer J, Jacobi F, Low N, Hofler M, Wittchen H. Pain associated with specific anxiety and depressive disorders in a nationally representative population sample. Soc Psychiatry Psychiatr Epidemiol 2010;45:89–104.
[11] Beitman BD, DeRosear L, Basha IM, Flaker G. Panic disorder in cardiology patients with atypical or non-anginal chest pain: a pilot study. J Anxiety Disord 1987;1:277–82.
[12] Bentler PM. Semantic space is approximately bipolar. J Psychol 1969;71:33–40.
[13] Blumer D, Heilbronn M. Chronic pain as a variant of depressive disease: the pain prone disorder. J Nerv Ment Dis 1981;170:381–406.
[14] Bruehl S, Chung OY, Burns JW. Differential effects of expressive anger regulation on chronic pain intensity in CRPS and non-CRPS limb pain patients. Pain 2003;104:647–54.
[15] Bruehl S, Chung OY, Burns JW. Trait anger and blood pressure recovery following acute pain: evidence for opioid-mediated effects. Int J Behav Med 2006;13:138–46.
[16] Bruehl S, Burns JW, Chung O, Chont M. Pain-related effects of trait anger expression: neural substrates and the role of endogenous opioid mechanisms. Neurosci Biobehav Rev 2009;33:475–91.
[17] Burns JW, Bruehl S. Anger management style, opioid analgesic use and chronic pain severity: a test of opioid-deficit hypothesis. J Behav Med 2005;28:555–63.
[18] Burns JW, Bruehl S, Caceres C. Anger management style, blood pressure reactivity, and acute pain sensitivity: evidence for "trait × situation" models. Ann Behav Med 2004;27:195–204.
[19] Carson JW, Keefe FJ, Goli V, Fras AM, Lynch TR, Thorp SR, Buechler JL. Forgiveness and chronic low back pain: a preliminary study examining the relationship of forgiveness to pain, anger, and psychological distress. J Pain 2005;6:84–91.
[20] Castro M, Kraychete D, Daltro C, Lopes J, Menezes R, Oliveira I. Comorbid anxiety and depression disorders in patients with chronic pain. Arq Neuropsiquiatr 2009;67:982–5.
[21] Cole MG, Dendukuri N. Risk factors for depression among elderly community subjects: a systematic review and meta-analysis. Am J Psychiatry 2003;160:1147–56.
[22] Demyttenaere K, Bruffaerts R, Lee S, Posada-Villa J, Kovess V, Angermeyer MC, Von Korff M. Mental disorders among persons with chronic back or neck pain: results from the world mental health surveys. Pain 2007;129:332–42.
[23] Diamond S. Depressive headaches. Headache 1964;4:255–8.
[24] Dobson KS. An analysis of anxiety and depression scales. J Pers Assess 1985;49:522–6.
[25] Dworkin SF, Von Korff M, LeResche L. Multiple pains and psychiatric disturbance: an epidemiologic investigation. Arch Gen Psychiatry 1990;47:239–44.

[26] Ehlert U, Heim C, Hellhammer DH. Chronic pelvic pain as a somatoform disorder. Psychother Psychosom 1999;68:87–94.

[27] Estlander A, Knaster P, Karlsson H, Kaprio J, Kalso E. Pain intensity influences the relationship between anger management style and depression. Pain 2008;140:387–92.

[28] Fernandez E. The role of affect in somatoform and factitious disorders. Curr Rev Pain 1998;2:109–14.

[29] Fernandez E. Anxiety, depression, and anger in pain: research findings and clinical options. Dallas, TX: Advanced Psychological Resources; 2002.

[30] Fernandez E, Kerns RD. Anxiety, depression, and anger: core components of negative affect in medical populations. In: Boyle GJ, Matthews D, Saklofske D, editors. International handbook of personality theory and testing: Vol. 1: Personality theories and models. London: Sage; 2008. p. 659–76.

[31] Fernandez E, Clark TS, Rudick-Davis D. A framework for conceptualization and assessment of affective disturbance in pain. In: Block AR, Kremer EF, E. Fernandez E, editors. Handbook of pain syndromes: a biopsychosocial perspective. Mahwah, NJ: Lawrence Erlbaum Associates; 1999. p. 123–47.

[32] Fernandez E, Wasan A. The anger of pain sufferers: attributions to agents and appraisals of wrongdoing. In: Potegal M, Stemmler G, Spielberger C, editors. The international handbook of anger: constituent and concomitant biological, psychological, and social processes. New York: Springer; 2010. p. 449–64.

[33] Fishbain DA, Goldberg M, Meagher B R, Steele R. Male and female chronic pain categorized by DSM-III psychiatric diagnostic criteria. Pain 1986;26:181–97.

[34] Gatchel RJ. Comorbidity of chronic pain and mental health disorders: the biopsychosocial perspective. Am Psychol 2004;59:795–805.

[35] Gatchel RJ, Dersh J. Psychological disorders and chronic pain: are there cause and effect relationships? In: Turk DC, Gatchel RJ, editors. Psychological approaches to pain management: a practitioner's handbook, 2nd ed. New York: Guilford Press; 2002.

[36] Geerlings SW, Twisk JWR, Beekman ATF, Deeg DJH, Van Tilburg W. Longitudinal relationship between pain and depression in older adults: sex, age, and physical disability. Soc Psychiatry Psychiatr Epidemiol 2002;37:23–30.

[37] Giamberardino MA, Costantini R, Affaitati G, Fabrizio A, Lapenna D, Tafuri E, Mezzetti A. Viscero-visceral hyperalgesia: characterization in different clinical models. Pain 2010;151:307–22.

[38] Gormsen L, Rosenberg R, Bach FW, Jensen TS. Depression, anxiety, health-related quality of life and pain in patients with chronic fibromyalgia and neuropathic pain. Eur J Pain 2010;14:127. e1–8.

[39] Graham JE, Lobel M, Glass P, Lokshina I. Effects of written anger expression in chronic pain patients: making meaning from pain. J Behav Med 2008;31:201–12.

[40] Heim HM, Oei TP. Comparison of prostate cancer patients with and without pain. Pain 1993;53:159–62.

[41] Kerns RD, Rosenberg R, Jacob MC. Anger expression and chronic pain. J Behav Med 1994;17:57–67.

[42] Kessler R, Coccaro E, Maurizio F. The prevalence and correlates of DSM-IV intermittent explosive disorders. Directions Psychiatry 2007;27:221–9.

[43] Kristjansdottir GK. The relationships between pains and various discomforts in schoolchildren. Childhood 1997;4:491–504.

[44] Lindsay PG, Wyckoff M. The depression-pain syndrome and its response to antidepressants. Psychosomatics 1981;22:571–3,576–7.

[45] Lombardo ER, Tan G, Jensen MP, Anderson KO. Anger management style and associations with self-efficacy and pain in male veterans. J Pain 2005;6:765–70.

[46] Love AW. Depression in chronic low back pain patients: diagnostic efficiency of three self-report questionnaires. J Clin Psychol 1987;43:84–9.

[47] Magni G, Schifano F, de Leo D. Pain as a symptom in elderly depressed patients: relationship to diagnostic subgroups. Eur Arch Psychiatry Neurol Sci 1985;235:143–5.

[48] Meeks T, Dunn L, Kim D, Golshan S, Sewell D, Atkinson J, Lebowitz B. Chronic pain and depression among geriatric psychiatry inpatients. Int J Geriatr Psychiatry 2008;23:637.

[49] Miller LR, Cano A. Comorbid chronic pain and depression: who is at risk? J Pain 2009;10:619–27.

[50] Okifuji A, Turk DC, Curran SL. Anger in chronic pain: Investigations of anger targets and intensity. J Psychosom Res 1999;47:1–12.

[51] Otis JD, Keane TM, Kerns RD. An examination of the relationship between chronic pain and post-traumatic stress disorder. J Rehabil Res Dev 2003;40:397–406.

[52] Parmelee PA, Harralson TL, Smith LA, Schumacher HR. Necessary and discretionary activities in knee osteoarthritis: Do they mediate the pain-depression relationship? Pain Med 2007;8:449–61.

[53] Polatin PB, Kinney RK, Gatchel RJ, Fogarty WT. Prevalence of psychopathology in acute and chronic low back pain patients. J Occup Rehabil 1993;3:95–103.

[54] Romano JM, Turner JA. Chronic pain and depression: Does the evidence support a relationship? Psychol Bull 1985;97:18–34.

[55] Russell JA, Carroll JM. On the bipolarity of positive and negative affect. Psychol Bull 1999;125:3–30.

[56] Sanderson WC, DiNardo, Rapee RM, Barlow DH. Syndrome comorbidity in patients diagnosed with a DSM-III-R anxiety disorder. J Abnorm Psychol 1990;99:308–12.

[57] Sagduyu A, Sahiner T. Migren ve gerilim tipi bas agrisi tanisi alanlarda ruhsal bozukluklar. Turk Psikiyatri Derg 1997;8:45–9.

[58] Schmidt NB, Santiago HT, Trakowski JH, Kendren JM. Pain in patients with panic disorder: Relation to symptoms, cognitive characteristics and treatment outcome. Pain Res Manag 2002;7:134–41.

[59] Sherbourne CD, Asch SM, Shugarman LR, Goebel JR, Lanto AB, Rubenstein LV, Wen L, Zubkoff L, Lorenz KA. Early identification of co-occuring pain, depression, and anxiety. J Gen Intern Med 2009;24:620–5.

[60] Smith BW, Zautra AJ. The effects of anxiety and depression on weekly pain in women with arthritis. Pain 2008;138:354–61.

[61] Smith GR. The epidemiology and treatment of depression when it coexists with somatoform disorders, somatization, or pain. Gen Hosp Psychiatry 1992;14:265–72.

[62] Srinivasan K, Joseph W. A study of lifetime prevalence of anxiety and depressive disorders in patients presenting with chest pain to emergency medicine. Gen Hosp Psychiatry 2004;26:470–4.

[63] Sullivan MJL, D'Eon J. Relation between catastrophizing and depression in chronic pain patients. J Abnorm Psychol 1990;99:260–3.

[64] Tsang A, Von Korff M, Lee S, Alonso J, Karam E, Angermeyer MC, Borges GLG, Bromet EJ, de Girolamo G, de Graff R, Gureje O, Lepine JP, Haro JM, Levinson D, Browne MAO, Posada-Villa J, Seedat S, Watanabe M. Common chronic pain conditions in developed and developing countries: gender and age differences and comorbidity with depression-anxiety disorders. J Pain 2008;9:883–91.

[65] Turk DC, Fernandez E. On the putative uniqueness of cancer pain: do psychological principles apply? Behav Res Ther 1990;28:1–13.

[66] Turner JA, Romano JM. Self-report screening measures for depression in chronic pain patients. J Clin Psychol 1984;40:909–13.

[67] Van Middendorp H, Lumley MA, Moerbeek M, Jacobs JWG, Bijlsma JWJ, Geenen R. Effects of anger and anger regulation styles on pain in daily life of women with fibromyalgia: a diary study. Eur J Pain 2010;14:176–82.

[68] Violon A. The onset of facial pain: a psychological study. Psychother Psychosom 1980;34:11–6.

[69] Von Knorring L, Perris C, Eisemann M, Eriksson U, Perris H. Pain as a symptom in depressive disorders: I. Relationship to diagnostic subgroup and depressive symptomatology. Pain 1983;15:19–26.

[70] Wasan A, Fernandez E, Jamison RN, Bhattacharya N. Association of anxiety and depression with reported disease severity in patients undergoing evaluation for chronic rhinosinusitis. Ann Otol Rhinol Laryngol 2007;116:491–7.

[71] Weisberg J, Boatwright B. Mood, anxiety, and personality traits and states in chronic pain. Pain 2007;133:1–2.

[72] Wells KB, Stewart A, Hays RD, Burnam MA, Rogers W, Daniels M, Berry S, Greenfield S, Ware J. The functioning and well-being of depressed patients. Results from the Medical Outcomes Study. JAMA 1989;262:914–9.

[73] Worthington JJ, Pollack MH, Otto MW, Gould RA. Panic disorder in emergency ward patients with chest pain. J Nerv Ment Dis 1997;185:274–6.

Correspondence to: Ephrem Fernandez, PhD, Department of Psychology, University of Texas at San Antonio, San Antonio, TX 78249, USA. Email: ephrem.fernandez@utsa.edu.

Myofascial Pain Syndrome in Headache Patients

César Fernández-de-las-Peñas,[a,b,c] Ana Isabel de-la-Llave-Rincón,[a,b] and Cristina Alonso-Blanco[d]

[a]Department of Physical Therapy, Occupational Therapy, Physical Medicine and Rehabilitation, [b]Esthesiology Laboratory, Rey Juan Carlos University, Alcorcón, Madrid, Spain; [c]Centre for Sensory-Motor Interaction, Department of Health Science and Technology, Aalborg University, Aalborg, Denmark; [d]Department of Nursing, Rey Juan Carlos University, Alcorcón, Madrid, Spain

Headache is the most common problem seen in clinical practice by many health care professionals, with tension-type headache and migraine being the most common forms [3]. Globally, the percentage of adults with headache is 10% for migraine, 38% for tension-type headache, and 3% for chronic daily headache [39]. Headache causes substantial levels of disability, not only to patients and their families, but also to society as a whole because of its very high prevalence in the general population [55]. In the last decade, increasing knowledge has emerged on the role of myofascial pain in headaches [31]. In fact, because the mechanisms of pain in both headache and fibromyalgia involve sensitization of the central nervous system (CNS) [40], a common pathophysiological hypothesis has been proposed for both conditions. This hypothesis also extends to patients with myofascial pain syndrome because they exhibit similar features (Fig. 1) [30]. This chapter will show how trigger points contribute to headache, particularly migraine and tension-type headache, by sensitizing the CNS.

Pain Comorbidities: Understanding and Treating the Complex Patient
edited by Maria Adele Giamberardino and Troels Staehelin Jensen
IASP Press, Seattle, © 2012

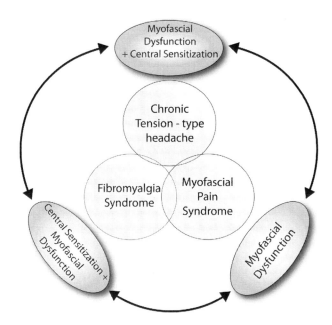

Fig. 1. A common pathophysiological hypothesis for tension-type headache, fibromyalgia syndrome, and myofascial pain syndrome.

Clinical Features of Muscle Referred Pain

1) Referred pain is described as diffuse, burning, tightening, or pressing, with a duration ranging from just a few seconds to hours or days.
2) Referred pain can spread in cranial/caudal or ventral/dorsal directions.
3) The intensity of referred pain and the extent of the area of referred pain are positively correlated with the degree of sensitization of the CNS.
4) Muscle referred pain can be accompanied by other symptoms, such as numbness, stiffness, weakness, fatigue, or motor dysfunction.

Clinical Presentation of Myofascial Pain Syndrome

Myofascial pain syndrome is characterized by trigger points (TrPs). A TrP is defined as a hyperirritable spot situated within a taut band of skeletal muscle that is painful on compression, stretching, or contraction and responds to stimulation with a specific pattern of referred pain [52]. There are two types of TrPs: active and latent. From a clinical viewpoint, active TrPs cause clinical symptoms, and when these points are stimulated, they produce local and referred pain that reproduces the spontaneous pain reported by the patient. Patients with headache may have active TrPs with a typical pattern of referred pain. Stimulation of the active TrPs evokes the same sensations that the patient perceives during spontaneous headache attacks or may even reproduce the patient's typical headache. Latent TrPs evoke referred pain with mechanical stimulation, contraction, or stretching, but this pain does not reproduce any symptoms familiar to the subject. Both active and latent TrPs can cause motor dysfunctions [41].

Trigger point diagnosis involves taking a specific history related to pain complaints and identifying several features during physical examination: (a) a palpable taut band in a skeletal muscle; (b) a tender spot in the taut band; (c) a palpable or visible local twitch response on snapping palpation, or needling, of the TrP; and (d) referred pain elicited by stimulation or palpation of the tender spot [52]. To be reliable, TrP diagnosis requires adequate manual skills, training, and clinical practice [48]. Gerwin et al. [34] found that the above criteria yielded good interexaminer reliability ranging from 0.84 to 0.88. Nevertheless, there is controversy on the proper diagnostic criteria for TrPs and their reliability [42]. Referred pain is one of the cardinal signs in TrP diagnosis. Some authors have described the referred pain patterns from several head and neck muscles that have the potential to refer pain to the head [52,56]. However, although referred pain patterns have great value for clinicians, these patterns can be different among subjects. In fact, some subjects have more extensive patterns of referred pain than others, and the extensiveness of referred pain is dependent on the degree of activity of the TrP and how much pressure is applied to it. Fig. 2 shows the referred pain patterns most commonly elicited by TrPs in neck and shoulder muscles.

The most credible etiological suggestion for TrP pathogenesis is the *integrated hypothesis* [52]. This hypothesis proposes that abnormal depolarization of the post-junction membrane of motor endplates, enhanced by sustained muscular contraction, gives rise to a localized hypoxic "ATP energy crisis" associated with sensory and autonomic processes that are sustained by sensitization mechanisms [43]. Gerwin et al. [33] have suggested that TrP pathogenesis may result when muscle fibers are injured

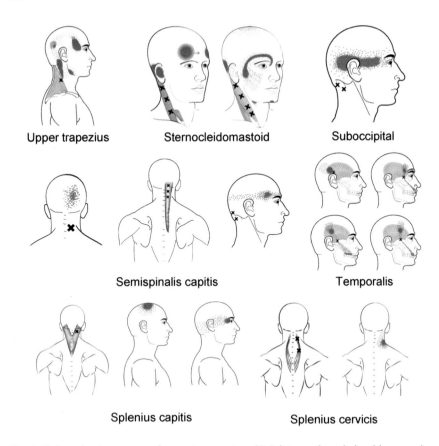

Fig. 2. Referred pain patterns from trigger points (TrPs) in neck and shoulder muscles: upper trapezius, sternocleidomastoid, suboccipital, splenius capitis, semispinalis capitis, splenius cervicis, and temporalis.

or overloaded, leading to endogenous (involuntary) shortening of muscle fibers, loss of oxygen supply, loss of nutrient supply, and increased metabolic demand in local tissues [51]. Readers are referred to other textbooks for more details on TrP pathogenesis [9,52].

Myofascial Trigger Points in Headache

To understand the relevance of TrP referred pain in headache, we should discuss the concept of pericranial tenderness. The most prominent finding in patients with headache is an increased tenderness to palpation of pericranial tissues, not only in muscles [19,21], but also in nerves [13,18].

Nevertheless, whether this local sensitivity is a primary factor (cause) or a secondary factor (consequence) in headache is under debate. A 12-year follow-up longitudinal study has demonstrated that individuals who develop chronic headache have normal tenderness scores before the beginning of pain, suggesting that mechanical sensitivity is a consequence of headache rather than a risk factor for its development [5].

The presence of mechanical pain sensitivity supports the role of both peripheral and central processes [4] in the development of chronic headache. However, since central sensitization is generated by prolonged nociceptive inputs from the periphery [44] and is dynamically influenced by the activity and location of these nociceptive inputs [37], the role of peripheral mechanisms in the pathophysiology of headache is still a matter of debate. In this context, the following questions have particular relevance: Can TrPs contribute to these sensitization processes in chronic headache? Can TrPs be involved in the pathogenesis of headache? Can TrPs precipitate a migraine attack?

Both bradykinin and serotonin are well-known stimulants of muscle nociceptors [45]. Active muscle TrPs are associated with higher levels of chemical mediators, such as bradykinin, calcitonin gene-related peptide, substance P, tumor necrosis factor-α, and interleukin-1β, not only in their immediate vicinity [50], but also in distant pain-free areas [49]. An active muscle TrP could thus sensitize peripheral nociceptors, which could contribute to central sensitization and chronic pain [30]. In agreement with this line of reasoning, a recent study has demonstrated that segmental central sensitization increases TrP activity [54]. This study supports the notion that central sensitization promotes, increases, or perpetuates TrP activity, but it does not show that the cause of TrP formation is central sensitization.

In the last few decades, an increasing number of studies have investigated the relevance of TrPs in headache, particularly tension-type headache and migraine. In fact, several clinical studies conducted by different research groups have demonstrated the relevance of active TrPs [31]. In a series of blinded, controlled studies, Fernández-de-las-Peñas et al. found that active TrPs are highly prevalent in patients with tension-type headache and migraine. In individuals with chronic tension-type headache, active TrPs were found in the superior oblique muscles (86%) [22], the suboccipitals (65%) [10], the upper trapezius (60%) [28], the temporalis muscles (60%) [16,29], the sternocleidomastoid (50%) [11], and the lateral rectus muscles (60%) [24]. In patients with episodic tension-type headache, the location of active TrPs is extremely similar to their location in the chronic form [12,14,26]. Nevertheless, a recent study determined that active TrPs are more prevalent in chronic tension-type headache than in the episodic form [53]. In addition, these studies also found that active TrPs were associated with more severe headache in patients with chronic, but not episodic, tension-type headache, which may be considered to indicate a temporal integration of nociceptive inputs from active muscle TrPs [31]. Finally, a recent study has also found that children with chronic tension-type headache have active TrPs in the suboccipital (80%), superior oblique (30%), temporalis (60%), sternocleidomastoid (20%), and upper trapezius (20%) muscles [27].

Individuals with unilateral migraine had active TrPs in the upper trapezius (30%), sternocleidomastoid (45%), temporalis (40%), and superior oblique (50%) muscles. The TrPs were located ipsilateral to migraine attacks rather than on the nonsymptomatic side [23,25]. Similarly, patients with bilateral migraine had active TrPs within the temporalis and suboccipital muscles bilaterally [7]. Finally, some case series have reported the presence of active TrPs in patients with cervicogenic headache [38,47] and cluster headache [8].

How Can Trigger Points Contribute to Headaches?

Olesen proposed that headache might result from an excess of nociceptive inputs from peripheral structures [46]. The trigeminal nucleus caudalis plays a central role in this model because the perceived intensity of headache would result from the sum of nociceptive inputs from cranial and extracranial tissues converging on the neurons of the nucleus caudalis. Bendtsen suggested that the barrage of peripheral nociceptive inputs could be responsible for the development of central sensitization [1]. Fernández-de-las-Peñas et al. formulated a pain model for tension-type headache involving peripheral sensitization of nociceptors by active TrPs, as well as central sensitization. Active TrPs located in muscles innervated by cervical spinal nerves C1–C3 (upper trapezius, sternocleidomastoid, and suboccipital muscles) and by the trigeminal nerve (temporalis, masseter, and extraocular muscles) may be responsible for peripheral nociceptive inputs. They may send a continuous afferent barrage toward the trigeminal nucleus caudalis, sensitizing the CNS [20]. In this pain model, muscle tenderness is the consequence of tension-type headache, and TrPs (leading to referred pain) are one of the main causes (but not the only cause) of this type of headache [15]. It seems plausible that active TrPs are related to the origin of tension-type headache and play a role in sensitization; however, there is no clear evidence to claim that either peripheral or central sensitization is the major factor in tension-type headache, because both sensitization mechanisms probably occur at the same time.

A different hypothesis can be formulated in the case of migraine, because an association of TrPs with migraine does not constitute a causal relationship. The presence of TrPs indicates that peripheral nociceptive input to the trigeminal nucleus can act as a migraine trigger, but not as a causative factor. A link between pain generators in the neck, head, and shoulder muscles and migraine attacks may be the activation of the trigeminal nucleus caudalis, leading to the activation of the trigeminovascular system. In this instance, TrPs located in any muscle innervated by the trigeminal nerve or by the upper cervical nerves may be considered "thorns" that can precipitate, perpetuate, or aggravate migraine in some predisposed individuals. Obviously, other triggers also exist for migraine.

Management of Trigger Points for Headache

Pharmacological Studies

Bendtsen and Jensen demonstrated that amitriptyline reduces both headache and pericranial myofascial tenderness in patients with chronic tension-type headache [2]. The decrease in myofascial tenderness during treatment with amitriptyline may be caused by a segmental reduction of central sensitization in combination with an enhanced efficacy of noradrenergic or serotonergic descending inhibition [2].

Nonpharmacological Studies

There is preliminary evidence for the effectiveness of TrP treatment in patients with migraine. Calandre et al. reported resolution of migraine after treating TrPs in neck and shoulder muscles with lidocaine or saline injections [6]. García-Leiva et al. found that TrP injection with ropivacaine (10 mg) was also effective in reducing the frequency and intensity of migraine [32]. Finally, another study showed that deactivation of active TrPs in migraine not only reduced the number and intensity of headache attacks, but also decreased somatic tissue hypersensitivity, as measured through electrical pain thresholds in the headache pain area [35].

Similarly, Harden et al. reported that patients with chronic tension-type headache who received botulinum toxin A injection in active muscle TrPs experienced greater reductions in headache frequency and intensity over the short term [36]. The effectiveness of manual deactivation of TrPs in tension-type headache has never been formally investigated. Starting from the premise that not all patients with tension-type headache will benefit to the same degree from a specific intervention, in this case manual TrP therapy, Fernández-de-las-Peñas et al. elaborated a clinical prediction rule to identify women with chronic tension-type headache who would experience short-term success with manual TrP therapy [16]. Four variables were identified for immediate short-term relief (headache duration of less than 8.5 hours/day, headache frequency of less than 5.5 days/week, bodily pain rated at less than 47 on a scale of 0–100, and vitality rated at less than 47.5 on a scale of 0–100), and two variables were identified for success at a 1-month follow-up (headache frequency of less than 5.5 days/week, and bodily pain rated at less than 47) [16]. If all variables were present, the chance of experiencing immediately successful treatment improved from 54% to 87.4%.

Fernández-de-las-Peñas et al. determined a second clinical prediction rule, based on a study in which women with tension-type headache received a multimodal physical therapy session including TrP therapies and joint mobilization of the cervical and thoracic spine. The authors identified the following eight variables: mean age of less than 44.5 years, left sternocleidomastoid TrPs, suboccipital TrPs, left superior oblique TrPs, cervical rotation to the left of more than 69°, a total tenderness score of less than 20.5, a score of less than 18.5 on the Neck Disability Index, and a referred pain area from a TrP in the right upper trapezius muscle of greater than 42.23 (arbitrary units) [17]. If five of the eight variables were present, the chance of experiencing an immediately successful treatment improved from 47% to 86.3% [17]. These clinical rules support the role of TrPs in the management of tension-type headache; however, further studies validating current data are needed.

Conclusion

It seems that referred pain from trigger points plays an important role in the pathogenesis of some primary headaches, including tension-type and migraine headache. In tension-type headache, it is probable that pain can be explained, at least partially, by the referred pain elicited by active TrPs. In migraine, TrPs may be a trigger factor for initiating or perpetuating a migraine attack. There is preliminary evidence showing that deactivation of TrPs may be effective in reducing migraine and tension-type headache.

References

[1]   Bendtsen L. Central sensitization in tension-type headache: possible pathophysiological mechanisms. Cephalalgia 2000; 29:486–508.
[2]   Bendtsen L, Jensen R. Amitriptyline reduces myofascial tenderness in patients with chronic tension-type headache. Cephalalgia 2000;20:603–10.
[3]   Bendtsen L, Jensen R. Tension-type headache: the most common, but also the most neglected headache disorder. Curr Opin Neurol 2006;19:305–9.
[4]   Bendtsen L, Schoenen J. Synthesis of tension type headache mechanisms. In: Olesen J, Goasdby P, Ramdan NM, Tfelt-Hansen P, Welch KA. The headaches, 3rd ed. Philadelphia: Lippincott Williams & Wilkins; 2006.
[5]   Buchgreitz L, Lyngberg AC, Bendtsen L, Jensen R. Increased pain sensitivity is not a risk factor but a consequence of frequent headache: a population-based follow-up study. Pain 2008;137:623–30.
[6]   Calandre EP, Hidalgo J, García-Leiva JM, Rico-Villademoros F. Effectiveness of prophylactic trigger point inactivation in chronic migraine and chronic daily headache with migraine features. Cephalalgia 2003;23:713.
[7]   Calandre EP, Hidalgo J, García-Leiva JM, Rico-Villademoros F. Trigger point evaluation in migraine patients: an indication of peripheral sensitization linked to migraine predisposition? Eur J Neurol 2006;13:244–9.
[8]   Calandre EP, Hidalgo J, Garcia-Leiva JM, Rico-Villademoros F, Delgado-Rodriguez A. Myofascial trigger points in cluster headache patients: a case series. Head Face Med 2008;4:32.
[9]   Dommerholt J, Huijbregts P. Myofascial trigger points: pathophysiology and evidence-informed diagnosis and management. Boston: Jones & Bartlett; 2011.
[10] Fernández-de-las-Peñas C, Alonso-Blanco C, Cuadrado ML, Gerwin RD, Pareja JA. Trigger points in the suboccipital muscles and forward head posture in tension-type headache. Headache 2006;46:454–60.

[11] Fernández-de-las-Peñas C, Alonso-Blanco C, Cuadrado ML, Gerwin RD, Pareja JA. Myofascial trigger points and their relationship with headache clinical parameters in chronic tension-type headache. Headache 2006;46:1264–72.

[12] Fernández-de-las-Peñas C, Alonso-Blanco C, Cuadrado ML, Pareja JA. Myofascial trigger points in the suboccipital muscles in episodic tension-type headache. Man Ther 2006;11:225–30.

[13] Fernández-de-las-Peñas C, Arendt-Nielsen L, Cuadrado ML, Pareja JA. Generalized mechanical pain sensitivity over nerve tissues in patients with strictly unilateral migraine. Clin J Pain 2009;25:401–6.

[14] Fernández-de-las-Peñas C, Arendt-Nielsen L, Simons DG. Contributions of myofascial trigger points to chronic tension-type headache. J Man Manip Ther 2006;14:222–31.

[15] Fernández-de-las-Peñas C, Arendt-Nielsen L, Simons DG, Cuadrado ML, Pareja JA. Sensitization in tension type headache: a pain model. In: Fernández-de-las-Peñas C, Arendt-Nielsen L, Gerwin R, editors. Tension-type and cervicogenic headache: pathophysiology, diagnosis and treatment. Baltimore: Jones & Bartlett; 2010. p. 97–106.

[16] Fernández-de-las-Peñas C, Cleland JA, Cuadrado ML, Pareja JA. Predictor variables for identifying patients with chronic tension-type headache who are likely to achieve short-term success with muscle trigger point therapy. Cephalalgia 2008;28:264–75.

[17] Fernández-de-las-Peñas C, Cleland JA, Palomeque-del-Cerro L, Caminero AB, Guillem-Mesado A, Jiménez-García R. Development of a clinical prediction rule for identifying women with tension-type headache who are likely to achieve short-term success with joint mobilization and muscle trigger point therapy. Headache 2011;51:246–61.

[18] Fernández-de-las-Peñas C, Coppieters MW, Cuadrado ML, Pareja JA. Patients with chronic tension-type headache demonstrate increased mechano-sensitivity of the supra-orbital nerve. Headache 2008;48:570–7.

[19] Fernández-de-las-Peñas C, Cuadrado ML, Arendt-Nielsen L, Pareja JA. Side-to-side differences in pressure pain thresholds and pericranial muscle tenderness in strictly unilateral migraine. Eur J Neurol 2008;15:162–8.

[20] Fernández-de-las-Peñas C, Cuadrado ML, Arendt-Nielsen L, Simons DG, Pareja JA. Myofascial trigger points and sensitisation: an updated pain model for tension-type headache. Cephalalgia 2007;27:383–93.

[21] Fernández-de-las-Peñas C, Cuadrado ML, Ge HY, Arendt-Nielsen L, Pareja JA. Increased pericranial tenderness, decreased pressure pain threshold, and headache clinical parameters in chronic tension-type headache patients. Clin J Pain 2007;23:346–52.

[22] Fernández-de-las-Peñas C, Cuadrado ML, Gerwin RD, Pareja JA. Referred pain from the trochlear region in tension-type headache: a myofascial trigger point from the superior oblique muscle. Headache 2005;45:731–7.

[23] Fernández-de-las-Peñas C, Cuadrado ML, Gerwin R, Pareja JA. Myofascial disorders in the trochlear region in unilateral migraine: a possible initiating or perpetuating factor. Clin J Pain 2006;22:548–53.

[24] Fernández-de-las-Peñas C, Cuadrado ML, Gerwin RD, Pareja JA. Referred pain from the lateral rectus muscle in subjects with chronic tension-type headache. Pain Med 2009;10:43–8.

[25] Fernández-de-las-Peñas C, Cuadrado ML, Pareja JA. Myofascial trigger points, neck mobility and forward head posture in unilateral migraine. Cephalalgia 2006;26:1061–70.

[26] Fernández-de-las-Peñas C, Cuadrado ML, Pareja JA. Myofascial trigger points, neck mobility and forward head posture in episodic tension-type headache. Headache 2007;47:662–72.

[27] Fernández-de-Las-Peñas C, Fernández-Mayoralas DM, Ortega-Santiago R, Ambite-Quesada S, Palacios-Ceña D, Pareja JA. Referred pain from myofascial trigger points in head and neck-shoulder muscles reproduces head pain features in children with chronic tension type headache. J Headache Pain 2011;12:35–43.

[28] Fernández-de-las-Peñas C, Ge H, Arendt-Nielsen L, Cuadrado ML, Pareja JA. Referred pain from trapezius muscle trigger point shares similar characteristics with chronic tension-type headache. Eur J Pain 2007;11:475–82.

[29] Fernández-de-las-Peñas C, Ge H, Arendt-Nielsen L, Cuadrado ML, Pareja JA. The local and referred pain from myofascial trigger points in the temporalis muscle contributes to pain profile in chronic tension-type headache. Clin J Pain 2007;23:786–92.

[30] Fernandez-de-Las-Penas C, Schoenen J. Chronic tension-type headache: what is new? Curr Opin Neurol 2009;22:254–61.

[31] Fernández-de-las-Peñas C, Simons DG, Gerwin RD, Cuadrado ML, Pareja JA. Muscle trigger points in tension type headache. In: Fernández-de-las-Peñas C, Arendt-Nielsen L, Gerwin R, editors. Tension-type and cervicogenic headache: pathophysiology, diagnosis and treatment. Baltimore: Jones & Bartlett; 2010. p. 61–76.

[32] García-Leiva JM, Hidalgo J, Rico-Villademoros F, Moreno V, Calandre EP. Effectiveness of ropivacaine trigger points inactivation in the prophylactic management of patients with severe migraine. Pain Med 2007;8:65–70.

[33] Gerwin RD, Dommerholt D, Shah JP. An expansion of Simons' integrated hypothesis of trigger point formation. Curr Pain Head Report 2004;8:468–75.

[34] Gerwin RD, Shannon S, Hong CZ, Hubbard D, Gevirtz R. Inter-rater reliability in myofascial trigger point examination. Pain 1997;69:65–73.

[35] Giamberardino MA, Tafuri E, Savini A, Fabrizio A, Affaitati G, Lerza R, Di Ianni L, Lapenna D, Mezzetti A. Contribution of myofascial trigger points to migraine symptoms. J Pain 2007;8:869–78.

[36] Harden RN, Cottrill J, Gagnon CM, Smitherman TA, Weinland SR, Tann B, Joseph P, Lee TS, Houle TT. Botulinum toxin a in the treatment of chronic tension-type headache with cervical myofascial trigger points: a randomized, double-blind, placebo-controlled pilot study. Headache 2009;49:732–43.

[37] Herren-Gerber R, Weiss S, Arendt-Nielsen L, Petersen-Felix S, Di Stefano G, Radanov BP, Curatolo M. Modulation of central hypersensitivity by nociceptive input in chronic pain after whiplash injury. Pain Med 2004;5;366–76.

[38] Jaeger B. Are cervicogenic headaches due to myofascial pain and cervical spine dysfunction? Cephalalgia 1989;9:157–64.

[39] Jensen R, Stovner LJ. Epidemiology and co-morbidity of headache. Lancet Neurol 2008;7:354–61.

[40] Lenaerts ME, Gill PS. At the crossroads between tension-type headache and fibromyalgia. Curr Pain Headache Rep 2006;10:463–6.

[41] Lucas KR. The impact of latent trigger points on regional muscle function. Curr Pain Headache Rep 2008;12:344–9.

[42] Lucas N, Macaskill P, Irwig L, Moran R, Bogduk N. Reliability of physical examination for diagnosis of myofascial trigger points: a systematic review of the literature. Clin J Pain 2007;25:80–9.

[43] McPartland JM, Simons DG. Myofascial trigger points: translating molecular theory into manual therapy. J Man Manipul Ther 2006;14:232–9.

[44] Mendell LM, Wall PD. Responses of single dorsal cord cells to peripheral cutaneous unmyelinated fibres. Nature 1965;206:97–9.

[45] Mense S. The pathogenesis of muscle pain. Curr Pain Headache Rep 2003;7:419–25.

[46] Olesen J. Clinical and patho-physiological observations in migraine and tension-type headache explained by integration of vascular, supraspinal and myofascial inputs. Pain 1991;46:125–32.

[47] Roth JK, Roth RS, Weintraub JR, Simons DG. Cervicogenic headache caused by myofascial trigger points in the sternocleidomastoid: a case report. Cephalalgia 2007;27:375–80.

[48] Sciotti VM, Mittak VL, DiMarco L, Ford LM, Plezbert J, Santipadri E, Wigglesworth J, Ball K. Clinical precision of myofascial trigger point location in the trapezius muscle. Pain 2001;93:259–66.

[49] Shah JP, Danoff JV, Desai MJ, Parikh S, Nakamura LY, Phillips TM, Gerber LH. Biochemicals associated with pain and inflammation are elevated in sites near to and remote from active myofascial trigger points. Arch Phys Med Rehabil 2008;89:16–23.

[50] Shah JP, Phillips TM, Danoff JV, Gerber L. An in vitro microanalytical technique for measuring the local biochemical milieu of human skeletal muscle. J Appl Physiol 2005;99:1977–84.

[51] Simons DG. Review of enigmatic MTrPs as a common cause of enigmatic musculoskeletal pain and dysfunction. J Electromyogr Kinesiol 2004;14:95–107.

[52] Simons DG, Travell J, Simons LS. Myofascial pain and dysfunction: the trigger point manual, volume 1, 2nd ed. Baltimore: Williams & Wilkins; 1999.

[53] Sohn JH, Choi HC, Lee SM, Jun AY. Differences in cervical musculoskeletal impairment between episodic and chronic tension-type headache. Cephalalgia 2010;30:1514–23.

[54] Srbely JZ, Dickey JP, Bent LR, Lee D, Lowerison M. Capsaicin-induced central sensitization evokes segmental increases in trigger point sensitivity in humans. J Pain 2010;11:636–43.

[55] Stovner L, Hagen K, Jensen R, Katsarava Z, Lipton R, Scher A, Steiner T, Zwart JA. The global burden of headache: a documentation of headache prevalence and disability worldwide. Cephalalgia 2007;27:193–210.

C. Fernández-de-las-Peñas et al.

[56] Wright EF. Referred craniofacial pain patterns in patients with temporomandibular disorder. J Am Dent Assoc 2000;131:1307–15.

Correspondence to: César Fernández de las Peñas, PT, PhD, Facultad de Ciencias de la Salud, Universidad Rey Juan Carlos, Avenida de Atenas s/n, 28922 Alcorcón, Madrid, Spain. Email: cesar.fernandez@urjc.es.

Concurrent Visceral Pain Syndromes: The Concept of Viscerovisceral Hyperalgesia

Maria Adele Giamberardino,[a] Giannapia Affaitati,[a] and Raffaele Costantini[b]

[a]Department of Medicine and Science of Aging and [b]Institute of Surgical Pathology, "G. D'Annunzio" University of Chieti, Italy

Pain from internal organs is among the most important forms of pain in the clinical setting [15,28,63]. Acute visceral pain represents a strong priority in internal medicine as it can be the expression of potentially life-threatening conditions, such as a myocardial infarction or an intestinal obstruction, making its prompt recognition and treatment mandatory. Chronic or recurrent visceral pains, on the other hand, are also of the utmost importance, because they affect a vast proportion of the general population and represent one of the main reasons why patients seek medical care [36]. Community surveys demonstrate, for example, that 20% of people have recurrent chest pain, 25% have intermittent abdominal pain, and 24% of women have persistent pelvic pain [4,5,24,73]. Of crucial importance is the fact that different forms of visceral pain frequently occur together. For instance, a history of angina is a significant predictive factor for the development of biliary stones in men, and irritable bowel syndrome (IBS) coexists with dysmenorrhea, endometriosis, or chronic pelvic pain in a high percentage of women. A significant co-occurrence is also observed between functional gastrointestinal disorders and various urinary tract pain conditions, such as interstitial cystitis (IC) [1,2,6,7,21,47,64].

This comorbidity often gives rise to significant interactions among the visceral organs in which various algogenic conditions mutually enhance pain symptoms, a phenomenon termed "viscerovisceral hyperalgesia," which can pose significant diagnostic problems and therapeutic challenges [28,32,63]. Though known for quite some time clinically, viscerovisceral hyperalgesia has been fully appreciated only in relatively recent times through controlled studies in patients [29]. In parallel, a significant amount of experimental research is currently being conducted to investigate its pathophysiology, an indispensable step toward better treatment approaches [11].

This chapter provides an introductory section on visceral pain features and then focuses on viscerovisceral hyperalgesia in terms of clinical characterization, analysis of possible mechanisms, and implications for therapy.

Visceral Pain Phenomena

Visceral nociception is expressed clinically in a number of phenomena. The most typical temporal sequence involves an initial phase of "true visceral pain," followed by referral of the symptom to somatic structures. True visceral pain is an indefinite sensation, vague, diffuse and poorly discriminated, as a result of the low density of innervation of viscera (compared to that of somatic structures) and the extensive functional divergence of the visceral afferent fibers in the central nervous system (CNS) [13,52]. True visceral pain is always located in the same site—whatever the viscus in question, the pain is felt at the midline, in the lowest sternal or epigastric region, anteriorly or posteriorly in the interscapular area and is typically accompanied by a number of neurovegetative signs, such as nausea, vomiting, sweating, pallor, changes in heart rate, and changes in the frequency of urination or defecation. Its intensity is variable, bearing no relationship to the extent of the internal damage. For example, extensive myocardial infarctions may induce very mild pain or even no pain at all but only give rise to neurovegetative signs (called "visceral pain equivalents"), while conditions such as IBS—lacking a documentable organic internal damage—can be extremely painful [57].

The duration of this phase is always transitory—lasting only minutes to hours—after which the pain either stops or is "referred" elsewhere. Occasionally, this phase of true visceral pain may be bypassed—or overlooked, given the lack of specificity of the symptoms—with "referred pain" occurring from the very beginning. The concept of referred pain, known since the time of Henry Head (who published in the late 19th century), implies pain perceived in an area other than that of the primary nociceptive insult [37]. A visceral stimulus thus induces pain in a somatic area distant from the affected organ, but normally situated within the same neuromeric field (i.e., the somatic area receiving the same innervation as the organ in question). Therefore, while true visceral pain is perceived in a common site irrespective of the organ involved, visceral referred pain is organ specific, with painful areas differing according to the organ affected. For example, referred cardiac pan is felt in the left side of the chest and the left arm/forearm, pain from the upper urinary tract in the ipsilateral lumbar region/flank, gallbladder pain in the upper right abdominal quadrant, and pain from the reproductive organs in the lowest abdominal quadrants. At the beginning of the process of referral, spontaneous pain may not be accompanied by any local hypersensitivity and is known as referred pain without hyperalgesia. This pain without hyperalgesia is typically the consequence of the extensive convergence of afferent information from both the viscera and the area of referral at various levels in the CNS, which is why higher brain centers misinterpret the visceral message as a message coming from the somatic periphery [13–15]. In time, secondary hyperalgesia tends to develop in the somatic tissues of the referred area (referred pain with hyperalgesia), as detected and quantified in various clinical conditions involving recurrent visceral pain—such as angina from ischemic heart disease, biliary and urinary colic from calculosis, and abdominal pain from IBS, dysmenorrhea, and endometriosis—by measuring pain thresholds to various stimuli, mostly mechanical and electrical but also including thermal and chemical stimuli [12,25,27,31,32,71,72]. The overall outcome of these studies shows that referred hyperalgesia, as demonstrated by a decreased pain threshold, is mostly present in muscle tissue and is accentuated by repetition of the visceral pain episodes. Not only does the hyperalgesia outlast the sponta-neous pain—since it is normally detectable in the intervals between pain episodes—but in most cases it also outlasts the primary triggering factor in the internal organ. In fact, it sometimes persists for a long time after the visceral noxious stimulus has ceased, as in the case of lumbar hyper-algesia that is still detectable several years after elimination of the stone in patients with urinary calculosis [70].

In acute inflammatory visceral pain, such as acute appendicitis or cholecystitis, referred hyperalgesia often tends to also involve the super-ficial somatic tissues (subcutaneous and cutaneous layers), but it resolves after elimination of the visceral trigger. In acute cholecystis, in fact, it dis-appears after cholecystectomy, unlike the persistence of some degree of hyperalgesia after stone elimination in urinary colic [65,66]. This finding probably indicates that repeated painful visceral inputs, as in colics, rather than isolated acute episodes, are needed to leave persistent hyperalgesic traces in the referred area. Central sensitization is the main mechanism behind referred hyperalgesia accompanying visceral pain states. As a con-sequence of the massive visceral afferent barrage, viscerosomatic conver-gent neurons become hyperactive and hyperexcitable. In this condition, the central effect of even normal sensory inputs coming from the somatic area of referral is facilitated (according to the convergence-facilitation theory) [14]. Viscerosomatic reflex arcs are also likely to contribute to the referred phenomena [41,57,76] (see also [28] for a more detailed discus-sion of these mechanisms).

Visceral hyperalgesia is another prominent phenomenon fre-quently manifesting in visceral nociception. It consists of local hypersen-sitivity of a specific internal organ, usually as a consequence of visceral inflammation that leads to both peripheral and central sensitization [23]. Common examples of visceral hyperalgesia are stomach pain upon inges-tion of food or fluids when the gastric mucosa is inflamed, pain upon uri-nary distension of the bladder in the course of cystitis, and intestinal pain during normal intestinal transit in cases of inflammatory conditions of the digestive tract. IBS and interstitial cystitis are regarded as paradigmatic examples of visceral hyperalgesia where the threshold for discomfort is lowered at the intestinal and bladder level, at least in a large proportion of affected patients [19,53,62,75].

While true visceral pain, referred pain, and visceral hyperalgesia have been recognized for a long time, viscerovisceral hyperalgesia was discovered more recently. The following sections describe clinical and experimental evidence for this phenomenon.

Viscerovisceral Hyperalgesia: Evidence from Clinical Studies

The considerable rise in life expectancy in the past 100 years, especially in developed countries, has made it increasingly likely for clinicians to observe patients affected with more than one visceral pain condition at the same time [36]. If the affected visceral organs share at least part of their central sensory projection, viscerovisceral hyperalgesia (VVH) may take place, in which the patient experiences an enhancement of both spontaneous pain and referred muscle hyperalgesia from all organs involved [23]. Recent clinical controlled studies by our group have documented the phenomenon in several concurrent syndromes from organs with partially overlapping innervation, including the heart and gallbladder (T5), the colon and female reproductive organs (T10–L1), and the urinary tract and female reproductive organs (T10–L1). In contrast, VVH was not found in concurrent syndromes arising from the gallbladder and left urinary tract—organs for which no common sensory projection has been ascertained. A summary of these studies, conducted in 229 patients and 40 healthy controls, is given below [29] (Tables I, II).

Heart-Gallbladder Interaction: Coronary Artery Disease Plus Gallbladder Calculosis

We conducted a study to compare patients of both sexes who had both symptomatic coronary artery disease (angina, Class III or IV) [68] and symptomatic gallbladder calculosis with patients who only had symptomatic coronary artery disease and patients who only had symptomatic gallstones. Patients with the two conditions had the same degree of coronary artery luminal narrowing at angiography ($\geq$50%) as patients with coronary artery disease alone and the same size of gallbladder stone as patients with gallbladder disease alone (10–40 mm). All coronary artery disease patients were taking the same long-term regimen of antiaggregants and nitrates.

Table I
Viscerovisceral interactions in patients: clinical expressions

Affected Organs	Overlapping Projection	Visceral Diseases	Symptoms in Comorbidity Compared to Single Visceral Diseases
1) Heart + gallbladder	T5	Coronary artery disease + gallbladder calculosis	Increased angina and biliary pain; increased referred muscle hyperalgesia from heart and gallbladder
2) Colon + uterus	T10–L1	IBS + dysmenorrhea	Increased intestinal and menstrual pain; increased referred muscle hyperalgesia from colon and uterus
3) Ureter + uterus	T10–L1	Ureteral calculosis + dysmenorrhea/ endometriosis	Increased urinary and menstrual pain; increased referred muscle hyperalgesia from ureter and uterus
4) Gallbladder + left upper urinary tract	Not documented	Gallbladder + left ureteral calculosis	No increase in biliary and urinary pain; no increase in referred muscle hyperalgesia from gallbladder and ureter

Besides reporting retrospective data relative to the month preceding their entry to the study protocol, patients were involved in a 1-month prospective study to record any typical angina (relieved by sublingual nitroderivatives) and biliary pain episodes and to note their mean and maximal intensity on a visual analogue scale (VAS), part of an ad hoc questionnaire. At the end of the month, we measured muscle pressure pain thresholds in the left anterior chest region (in the area of pain referral from the heart) and muscle electrical pain thresholds in the upper right abdominal quadrant (the cystic point, in the area of pain referral from the gallbladder) [25]. Electrical stimulation was not used in the pectoralis muscle so as to avoid any risk of interference with cardiac activity.

Biliary calculosis had a significant impact on symptoms from coronary artery disease. Patients with the two conditions, as compared to those with coronary artery disease alone, presented a significantly higher number and greater intensity of angina episodes at both retrospective and prospective evaluation. Pressure pain thresholds in the left chest area were significantly reduced with respect to normal in both groups, indicating referred hyperalgesia from the heart in all coronary artery disease patients; however, these thresholds were significantly lower in the group

Table II
Viscerovisceral interactions in patients: effects of treatment

Affected Organs	Visceral Diseases	Type of Treatment	Effects of Treatment on Pain Symptoms
1) Heart + gallbladder	Coronary artery disease + gallbladder calculosis	Cardiac revascularization	Disappearance of cardiac pain; reduction of biliary pain and referred muscle hyperalgesia from the gallbladder
		Cholecystectomy	Disappearance of biliary pain; reduction of angina pain and referred muscle hyperalgesia from the heart
2) Colon + uterus	IBS + dysmenorrhea	Dietary treatment of IBS	Improvement of intestinal pain; reduction of menstrual pain and referred muscle hyperalgesia from the uterus
		Hormonal treatment of dysmenorrhea	Disappearance of menstrual pain; reduction of intestinal pain and referred muscle hyperalgesia from the colon
3) Ureter + uterus	Ureteral calculosis + dysmenorrhea/ endometriosis	ESWL with complete stone elimination	Disappearance of urinary pain; reduction of menstrual pain and referred muscle hyperalgesia from the uterus
		ESWL without complete stone elimination	Persistence of urinary pain; no improvement in menstrual pain and referred muscle hyperalgesia from the uterus
		Hormonal treatment of dysmenorrhea	Disappearance of menstrual pain; reduction of urinary pain and referred muscle hyperalgesia from the ureter
		Laser treatment of endometriosis	Reduction of urinary pain and referred muscle hyperalgesia from the ureter
4) Gallbladder + left upper urinary tract	Gallbladder calculosis + left ureteral calculosis	Cholecystectomy	Disappearance of biliary pain; no improvement in urinary pain and referred muscle hyperalgesia from the ureter
		ESWL with complete stone elimination	Disappearance of urinary pain; no improvement in biliary pain and referred muscle hyperalgesia from the gallbladder

Abbreviations: ESWL, extracorporeal shock-wave lithotripsy; IBS, irritable bowel syndrome.

with gallbladder comorbidity as compared to the group with coronary disease alone.

In addition, cholecystectomy performed in a subgroup of the comorbid patients not only resolved the biliary pain, but also significantly reduced painful cardiac symptoms, in terms of a decrease in the number and intensity of angina episodes during a 1-month postintervention period as compared with the 1-month period before the intervention, as well as a reduction in referred hyperalgesia in the chest area, as shown by increased pressure pain thresholds.

Coronary artery disease also had a significant impact on symptoms from biliary calculosis. In fact, both retrospectively and prospectively, comorbid patients showed a significantly higher number and greater intensity of biliary colics and significantly lower electrical pain thresholds at the cystic point than did patients with biliary calculosis alone. In addition, when cardiac revascularization was performed in a subgroup of the patients with both heart and gallbladder disease, it completely resolved all cardiac pain symptoms and, at the same time, significantly reduced biliary symptoms (the number and intensity of biliary colics during a 1-month period after surgery as compared to a similar preoperative period) as well as referred hyperalgesia at the cystic point (electrical pain thresholds significantly increased).

In synthesis, cardiac and gallbladder pain comorbidity produces enhanced spontaneous pain and referred hyperalgesia from both the heart and the gallbladder, with treatment of heart disease also improving gallbladder symptoms and treatment of gallbladder disease also lessening cardiac symptoms.

Colon-Uterus Interaction: Irritable Bowel Syndrome Plus Dysmenorrhea

Female patients affected with both IBS and dysmenorrhea were compared to patients with IBS alone and patients with dysmenorrhea alone. Women with both conditions did not differ significantly regarding the amount of time they had been suffering from IBS and dysmenorrhea when compared to women with IBS alone or dysmenorrhea alone. All underwent a 1-year retrospective and a 1-year prospective assessment through an ad hoc questionnaire, to investigate characteristics of the pain caused by IBS and dysmenorrhea. At the end of the prospective study, abdominal electrical pain thresholds were measured in the referred areas of the colon and uterus (see [29] for a description of these areas).

IBS had a significant impact on symptoms from dysmenorrhea, since at both retrospective and prospective examination comorbid patients showed a significantly higher number of "painful menstrual cycles" (pain intensity at menses exceeding 70 mm on a VAS) and significantly lower electrical pain thresholds in the referred area from the uterus compared with patients with dysmenorrhea only. In addition, for a subgroup of patients with the two conditions who underwent a 6-month dietary regimen for IBS, along with a substantial improvement of IBS symptoms there was also a significant reduction of dysmenorrhea symptoms (the number of painful menstrual cycles during a 6-month post-treatment period vs. the 6-month pretreatment period). This subgroup of patients also had a significant reduction in referred muscle hyperalgesia in the abdominal area of pain referral from the uterus (as shown by increased electrical pain thresholds). The improvement of dysmenorrhea symptoms was proportional to the efficacy of IBS treatment.

Dysmenorrhea also showed a significant impact on IBS symptoms. In fact, both retrospectively and prospectively, compared with patients with IBS alone, the comorbid patients experienced significantly more spontaneous IBS pain (a greater number of "IBS pain days" and higher intensity of IBS pain) and presented significantly lower electrical pain thresholds in the abdominal referred area from the colon. In addition, in a subgroup of patients with the two conditions who underwent a 6-month hormonal treatment for dysmenorrhea, along with a complete resolution of the menstrual pain symptoms there was also a significant improvement of IBS pain (reduction of "IBS pain days" and IBS pain intensity for 6 months after treatment compared to the 6 months before treatment). There was also a significant increase in electrical pain thresholds in the referred abdominal area from the colon.

The interdependence of intestinal and menstrual symptoms was also indirectly confirmed by follow-up data in a subgroup of comorbid patients who chose to not undergo any therapy for either IBS or dysmenorrhea for a period of 6 months. These patients did not show any improvement in the direct or referred symptoms of either condition.

In synthesis, colon-uterus pain comorbidity produces enhanced spontaneous pain and referred hyperalgesia from both the intestine and the female reproductive organs. Treatment of the intestinal disease also improves menstrual symptoms, and treatment of the uterine pain condition also lessens intestinal pain.

Ureter-Uterus Interaction

Symptomatic Urinary Calculosis Plus Dysmenorrhea

Women of reproductive age were studied who had unilateral symptomatic urinary calculosis plus dysmenorrhea, unilateral calculosis alone, or dysmenorrhea alone. The three groups did not differ regarding urinary stone characteristics and the amount of time women had been having colics, nor the amount of time they had experienced dysmenorrhea. Participants were asked to report their spontaneous urinary and menstrual symptoms in a 1-year retrospective and 1-year prospective study, through an ad hoc questionnaire. At the end of the prospective study, all subjects underwent measurement of muscle pain thresholds in the referred areas from the upper urinary tract (the ipsilateral lumbar region, L1) and the uterus [29].

Dysmenorrhea showed a significant impact on symptoms from urinary calculosis. Both retrospectively and prospectively, comorbid women experienced a significantly higher number and greater intensity of urinary colics than women with calculosis alone. Lumbar pain thresholds to electrical stimulation were significantly lower than normal in all women with calculosis; however, those with concurrent dysmenorrhea had significantly lower values than those with calculosis alone. In addition, in a subgroup of comorbid women who underwent a 6-month hormonal treatment for dysmenorrhea, along with complete resolution of menstrual symptoms, a significant improvement was observed in urinary pain symptoms (in terms of a reduction of the number and intensity of colics over a 6-month post-treatment versus a 6-month pretreatment period), and there was a significant reduction of referred lumbar hyperalgesia (increased thresholds).

Urinary calculosis also showed a significant impact on symptoms from dysmenorrhea. In fact, both retrospectively and prospectively, women with both conditions experienced a significantly higher number of painful menstrual cycles than women with dysmenorrhea alone. In all dysmenorrheic women, muscle pain thresholds to electrical stimulation in the abdominal uterine referred area were significantly reduced with respect to normal, but in women with concurrent urinary calculosis values were significantly lower than in women with dysmenorrhea alone.

In addition, in a subgroup of comorbid women subjected to extracorporeal shock-wave lithotripsy (ESWL) for their urinary calculosis [45], which was followed by complete elimination of stone fragments through the urine, there was not only a complete resolution of urinary symptoms, but also a significant reduction of menstrual pain (the number of painful menstrual cycles over a 6-month period subsequent to elimination as compared to a 6-month period preceding treatment) and of referred abdominal muscle hyperalgesia from the uterus. In contrast, women who did not eliminate the stone fragments completely after ESWL continued to experience not only urinary colics but also menstrual symptoms similar to those preceding treatment.

Symptomatic Urinary Calculosis Plus Asymptomatic Endometriosis

Women with unilateral upper urinary calculosis plus asymptomatic endometriosis were compared to women with calculosis alone. In the comorbid group, endometriosis had been discovered by chance at laparoscopy performed for infertility reasons and was not causing pelvic pain. All patients were involved in a 6-month prospective study, in which they were asked to keep note of their urinary pain (the location, number, and current intensity of colics) on an ad hoc questionnaire. At the end of this period, all participants underwent electrical pain threshold measurement at lumbar level (L1), ipsilaterally to the affected urinary tract. Asymptomatic endometriosis showed a significant impact on symptoms from urinary calculosis because women with the two conditions, compared to those with calculosis alone, had significantly more numerous and intense urinary colics and significantly lower lumbar pain thresholds. After laser therapy for endometriosis was applied during a further laparoscopy [20], a substantial improvement was noted in the urinary symptoms, as shown by a significant reduction of the number and intensity of colics over a 6-month posttreatment period as compared to the 6 months before treatment, together with a significant increase in electrical pain thresholds at the lumbar level.

In synthesis, ureter-uterus pain comorbidity enhances pain symptoms and referred hyperalgesia from both the urinary tract and the female reproductive organs. The increase in urinary pain also occurs in the case of asymptomatic endometriosis, when the female pelvic condition is latent with respect to spontaneous pelvic pain. Treatment of the ureter disease also improves menstrual symptoms, while treatment of the uterine pain condition also lessens urinary pain.

Gallbladder-Left Upper Urinary Tract Interaction: Gallbladder Calculosis Plus Left Urinary Calculosis

The interaction between two viscera with no clearly documented sensory overlap was explored by examining, in patients of both sexes who had both symptomatic gallbladder calculosis and symptomatic left urinary calculosis, the impact of cholecystectomy on urinary symptoms or the impact of ESWL on biliary symptoms. The study included patients with these two comorbidities who were scheduled for either cholecystectomy or ESWL of urinary calculosis in the coming year. Participants completed a 6-month prospective study to monitor their biliary and urinary symptoms (the number and current intensity of pain episodes), at the end of which they underwent electrical pain threshold measurement in the left lumbar region (cholecystectomy patients) or at the cystic point (ESWL patients). One month after cholecystectomy or ESWL, participants were monitored for a further 6-month period for their symptoms, after which their thresholds were measured again. Cholecystectomy had no significant impact on urinary pain. In fact, while biliary painful symptoms disappeared after the intervention, no significant change was observed in the number and intensity of urinary colics or in lumbar pain thresholds. Similarly, ESWL had no significant impact on biliary pain. While urinary symptoms resolved after complete elimination of stone fragments, which occurred in all of the ESWL-treated patients, no change was observed in the number and intensity of biliary colics or in pain thresholds at the cystic point.

In synthesis, gallbladder-left urinary tract pain comorbidity does not produce any mutual enhancement of visceral pain symptoms, as indirectly shown by the fact that effective treatment of one condition does not improve symptoms from the other.

Summary

The results of this series of studies in patients clearly show a mutual enhancement of both direct and referred symptoms from a number of painful diseases from visceral domains sharing part of their central sensory projection—the heart and gallbladder, the digestive tract and female reproductive organs, and the urinary tract and female reproductive organs. The phenomenon still occurs if one of the two visceral conditions is latent with respect to spontaneous pain, as in asymptomatic endometriosis. The interdependence of the two visceral organs involved in each interaction is shown by the effects of treatments, with expressions of VVH appearing to be strictly modulated by inputs from the internal organs involved. Effective therapy of the disease in one organ will also decrease the typical symptoms from the other location, but if treatment of one disease is either ineffective or only minimally effective, there is either no change or a minimal change in the symptomatology from the other disease. The mutual exacerbation of symptoms described above appears particularly relevant clinically, because the concurrent presence of two painful diseases in internal organs, like the ones considered in the studies reported in this section, is rather frequent epidemiologically.

The result of a lack of mutual enhancement of symptoms between organs that have no documented overlapping sensory innervation suggests that a common sensory projection is an important factor in promoting the phenomenon of VVH, although further clinical studies need to be performed in this respect, for instance involving truly distant organs such as the heart and the urinary bladder.

Mechanisms of Viscerovisceral Hyperalgesia: Evidence from Experimental Studies

Phenomena of cross-sensitization between different internal organs have been shown experimentally in both humans and animals by several research groups. Brinkert et al. [10] showed hypersensitivity in the sigmoid colon and rectum in women with dysmenorrhea. Using mechanical (balloon) distension applied via a barostat they were able to detect significantly lower distension volumes for threshold discomfort, particularly in the sigmoid colon. Frøkjaer et al. [22] were able to experimentally induce duodenal and/or rectal hypersensitivity in healthy human volunteers after sensitizing the distal esophagus with perfusion of acid and saline.

In animal studies, experimentally induced gastroesophageal reflux in anesthetized rats enhanced the activity of upper thoracic spinal neurons receiving noxious cardiac input [59], colon inflammation produced signs of inflammation in the otherwise healthy bladder and uterus, and uterine inflammation sensitized primary afferents from the colon; experimental endometriosis caused vaginal hyperalgesia and reduced volume voiding thresholds of the bladder, in addition to exacerbating behaviors indicating pain from the ureter (see below) [7,17,44,51,77] (see also the chapter by Malykhina in this volume for a complete review of experimental studies on cross-sensitization).

Animal Model of Viscerovisceral Hyperalgesia Between Female Reproductive Organs and the Urinary Tract

Experimental endometriosis combined, in sequence, with an artificial ureteral stone in female rats (ENDO + stone) mimics the women's condition of VVH from asymptomatic endometriosis plus ureteral calculosis [29]. The stone model is induced by injecting dental cement into the upper third of one ureter. Rats with the artificial stone not only display spontaneous behavior indicative of direct visceral pain (multiple "ureteral crises" of different duration and complexity, reminiscent of urinary colics) over 4–5 days postoperatively, but also develop referred hypersensitivity of the ipsilateral lumbar oblique musculature over 7–10 days. This hypersensitivity, revealed by a significant decrease in the vocalization threshold to electrical and mechanical muscle stimulation, is proportional in extent to the amount of spontaneous pain behavior and is dose-dependently reduced by treatment with nonsteroidal anti-inflammatory drugs (NSAIDs) or other analgesics or spasmolytics [33,34,43].

The endometriosis model, originally set up to study infertility, is obtained by grafting pieces of autologous endometrium into different locations in the abdominal cavity, which causes fluid-filled cysts to form 2–3 weeks after the implant. Though presenting features that reflect a latent algogenic status at the pelvic level (the above-reported vaginal hyperalgesia and bladder hyperreactivity), endometriosis alone does not produce any spontaneous pain behavior or referred muscle hyperalgesia [8,48].

However, if endometriosis is combined with stone formation 3 weeks later (when cysts are already in place), the enhancement of pain indicators is impressive. In fact, rats in the ENDO + stone group compared to those in the stone-only group and sham-ENDO + stone group not only showed an exponential increase in the typical ureteral pain indices (the number and duration of ureteral crises and the extent of referred lumbar muscle hyperalgesia), but also displayed additional behaviors (in between the ureteral crises). These new behaviors were regarded as typical of uterine provenance, being similar to those observed in models of uterine nociception [74]. The combination of experimental endometriosis and artificial ureteral calculosis thus enhances urinary pain behavior and evokes behavior indicating pain from the female reproductive organs. As observed in women with asymptomatic endometriosis plus ureteral calculosis, treatment of only one condition in this model relieves symptoms from the other, i.e., administration of NSAIDs or tramadol to rats with endometriosis before stone formation prevented the post-stone enhancement of pain behavior [26]. ENDO + stone thus appears to be a reliable animal model of VVH, suitable for study of mechanisms of the phenomenon.

Considering the modalities of occurrence of VVH that have been ascertained so far in the clinic, a plausible hypothesis is that central mechanisms play an important role in its generation, based on the convergence of sensory information from the two affected organs and the relative areas of somatic referral at different levels in the CNS. The nociceptive input from one organ would sensitize viscero-viscerosomatic convergent neurons, so that the message coming from the second organ and from the somatic areas of pain referral would be facilitated [11,14,29]. As a matter of fact, in addition to viscerosomatic convergence, viscerovisceral convergences have been widely documented centrally among various internal organs, including the urinary tract, female reproductive organs, and colon, as well as the heart and the gallbladder [3,11,17,18,77]. Regarding pelvic organs in particular, convergence of sensory information from discrete pelvic structures occurs at different levels of the nervous system including the dorsal root ganglia, spinal cord, and brain [46,63].

This sensitization hypothesis is supported by electrophysiological data. Previous extracellular recordings at the spinal cord level in the stone-only model have shown signs of central sensitization, with increased activity and excitability of sensory neurons receiving convergent input from the ureter and the somatic area of referral [30,61]. In electrophysiological recordings in the ENDO + stone model, enhancement of these sensitization indices is significant, with increased neuronal activity and excitability, together with markedly enlarged somatic receptive fields, with respect to both stone-only rats and sham-ENDO + stone rats (unpublished data).

Ongoing studies in other experimental examples of cross-organ sensitization, however, suggest that peripheral mechanisms also may contribute to the generation of VVH, as pointed out by Brumovsky and Gebhart [5] in a recent review on the topic. Thus, cross-sensitization and, consequently, the clinical expression of visceral hyperalgesia would result from a series of events involving peripheral and central factors in concert. The authors propose the following sequence, taking an inflammatory process in any given organ as an example for initiation of cross-organ sensitization. Inflammation at one visceral organ would increase the excitability of dichotomizing and non-dichotomizing sensory neurons innervating the organ, leading to cross-inflammation of a nearby organ. Inflammatory mediators and/or electrical or neurochemical coupling between axons and cell bodies of sensory neurons would increase the excitability of afferent fibers innervating the non-diseased organ. The cell bodies of the affected sensory neurons would upregulate their expression of receptors and ion channels and increase the axonal transport of excitatory neurotransmitters, including neuropeptides. These molecules would be released in the affected organs to further promote inflammation and sensitization of receptive endings in the organs and increased release of excitatory neurotransmitters in the dorsal horn onto second-order neurons receiving convergent input from more than one visceral organ and also from somatic structures. The sensory input would thus be "amplified" through transmission by these neurons to higher centers of the nervous system. Changes in spinal or supraspinal glial-neuronal relations could also contribute to this amplification process, given that peripheral inflammation activates microglia in the spinal cord that release proinflammatory cytokines [50] and can influence the excitability of central neurons. Further studies in various experimental models are needed to fully elucidate the mechanisms behind VVH.

Gender Differences
in Viscerovisceral Hyperalgesia

Given the more complex nature of their reproductive function, women are undeniably more subject than men to manifest a number of "paraphysiological" visceral pains from "sex-specific" organs, such as mild to severe recurrent pain from the uterus (depending on whether they are dysmenorrheic) with the ovarian cycle, or labor or postpartum pain during their fertile years. They are also more prone to develop frank "pathological" pains from the same viscera, for instance endometriosis or states of chronic pelvic pain subsequent to ascending genital infections, which are more frequent in women than in men for anatomical reasons (women have a shorter urethra) [7,9,35,39,58,60]. Several visceral pain diseases from non-sex-specific organs are also more frequent in women, particularly "dysfunctional" syndromes such as IBS or interstitial cystitis, where no specific organic cause has been ascertained; this higher incidence would seem linked to a supposed higher susceptibility of the female sex to develop the sensitization phenomena that are at least partly responsible for the pain expressed in these conditions [2,38,62]. The hypothesis of women being more prone to sensitization seems to be supported by experimental findings of the development of larger referred pain areas in females with respect to males following experimental stimulation of internal organs, especially the gastrointestinal tract [54].

Several visceral pain diseases clearly prevail in men, such as coronary artery disease (at least before age 55), pancreatic disease, and duodenal ulcer [6,49]. However, the higher frequency in women of numerous pelvic pain conditions, mostly arising from organs that have an overlapping sensory innervation, renders it more probable for the female sex to present with phenomena indicating VVH [24]. An additional factor is the further exacerbation of visceral pain sensitivity in specific periods of the hormonal cycle in women during the fertile phase of life. Many types of pain are reported to increase perimenstrually, such as pain from the stomach, pain from variant angina, and urinary pain, in addition to intestinal pain from IBS (with increased rectal pain sensitivity at menses as compared to the other phases of the cycle). Urinary colics from calculosis also cluster periovulatorily if the women are dysmenorrheic [32,38,40,42,56].

Lastly, the tendency by many physicians to underestimate algogenic processes of the female reproductive organs simply because pain from this area is regarded as "normal" [60] is a further contributing factor to women's tendency to develop complex viscerovisceral interactions. Prolonged painful triggers from this domain predispose women to long-term hypersensitivity toward minimal algogenic inputs from other neuromerically connected organs.

Greater and earlier clinical attention to even mild painful processes from internal organs is of particular importance to prevent VVH in all patients, and particularly in women. This increased attention will ultimately lead to improved management of this important phenomenon in the future.

Conclusions

Viscerovisceral hyperalgesia has important implications for diagnosis and treatment of visceral pain. This widespread phenomenon—based on the high incidence of concurrent visceral diseases—may be at the origin of a number of unexplained, intricate situations in which pain symptoms from one organ appear excessively intense (disproportionate) in relation to the specific pain disease affecting that organ [55]. When facing these complex clinical contexts, the clinician should thus always suspect that those symptoms, no matter how typical they might seem of a specific organ, are the result of a summation process of inputs from multiple viscera. The message for the clinician is thus to systematically explore all the organs that share at least part of their central sensory projection with the organ that is the primary cause of pain, to look for VVH. This consideration is particularly important because VVH has been shown to occur even when one of two comorbid visceral diseases is latent with respect to spontaneous pain. Detection of all possible algogenic conditions in neuromerically connected structures allows a broadening of the range of interventions, since treatment of one condition may have a significant impact on symptoms from the others, reducing the burden of merely symptomatic therapy for visceral pain [29].

References

[1] Alagiri M, Cottiner S, Ratner V, Slade D, Hanno PM. Interstitial cystitis, unexplained associations with other chronic disease and pain syndromes. Urology 1997;49:52–7.

[2] Altman G, Cain KC, Motzer S, Jarrett M, Burr R, Heitkemper M. Increased symptoms in female IBS patients with dysmenorrhea and PMS. Gastroenterol Nurs 2006;29:4–11.

[3] Ammons WS, Blair RW, Foreman RD. Responses of primate T1–T5 spinothalamic neurons to gallbladder distension. Am J Physiol 1984;247:995–1002.

[4] Anand P, Aziz Q, Willert R, van Oudenhove L. Peripheral and central mechanisms of visceral sensitization in man. Neurogastroenterol Motil 2007;19:29–46.

[5] Baranowski AP. Chronic pelvic pain. Best Pract Res Clin Gastroenterol 2009;23:593–610.

[6] Bellasi A, Raggi P, Merz CN, Shaw LJ. New insights into ischemic heart disease in women. Clev Clin J Med 2007;74:585–94.

[7] Berkley KJ. A life of pelvic pain. Physiol Behav 2005;86:272–80.

[8] Berkley KJ, Cason A, Jacobs H, Bradshaw HB, Wood E. Vaginal hyperalgesia in a rat model of endometriosis. Neurosci Lett 2001;306:185–8.

[9] Berkley KJ, McAllister SL. Don't dismiss dysmenorrhea! Pain 2011;152:1940–1.

[10] Brinkert W, Dimcevski G, Arendt-Nielsen L, Drewes AM, Wilder-Smith OH. Dysmenorrhoea is associated with hypersensitivity in the sigmoid colon and rectum. Pain 2007;132:S46–51.

[11] Brumovsky PR, Gebhart GF. Visceral organ cross-sensitization: an integrated perspective. Auton Neurosci 2010:153;106–15.

[12] Caldarella MP, Giamberardino MA, Sacco F, Affaitati G, Milano A, Lerza R, Balatsinou C, Laterza F, Pierdomenico SD, Cuccurullo F, Neri M. Sensitivity disturbances in patients with irritable bowel syndrome and fibromyalgia. Am J Gastroenterol 2006;101:2782–9.

[13] Cervero F. Visceral pain: mechanisms of peripheral and central sensitization. Ann Med 1995;27:235–9.

[14] Cervero F. Visceral pain-central sensitization. Gut 2000;47:56–7.

[15] Cervero F. Mechanisms of visceral pain. In: Giamberardino MA, editor. Pain 2002—An updated review: refresher course syllabus. Seattle: IASP Press; 2002. p. 403–11.

[16] Cervero F, Laird JM. Understanding the signaling and transmission of visceral nociceptive events. J Neurobiol 2004;61:45–54.

[17] Chaban VV. Visceral sensory neurons that innervate both uterus and colon express nociceptive TRPV1 and P2X3 receptors in rats. Ethn Dis 2008;18:S220–4.

[18] Chaban V, Christensen A, Wakamatsu M, McDonald M, Rapkin A, McDonald J, Micevych P. The same dorsal root ganglion neurons innervate uterus and colon in the rat. Neuroreport 2007;18:209–12.

[19] DuPont AW, Pasricha PJ. Irritable bowel syndrome and functional abdominal pain syndromes. In: Pasricha PJ, Willis WD, Gebhart GF, editors. Chronic abdominal and visceral pain. New York: Informa Healthcare; 2007. p. 341–57.

[20] Eltabbakh GH, Bower NA. Laparoscopic surgery in endometriosis. Minerva Ginecol 2008;60:323–30.

[21] Festi D, Dormi A, Capodicasa S, Staniscia T, Attili AF, Loria P, Pazzi P, Gazzella G, Sama C, Roda E, Colecchia A. Incidence of gallstone disease in Italy: results from a multicenter, population-based Italian study (the MICOL project). World J Gastroenterol 2008;14:5282–9.

[22] Frøkjaer JB, Andersen SD, Gale J, Arendt-Nielsen L, Gregersen H, Drewes AM. An experimental study of viscero-visceral hyperalgesia using an ultrasound-based multimodal sensory testing approach. Pain 2005;119:191–200.

[23] Giamberardino MA. Visceral hyperalgesia. In: Devor M, Rowbotham MC, Wiesenfeld-Hallin Z, editors. Proceedings of the 9th World Congress on Pain. Progress in pain research and management, vol. 16. Seattle: IASP Press; 2000. p. 523–50.

[24] Giamberardino MA. Women and visceral pain: are the reproductive organs the main protagonists? Mini-review at the occasion of the "European Week against Pain in Women 2007". Eur J Pain 2008;12:257–60.

[25] Giamberardino MA, Affaitati G, Lerza R, Lapenna D, Costantini R, Vecchiet L. Relationship between pain symptoms and referred sensory and trophic changes in patients with gallbladder pathology. Pain 2005;114:239–49.

[26] Giamberardino MA, Berkley KJ, Affaitati G, Lerza R, Centurione L, Lapenna D, Vecchiet L. Influence of endometriosis on pain behaviors and muscle hyperalgesia induced by a ureteral calculosis in female rats. Pain 2002;95:247–57.

[27] Giamberardino MA, Berkley KJ, Iezzi S, de Bigontina P, Vecchiet L. Pain threshold variations in somatic wall tissues as a function of menstrual cycle, segmental site and tissue depth in non-dysmenorrheic women, dysmenorrheic women and men. Pain 1997;71:187–97.

[28] Giamberardino MA, Cervero F. The neural basis of referred visceral pain. In: Parischa PJ, Willis WD, Gebhart GF, editors. Chronic abdominal and visceral pain: theory and practice. New York: Informa Healthcare; 2007. p. 177–92.

[29] Giamberardino MA, Costantini R, Affaitati G, Fabrizio A, Lapenna D, Tafuri E, Mezzetti A. Viscero-visceral hyperalgesia: characterization in different clinical models. Pain 2010;151:307–22.

[30] Giamberardino MA, Dalal A, Valente R, Vecchiet L. Changes in activity of spinal cells with muscular input in rats with referred muscular hyperalgesia from ureteral calculosis. Neurosci Lett 1996;203:89–92.

[31] Giamberardino MA, de Bigontina P, Martegiani C, Vecchiet L. Effects of extracorporeal shock-wave lithotripsy on referred hyperalgesia from renal/ureteral calculosis. Pain 1994;56:77–83.

[32] Giamberardino MA, De Laurentis S, Affaitati G, Lerza R, Lapenna D, Vecchiet L. Modulation of pain and hyperalgesia from the urinary tract by algogenic conditions of the reproductive organs in women. Neurosci Lett 2001;304:61–4.

[33] Giamberardino MA, Valente R, de Bigontina P, Iezzi S, Vecchiet L. Effects of spasmolytics and/or non-steroidal antiinflammatories on muscle hyperalgesia of ureteral origin in rats. Eur J Pharmacol 1995;278:97–101.

[34] Giamberardino MA, Valente R, de Bigontina P, Vecchiet L. Artificial ureteral calculosis in rats: behavioural characterization of visceral pain episodes and their relationship with referred lumbar muscle hyperalgesia. Pain 1995;61:459–69.

[35] Haggerty CL, Ness RB. Epidemiology, pathogenesis and treatment of pelvic inflammatory disease. Expert Rev Anti Infect Ther 2006;4:235–47.

[36] Halder SLS, Locke GR III. Epidemiology and social impact of visceral pain. In: Giamberardino MA, editor. Visceral pain: clinical, pathophysiological and therapeutic aspects. Oxford: Oxford University Press; 2009. p. 1–8.

[37] Head H. On disturbances of sensation with especial reference to the pain of visceral disease. Brain 1896;19:11–276.

[38] Heitkemper MM, Jarrett ME. Update on irritable bowel syndrome and gender differences. Nutr Clin Pract 2008;23:275–83.

[39] Holdcroft A, Snidvongs S, Cason A, Dore CJ, Berkley KJ. Pain and uterine contractions during breast feeding in the immediate postpartum period increase with parity. Pain 2003;104:589–96.

[40] Houghton LA, Lea R, Jackson N, Whorwell PJ. The menstrual cycle affects rectal sensitivity in patients with irritable bowel syndrome but not healthy volunteers. Gut 2002;50:471–4.

[41] Jänig W, Häbler H-J. Visceral-autonomic integration. In: Gebhart GF, editor. Visceral pain. Progress in pain research and management, vol. 5. Seattle: IASP Press; 1995. p. 311–48.

[42] Kawano H, Motoyama T, Ohgushi M, Kugiyama K, Ogawa H, Yasue H. Menstrual cyclic variation of myocardial ischemia in premenopausal women with variant angina. Ann Intern Med 2001;135:977–81.

[43] Laird JM, Roza C, Olivar T. Antinociceptive activity of metamizol in rats with experimental ureteric calculosis: central and peripheral components. Inflamm Res 1998;47:389–95.

[44] Li J, Micevych P, McDonald J, Rapkin A, Chaban V. Inflammation in the uterus induces phosphorylated extracellular signal-regulated kinase and substance P immunoreactivity in dorsal root ganglia neurons innervating both uterus and colon in rats. J Neurosci Res 2008;86:2746–52.

[45] Madaan S, Joyce AD. Limitations of extracorporeal shock wave lithotripsy. Curr Opin Urol 2007;17:109–13.

[46] Malykhina AP. Neural mechanisms of pelvic organ cross-sensitization. Neuroscience 2007;149: 660–72.

[47] Malykhina AP, Qin C, Greenwood-van Meerveld B, Foreman RD, Lupu F, Akbarali HI. Hyperexcitability of convergent colon and bladder dorsal root ganglion neurons after colonic inflammation: mechanism for pelvic organ cross-talk. Neurogastroenterol Motil 2006;18:936–48.

[48] McAllister SL, McGinty KA, Resuehr D, Berkley KJ. Endometriosis-induced vaginal hyperalgesia in the rat: role of the ectopic growths and their innervation. Pain 2009;147:255–64.

[49] Merskey H, Bogduk N, editors. Classification of chronic pain: descriptions of chronic pain syndromes and definitions of pain terms, 2nd ed. Seattle: IASP Press; 1994.

[50] Milligan ED, Watkins LR. Pathological and protective roles of glia in chronic pain. Nat Rev Neurosci 2009;10:23–36.

[51] Morrison T, Dmitrieva N, Winnard KP, Berkley KJ. Opposing viscerovisceral effects of surgically induced endometriosis and a control abdominal surgery on the rat bladder. Fertil Steril 2006; 86:1067–73.

[52] Ness TJ, Gebhart GF. Visceral pain: a review of experimental studies. Pain 1990;41:167–34.

[53] Parsons JK, Kurth K, Sant GR. Epidemiologic issues in interstitial cystitis. Urology 2007;69:5–8.

[54] Pedersen J, Reddy H, Funch-Jensen P, Arendt-Nielsen L, Gregersen H, Drewes AM. Cold and heat pain assessment of the human oesophagus after experimental sensitisation with acid. Pain 2004;110:393–9.

[55] Pezzone MA, Liang R, Fraser MO. A model of neural cross-talk and irritation in the pelvis: implications for the overlap of chronic pelvic pain disorders. Gastroenterology 2005; 128:1953–64.

[56] Powell-Boone T, Ness TJ, Cannon R, Lloyd LK, Weigent DA, Fillingim RB. Menstrual cycle affects bladder pain sensation in subjects with interstitial cystitis. J Urol 2005;174:1832–6.

[57] Procacci P, Zoppi M, Maresca M. Clinical approach to visceral sensation. In: Cervero F, Morrison JFB, editors. Visceral sensation. Progress in brain research. Amsterdam: Elsevier; 1986. p. 21–8.

[58] Proctor M, Farquhar C. Diagnosis and management of dysmenorrhoea. BMJ 2006; 332:1134–8.

[59] Qin C, Malykhina AP, Thompson AM, Farber JP, Foreman RD. Cross-organ sensitization of thoracic spinal neurons receiving noxious cardiac input in rats with gastroesophageal reflux. Am J Physiol Gastrointest Liver Physiol 2010;298:934–42.

[60] Reddish S. Dysmenorrhea. Aust Family Phys 2006;35:842–9.

[61] Roza C, Laird JMA, Cervero F. Spinal mechanisms underlying persistent pain and referred hyperalgesia in rats with an experimental ureteric stone. J Neurophysiol 1998;79:1603–12.

[62] Rudick CN, Pavlov VI, Chen MC, Klumpp DJ. Gender specific pelvic pain severity in neurogenic cystitis. J Urol 2012;187:715–24.

[63] Sengupta JN. Visceral pain: the neurophysiological mechanism. Handb Exp Pharmacol 2009;194:131–74.

[64] Stanford EJ, Dell JR, Parsons CL. The emerging presence of interstitial cystitis in gynecologic patients with chronic pelvic pain. Urology 2007;69:53–9.

[65] Stawowy M, Bluhme C, Arendt-Nielsen L, Drewes AM, Funch-Jensen P. Somatosensory changes in the referred pain area in patients with acute cholecystitis before and after treatment with laparoscopic or open cholecystectomy. Scand J Gastroenterol 2004;39:988–93.

[66] Stawowy M, Rossel P, Bluhme C, Funch-Jensen P, Arendt-Nielsen L, Drewes AM. Somatosensory changes in the referred pain area following acute inflammation of the appendix. Eur J Gastroenterol Hepatol 2002;14:1079–84.

[67] Stratton P, Berkley KJ. Chronic pelvic pain and endometriosis: translational evidence of the relationship and implications. Hum Reprod Update 2011;17:327–46.

[68] The Criteria Committee of the New York Heart Association. Nomenclature and criteria for diagnosis of diseases of the heart and great vessels, 9th ed. Boston: Little, Brown and Co.; 1994. p. 253–6.

[69] Tietjen GE, Bushnell CD, Herial NA, Utley C, White L, Hafeez F. Endometriosis is associated with prevalence of comorbid conditions in migraine. Headache 2007;47:1069–78.

[70] Vecchiet L, Giamberardino MA, de Bigontina P. Referred pain from viscera: when the symptom persists despite the extinction of the visceral focus. Adv Pain Res Ther 1992;20:101–10.

[71] Vecchiet L, Giamberardino MA, Dragani L, Albe-Fessard D. Pain from renal/ureteral calculosis: evaluation of sensory thresholds in the lumbar area. Pain 1989;36:289–95.

[72] Vecchiet L, Giamberardino MA, Dragani L, Galletti R, Albe-Fessard D. Referred muscular hyperalgesia from viscera: clinical approach. Adv Pain Res Ther 1990;13:175–82.

[73] Vercellini P, Somigliana E, Viganò P, Abbiati A, Barbara G, Fedele L. Chronic pelvic pain in women: etiology, pathogenesis and diagnostic approach. Gynecol Endocrinol 2009;25:149–58.

[74] Wesselmann U, Czakanski PP, Affaitati G, Giamberardino MA. Uterine inflammation as a noxious visceral stimulus: behavioral characterization in the rat. Neurosci Lett 1998;246:73–6.

[75] Wilder-Smith CH. The balancing act: endogenous modulation of pain in functional gastrointestinal disorders. Gut 2011;60:1589–99.

[76] Willis WD Jr. Dorsal root potentials and dorsal root reflexes: a double-edged sword. Exp Brain Res 1999;124:395–421.
[77] Winnard KP, Dmitrieva N, Berkley KJ. Cross-organ interactions between reproductive, gastro-intestinal, and urinary tracts: modulation by estrous stage and involvement of the hypogastric nerve. Am J Physiol Regul Integr Comp Physiol 2006;291:R1592–601.

Correspondence to: Maria Adele Giamberardino, MD, Via Carlo de Tocco n. 3, 66100 Chieti, Italy. Email: mag@unich.it.

Visceral Pain and Headache in Fibromyalgia

Robert D. Gerwin

Department of Neurology, Johns Hopkins University School of Medicine, Baltimore, Maryland, USA; Pain and Rehabilitation Medicine, Bethesda, Maryland, USA

Fibromyalgia syndrome (FMS) is a chronic, widespread pain condition that is fundamentally a disorder of pain processing, with important aspects of both central pain modulation dysfunction [12,22,70] and persistent peripheral nociceptive input [1,69]. Evidence demonstrates that central pain processing in both the spinal cord and the brain is abnormal in FMS. Central sensitization, resulting from neuroplastic changes in dorsal horn neurons, is a prominent feature [22]. Activation of supratentorial centers—the primary and secondary somatosensory cortices, amygdala, thalamus, lentiform nucleus, and anterior cingulate cortex (ACC)—is associated with the pain experience itself, as well as with anticipation of pain [41] and with the hypersensitivity and allodynia typical of fibromyalgia. Peripheral nociceptive afferent input maintains central sensitization [70]. These phenomena are key to understanding the frequent association of comorbid visceral disorders with fibromyalgia.

The recognition that central sensitization and dysfunction of central pain modulation are prominent in FMS has led to interest in the relationship of this syndrome to other central sensitization disorders such

Pain Comorbidities: Understanding and Treating the Complex Patient
edited by Maria Adele Giamberardino and Troels Staehelin Jensen
IASP Press, Seattle, © 2012

331

as irritable bowel syndrome (IBS), irritable or painful bladder syndrome, and a variety of other so-called "functional" syndromes. Medical and allied health fields have both become intensely interested in this relationship [38].

Chronic pelvic pain (CPP) and somatic syndromes such as FMS and irritable bowel and bladder syndromes share many of the same characteristics [79]. CPP has no identifiable pelvic pathology in 30% of cases; rather, it is a functional disorder of central pain dysmodulation. A person with a visceral pain syndrome causing CPP is likely to have at least one additional visceral pain syndrome. CPP is associated with nonvisceral pain syndromes as well, notably FMS and complex regional pain syndrome [40]. The fact that FMS, chronic visceral pain, and migraine headache all show central sensitization and hypersensitivity suggests that they have a common trigger. One possibility is that, through central sensitization and hypersensitivity, all sensations from viscera are magnified. Additionally, convergence of multiple distinct nociceptive inputs onto one nociceptive neuron can lead to pain felt in both somatic (body wall) and visceral structures. There is also a common cortical sensory network underlying cutaneous and visceral pain [72]. Differential activation of insular, somatosensory, motor, and prefrontal cortices is likely to account for the ability to differentiate visceral and motor responses to visceral pain stimulation. Neuroplastic changes in second-degree neurons lead to activation of existing, but normally nonfunctioning, synaptic connections, which results in convergence of somatic and visceral sensation onto one nociceptive neuron [50].

Central sensitization is also important in migraine headache and related scalp allodynia. Migraine is associated with other conditions in which—as in the case of FMS—central sensitization is thought to be an important etiological factor, such as IBS, interstitial cystitis, CPP, and endometriosis [74]. Central sensitization is the common thread that runs through all of the conditions that will be discussed in this chapter.

This chapter is concerned with the visceral and headache comorbidities of FMS. Patients with FMS have an increased risk for functional disorders (Table I). In addition, those with one functional disorder are more likely to have another functional disorder [19]. A brief review of the nature of pain in FMS will be followed by a review of the epidemiology of the most important visceral and headache comorbid syndromes, and finally by a discussion of each of the major comorbid pain syndromes.

Table I
Characteristics of fibromyalgia

1. Chronic widespread pain
2. Widespread tenderness
3. Fatigue
4. Sleep disorders (nonrestorative sleep)
5. Morning stiffness
6. Bowel disorders (irritable bowel syndrome)
7. Irritable bladder/painful bladder
8. Temporomandibular joint disorder
9. Endometriosis
10. Headache

Pain in Fibromyalgia

Pain is a complex sensation that embodies sensory perception, spatial stimulus localization, intensity determination, an affective/emotional response that reflects personal experience, and a cognitive component that interprets the meaning of the painful experience [41]. The characteristic features of FMS are first and foremost pain and widespread tenderness. A number of associated clinical features are common (Table II). Pain is only one, but the most important, manifestation of FMS, without which the condition cannot be diagnosed. However, the mechanisms that lead to pain in FMS do not explain the entirety of the syndrome.

Table II
Common visceral comorbidity disorders
that occur in fibromyalgia

1. Interstitial cystitis (painful bladder syndrome)
2. Irritable bladder and cystitis
3. Dysmenorrhea and premenstrual syndrome
4. Endometriosis
5. Vulvovestibulitis
6. Prostatitis
7. Irritable bowel syndrome

The typical presentation of FMS is that of a woman complaining of generalized or allover pain, fatigue, poor sleep, and a variety of comorbid conditions that reduce her quality of life (Table I) [63]. The ratio of women to men with FMS is about 8:1, although a retrospective review of insurance diagnoses (using the ICD-9 code 729.1) found the ratio to be only 1.64:1 [81]. The diagnostic criteria in this study were not controlled. Nevertheless, it is clear that women are overrepresented among FMS patients.

Central Modulation of Pain

Pain in FMS is the result of a dysfunction of central pain modulation, resulting in central hypersensitivity [22] and inadequate inhibition of ascending nociceptive input in the spinothalamic tract by the descending supraspinal inhibitory control system [12]. Descending facilitatory mechanisms are also enhanced. The failure of the descending pain inhibitory system may reflect deficiencies in serotonergic and noradrenergic neurotransmission in central pain pathways [16]. Elevated levels of substance P in the cerebrospinal fluid of FMS patients support the concept of a central pain-processing dysfunction [62]. Elevated local neurotransmitter and cytokine levels in FMS are consistent with the model of nociceptive input and peripheral sensitization leading to central sensitization [27,65]. Once central sensitization has taken place, only minimal nociceptive input is required to maintain it. Hypersensitivity is not restricted to nociception or pain, but crosses modalities that include touch, vibration, thermal stimulation, and sound. Central sensitization is considered to be the cause of many comorbid painful conditions in FMS.

Contribution of Peripheral Pain

Peripheral nociceptive input in fibromyalgia contributes to the initiation and/or maintenance of central sensitization [70,71]. An important implication is that treating peripheral sources of afferent nociceptive input such as myofascial trigger points, which are commonly seen in FMS, as described below, may lessen pain and result in clinical improvement. In addition, activity of pain-related regions in the brain is enhanced in chronic viscerosomatic pain [56].

Myofascial Trigger Points

Trigger points, the central feature of myofascial pain syndrome, have recently been found to be prominent in FMS [5,25]. The association of somatic pain with visceral pain syndromes has led to the concept of viscerosomatic pain syndromes [26,30]. Myofascial trigger points form in the body wall, specifically in muscle tissue, in response to the visceral pain that occurs in painful bladder syndromes, chronic noninfectious prostatitis, endometriosis [36], IBS, and other conditions. Trigger points in the body wall musculature can cause referred pain syndromes that mimic visceral pain, such as the pain of ureterolithiasis [28] or irritable bladder syndrome. Despite the paucity of studies in this area, our experience has been that treatment of the visceral pain reduces the somatic myofascial pain syndrome findings, and treatment of the myofascial trigger points decreases visceral pain and improves visceral organ function.

Operant Conditioning in Fibromyalgia

Operant conditioning is a process in which rewarded or punished behavior leads to either habituation or sensitization. Pain sensitivity can be increased or decreased by positive or negative feedback of pain behaviors, transforming acute pain into chronic pain. Persons who had both FMS and IBS were expected to be more responsive to operant training than those with FMS alone, or than healthy controls with no pain. Contrary to this expectation, subjects with both FMS and IBS had impaired operant learning, similar to persons with chronic low back pain and those with complex regional pain syndrome [9]. The conclusion is that visceral pain is processed differently from somatic pain.

Common Visceral Comorbid Conditions in Fibromyalgia

Common comorbid conditions in FMS include IBS, painful bladder syndrome (interstitial cystitis/irritable bladder), dysmenorrhea, vulvovestibulitis, pain associated with endometriosis, and noninfectious chronic prostatitis. In each of these conditions, FMS is more common than in control populations. Likewise, each of these conditions is more common in patients with FMS. Migraine headache is also more common in FMS populations, and FMS is more common in migraine patients.

Fibromyalgia and all of the comorbid conditions to which FMS patients are susceptible occur more commonly in females than in males.

Most pain disorders worsen during the late luteal and early follicular phases of the menstrual cycle, suggesting that fluctuations in ovarian hormones have an effect on pain perception [47].

Genito-urinary Pain Syndromes

Women with FMS are significantly more likely to have a wide variety of genito-urinary disorders in general when compared to women without FMS, including premenstrual syndrome, dysmenorrhea, vulvovestibulitis, breast cysts, and cystitis [66]. In general, women with FMS are more likely to have pelvic visceral pain syndromes. These syndromes include bowel and bladder dysfunctions and dysfunctions related to the reproductive organs, such as endometriosis. Women with endometriosis are more likely to have FMS than normal controls (5.9% versus 3.4%, $P < 0.0001$) [67]. Allergies, asthma, eczema, and autoimmune disease in women coexist with endometriosis and FMS, suggesting that there is an abnormality in immune response in FMS. Prostatitis is the equivalent condition in men.

Sexual abuse is intuitively linked to conditions associated with genito-urinary chronic pain syndromes and to FMS, in keeping with the concept that many patients with FMS report a history of traumatic events prior to the onset of FMS. A meta-analysis dealing with sexual abuse and somatic disorders gave both expected and unexpected results [53]. Not surprisingly, sexual abuse was significantly associated with nonspecific chronic pain (odds ratio [OR], 2.20; 95% confidence interval [CI], 1.54–3.15; 1 study), and with CPP (OR, 2.73; 95% CI, 1.73–4.30; 10 studies). There was also a significant association with a lifetime diagnosis of functional gastrointestinal (GI) disorders (OR, 2.43; 95% CI, 1.36–4.31; 5 studies). However, despite the high association with genito-urinary syndromes and other somatic pain syndromes, there was no statistically significant association of sexual abuse with FMS in four studies (OR, 1.61; 95% CI, 0.85–3.070) [11,15,73,74]. However, in two studies that looked specifically at rape as sexual abuse, there was a significant association between rape and FMS (OR, 3.35; 95% CI, 1.51–7.46) [15,74]. Ciccone et al. [15] suggested that post-traumatic stress disorder (PTSD) in rape victims was the causative factor leading to FMS, since rape alone was not predictive of FMS when PTSD was controlled for in a logistic regression model. Hypothalamic-pituitary-adrenal axis (HPA) dysfunction as a result of sexual abuse has been suggested to play a role in the later development of somatic pain syndromes such as FMS [32,85].

Interstitial Cystitis and Irritable Bladder

Fibromyalgia is directly and reciprocally linked to one or more comorbid urologic conditions [60]. It was diagnosed in 9–12% of interstitial cystitis (IC) patients, and 23–27% of FMS patients had symptoms consistent with IC. IBS, FMS, and chronic fatigue syndrome (CFS) all occur more frequently in patients with IC than in control subjects. Fibromyalgia occurred in 17.7% of IC subjects compared to 2.6% of control subjects. Multiple comorbid conditions associated with IC, as opposed to just one associated condition plus IC, were related to increased stress, pain, depression, and sleep disturbance. The presence of IC alone, IC plus one associated comorbid condition, and IC plus multiple associated disorders raises the possibility that there may be a progression from organ-centered disease to regional to systemic disease [52]. Subjects with IC and multiple non-bladder-related syndromes were more likely to have FMS, CFS, and/or IBS than persons with IC and few associated non-bladder-related syndromes [80].

Women with irritable bladder or bladder pain, as well as women with IC, are more likely to have sexual dysfunction than women without these conditions. Specifically, the RAND Interstitial Cystitis Epidemiology study showed that women with urinary frequency greater than 10 times/day, pain-related urgency, pressure, or discomfort, and pain associated with bladder distension have high levels of sexual dysfunction [10]. Of those with a current sexual partner (75% of the 1469 women meeting the above criteria), 88% reported one or more general sexual dysfunction symptoms.

Alpha-2-delta ligand inhibitors, effective in treating symptoms of FMS, reduce rectal hypersensitivity [24] and are worthy of further investigation in IBS management. A 5-hydroxytryptamine-4 partial agonist improved symptoms of both IBS and FMS in patients with both conditions [57].

Vulvodynia/Vestibulitis

Vulvodynia is not a visceral pain syndrome per se, but it is so closely related to visceral genitourinary syndromes that it is considered here. It is characterized by a number of distressing symptoms, including pain at rest and on contact (sexual contact or tight-fitting clothing), burning, itching, redness, and inflammation [31]. The pathophysiology of vestibulitis has three interdependent components: the vestibular mucosa, the pelvic floor musculature, and a dysregulation of central pain modulation similar to that seen in FMS [86].

Nongenital musculoskeletal pelvic floor pain is often associated with genital pain, such as vulvovestibular pain [61]. The diagnosis of vestibulitis, the most common type of chronic vulvovaginal pain, is based on a report of pain during intercourse and vestibular sensitivity on clinical examination [61].

Phone surveys show a significant association of vulvodynia with FMS (OR, 3.84; 95% CI, 1.54–9.55) and IBS (OR, 3.11; 95% CI, 1.6–6.05) [6,31]. A phone survey of 2127 U.S. households identified 100 women with vulvar pain. The odds ratio for repeated urinary tract infections in these women is 6.15 (95% CI, 3.51–10.77) and for yeast infections 4.24 (95% CI, 2.47–7.28). Comorbid conditions of importance associated with vulvodynia in these subjects include FMS (OR, 2.15; 95% CI, 1.06–4.36) and IBS (OR, 1.86; 95% CI, 1.07–3.23). Depression and CFS were also significantly associated with vulvodynia. Dyspareunia and vestibular hypersensitivity, along with a severe impact on sex life, were prominent complaints in addition to vulvar pain [6,7].

Prostatitis

Chronic prostatitis is a common disorder, affecting up to 11.5% of men younger than 50 years of age and 8.5% of men 50 years of age or older [51]. It is one of the causes of CPP in men, although men may also have CPP as a result of IBS or irritable or painful bladder syndrome. Chronic prostatitis is usually divided into infectious and noninfectious prostatitis, based on the results of repeated cultures. However, "noninfectious" prostatitis may have biofilm infections that do not yield positive cultures and do not respond to ordinary antibiotic treatment. Both categories of chronic prostatitis may cause CPP. The condition is characterized by pelvic pain and urinary tract symptoms. Sitting is painful. Myofascial trigger points are commonly found in the pelvic floor muscles, including the levator ani muscles, and in the gluteal muscles, including the piriformis. The adductor muscles of the thigh are also commonly affected. The outcomes of medical treatment are poor. Depression and somatization are common. Chronic prostatitis has an important impact on work. There is no accepted treatment, but treatment of the comorbid trigger points and adjuvant pharmacological treatment with pregabalin or duloxetine, both approved by the U.S. Food and Drug Administration (FDA) for the treatment of FMS, can be beneficial.

Irritable Bowel Syndrome

Patients with FMS have a high incidence of IBS, and IBS patients are also more likely to have comorbid conditions, including FMS, CFS, and CPP, any one of which may occur in up to 65% of IBS patients [58]. The prevalence of IBS is 10–20%; it is more common in women seeking care for FMS than in men [76]. There are three interacting components to IBS: psychosocial factors, altered motility, and heightened sensory function [76]. Visceral hyperalgesia is caused by altered visceral receptor sensitivity and by altered central sensory modulation [3]. Plasma levels of interleukin-6 (IL-6) and IL-8 are increased in IBS patients. In patients who also have extraintestinal comorbidities such as FMS, IL-1β and tumor necrosis factor (TNF)-α are also increased [64]. Abdominal pain is the most disruptive IBS symptom [13]. FMS has a strong association with IBS, with a median 49% of FMS subjects having IBS [82]. Lubano [42] found FMS in 20% of IBS patients, but the IBS patients with FMS were those with more severe IBS, so that the association may be related to severity and not random within the IBS population. In another study, the prevalence of IBS in patients with FMS ranged from 30–35% up to 70% [68]. Somatosensory processing in IBS is increased both for visceral hyperalgesia and cutaneous heat hyperalgesia, activating the same neural regions in both, supporting the hypothesis that there is increased afferent activity in ascending pathways to the brain [77]. Fibromyalgia and IBS are both considered functional disorders with altered somatic or visceral sensory perception. Pain is a prominent symptom in both conditions. Multivariate analyses suggest that the two conditions are distinct entities and not manifestations of a common somatization disorder [82]. Somatic body wall sensitivity is greater (body wall hypersensitivity or lower threshold to nociceptive responses when given a nociceptive stimulus) in subjects with IBS, FMS, and a combination of IBS and FMS, when compared to normal controls [14].

There is a high prevalence of IBS among FMS subjects when one considers IBS as a comorbid condition of FMS, instead of FMS as a comorbid condition of IBS, confirming the great degree of overlap between these conditions. Functional GI disorders were more than twice as common in FMS patients than in control subjects [4]. At least one functional GI disorder was found in 98% of FMS subjects, compared to 39% of control subjects. IBS was the most common functional GI disorder in FMS patients. Psychological distress scores were significantly higher in IBS patients, particularly those with fecal incontinence, than in controls. IBS occurred frequently in FMS patients, ranging from 63% by ROME I criteria to 81% by ROME II criteria, compared to only 15% and 24%, respectively, in controls ($P < 0.001$). The odds ratio that IBS would be found in Swedish subjects with chronic widespread pain (a surrogate diagnosis for FMS) was 5.15 (95% CI, 4.55–5.88) [37]. Depression in the FMS patients and in those with both FMS and IBS was consistent with other reports of depression in FMS, in the range of 30–40%.

Irritable bowel syndrome is common in the United States, occurring in 13.1% of white Americans and 7.9% of African Americans [83]. There is a statistically insignificant trend toward IBS occurring more frequently among younger subjects under the age of 50 (9.5%) compared to those over the age of 50 (9.9%). In a study in India [45], the overall prevalence of IBS was 4% (95% CI, 3.5–4.6), but prevalence increased with age and was maximal (5.8%) in the 51–60-year age group. IBS was also significantly more common in females than in males (4.8% vs. 3.2%, $P = 0.008$). Thus, both age and gender stratification in IBS prevalence emerged in this study.

The association between IBS and FMS makes IBS an important condition to consider in subjects with FMS. The question has been raised as to whether the female preponderance in IBS is related to the association of IBS with FMS, where there is a predominance of females. Subjects with comorbid IBS and FMS are overwhelmingly female (83.4%, F:M = 5:1), whereas IBS without FMS is more often found in men than in women (59.4%, F:M = 2:3) [2]. This finding suggests that IBS is not really a woman's disorder, as some have suggested.

The ACC is activated on functional MRI scans in normal subjects with painful bowel stimulation, where symptom intensity and regional activity are strongly correlated. However, subjects with IBS showed activation of the left prefrontal cortex, indicating an altered response to visceral pain [41].

Post-traumatic stress disorder has been linked to both IBS and FMS, suggesting a potential common underlying predisposing or potentiating factor. PTSD was reported in 57% of a limited sample of FMS patients [18], but only 7.8% of IBS patients met the diagnostic criteria for PTSD [17], suggesting that despite a history of traumatic experiences in both conditions, PTSD may be more important in chronic widespread pain conditions such as FMS than in organ-specific pain conditions such as IBS. These studies did not indicate whether PTSD increased the likelihood of developing a comorbid condition when a patient had either IBS or FMS.

Pain in IBS is often preceded by an inflammatory or infectious bowel disorder that heals completely, leaving the colon histopathologically normal. However, IBS patients develop a widespread hyperalgesia in cutaneous and somatic tissues that is centrally mediated. It is maintained by low-intensity, tonic nociceptive input from visceral organs. Rectal lidocaine gel diminishes or abolishes local rectal pain, showing the importance of peripheral factors in pain maintenance, and it also decreases or eliminates centrally mediated mechanical and thermal pain in distant structures such as the foot [56].

Migraine and Fibromyalgia

Migraine headache is the result of dysfunctional activation of the trigeminovascular complex, resulting in an intracranial sterile, neurogenic, perivascular edema. Activated mast cells release proinflammatory mediators including cytokines and histamine [86]. Altered brain excitation occurs in chronic migraine; cutaneous allodynia reflects central sensitization. Chronically sensitized nociceptive neurons may play a critical role in chronic migraine [48]. Migraine without aura is associated with vasodilation of the middle meningeal artery and the middle cerebral artery. Headache relief with sumatriptan therapy is associated with vasoconstriction of only the middle meningeal artery [8]. Among many mechanical, metabolic, and chemical triggers of trigeminovascular system activation are the myofascial trigger points, which also refer pain to areas of headache [29].

Fibromyalgia and migraine headache are closely associated [21]. Migraine is more common in women, as is FMS. There is both an increased incidence of migraine in women with FMS, and an increased incidence of FMS in migraineurs. Migraine occurred in 48% of a sample of FMS patients with headache and predated FMS symptoms by an average of 7 years [46]. Among 34 somatic comorbid disorders potentially associated with migraine, FMS was one of the two most common comorbid conditions, with or without migraine aura, the other being hypothyroidism (also a common comorbid condition of FMS) [42]. FMS was found in 35.6% of patients with transformed migraine [55]. It was present in 36.4% of 217 consecutive headache patients [21], most commonly in chronic migraine and chronic tension-type headache patients. Out of 100 consecutive migraine patients, 22.2% met the diagnostic criteria for FMS [35]. Tietjen et al. [75] identified three comorbidity groups in a headache clinic population of 223 migraineurs. Group 1 was defined by hypertension, hyperlipidemia, diabetes mellitus, and hypothyroidism. Males were more prevalent in this group than in group 2, which was defined by depression, anxiety, and FMS. Males comprised 26% of group 1 patients (versus 74% females) ($P < 0.5$). Group 2 was predominantly female (91% female versus 9% male). The group with FMS, depression, and anxiety had greater disability ($P < 0.05$) and a lower quality of life ($P < 0.001$), and they reported more sexual, physical, and emotional abuse. Childhood abuse has been linked to overactivity of the HPA system [33], a finding that has often been linked to FMS.

Enhanced cortisol release has been found only in those FMS patients with a major depressive disorder, suggesting that altered HPA axis function is associated with affective disorders in FMS [85]. Both enhanced and suppressed HPA axis activity has been reported in FMS [59,84], and there have been mixed responses in other related disorders, including CFS. Increased cortisol release with a maintained circadian rhythm of cortisol production has also been reported in migraine, but it was thought to be related to the stress of muscle pain, as it coincided with sympathoneural activation and was corrected with recovery from pain [43,54].

Alterations of the HPA axis in migraine are not likely to be primary abnormalities, but are more likely to be secondary to the effects of migraine itself, whereas in FMS, HPA axis alteration may be of etiological importance in a subset of patients, particularly those with a history of abuse and depression.

There are further commonalities between migraine and FMS. Both conditions show reduced habituation of cortical areas related to nociceptive perception [20]. Reduced habituation means that there is a decrease in cortical recruitment in response to continued nociceptive stimulation. Thus, pain becomes persistent in the face of continued stimulation, the clinical condition seen in FMS. Depression correlates well with the habituation index of the two evoked potential complexes P2 and N2–P2, showing that habituation is a complex phenomenon and is not simply related to abnormal central processing of pain [20].

Pharmacological management of FMS and migraine shares many commonalities, such as the prophylactic effect of serotonin-norepinephrine reuptake inhibitors and of the calcium channel $\alpha_2\delta$-ligand inhibitors, but one cannot argue backwards from treatment effects to propose a common etiological mechanism, as the same drug may have different mechanisms of action in different conditions.

Conclusion

Fibromyalgia and its comorbidities share common dysfunctions in central pain modulation that increase the likelihood of multiple comorbid disorders. Central sensitization is key to FMS and to the multiple comorbid conditions considered here. The clinical presentation may be FMS alone, or any one of the associated conditions described, or a complex presentation of multiple conditions that may or may not include FMS. A thoughtful evaluation can uncover comorbid conditions, leading to more comprehensive and effective treatment.

References

[1]   Affaitati G, Costantini R, Fabrizio A, Lapenna D, Tafuri E, Giamberardino MA. Effects of treatment of peripheral pain generators in fibromyalgia patients. Eur J Pain 2011;15:61–9.
[2]   Akkus S, Senol A, Ayvacioglu NB, Tunc E, Eren I, Isler M. Is female predominance in irritable bowel syndrome related to fibromyalgia? Rheumatol Int 2004;24:106–9.
[3]   Alaradi O, Barkin JS. Irritable bowel syndrome: update on pathogenesis and management. Med Princ Pract 2002;11:2–17.

[4]   Almansa C, Rey E, Sánchez RG, Sánchez AA, Diaz-Rubio M. Prevalence of functional gastroin-
      testinal disorders in patients in patients with fibromyalgia and the role of psychologic distress.
      Clin Gastroenterol Hepatol 2009;7:438–45.
[5]   Alonso-Blanco C, Fernández-de-las-Peñas C, Morales-Caberzas M, Zarco-Moreno P, Ge HY,
      Florez-Garcia M. Multiple active myofascial trigger points reproduce the overall spontaneous
      pain pattern in women with fibromyalgia and are related to widespread mechanical hypersensi-
      tivity. Clin J Pain 2011;27:405–13.
[6]   Arnold LD, Bachmann GA, Kelly S, Rosen R, Rhoads GG. Vulvodynia: characteristics and as-
      sociations with comorbidities and quality of life. Obstet Gynecol 2006;107:617–24.
[7]   Arnold LD, Bachmann GA, Rosen R, Rhoads GG. Assessment of vulvodynia symptoms in a
      sample of U.S. women: a prevalence survey with a nested case control study. Am J Obstet Gyne-
      col 2007;196:128.e1–6.
[8]   Asghar MS, Hansen AE, Amin FM, van der Geest RJ, Koning P, Larsson HB, Olesen H, Ashina
      M. Evidence for a vascular factor in migraine. Ann Neurol 2011;69:635–45.
[9]   Becker S, Kleinböhl D, Baus D, Hölzl R. Operant learning of perceptual sensitization and ha-
      bituation is impaired in fibromyalgia patients with and without irritable bowel syndrome. Pain
      2011;152:1408–17.
[10] Bogart LM, Suttorp MJ, Elliott MN, Clemens JQ, Berry SH. Prevalence and correlates of
      sexual dysfunction among women with bladder pain syndrome/interstitial cystitis. Urology
      2011;77:576–80.
[11] Boisset-Pioro MH, Esdalle JM, Fitzcharles MA. Sexual and physical abuse in women with fibro-
      myalgia syndrome. Arthritis Rheum 1995;38:235–41.
[12] Bradley LA. Pathophysiology or fibromyalgia. Am J Med 2009;122(12 Suppl):S22–30.
[13] Cain KC, Headstrom P, Jarrett ME, Motzer SA, Park H, Burr RL, Surawicz CM, Heitkemper
      MM. Abdominal pain impacts quality of life in women with irritable bowel syndrome. Am J
      Gastroenterol 2006;10:124–32.
[14] Calderella MP, Giamberardino MA, Sacco F, Affaitati G, Milano A, Lerza R, Balatsinou C, Lat-
      erza F, Pierdomenico SD, Cuccurullo F, Neri M. Sensitivity disturbances in patients with irritable
      bowel syndrome and fibromyalgia. Am J Gastroenterol 2006;101:2782–9.
[15] Ciccone DS, Elliot DK, Chandler HK, Nayak S, Raphael KG. Sexual and physical abuse in women
      with fibromyalgia syndrome: a test of the trauma hypothesis. Clin J Pain 2005;21:378–86.
[16] Clauw DJ. Fibromyalgia: an overview. Am J Med 2009;122(12 Suppl): S3-13.
[17] Cohen H, Jolkowitz A, Buskila D, Pelles-Avraham S, Kaplan Z, Neumann L, Sperber AD. Post-
      traumatic stress disorder and other co-morbidities in a sample population of patients with ir-
      ritable bowel syndrome. Eur J Intern Med 2006;17:567–71.
[18] Cohen H, Neumann L, Haiman Y, Matar MA, Press J, Buskila D. Prevalence of post-traumatic
      stress disorder in fibromyalgia patients: overlapping syndromes or post-traumatic fibromyalgia
      syndrome? Semin Arthritis Rheum 2002;32:38–50.
[19] Cole JA, Rothman KJ, Cabral HJ, Zhang Y, Farraye FA. Migraine, fibromyalgia, and depression
      among people with IBS: a prevalence study. BMC Gastroenterol 2006;6:26.
[20] de Tommaso M, Federici A, Santostasi R, Calabrese R, Vecchio E, Lapadula G, Iannone F, Lam-
      berti P. Laser-evoked potentials habituation in fibromyalgia. J Pain 2011:12:116–24.
[21] de Tommaso M, Sardaro M, Serpino C, Costantini F, Vecchio E, Prudenzano M, Lamberti P,
      Livrea P. Fibromyalgia comorbidity in primary headaches. Cephalalgia 2009;29:453–64.
[22] Desmeules JA, Cedraschi C Rapiti E, Baumgartner E, Finckh A, Cohen P, Dayer P, Vischer TL.
      Neurophysiologic evidence for a central sensitization in patients with fibromyalgia. Arthritis
      Rheum 2003;48:1420–9.
[23] Evans RW, de Tommaso M. Migraine and fibromyalgia. Headache 2011;51:295–9.
[24] Gale JD, Houghton LA. Alpha 2 delta ($\alpha_2\delta$) ligands, gabapentin and pregabalin: what is the evi-
      dence for potential use of these ligands in irritable bowel syndrome. Front Pharmacol 2011,2:28.
[25] Ge HY, Wang Y, Danneskiold-Samsøe B, Graven-Nielsen T, Arendt-Nielsen L. The predeter-
      mined sites of examination for tender points in fibromyalgia syndrome are frequently associated
      with myofascial trigger points. J Pain 2010;11:644–51.
[26] Gerwin RD. Myofascial and visceral pain syndromes: visceral-somatic pain representations. J
      Musculoskel Pain 2002;10:165–75.
[27] Gerwin RD, Dommerholt J, Shah J. An expansion of Simons' integrated hypothesis of trigger
      point formation. Curr Pain Headache Rep 2004;8:468–75.

[28] Giamberardino MA, Affaitati G, Lerza R, Fanò G, Fulle S, Belia S, Lapenna D, Vecchiet L. Evaluation of indices of skeletal muscle contraction in areas of referred hyperalgesia from an artificial ureteric stone in rats. Neurosci Lett 2003;338:212–6.

[29] Giamberardino MA, Tafuri E, Savini A, Fabrizo A, Affaitati G, Lerza R, Di Ianni L, Lapenna D, Mezzetti A. Contribution of myofascial trigger points to migraine symptoms. J Pain 2007;8:869–78.

[30] Giamberardino MA, Vecchiet L. Visceral pain, referred hyperalgesia and outcome: new concepts. Eur J Anesthesiol Suppl 1995;10:61–6.

[31] Gordon AS, Panahian JM, McComb F, Melegari C, Sharp S. Characteristics of women with vulvar pain disorders: responses to a Web-based survey. J Sex Marit Ther 2003;29(Suppl 1):45–58.

[32] Griep EN, Boersma JA, Lentjes EG, Prins AP, van der Korst JK, de Kloet ER. Function of the hypothalamic-pituitary-adrenal axis in patients with fibromyalgia and low back pain. J Rheumatol 1998;25:1374–81.

[33] Heim C, Newport DJ Heit S Graham YP, Wilcox M, Bonsall R, Miller AH, Nemeroff CB. Pituitary-adrenal and autonomic responses to stress in women after sexual and physical abuse in childhood. JAMA 2000;284:592–7.

[34] Hudson JL, Pope HG Jr. Does childhood sexual abuse cause fibromyalgia? Arthritis Rheum 1995;38:161–3.

[35] Ifergane F, Buskila D, Simiseshvely N, Zeev K, Cohen H. Prevalence of fibromyalgia syndrome in migraine patients. Cephalalgia 2006;26:451–6.

[36] Jarrell J. Endometriosis and abdominal myofascial pain in adults and adolescents. Curr Pain Headache Rep 2011;15:368–76.

[37] Kato K, Sullivan PF, Evengård B, Pedersen NL. Chronic widespread pain and its comorbidities. Arch Int Med 2006;166:1649–54.

[38] Kindler LL, Bennet RM, Jones KD. Central sensitivity syndromes: mounting pathophysiologic evidence to link fibromyalgia with other common chronic pain disorders. Pain Manag Nurs 2011;12:15–24.

[39] Kurland JE, Coyle WJ, Winkler A, Zable E. Prevalence of irritable bowel syndrome and depression in fibromyalgia. Dig Dis Sci 2006;51:454–60.

[40] Labat JJ, Riant T, Delavierre D, Sibert L, Watier A, Rigaud J. [Global approach to chronic pelvic and perineal pain: from the concept of organ pain to that of dysfunction of visceral pain regulation systems.] Prog Urol 2010;20:1027–34.

[41] Ladabaum U, Minoshima S, Owyang C. Pathology of visceral pain: molecular mechanism and therapeutic implications v. central nervous system processing of somatic and visceral sensory signals. Am J Physiol Gastrointest Liver Physiol 2000;279:G1–6.

[42] Le H, Tflet-Hansen P, Russell MB, Skythe A, Kyvik KO, Olesen J. Co-morbidity of migraine with somatic disease in a large population-based study. Cephalalgia 2011;31:43–64.

[43] Leistad RB, Stovner LJ, White LR, Nilsen KB, Westgaard RH, Sand T. Noradrenalin and cortisol changes in response to low-grade cognitive stress differ in migraine and tension-type headache. J Headache Pain 2007;8:157–66.

[44] Lubrano E, Iovino P, Tremolaterra F, Parsons WJ, Ciacci C, Massacca G. Fibromyalgia in patients with irritable bowel syndrome. An association with the severity of the intestinal disorder. Int J Colorectal Dis 2001;16:211–5.

[45] Makharia GK, Verma AK, Amarchand R, Goswami A, Singh P, Aqnihotri A, Suhail F, Krishnan A. Prevalence of irritable bowel syndrome: a community based study from northern India. J Neurogastroenterol Motil 2011;17:82–7.

[46] Marcus DA, Bernstein C, Rudy TE. Fibromyalgia and headache: an epidemiological study supporting migraine as part of the fibromyalgia syndrome. Clin Rheumatol 2005;24:595–601.

[47] Martin VT. Ovarian hormones and pain response: a review of clinical and basic science studies. Gend Med 2009;6(Suppl 2):S168–92.

[48] Mathew NT. Pathophysiology of chronic migraine and mode of action of preventive medications. Headache 2011;51(Suppl 2): S84–92.

[49] Minocha A, Johnson WD, Abell TL, Wigington WC. Prevalence, sociodemography, and quality of life of older versus younger patients with irritable bowel syndrome: a population-based study. Dig Dis Sci 2006;51:446–53.

[50] Moshiree B, Price DD, Robinson ME, Gaible R, Verne GN. Thermal and visceral hypersensitivity in irritable bowel syndrome patients with and without fibromyalgia. Clin J Pain 2007;23:323–30.

[51] Nickel JC, Downey J, Hunter D, Clark J. Prevalence of prostatitis-like symptoms in a population based study using the National Institutes of Health chronic prostatitis symptom index. J Urol 2001;185:842–5.

[52] Nickel JC, Tripp DA, Pontari M, Moldwin R, Mayer S, Carr LK, Doggweiler R, Yang CC, Mishra N, Nordling J. Interstitial cystitis/painful bladder syndrome and associated medical conditions with an emphasis on irritable bowel syndrome, fibromyalgia and chronic fatigue syndrome. J Urol 2010;184:1358–63.

[53] Paras ML, Murad MH, Chen LP, Goranson EN, Sattler AL, Colbenson KM, Elamin MB, Seime RJ, Prokop LJ, Zirakzadeh A. Sexual abuse and lifetime diagnosis of somatic disorders. A systematic review and meta-analysis. JAMA 2009;302:550–61.

[54] Patacchioli FR, Monnazzi P, Simeoni S, De Filippis S, Salvatori I, Coloprisco G, Martelletti P. Salivary cortisol, dehydroepiandrosterone-sulphate (DHEA-S) and testosterone in women with chronic migraine. J Headache Pain 2006;7:90–4.

[55] Peres MF, Young WB, Kaup AO, Zukerman E, Silberstein SD. Fibromyalgia is common in patients with transformed migraine. Neurology 2001;9:1326–8.

[56] Price DD, Craggs JG, Zhou QQ, Verne GN, Perlstein WM, Robinson WE. Widespread hyperalgesia in irritable syndrome is dynamically maintained by tonic visceral impulse input and placebo/nocebo factors: evidence from human psychophysics, animal models, and neuroimaging. Neuroimage 2009;47:995–1001.

[57] Reitblat T, Zamir D, Polishchuck I, Nonshatko G, Malnick S, Kalichman L. Patients treated by tegaserod for irritable bowel syndrome with constipation showed significant improvement in fibromyalgia symptoms. A pilot study. Clin Rheumatol 2009;28:1079–82.

[58] Riedl A, Schmidtmann M, Stengel A, Goebel M, Wisser AS, Klapp BF, Monnikes H. Somatic comorbidities of irritable bowel syndrome: a systematic analysis. J Psychosom Res 2008;64:573–82.

[59] Riva R, Mork PJ, Westgaard RH, Lundberg U. Comparison of the cortisol awakening response in women with shoulder and neck pain and women with fibromyalgia. Psychoneuroendocrinology 2012;37:299–306.

[60] Rodriguez MAB, Afari, Buchwald D, for the National Institute of Diabetes and Digestive and Kidney Diseases Working Group on Urological Chronic Pelvic Pain. A review of the evidence for overlap between urological and non-urological unexplained clinical conditions. J Urol 2009;182:2123–31.

[61] Rosenberg TY. Musculoskeletal pain and sexual function in women. J Sex Med 2010;7:645–53.

[62] Russell IJ, Orr MD, Littman B, Vipraio GA, Alboukred D, Michalek JE, Lopez Y, Mackillip F. Elevated cerebrospinal fluid levels of substance P in patients with the fibromyalgia syndrome. Arthritis Rheum 1994;37:1593–601.

[63] Schaefer C, Chandran A, Hufstader M, Baik R, McNett M, Goldenberg D, Gerwin R, Zlateva G. The comparative burden of mild, moderate and severe fibromyalgia: results from a cross-sectional survey in the United States. Health Qual Life Outcomes 2011;9:71.

[64] Scully P, McKernan DP, Keohane J, Groeger D, Shanahan F, Dinan TG, Quigley EM. Plasma cytokine profiles in females with irritable bowel syndrome and extra-intestinal co-morbidity. Am J Gastroenterol 2010;105:2235–43.

[65] Shah J, Danoff JB, Desai MJ, Parikh S, Nakamura LY, Phillips TM, Gerber LH. Biochemicals associated with pain and inflammation are elevated in sites near to and remote from active myofascial trigger points. Arch Phys Med Rehabil 2008;89:16–23.

[66] Shaver JL, Wilbur J, Robinson FP, Wang E, Buntin MS. Women's health issues with fibromyalgia syndrome. J Womens Health (Larchmt) 2006;15:1035–45.

[67] Sinaii N, Cleary SD, Ballweg ML, Nieman LK, Stratton P. High rates of autoimmune and endocrine disorders, fibromyalgia, chronic fatigue syndrome and atopic diseases among women with endometriosis: a survey analysis. Hum Reprod 2002;17:2715–24.

[68] Sperber A, Dekel R. Irritable bowel syndrome and co-morbid gastrointestinal and extra-gastrointestinal functional syndromes. J Neurogastroenterol Motil 2010;16:113–8.

[69] Staud R. Biology and therapy of fibromyalgia: pain in fibromyalgia syndrome. Arthritis Res Ther 2006;8:208.

[70] Staud R, Nagel S, Robinson ME, Price DD. Enhanced central pain processing of fibromyalgia patients is maintained by muscle afferent input: a randomized, double-blind, placebo-controlled study. Pain 2009;145:96–104.

[71] Staud R, Rodriguez ME. Mechanisms of disease: pain in fibromyalgia. Nat Clin Pract Rheumatol 2006;2:90–8.

[72] Strigo IA, Bolvin M, Bushnell MC. Differentiation of visceral and cutaneous pain in the human brain. J Neurophysiol 2003;89:3294–303.
[73] Taylor ML, Trotter DR, Csuka ME. The prevalence of sexual abuse in women with fibromyalgia. Arthritis Rheum 1995;38:229–34.
[74] Tietjen GE, Conway A, Utley C, Herial NA. Migraine is associated with menorrhagia and endometriosis. Headache 2006;46:422–8.
[75] Tietjen GE, Herial NA, Hardgrove J, Utley C, White L. Migraine comorbidity constellations. Headache 2007;47:857–65.
[76] Torii A, Toda G. Management of irritable bowel syndrome. Intern Med 2004;43:353–9.
[77] Verne GN, Himes NC, Robinson ME, Gopinath KS, Briggs RW, Crosson B, Price DD. Central representation of visceral and cutaneous hypersensitivity in the irritable bowel syndrome. Pain 2003;103:99–110.
[78] Walker EA, Keegan D, Gardner G, Sullivan M, Bernstein D, Katon WJ. Psychosocial factors in fibromyalgia compared with rheumatoid arthritis. II: Sexual, physical and emotional abuse and neglect. Psychosom Med 1997;59:572–7.
[79] Warren JW, Morozov V, Howard FM. Could chronic pelvic pain be a functional somatic syndrome? Am J Obstet Gynecol 2011;205:199.e1–5.
[80] Warren JW, Wesselmann U, Morozov V, Langenberg PW. Numbers and types of nonbladder syndromes as risk factors for interstitial cystitis/painful bladder syndrome. Urology 2011;77:313–9.
[81] Weir PT, Harlan GA, Nkoy FL, Jones SS, Hegmann KT, Gren LH, Lyon JL. The incidence of fibromyalgia and its associated comorbidities: a population-based retrospective cohort based on International Classification of Diseases, 9th Revision codes. J Clin Rheumatol 2006;12:124–8.
[82] Whitehead WE, Palsson O, Jones KR. Systemic review of the comorbidity of irritable bowel syndrome with other disorders: what are the causes and implications? Gastroenterology 2002;122:1140–56.
[83] Wigington WC, Johnson WD, Minocha A. Epidemiology of irritable bowel syndrome among African Americans as compared with whites: a population-based study. Clin Gastroenterol Hepatol 2005;3:647–53.
[84] Wingenfeld K, Heim C, Schmidt I, Wagner D, Meinischmidt G, Helljammer DH. HPA axis reactivity and lymphocyte glucocorticoid sensitivity in fibromyalgia syndrome and chronic pelvic pain. Psychosom Med 2008;70:65–72.
[85] Wingenfeld K, Nutzinger D, Kauth J, Hellhammer DH, Lautenbacher S. Salivary cortisol release and hypothalamic pituitary adrenal axis feedback sensitivity in fibromyalgia is associated with depression and not with pain. J Pain 2010;11:1195–202.
[86] Xanthos DN, Gaderer S, Drdla R, Nuro E, Abramova A, Ellmeier W, Sandkühler J. Central nervous system mast cells in peripheral inflammatory nociception. Mol Pain 2011;7:42.
[87] Zolnoun D, Hartmann K, Lamvu G, As-Sanie S, Maixner W, Steege J. A conceptual model for the pathophysiology of vulvar vestibulitis syndrome. Obstet Gynecol Surv 2006;61:395–401.

Correspondence to: Robert D. Gerwin, MD, Department of Neurology, Johns Hopkins University School of Medicine, Baltimore, MD 21287, USA. Email: gerwin@painpoints.com.

Muscular Pain Comorbidities in Joint Diseases

18

Thomas Graven-Nielsen,[a] Henning Bliddal,[b]
and Lars Arendt-Nielsen[a]

[a]Center for Sensory-Motor Interaction, Laboratory for Musculoskeletal Pain and Motor Control, Aalborg University, Aalborg, Denmark; [b]The Parker Institute, Frederiksberg Hospital, Frederiksberg, Denmark

Chronification of pain and widespread musculoskeletal pain are significant clinical problems. One important issue is the interaction between joint diseases and comorbid pain manifestations in other structures such as muscles or distant joints. For the deeper structures, comorbidities are often neglected due to the diffuse pain characteristics. Distinction between primary and comorbid pain conditions is required to improve diagnostics and guide relevant management.

Pain from joints or adjacent muscles may be impossible to distinguish. Joint damage or inflammation may affect the surrounding soft tissues such as muscle or ligaments. Another challenge is referred pain, which may be a confounding factor in the diagnosis of regional pain conditions. Widespread pain may be another complication of the rheumatological joint diseases typically seen in patients with rheumatoid arthritis or systemic lupus. The clinical symptom of joint and muscle pain may overlap considerably among different pain conditions, representing a frequent problem when physicians are making a diagnosis. Valuable information for distinguishing patterns of pain from muscle, ligaments, and joints

Pain Comorbidities: Understanding and Treating the Complex Patient
edited by Maria Adele Giamberardino and Troels Staehelin Jensen
IASP Press, Seattle, © 2012

349

has recently been presented that has improved current knowledge of the manifestations of these pain conditions. In addition to the neuronal pain mechanisms relevant for pain distribution and sensitization, joint diseases often result in reduced joint function, which may affect other structures because of changes in biomechanical loading. This situation can potentially initiate pain and sensitization mechanisms distant to the diseased joint. For example, trauma on the medial compartment of the tibiofemoral knee joint may precipitate painful changes in the myotendinous part of the muscles (pes anserinus), which is typical of knee osteoarthritis (OA). The effect of a change in biomechanical loading due to joint diseases is not the scope of this chapter, but it should be regarded as a comorbid factor in joint diseases.

This chapter will focus on comorbid manifestations of joint pain, the potential mechanisms involved, and assessment methods. A joint pain comorbidity is defined as a pain manifestation (or disease) located outside the affected joint that can potentially aggravate other pain mechanisms by neuronal convergence or spreading sensitization.

Painful Joint Diseases and Comorbidities

Joint pain is a significant clinical problem [17,26,100]. Conditions affecting the joints may be secondary to trauma, infections, or other noxious effects on the joints, or they may arise as idiopathic joint diseases with no obvious precipitating factor. OA is by far the most common disease, while rheumatoid arthritis is a differential diagnosis in joint pain among younger patients.

Joint diseases affect joint function, but they are not always associated with joint pain. Thus, rheumatoid arthritis may continue subclinically and create erosions in spite of presumed remission [18], and even at advanced stages of OA, about half of those affected have no complaints of joint pain [9].

While its etiology is unclear, OA involves all joint tissues, including the articular cartilage, subchondral bone, and soft tissues in and around the joint. Peripheral sensitization of the nociceptors is likely and can arise from inflamed synovium and damaged subchondral bone. Radiographic changes have only a weak correlation with pain in OA [6,36], but with magnetic resonance imaging (MRI), signs of inflammation are closely associated with the clinical symptoms [12,54]. Nonetheless, a substantial number of patients (4–14%) with knee pain have normal X-rays [27,37,68]. Moreover, hyperalgesia to pressure stimulation around the OA knee is not related to radiographic scores (Fig. 1).

Pain patterns from joints have been extensively studied, typically by joint provocation followed by recordings of the referred pain areas. As an example, the pain patterns from the cervical zygapophysial joints were assessed by distending the joint capsule in healthy volunteers with injections of contrast medium under fluoroscopic control [33]. The opposite approach was used in patients where the referred pain areas from the zygapophysial joint pain were eliminated by selective nerve blocks [23]. The referred pain areas from zygapophysial joints show that these areas may coexist with pain areas typically considered as referred pain from myofascial trigger points, and regions of pain in the myofascial pain syndrome can actually originate from joints rather than from muscles. Although this situation represents a diagnostic challenge for identification of the source of pain, it also suggests the possibility of joint pain being comorbid with a myofascial pain syndrome. It has been hypothesized that assessment of mechanical pain sensitivity can distinguish symptomatically between

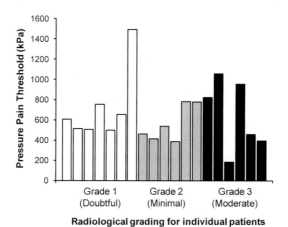

Fig. 1. Examples of pressure pain thresholds assessed on the knee in patients with osteoarthritis, illustrated with respect to the radiological Kellgren-Lawrence score. The figure clearly illustrates that there is no association between the severity of hyperalgesia and the extent of joint damage.

painful and healthy cervical zygapophysial joints. However, a recent study found that reduced pressure pain thresholds were not diagnostic for cervical zygapophysial joint pain [89]. The referred pain distribution from the thoracic and the lumbar zygapophysial joints, the atlanto-axial and atlanto-occipital joints, and other joints has previously been mapped [30,32,38]. Colocation of referred pain from adjacent joints was consistently reported, preventing clinical identification of symptomatic joints based purely on pain localization.

Diskogenic pain is highly relevant in chronic musculoskeletal disorders. In patients with diskogenic pain, electrothermal stimulation of the lumbar intervertebral disks evoked pain distributed from the low back to the buttocks, the hips, and the distal leg areas [77]. Progressively increasing heat stimulation intensities initially induced pain in the back and later developed into pain spreading distally to the legs. Low back pain patients often report a similar manifestation with pain in the legs and feet, especially with high pain intensity. Unfortunately, it has not been possible to establish a uniform pain distribution for each individual disk. Nevertheless, the extensive referred pain areas from nociceptive disk structures may cause a diagnostic problem with regard to other possible causes of pain (e.g., nerve root compression) and may lead to other pain manifestations in the lower legs such as referred hyperalgesia.

Inflammatory conditions of joints are accompanied by reports of joint pain as well as pain in the surrounding soft tissue due to spreading of the inflammation [80]. Such scenarios with pain from both joint and muscle tissue make it difficult to distinguish the joint as the primary nociceptive locus. Pain in the shoulder and surrounding areas is one example that can occur in several diseases, with a comparable pain distribution (Table I).

Inflammatory vascular disease, for instance polymyalgia or temporal arteritis, is a confounding factor for the condition of shoulder pain and represents a challenging differential diagnosis [20]. In degenerative joint diseases, some degrees of soft tissue involvement are also found, which are accompanied by varying degrees of pain. There is an interesting lack of association between pain and radiographic joint changes in osteoarthritis [36]; a comorbid soft tissue problem is one explanation that offers further perspectives for nonsurgical disease modification, even within conditions of cartilage and bone degeneration [1]. Typical pain areas from

Table I
Symptoms and pain in selected joint diseases

Tendinitis and bursitis related to the rotator cuff (shoulder)
Reduced active abduction and referred pain distributed to the lateral part of the upper arm.

Capsulitis (shoulder)
As above, plus reduced active and passive movement in all directions.

Arthritis (shoulder)
In addition to the above, local signs of inflammation and pain at rest.

Polymyalgia rheumatica (shoulder)
Reduced active abduction. Pain frequently occurs in the trapezius muscle from the shoulder in the direction of the neck and lateral part of the upper arm.

Osteoarthritis, light (knee)
Post-exercise pain.

Osteoarthritis, moderate (knee)
Pain triad: pain at the beginning of exercise, relative relief with ambulation, and renewed pain upon continued activity. Relatively short period of morning stiffness.

Osteoarthritis, severe (knee)
As above, plus pain at rest.

Arthritis (knee)
Pain at rest and on movement, stiffness after rest, long period of morning stiffness.

knee OA joints are illustrated in Fig. 2. Common joint disorders associated with comorbid issues (e.g., muscle pain and other diseases) in the shoulder and knees are presented in Table I.

Fundamental Aspects of Muscle and Joint Pain

Excitation of polymodal muscle nociceptors related to group III and IV ($A\delta$ and C) afferent nerve fibers is associated with perception of acute musculoskeletal pain [72]. Following nociceptor activation, the release of neuropeptides may cause sensitization of the nociceptors, with hyperalgesia as the perceptual correlate. Prolonged activity of nociceptors may further sensitize second-order neurons (central sensitization), resulting in facilitated responses to non-noxious and noxious stimulation and expansion of receptive fields [72,88].

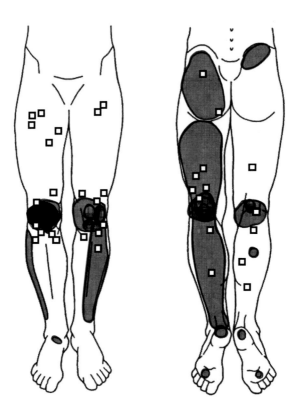

Fig. 2. Distribution of habitual pain in osteoarthritis patients. Individual pain areas from 14 patients are shaded in gray and superimposed (i.e., common pain areas are visualized as a darker gray). Examples of latent myofascial trigger points are indicated with open squares. The frequency of latent myofascial trigger points was significantly higher than in matched control subjects. Based on data from Bajaj et al. [10,11].

The joint is innervated by afferent nerves, including group II–IV fibers (Aβ, Aδ, and C fibers) [84]. Corpuscular endings related to group II fibers are identified in ligaments and in the fibrous capsule, whereas all joint structures are innervated by free nerve endings (group III and IV fibers), although not the cartilage. Silent nociceptors, a set of group IV fibers that do not respond to noxious mechanical stimuli under normal conditions, are active in inflammatory conditions [86]. Animal OA models and joint inflammation models have provided the most information on the basic neurobiology of joint pain. The animal joint models cannot be translated into human models. Nonetheless, there are human studies focusing on pain mechanisms related to structures surrounding the joints. Intense and prolonged nociceptive input from the OA knee joint in animals may result in central sensitization [70]. The dorsal horn neurons are strongly controlled by the descending inhibitory pathways. Potential impairments of descending control will cause similar manifestations as central sensitization, including a reduced excitation threshold of spinal cord neurons to joint nociceptive input, increased receptive fields, and increased ongoing discharges of neurons [83].

Sluka demonstrated that muscle tissue and joint tissue in rats have different sensory responses to experimental nociception, with prolonged allodynia in joint compared to muscle tissue [92]. It would appear reasonable to presume that human muscle and other deep tissue (e.g., tendons and the tendon-bone junction) have a similar difference in sensory manifestations to experimental pain stimulation. Experimental pain induced by mechanical, thermal and chemical stimuli has been demonstrated to arise from several human joint structures including ligaments, fibrous capsule, adipose tissue, meniscus, periosteum, and synovial layer, but not cartilage [34,62,69].

Quantitative Assessment of Musculoskeletal Pain

Quantitative sensory assessments of musculoskeletal pain require two different disciplines. The first is a standardized stimulation of deep-tissue nociceptors, and the second is a quantification of the evoked pain sensation. This experimental approach is useful for quantifying pain manifestations related to the primary joint disease and secondary (comorbid) effects.

The perception of pain is multidimensional, which calls for a detailed quantitative sensory testing approach; the complex perception of pain cannot be described with an assessment based on one modality of standardized stimulation. Application of different stimulus modalities and quantitative assessment of various pain mechanisms will provide details of the pain system in normal as well as in pathophysiological situations. A highly controlled and short-lasting experimental pain stimulus obviously results in a different pain experience compared to a chronic pain condition, but the experimental approach does show the status of basic pain mechanisms.

Assessment Methods

Quantitative pain assessment is performed by different methodologies, which always involve psychophysics. Although this section will focus on psychophysical methods, electrophysiological or imaging approaches are also useful for quantitative purposes. Response-dependent and stimulus-dependent techniques are used to determine psychophysical reactions [45]. Response-dependent techniques are based on stimulations with different stimulation intensities, after which subjects score the sensation on scales such as visual analogue scales (VAS) or verbal descriptor scales. Questionnaires (such as the McGill Pain Questionnaire) may also be useful for assessing the intensity and quality of pain [45].

Detection threshold, pain threshold, or pain tolerance is determined with stimulus-dependent methods, in which the stimulus intensity is changed until a specific perception is detected. In stimulus-dependent methods, scoring systems are avoided, and the thresholds are defined in physical units. Regardless of the technique used, it is important to characterize nonpainful as well as painful sensations by stimulus-response functions in order to characterize allodynic and hyperalgesic muscle and joint responses. Somatosensory sensitivity and pain must be assessed in the local pain area (e.g., a painful joint) and in remote areas where a direct peripheral sensitization effect (spreading sensitization) is not likely to occur as a result of the local pain condition.

For assessments of localized, regional, and widespread pain in clinical studies, detailed profiling of the usual pain intensity, distribution, and quality is needed. Scales (e.g., VAS), pain drawings, and questionnaires (e.g., the McGill Pain Questionnaire) are appropriate. Assessment of other aspects of the pain experience, such as unpleasantness or soreness, is also relevant. Moreover, as musculoskeletal pain and indeed joint pain have implications for many aspects of daily life, there are several adequate questionnaires for assessment of functional implications (e.g., the General Function Score, Roland and Morris Disability Scale, and Oswestry Pain Disability Index) [98]. One of the instruments used most extensively to evaluate health status in hip and knee osteoarthritis is the Western Ontario and McMaster Universities' Osteoarthritis Index (WOMAC); importantly, it evaluates pain during various tasks [16].

Stimulus Modalities for Pain Sensitivity Assessment

Several methods for evoking standardized experimental pain can be used for quantitative assessment of the pain sensitivity of deep tissue. Pressure stimulation (pressure algometry) to excite nociceptors in deep tissue is a method that is widely used and validated [22,58]. A topographical mapping technique was recently developed [6], where pain sensitivity maps of the knee, neck, spine, head, or specific muscles can be obtained by recording pain responses from many different sites (Fig. 3). Manually applied pressure stimulation is associated with some variability, which can be minimized by computer-controlled pressure; stimulus-response functions relating pressure intensity with the pain response can easily be established [52]. The volume of tissue stimulated with manual pressure algometry is relatively small. A larger volume of deep tissue is stimulated with the computer-controlled cuff-algometry technique, which is also less influenced by local variations in pain sensitivity. The cuff algometry technique is based on inflation of a tourniquet mounted around

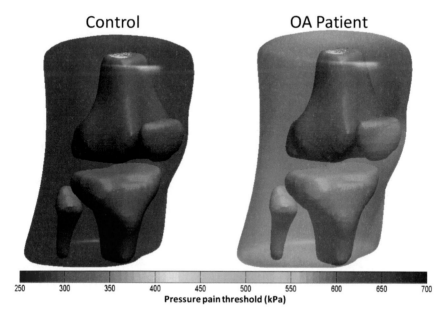

Fig. 3. Mapping of pain sensitivity. Pressure pain thresholds were assessed on several sites around the knee in a nonsymptomatic healthy subject and in a patient with osteoarthritis (OA) pain. A novel mapping approach illustrates the individual pattern of sensitivity changes in patients. Based on data from Arendt-Nielsen et al. [6].

an extremity, followed by the determination of pain threshold or stimulus-response functions [60,81]. In the lower legs, significantly lower pain thresholds and tolerances were recorded by cuff algometry in fibromyalgia patients compared with controls [60].

Other models may also be useful for stimulation of deep tissue. A widely used method is the injection of algesic substances (e.g., capsaicin, glutamate, acidic saline, and hypertonic saline [47]), allowing a more tonic pain stimulation and providing the ability to assess local and referred pain patterns. Some muscles, such as the tibialis anterior muscle, show distinct referred pain areas, and enlargement of the referred pain area may indicate a condition of central sensitization [48]. Muscle pain modalities based on different forms of exercise (e.g., strong, ischemic, or eccentric contractions) or external stimuli of nonmechanical modalities such as electrical or thermal stimulation [47], are used less frequently for assessment of musculoskeletal pain patients.

Deep-Tissue Hyperalgesia

Clinical examples of deep-tissue hyperalgesia are tender points and trigger points. According to the tender point count criteria for fibromyalgia, 11 of a total of 18 anatomically defined sites should be sore to a 4-kg pressure stimulation, although tender points are often assessed by manual palpation [101]. In contrast, trigger points are not described by a specific anatomical location but are muscle sites located in taut bands of muscle fibers with a hard and hypersensitive locus [90]. Trigger point stimulation by palpation or pressure algometry typically evokes referred pain, which is not the case for stimulation of tender points. Recently, a novel methodology has been developed to visualize the taut band related to trigger points in muscles [21]. Tender and trigger point assessment may involve pressure algometry to record pain thresholds [19,99], which is a more standardized approach than manual palpation. Nonetheless, the overlap of sites with reduced pressure pain thresholds and sites palpated with tender points in healthy subjects is poor [3].

The tenderness associated with muscle damage is most likely explained by sensitization of the deep-tissue nociceptors by the algesic substances that are released. Sensitized deep-tissue nociceptors are characterized by a decreased mechanical excitation threshold and an increased firing activity following suprathreshold stimulation [72]. Peripheral sensitization is unlikely to be the mechanism explaining widespread deep-tissue hyperalgesia in conditions like fibromyalgia; central sensitization is more likely to explain such findings. Interestingly, a detailed trigger point examination in fibromyalgia patients showed an increased number of trigger points in patients compared with controls [39,40], suggesting that more trigger points may be a result of central sensitization. Interestingly, capsaicin-induced sensitization of the C5 dermatome (the arm) reduced the pressure pain threshold (hyperalgesia) in the infraspinatus muscle (C5–6) [94], illustrating the segmental interaction that may be crucial for understanding comorbid symptoms.

Hyperalgesia as a Comorbid Finding in Joint Pain Patients

Recently there has been a focus on the peripatellar hypersensitivity detected in OA patients compared with healthy control subjects [6]. Interestingly, the most sensitive site around the osteoarthritic knee was located on the medial side in the patients with the highest habitual pain intensity [6], in accord with the medial compartment structures being predominantly involved in the osteoarthritic process [24]. The load on the medial compartment in painful arthritic knees is also higher than in asymptomatic knees [97]. Nociceptive activity from the joint capsule (stretching), the synovium (inflammation), and corroded subchondral bone [29] may eventually lead to facilitated central pain mechanisms. Peripheral sensitization of receptors is found within the first few hours after onset of inflammation. At that time, the central neurons show increased responses to noxious and innocuous stimulation of the joint and lower the mechanical threshold to stimuli [84]. If the pressure stimulation and clinical nociceptive locus stimulate different groups of nociceptors, the hyperalgesia detected in OA patients may also be due to a central summation or facilitatory mechanism. Facilitation of previously ineffective dorsal horn synaptic connections and spatial summation of neuronal activity might be of importance [43,50]. Imamura et al. [57] and Arendt-Nielsen et al. [6] reported that peripatellar hyperalgesia to pressure was mainly expressed in patients with severe knee pain, indicating a relationship between the tenderness in the encapsulated tissue and the intraarticular lesion in patients with knee OA.

Hyperalgesia to pressure stimulation outside the symptomatic joint has been reported in patients with OA in either the carpometacarpal joints [35], knee [6], or hip [65]. Spreading of the sensitization to the contralateral knee has also been observed in patients with knee OA [6], most likely because some patients have bilateral symptoms, and in addition, contralateral subclinical changes may exist in patients with only one symptomatic knee. In chronic diseases such as knee OA, it is also possible that the central neuronal systems are sensitized bilaterally. In such scenarios, the clinical pain manifestations start to spread together with spreading sensitization. For example, a joint pain patient may begin to complain of pain in other regions, the pain could potentially become widespread, and comorbid pain conditions may develop. In patients with low back pain (due to a herniated disk), a similar widespread hyperalgesia to pressure has been detected, with reduced pressure pain threshold in the tibialis anterior muscle [79]. The spreading hyperalgesia seems to be dependent on tonic pain for some time, as 10 minutes of electrical stimulation on the lumbar facet joint (L3–4) did not evoke hyperalgesia outside the stimulation area [78].

Recently, the first use of cuff algometry in patients with arthritis demonstrated the feasibility of using this method on the lower leg to measure hyperalgesia in knee OA patients [53]. Spreading sensitization was found that was similar to that observed with the use of conventional pressure algometry on the tibialis anterior muscle, with cuff pressure pain thresholds being significantly lower in OA patients compared to controls.

A higher frequency of latent myofascial trigger points was detected in the lower leg of OA patients compared with healthy controls [11], and such a comorbid condition might be explained by a generalized reduced threshold for eliciting a painful perception due to central sensitization. Interestingly, the habitual OA pain areas do not consistently include the latent myofascial trigger points (Fig. 2). Given that the etiology of myofascial trigger points is not clear, peripheral factors contributing to the frequent development of trigger points cannot be excluded, although it seems unlikely.

Temporal Summation of Pain

Repeated somatosensory stimulations with the same intensity evoke a perception of progressively increasing pain. This phenomenon is defined as "temporal summation of pain" and probably parallels the initial phase of the neuronal wind-up process reported in animals [5]. Short intervals between sequential stimuli at a constant strength (e.g., 10 stimuli with a 1-second interstimulus interval) are needed to evoke temporal summation. The temporal summation pain threshold is defined as the strength of the 10 stimuli resulting in a progressive increase in pain perception during the series of stimuli. In clinical and experimental studies, electrical, chemical, pressure, and focused ultrasound repeated stimuli have been used to assess the temporal summation of deep-tissue pain [49,93,102]. Computer-controlled sequential pressure stimulation on the muscles evoked temporal summation more efficiently compared to sequential stimulation on the skin [74]. Temporal summation of pain is facilitated in different groups of chronic musculoskeletal pain patients, and the involvement of central sensitization has been proposed as an explanation for the findings [6,93,95,96]. In healthy subjects, experimental muscle soreness has also been reported to facilitate the temporal summation of pressure-induced muscle pain [75], indicating that the time window for the nociceptive activity needed to cause central sensitization is relatively short. Facilitated temporal summation of the nociceptive withdrawal reflex elicited by repeated cutaneous electrical stimulation has also been used as an indicator for central sensitization in fibromyalgia patients and whiplash pain patients [13]. In some patients, minor nociceptive activity is plausible without confirmed tissue damage, and facilitated temporal summation is likely to explain the pain perceived in such cases.

Facilitated Temporal Summation of Muscle Pain as a Comorbid Finding in Joint Pain Patients

A recent study found that temporal summation assessed by pressure stimulation on the knee and tibialis anterior muscle was significantly facilitated in knee OA patients compared with controls [6]. Interestingly, patients with high-intensity habitual knee pain showed greater temporal summation of muscle pain than OA patients who were less affected. The duration of OA pain was correlated to the degree of temporal summation of pain [6], suggesting that the plasticity involved is a progressive process.

There is no distinct overlap between nerves innervating the knee (L2–L4) and the tibialis anterior muscle (L5–S1). However, expansion of receptive fields due to deep-tissue noxious input has been found in several animal pain models [55,88], and such neuronal hyperexcitability in the L2–L4 segments evoked by the knee OA lesion may spread to adjacent spinal segments, accounting for the facilitated temporal summation found when the tibialis anterior muscle is stimulated [6]. An intriguing finding was facilitated by temporal summation assessed contralaterally to the more affected knee [6], but this finding may be due to the fact that most patients with knee OA have OA symptoms in both knees, although one knee may be less severely affected than the other. An alternative or additional explanatory component is that the same neurons sensitized by the more severely affected knee contribute to enhanced temporal summation on the contralateral side because some neurons have bilateral receptive fields [85].

Referred Pain

Referred pain from a localized painful structure is often associated with musculoskeletal and visceral pain syndromes. Referred pain is based on a central mechanism and is frequently used diagnostically. Referred pain is defined as pain located in structures away from the source of nociception. With joint pain some typical syndromes are encountered; OA in the hip joint is often accompanied by complaints of knee pain (and vice versa), which may in some cases be the only symptom, and a common shoulder disorder, tendinitis of the supraspinatus muscle, may cause elbow pain. In many conditions it is not possible to distinguish between spread of pain and a combination of pain from referred and local pain areas. Joint pain mechanisms might be involved in the spread of pain and referred pain. Musculoskeletal referred pain is frequently perceived in deep structures (e.g., joints), whereas visceral referred pain is perceived both superficially and deeply.

Referred pain is a well-described phenomenon in many clinical and experimental conditions, although the neurophysiological mechanisms involved in referred pain are not fully described. A central mechanism is highly likely because referred pain can be evoked in areas with an effective regional anesthetic block. The effect of sensory information from the referred pain area is unclear because the intensity of referred pain is either unaffected or reduced when the referred pain structures are anesthetized [47,66].

The size and location of referred pain may reflect sensitization of central neural mechanisms. Animal studies have shown that muscle nociception results in development of new receptive fields and expansion of existing receptive fields [55]. The dorsal horn neurons receive widespread collateral synaptic connections from many deep-tissue nociceptive afferent fibers [72]. Functional synaptic connections exist on dorsal horn neurons, and some have latent synaptic connections in nonpainful conditions. After a strong nociceptive input, latent synapses may become functional, which would expand the degree of convergence of afferent information from different structures. Such neural reorganization has been confirmed in animal studies where new receptive fields were developed after intramuscular injection of bradykinin into the tibialis anterior [55]. The receptive fields that develop due to central sensitization may be involved in the mechanism mediating referred pain [47,71]. Human studies have demonstrated that the referred pain mechanism is a time-dependent process, because there is a short (approx. 20–40-second) delay between the perception of referred pain and local pain. Development of new receptive fields or unmasking of latent synapses may account for the delay in referred pain found in human studies. Interestingly, more subjects develop referred pain after prolonged painful pressure stimulation on the tibialis anterior compared with brief pressure stimulations at the same intensity [43], suggesting that a critical time period of nociceptive input is required for eliciting referred pain or that temporal summation is a key component of the referred pain mechanism. Another finding suggesting the involvement of central sensitization in the mechanism of referred pain is the reduced number of healthy subjects developing referred pain by experimental muscle pain when treated with an N-methyl D-aspartate (NMDA) antagonist (ketamine) compared with placebo [87].

Referred Pain as a Confounding Issue in Patients with Joint Pain

Referred pain from myofascial trigger points in myofascial pain patients illustrates an extensive mapping of referred pain patterns from many skeletal muscles [90]. A similar overlap in joint-related referred pain is likely.

In patients with pain conditions such as low back pain, osteoarthritis (Fig. 4), tennis elbow pain, fibromyalgia, and whiplash pain, experimentally induced referred pain areas are enlarged in comparison with similar assessments in control subjects without pain (for a review, see [4,48]). The expanded referred pain areas in patients were found after pain was induced in the tibialis anterior muscle; this muscle is normally not described as being habitually painful in patients. The referred pain from the tibialis anterior muscle is typically described as pain perceived in the ankle area in healthy subjects, but in some patients proximal referred pain has been reported. In line with the proximal spread of referred pain in pain patients, it has been demonstrated that myositis in animals causes sensitization of dorsal horn neurons that mainly spreads proximally [56]. The expanded areas of referred pain suggest that central

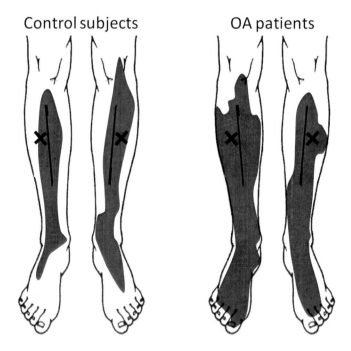

Fig. 4. Pain distribution after injection of a small bolus of hypertonic saline into the tibialis anterior muscles in healthy control subjects and osteoarthritis (OA) patients. The gray shaded area illustrates the overall area of pain, including all the individual pain distributions from 15 patients and 15 controls. Significantly larger referred pain areas and higher pain intensities were found in OA patients compared with control subjects. Based on data from Bajaj et al. [10,11].

neuronal mechanisms are sensitized in chronic musculoskeletal pain patients. Accordingly, if the increased referred pain areas in pain patients are re-assessed when antagonized by ketamine, referred pain areas are reduced and partly normalized [51].

Descending Control of Pain

An imbalance between descending facilitation and inhibition may implicate an increased excitability of central neuronal mechanisms manifested as central sensitization. Descending control can be assessed experimentally and is termed "conditioned pain modulation" (CPM) or "diffuse noxious inhibitory control" (DNIC). Descending inhibitory effects are evoked by painful heterotopic conditioning stimuli (thermal, mechanical, electrical, or chemical), resulting in decreased pain perception induced by painful stimulation given elsewhere in the body than the heterotopic stimulus. Acute experimental muscle pain impairs CPM efficacy in humans [7], indicating that musculoskeletal pain per se may negatively affect the potency of descending pain control. Reduced efficacy of endogenous pain modulation has been demonstrated in musculoskeletal pain conditions such as fibromyalgia [61,64], temporomandibular disorder [63], and chronic tension-type headache [82]. A dysfunction of descending pain modulation mechanisms may contribute to the clinical manifestations of widespread pain as a comorbid finding added to the original source of pain [8]. Activation of the rostral anterior cingulate cortex in fibromyalgia patients was recently shown to be reduced compared with healthy control subjects, and since this brain structure is probably essential in descending pain control, alterations in its activation may contribute to an imbalance in descending control [59]. Partly in contrast is the finding that opioid receptors in the rostral ventromedial medulla (RVM) do not seem to be involved in the descending analgesia produced in rats with muscle inflammation [28].

Abnormal Descending Pain Control as a Confounding Issue in Joint Pain Patients

After hip joint replacement in OA patients, Kosek and Orderberg [65] found that CPM was restored when patients became free of pain. In a study including knee OA patients, no significant increase in pressure pain thresholds over the peripatellar region was found during CPM compared with control subjects [6], extending the findings from hip OA patients. Interestingly, the mechanism of descending inhibition is intact in patients with short-term and long-term rheumatoid arthritis compared to controls [67]. Finally, a study on chronic monoarthritic animals found that CPM effects are impaired [25], corroborating some of the human findings.

From Acute Joint Pain to Chronic Widespread Pain and Spreading Sensitization

At present only hypothetical models are available to explain the transition to widespread pain from localized pain due to joint tissue damage or other challenges. The initial joint tissue damage will excite and sensitize joint nociceptors, potentially causing a sufficient nociceptive barrage of input to the central pain systems to result in central sensitization of neurons within the dorsal horn or at higher brain centers. The time needed for this transition is not known, although experimental muscle soreness models have indicated that one day of muscle soreness is sufficient to cause signs of central sensitization, such as facilitated temporal summation and spreading hyperalgesia [2,76]. In clinical settings, expanded referred pain areas from muscle pain stimulation have been shown in patients who have had tennis elbow pain for approximately 6 months [91]. In joint pain conditions, the above hypothesis may implicate a sequence where (1) peripheral joint nociceptors are excited and sensitized due to tissue damage, (2) ipsilateral second-order neurons at the same segmental site as the affected joint are sensitized, (3) segmental contralateral second-order neurons are sensitized, and (4) neuronal sensitization spreads extrasegmentally [48]. As already noted, an imbalance between descending inhibition and facilitation may implicate central sensitization. In parallel or in consequence, the higher brain centers may be reorganized after the sensitization of second-order neurons. Reorganized cerebral activation patterns have been detected by functional magnetic resonance imaging (fMRI) in fibromyalgia patients [46] and low back pain patients [44] compared with healthy controls. In line with the above proposal is the finding that more and more sensory abnormalities occur as the clinical pain condition progresses from one stage to the other [19], with widespread hyperalgesia occurring in chronic conditions.

Assessment of Primary and Secondary Sources of Pain

The identification of the primary source of pain and sensitization is challenging, particularly when the currently available diagnostic tools are unable to detect evident pathology outside painful joints. It is often difficult to identify whether pain felt at muscles or joints is due to a pathology (or dysfunction) of that particular structure or represents referred pain, where the origin is in another anatomical structure, such as a proximal joint. Clinical examinations are not always conclusive; for example, tenderness on palpation can be the result of both primary muscle pain (peripheral sensitization) and referred pain from an affected joint (central sensitization). A recent study showed that an experimental trigger point induced by an intramuscular injection of nerve growth factor evoked spreading sensitization/hyperalgesia in the neighboring muscle due to a facilitated central mechanism [41]. However, if the experimental trigger point was subsequently anesthetized, the spreading hyperalgesia was maintained. This finding complicates the interpretation of diagnostic blocking tests. An open question is the potential interaction between joint pain and visceral pain. Basic studies provide several examples of muscle-visceral [73] and visceral-somatic nociceptive interactions [42], but the relevance for joint-visceral, and visceral-joint interactions still needs to be evaluated. Acceptable sensitivity and specificity of a diagnostic test against a gold standard is required for a diagnostic test to be valid. There is a lack of validated diagnostic tools for distinguishing between primary and referred deep-tissue pain. Certain joint pain conditions can, however, be reliably diagnosed. In peripheral joints or similarly well-defined anatomical structures, the origin of the pain referral may be substantiated by abolishing pain after injection of local anesthetics into the suspected source. In particular, double-blind controlled blocks of the nerves that supply the zygapophysial joints can be diagnostically used to define pain from these joints [14,15,31,89].

Conclusion

Comorbid joint pain conditions are highly important. The pain itself, as well as the sensitization of joint nociceptors, as a robust source of central sensitization, are especially important factors to account for in the diagnostic procedure. Standardized assessments of pressure pain sensitivity inside and outside the affected joint, temporal summation of pain, and descending inhibitory pain modulations will add valuable contributions to understanding central sensitization as a confounding factor. Referred pain from joints is a challenge because it may mimic a localized source of pain. Further development of standardized sensory assessment protocols is needed to optimize diagnostic approaches, as well as drug effects, and provide rational treatment strategies.

References

[1]   Abramson SB, Attur M, Yazici Y. Prospects for disease modification in osteoarthritis. Nat Clin Pract Rheumatol 2006;2:304–12.
[2]   Andersen H, Arendt-Nielsen L, Svensson P, Danneskiold-Samsoe B, Graven-Nielsen T. Spatial and temporal aspects of muscle hyperalgesia induced by nerve growth factor in humans. Exp Brain Res 2008;191:371–82.
[3]   Andersen H, Ge HY, Arendt-Nielsen L, Danneskiold-Samsoe B, Graven-Nielsen T. Increased trapezius pain sensitivity is not associated with increased tissue hardness. J Pain 2010;11:491–9.
[4]   Arendt-Nielsen L, Graven-Nielsen T. Central sensitization in fibromyalgia and other musculoskeletal disorders. Curr Pain Headache Rep 2003;7:355–61.
[5]   Arendt-Nielsen L, Graven-Nielsen T. Translational aspects of musculoskeletal pain: from animals to patients. In: Graven-Nielsen T, Arendt-Nielsen L, Mense S, editors. Fundamentals of musculoskeletal pain. Seattle: IASP Press; 2008. p. 347–66.
[6]   Arendt-Nielsen L, Nie H, Laursen MB, Laursen BS, Madeleine P, Simonsen OH, Graven-Nielsen T. Sensitization in patients with painful knee osteoarthritis. Pain 2010;149:573–81.
[7]   Arendt-Nielsen L, Sluka KA, Nie HL. Experimental muscle pain impairs descending inhibition. Pain 2008;140:465–71.
[8]   Arendt-Nielsen L, Yarnitsky D. Experimental and clinical applications of quantitative sensory testing applied to skin, muscles and viscera. J Pain 2009;10:556–72.
[9]   Bagge E, Bjelle A, Eden S, Svanborg A. Osteoarthritis in the elderly: clinical and radiological findings in 79 and 85 year olds. Ann Rheum Dis 1991;50:535–9.
[10] Bajaj P, Bajaj P, Graven-Nielsen T, Arendt-Nielsen L. Osteoarthritis and its association with muscle hyperalgesia: an experimental controlled study. Pain 2001;93:107–14.
[11] Bajaj P, Graven-Nielsen T, Arendt-Nielsen L. Trigger points in patients with lower limb osteoarthritis. J Musculoskel Pain 2001;9:17–33.
[12] Baker K, Grainger A, Niu J, Clancy M, Guermazi A, Crema M, Hughes L, Buckwalter J, Wooley A, Nevitt M, Felson DT. Relation of synovitis to knee pain using contrast-enhanced MRIs. Ann Rheum Dis 2010;69:1779–83.
[13] Banic B, Petersen-Felix S, Andersen OK, Radanov BP, Villiger PM, Arendt-Nielsen L, Curatolo M. Evidence for spinal cord hypersensitivity in chronic pain after whiplash injury and in fibromyalgia. Pain 2004;107:7–15.
[14] Barnsley L, Bogduk N. Medial branch blocks are specific for the diagnosis of cervical zygapophyseal joint pain. Reg Anesth 1993;18:343–50.

[15] Barnsley L, Lord S, Bogduk N. Comparative local anaesthetic blocks in the diagnosis of cervical zygapophysial joint pain. Pain 1993;55:99–106.

[16] Bellamy N, Buchanan WW, Goldsmith CH, Campbell J, Stitt LW. Validation study of WOMAC: A health status instrument for measuring clinically important patient relevant outcomes to antirheumatic drug therapy in patients with osteoarthritis of the hip or knee. J Rheumatol 1988;15:1833–40.

[17] Breivik H, Collett B, Ventafridda V, Cohen R, Gallacher D. Survey of chronic pain in Europe: prevalence, impact on daily life, and treatment. Eur J Pain 2006;10:287–333.

[18] Brown AK, Quinn MA, Karim Z, Conaghan PG, Peterfy CG, Hensor E, Wakefield RJ, O'Connor PJ, Emery P. Presence of significant synovitis in rheumatoid arthritis patients with disease-modifying antirheumatic drug-induced clinical remission: evidence from an imaging study may explain structural progression. Arthritis Rheum 2006;54:3761–73.

[19] Carli G, Suman AL, Biasi G, Marcolongo R. Reactivity to superficial and deep stimuli in patients with chronic musculoskeletal pain. Pain 2002;100:259–69.

[20] Ceccato F, Roverano SG, Papasidero S, Barrionuevo A, Rillo OL, Paira SO. Peripheral musculoskeletal manifestations in polymyalgia rheumatica. J Clin Rheumatol 2006;12:167–71.

[21] Chen Q, Basford J, An KN. Ability of magnetic resonance elastography to assess taut bands. Clin Biomech (Bristol, Avon) 2008;23:623–9.

[22] Chesterton LS, Sim J, Wright CC, Foster NE. Interrater reliability of algometry in measuring pressure pain thresholds in healthy humans, using multiple raters. Clin J Pain 2007;23:760–6.

[23] Cooper G, Bailey B, Bogduk N. Cervical zygapophysial joint pain maps. Pain Med 2007;8:344–53.

[24] Creamer P, Lethbridge-Cejku M, Hochberg MC. Where does it hurt? Pain localization in osteoarthritis of the knee. Osteoarthritis Cartilage 1998;6:318–23.

[25] Danziger N, Weil-Fugazza J, Le BD, Bouhassira D. Alteration of descending modulation of nociception during the course of monoarthritis in the rat. J Neurosci 1999;19:2394–400.

[26] Davidsen M, Kjoller M, Helweg-Larsen K. The Danish National Cohort Study (DANCOS). Scand J Public Health 2011;39:131–5.

[27] Davis MA, Ettinger WH, Neuhaus JM, Barclay JD, Segal MR. Correlates of knee pain among US adults with and without radiographic knee osteoarthritis. J Rheumatol 1992;19:1943–9.

[28] de Resende MA, Silva LF, Sato K, Arendt-Nielsen L, Sluka KA. Blockade of opioid receptors in the medullary reticularis nucleus dorsalis, but not the rostral ventromedial medulla, prevents analgesia produced by diffuse noxious inhibitory control in rats with muscle inflammation. J Pain 2011;12:687–97.

[29] Dieppe PA. Relationship between symptoms and structural change in osteoarthritis: what are the important targets for therapy? J Rheumatol 2005;32:1147–9.

[30] Dreyfuss P, Michaelsen M, Fletcher D. Atlanto-occipital and lateral atlanto-axial joint pain patterns. Spine 1994;19:1125–31.

[31] Dreyfuss P, Schwarzer AC, Lau P, Bogduk N. Specificity of lumbar medial branch and L5 dorsal ramus blocks. A computed tomography study. Spine 1997;22:895–902.

[32] Dreyfuss P, Tibiletti C, Dreyer SJ. Thoracic zygapophyseal joint pain patterns. A study in normal volunteers. Spine 1994;19:807–11.

[33] Dwyer A, Aprill C, Bogduk N. Cervical zygapophyseal joint pain patterns. I: A study in normal volunteers. Spine 1990;15:453–7.

[34] Dye SF, Vaupel GL, Dye CC. Conscious neurosensory mapping of the internal structures of the human knee without intraarticular anesthesia. Am J Sports Med 1998;26:773–7.

[35] Farrell M, Gibson S, McMeeken J, Helme R. Pain and hyperalgesia in osteoarthritis of the hands. J Rheumatol 2000;27:441–7.

[36] Felson DT. The sources of pain in knee osteoarthritis. Curr Opin Rheumatol 2005;17:624–8.

[37] Felson DT, Naimark A, Anderson J, Kazis L, Castelli W, Meenan RF. The prevalence of knee osteoarthritis in the elderly. The Framingham Osteoarthritis Study. Arthritis Rheum 1987;30:914–8.

[38] Fukui S, Ohseto K, Shiotani M, Ohno K, Karasawa H, Naganuma Y. Distribution of referred pain from the lumbar zygapophyseal joints and dorsal rami. Clin J Pain 1997;13:303–7.

[39] Ge HY, Nie H, Madeleine P, Danneskiold-Samsoe B, Graven-Nielsen T, Arendt-Nielsen L. Contribution of the local and referred pain from active myofascial trigger points in fibromyalgia syndrome. Pain 2009;147:233–40.

[40] Ge HY, Wang Y, Danneskiold-Samsoe B, Graven-Nielsen T, Arendt-Nielsen L. The predetermined sites of examination for tender points in fibromyalgia syndrome are frequently associated with myofascial trigger points. J Pain 2010;11:644–51.

[41] Gerber RK, Nie H, Arendt-Nielsen L, Curatolo M, Graven-Nielsen T. Local pain and spreading hyperalgesia induced by intramuscular injection of nerve growth factor are not reduced by local anesthesia of the muscle. Clin J Pain 2011;27:240–7.

[42] Giamberardino MA. Referred muscle pain/hyperalgesia and central sensitisation. J Rehabil Med 2003;85–8.

[43] Gibson W, Arendt-Nielsen L, Graven-Nielsen T. Referred pain and hyperalgesia in human tendon and muscle belly tissue. Pain 2006;120:113–23.

[44] Giesecke T, Gracely RH, Grant MA, Nachemson A, Petzke F, Williams DA, Clauw DJ. Evidence of augmented central pain processing in idiopathic chronic low back pain. Arthritis Rheum 2004;50:613–23.

[45] Gracely RH. Studies of pain in human subjects. In: McMahon SB, Koltzenburg M, editors. Textbook of pain. Elsevier, Churchill Livingstone; 2006. p. 267–89.

[46] Gracely RH, Petzke F, Wolf JM, Clauw DJ. Functional magnetic resonance imaging evidence of augmented pain processing in fibromyalgia. Arthritis Rheum 2002;46:1333–43.

[47] Graven-Nielsen T. Fundamentals of muscle pain, referred pain, and deep tissue hyperalgesia. Scand J Rheumatol 2006;35(Suppl 122):1–43.

[48] Graven-Nielsen T, Arendt-Nielsen L. Assessment of mechanisms in localized and widespread musculoskeletal pain. Nat Rev Rheumatol 2010;6:599–606.

[49] Graven-Nielsen T, Arendt-Nielsen L, Svensson P, Jensen TS. Quantification of local and referred muscle pain in humans after sequential i.m. injections of hypertonic saline. Pain 1997;69:111–7.

[50] Graven-Nielsen T, Jansson Y, Segerdahl M, Kristensen JD, Mense S, Arendt-Nielsen L. Experimental pain by ischaemic contractions compared with pain by intramuscular infusions of adenosine and hypertonic saline. Eur J Pain 2003;7:93–102.

[51] Graven-Nielsen T, Kendall SA, Henriksson KG, Bengtsson M, Sörensen J, Johnson A, Gerdle B, Arendt-Nielsen L. Ketamine reduces muscle pain, temporal summation, and referred pain in fibromyalgia patients. Pain 2000;85:483–91.

[52] Graven-Nielsen T, Mense S, Arendt-Nielsen L. Painful and non-painful pressure sensations from human skeletal muscle. Exp Brain Res 2004;159:273–83.

[53] Graven-Nielsen T, Wodehouse T, Langford RM, Arendt-Nielsen L, Kidd BL. Normalisation of widespread hyperesthesia and facilitated spatial summation of deep-tissue pain in knee osteoarthritis patients after knee replacement. Arthritis Rheum 2012; in press.

[54] Hill CL, Hunter DJ, Niu J, Clancy M, Guermazi A, Genant H, Gale D, Grainger A, Conaghan P, Felson DT. Synovitis detected on magnetic resonance imaging and its relation to pain and cartilage loss in knee osteoarthritis. Ann Rheum Dis 2007;66:1599–603.

[55] Hoheisel U, Mense S, Simons DG, Yu XM. Appearance of new receptive fields in rat dorsal horn neurons following noxious stimulation of skeletal muscle: a model for referral of muscle pain? Neurosci Lett 1993;153:9–12.

[56] Hoheisel U, Sander B, Mense S. Myositis-induced functional reorganisation of the rat dorsal horn: effects of spinal superfusion with antagonists to neurokinin and glutamate receptors. Pain 1997;69:219–30.

[57] Imamura M, Imamura ST, Kaziyama HH, Targino RA, Hsing WT, de Souza LP, Cutait MM, Fregni F, Camanho GL. Impact of nervous system hyperalgesia on pain, disability, and quality of life in patients with knee osteoarthritis: a controlled analysis. Arthritis Rheum 2008;59:1424–31.

[58] Jensen K, Andersen HØ, Olesen J, Lindblom U. Pressure-pain threshold in human temporal region. Evaluation of a new pressure algometer. Pain 1986;25:313–23.

[59] Jensen KB, Kosek E, Petzke F, Carville S, Fransson P, Marcus H, Williams SC, Choy E, Giesecke T, Mainguy Y, Gracely R, Ingvar M. Evidence of dysfunctional pain inhibition in fibromyalgia reflected in rACC during provoked pain. Pain 2009;144:95–100.

[60] Jespersen A, Dreyer L, Kendall S, Graven-Nielsen T, Arendt-Nielsen L, Bliddal H, Danneskiold-Samsoe B. Computerized cuff pressure algometry: a new method to assess deep-tissue hypersensitivity in fibromyalgia. Pain 2007;131:57–62.

[61] Julien N, Goffaux P, Arsenault P, Marchand S. Widespread pain in fibromyalgia is related to a deficit of endogenous pain inhibition. Pain 2005;114:295–302.

[62] Kellgren JH, Samuel EP. The sensitivity and innervation of the articular capsule. J Bone Joint Surg 1950;4:193–205.

[63] King CD, Wong F, Currie T, Mauderli AP, Fillingim RB, Riley JL III. Deficiency in endogenous modulation of prolonged heat pain in patients with irritable bowel syndrome and temporomandibular disorder. Pain 2009;143:172–8.

[64] Kosek E, Hansson P. Modulatory influence on somatosensory perception from vibration and heterotopic noxious conditioning stimulation (HNCS) in fibromyalgia patients and healthy subjects. Pain 1997;70:41–51.

[65] Kosek E, Ordeberg G. Lack of pressure pain modulation by heterotopic noxious conditioning stimulation in patients with painful osteoarthritis before, but not following, surgical pain relief. Pain 2000;88:69–78.

[66] Laursen RJ, Graven-Nielsen T, Jensen TS, Arendt-Nielsen L. The effect of compression and regional anaesthetic block on referred pain intensity in humans. Pain 1999;80:257–63.

[67] Leffler AS, Kosek E, Lerndal T, Nordmark B, Hansson P. Somatosensory perception and function of diffuse noxious inhibitory controls (DNIC) in patients suffering from rheumatoid arthritis. Eur J Pain 2002;6:161–76.

[68] Lethbridge-Cejku M, Scott WW Jr, Reichle R, Ettinger WH, Zonderman A, Costa P, Plato CC, Tobin JD, Hochberg MC. Association of radiographic features of osteoarthritis of the knee with knee pain: data from the Baltimore Longitudinal Study of Aging. Arthritis Care Res 1995;8:182–8.

[69] Lewis T. Pain. New York: Macmillan; 1942.

[70] Martindale JC, Wilson AW, Reeve AJ, Chessell IP, Headley PM. Chronic secondary hypersensitivity of dorsal horn neurones following inflammation of the knee joint. Pain 2007;133:79–86.

[71] Mense S. Referral of muscle pain. New aspects. APS J 1994;3:1–9.

[72] Mense S, Simons DG. Muscle pain. Understanding its nature, diagnosis, and treatment. Philadelphia: Lippincott Williams & Wilkins; 2001.

[73] Miranda A, Peles S, Rudolph C, Shaker R, Sengupta JN. Altered visceral sensation in response to somatic pain in the rat. Gastroenterology 2004;126:1082–9.

[74] Nie H, Arendt-Nielsen L, Andersen H, Graven-Nielsen T. Temporal summation of pain evoked by mechanical stimulation in deep and superficial tissue. J Pain 2005;6:348–55.

[75] Nie H, Arendt-Nielsen L, Madeleine P, Graven-Nielsen T. Enhanced temporal summation of pressure pain in the trapezius muscle after delayed onset muscle soreness. Exp Brain Res 2006;170:182–90.

[76] Nie H, Madeleine P, Arendt-Nielsen L, Graven-Nielsen T. Temporal summation of pressure pain during muscle hyperalgesia evoked by nerve growth factor and eccentric contractions. Eur J Pain 2009;13:704–10.

[77] O'Neill CW, Kurgansky ME, Derby R, Ryan DP. Disc stimulation and patterns of referred pain. Spine 2002;27:2776–81.

[78] O'Neill S, Graven-Nielsen T, Manniche C, Arendt-Nielsen L. Ultrasound guided, painful electrical stimulation of lumbar facet joint structures: an experimental model of acute low back pain. Pain 2009;144:76–83.

[79] O'Neill S, Manniche C, Graven-Nielsen T, Arendt-Nielsen L. Generalized deep-tissue hyperalgesia in patients with chronic low-back pain. Eur J Pain 2007;11:415–20.

[80] Østergaard M, Szkudlarek M. Magnetic resonance imaging of soft tissue changes in rheumatoid arthritis wrist joints. Semin Musculoskelet Radiol 2001;5:257–74.

[81] Polianskis R, Graven-Nielsen T, Arendt-Nielsen L. Spatial and temporal aspects of deep tissue pain assessed by cuff algometry. Pain 2002;100:19–26.

[82] Sandrini G, Rossi P, Milanov I, Serrao M, Cecchini AP, Nappi G. Abnormal modulatory influence of diffuse noxious inhibitory controls in migraine and chronic tension-type headache patients. Cephalalgia 2006;26:782–9.

[83] Schaible HG. Spinal mechanisms contributing to joint pain. Novartis Found Symp 2004;260:4–22; discussion 22–7, 100–4, 277–9.

[84] Schaible HG, Richter F, Ebersberger A, Boettger MK, Vanegas H, Natura G, Vazquez E, Segond von BG. Joint pain. Exp Brain Res 2009;196:153–62.

[85] Schaible HG, Grubb BD. Afferent and spinal mechanisms of joint pain. Pain 1993;55:5–54.

[86] Schaible HG, Schmidt RF. Activation of groups III and IV sensory units in medial articular nerve by local mechanical stimulation of knee joint. J Neurophysiol 1983;49:35–44.

[87] Schulte H, Graven-Nielsen T, Sollevi A, Jansson Y, Arendt-Nielsen L, Segerdahl M. Pharmacological modulation of experimental phasic and tonic muscle pain by morphine, alfentanil and ketamine in healthy volunteers. Acta Anaesthesiol Scand 2003;47:1020–30.

[88] Sessle BJ, Hu JW, Yu X-M. Brainstem mechanisms of referred pain and hyperalgesia in the orofacial and temporomandibular region. In: Vecchiet L, Albe-Fessard D, Lindblom U, Giamberardino MA, editors. New trends in referred pain and hyperalgesia. Elsevier Science; 1993. p. 59–71.

[89] Siegenthaler A, Eichenberger U, Schmidlin K, Arendt-Nielsen L, Curatolo M. What does local tenderness say about the origin of pain? An investigation of cervical zygapophysial joint pain. Anesth Analg 2010;110:923–7.

[90] Simons DG, Travell JG, Simons L. Myofascial pain and dysfunction. The trigger point manual. Philadelphia: Lippincott Williams & Wilkins; 1999.

[91] Slater H, Arendt-Nielsen L, Wright A, Graven-Nielsen T. Sensory and motor effects of experimental muscle pain in patients with lateral epicondylalgia and controls with delayed onset muscle soreness. Pain 2005;114:118–30.

[92] Sluka KA. Stimulation of deep somatic tissue with capsaicin produces long-lasting mechanical allodynia and heat hypoalgesia that depends on early activation of the cAMP pathway. J Neurosci 2002;22:5687–93.

[93] Sörensen J, Graven-Nielsen T, Henriksson KG, Bengtsson M, Arendt-Nielsen L. Hyperexcitability in fibromyalgia. J Rheumatol 1998;25:152–5.

[94] Srbely JZ, Dickey JP, Bent LR, Lee D, Lowerison M. Capsaicin-induced central sensitization evokes segmental increases in trigger point sensitivity in humans. J Pain 2010;11:636–43.

[95] Staud R, Cannon RC, Mauderli AP, Robinson ME, Price DD, Vierck CJ Jr. Temporal summation of pain from mechanical stimulation of muscle tissue in normal controls and subjects with fibromyalgia syndrome. Pain 2003;102:87–95.

[96] Staud R, Craggs JG, Perlstein WM, Robinson ME, Price DD. Brain activity associated with slow temporal summation of C-fiber evoked pain in fibromyalgia patients and healthy controls. Eur J Pain 2008;12:1078–89.

[97] Thorp LE, Sumner DR, Wimmer MA, Block JA. Relationship between pain and medial knee joint loading in mild radiographic knee osteoarthritis. Arthritis Rheum 2007;57:1254–60.

[98] Turk DC, Melzack R. Handbook of pain assessment. New York: Guilford; 1992.

[99] Vanderweeën L, Oostendorp RA, Vaes P, Duquet W. Pressure algometry in manual therapy. Man Ther 1996;1:258–65.

[100] Vavken P, Dorotka R. The burden of musculoskeletal disease and its determination by urbanicity, socioeconomic status, age, and gender: results from 14,507 subjects. Arthritis Care Res (Hoboken) 2011;63:1558–64.

[101] Wolfe F, Smythe HA, Yunus MB, Bennett RM, Bombardier C, Goldenberg DL, Tugwell P, Campbell SM, Abeles M, Clark P. The American College of Rheumatology 1990 Criteria for the Classification of Fibromyalgia. Report of the Multicenter Criteria Committee. Arthritis Rheum 1990;33:160–72.

[102] Wright A, Graven-Nielsen T, Davies II, Arendt-Nielsen L. Temporal summation of pain from skin, muscle and joint following nociceptive ultrasonic stimulation in humans. Exp Brain Res 2002;144:475–82.

Correspondence to: Thomas Graven-Nielsen, DMSc, PhD, Center for Sensory-Motor Interaction, Department of Health Science and Technology, Faculty of Medicine, Aalborg University, Fredrik Bajers Vej 7D-3, DK-9220 Aalborg E, Denmark. Email: tgn@hst.aau.dk.

Part III

Management Aspects

19

The Multidisciplinary Pain Center: Treating Comorbidities

John D. Loeser

Department of Neurological Surgery, University of Washington, Seattle, Washington, USA

The goal of multidisciplinary pain centers is to rehabilitate patients with chronic pain so that they may lead more normal lifestyles. Although multidisciplinary pain centers have received appropriate recognition for their nomenclature, and the patients referred to these centers for care all share the complaint of chronic pain refractory to routine health care, those of us who treat these patients really do not focus our care on the complaint of pain [5]. Instead, most of our diagnostic and treatment energies are targeted at reducing the comorbidities that almost invariably can be identified in the patient with chronic pain [7,18]. Since the publication of the Melzack-Wall gate hypothesis in 1965, it has been recognized that the brain modulates sensory information, including the perception of pain [13]. Both physical and mental activities play a role in this process, and this is why dealing with comorbidities plays such an important role. What has been learned in the 50 years since the birth of multidisciplinary pain centers is that the complaint of pain almost always decreases as the comorbidities are successfully managed. Indeed, a fundamental difference between a patient with acute pain and a patient with chronic pain is the importance of

Pain Comorbidities: Understanding and Treating the Complex Patient
edited by Maria Adele Giamberardino and Troels Staehelin Jensen
IASP Press, Seattle, © 2012

dealing with the comorbidities, as these are often the major determinants of the persistence of chronic pain complaints and disabilities. It is often counterproductive to focus upon the chronic pain patient's complaint of pain, which commonly leads to the relentless pursuit of a broken part of the body that contains the "pain generator"—something that usually does not exist in the chronic pain patient. It is essential, therefore, to focus treatment programs upon the things that prevent the patient from enjoying a normal lifestyle. "The complaint of pain is an interesting social communication, the meaning of which remains to be determined," was one of Bill Fordyce's important contributions to our understanding of the chronic pain patient. Experience in many multidisciplinary pain centers has been that patients report a 20–40% decrease in pain from the onset of treatment to the end of the program, in spite of the fact that medications have been reduced or eliminated, physical activity has increased, and return to work has occurred [2]. Total elimination of pain is rare, but significant reduction of the impact of the comorbidities is common.

The most frequent comorbidities seen in chronic pain patients include deactivation; depression; sleep disturbance; drug misuse; disability; catastrophizing; misinformation from providers, friends and relatives, and public media; and inappropriate beliefs about the body. Successful rehabilitation of the chronic pain patient must effectively address each comorbidity, and accurate diagnoses of all comorbidities must be obtained at the time of admission to a treatment program [9]. If good responses to the treatment of the comorbidities are seen, it is highly likely that the complaints of pain will diminish. Reflecting common problems with these comorbidities, the goals of multidisciplinary pain management have been stated as:

- Identify and treat unresolved medical issues
- Eliminate inappropriate medications
- Institute desirable medications on a time-contingent basis
- Improve aerobic conditioning, endurance, strength, and flexibility
- Eliminate excessive guarding behaviors that interfere with normal activities
- Improve coping skills and psychological well-being
- Improve quality of sleep
- Alleviate depression

- Assess patient resources and identify vocational and recreational opportunities
- Educate the patient about pain anatomy, physiology, psychology, and discriminating hurt from harm
- Educate the patient about prudent health care consumption
- Assist the patient in establishing reasonable goals and maintaining treatment gains [17].

Almost all multidisciplinary pain centers treat patients in a group format, which is far more efficient from the providers' viewpoint and reduces costs for the patients and their insurance companies. It also takes advantage of the reinforcers present in group activities. Most chronic pain patients enjoy being part of a treatment group and benefit from the interactions with other patients. Treatment programs and their theoretical bases have been described in multiple publications [3,7,10]. It is important to operationalize all aspects of the patient's functioning so that performance can be monitored and treatments tailored to the issues manifested by the patient. One size does not fit all. Multidisciplinary pain centers focus upon the measurement of all types of activities and documentation of changes. We do not pay much attention to what the patient feels; instead we focus upon what the patient does. Behaviors are measurable; feelings are personal and private and are only inferred from what the patient does or says.

Deactivation

Chronic pain patients are usually physically deactivated; they have lost strength, flexibility, and endurance. They often believe that their pain condition precludes exercise and that using their bodies will damage their tissues further. In contrast, no organ system in the body benefits from inactivity [1]. One of the first tasks, therefore, for a treatment program is to teach the patient that "hurt" and "harm" are not synonyms. Using the painful region of the body will not damage it further. Indeed, we have seen over and over again that gradual increases in exercise are associated with reduced pain complaints. Patients are often reluctant to accept this phenomenon; arguing with them is not a prudent course of action, whereas demonstrating this phenomenon with each patient's own physical activity is a better action plan. The use of behavioral medicine principles is essential to improve physical well-being. The primary strategy for accomplishing the goal of increased physical activity begins with asking patients to demonstrate how much of an activity they can do before pain, weakness, or fatigue makes them stop. This strategy can be applied to walking laps, doing sit-ups, or any other repetitive activity that can be quantified by the number of repetitions or the duration of the activity. One then selects a slightly lower level of activity and asks the patient to perform this amount on a twice-daily basis. Each subsequent repetition of the activity is gradually incremented on a daily basis by adding repetitions, duration of activity, or distance traveled. The patient is rewarded for achieving the goal by strong verbal support from the treatment team and peers. The patient should keep a daily log of activity that can be placed on a simple graph that plots both target goals and actual accomplishments. Walking a fixed distance on a timed basis ("speed laps") is an excellent activity to work with, because increasing speed is automatically associated with reduced limping or other pain behaviors. As physical performance increases, more complex activities that simulate the workplace environment can be introduced.

Physical activities include generalized conditioning that is independent of the region of pain and specific exercises that are relevant to the painful area. Such activities are always undertaken on a time, number of repetitions, or distance contingency; stopping is never contingent upon pain. Patients quickly learn that one can do more and hurt less, which contrasts to their commonly held belief that activity will increase their pain. Goals are always set on the basis of past performance, with a planned gradual increase. Once a satisfactory level of activity has been reached, that level is maintained on a daily basis, for we are not interested in pushing performance to Olympian levels. An adequate level of physical conditioning is required to carry out routine daily activities at home or at work, and that level is generally the target for each patient. Patients learn that activity is possible without damaging their bodies or increasing their pain. Disuse, weakness, atrophy of muscle, and loss of bone mass are all comorbidities of being a chronic pain patient, and they must be overcome if a successful outcome is to occur.

Physicians, nurses, and physical and occupational therapists all play a role in addressing the need for increasing the patient's physical activities. Only active physical therapies are utilized; passive modalities may entertain the patient and provide temporary symptom remission, but they do not lead to improvements in physical conditioning. Biofeedback is often a useful treatment strategy, for patients can learn that they are capable of controlling bodily functions and influencing relaxation. Thus, the patient does the work; the health care providers offer education, guidance, and encouragement. Long-term follow-up is always part of the treatment program, because the gains made in treatment can easily be lost if the patient again becomes inactive. The importance of a provider who uses cognitive and behavioral principles to assist patients in achieving their goals cannot be overemphasized [19].

Depression

Depression is almost always a component of the chronic pain patient's dysfunctional status. The degree of depression is quite variable, but profoundly depressed states are not common in this setting. It is unfortunately true that depression is often overlooked by health care providers who are focusing on other symptoms and signs. Depression can be evaluated by interviewing patients and by the use of standardized test instruments, such as the Beck Depression Index or Center for Epidemiologic Studies Depression Scale (CES-D). Every chronic pain patient accepted for multidisciplinary pain management needs to have a careful assessment for depression. If depression is detected, a treatment plan must be developed that addresses this common cause of disability. The development of a physical activity program is often helpful in this respect. Eliminating medications that have a depressant effect can be another useful component of the plan. If the patient is not already on an antidepressant medication, an appropriate drug can be added to the treatment program. If the patient is already on an antidepressant, consideration must be given to altering the dose or drug as appropriate. It must be remembered that it takes many weeks for the effects of an antidepressant to be manifested. Finally, cognitive/behavioral strategies to treat depression should be implemented.

Explanatory models for depression include the loss of social and personal reinforcers because of inactivity or joblessness, or loss of restorative sleep, or the side effects of medications. Psychological strategies are aimed primarily at changing behaviors rather than altering personality. Depression is a comorbidity that interferes with all other aspects of the patient's improvement in functional status, and it must be addressed in any successful treatment plan.

Sleep Disturbance

Many chronic pain patients report nonrestorative sleep and difficulty falling asleep and staying asleep [14]. This problem can, of course, be due to the pain itself, or it can be related to depression or to the side effects of medication. It can also result from inactivity during the daytime so that the patient is not fatigued by bedtime. Addressing depression and physical inactivity as well as removing unbeneficial medications may all contribute to the improvement of sleep. Teaching patients skills for the improvement of sleep hygiene can also be effective. One of the most useful skills to learn is self-hypnosis for inducing sleep [6]. In general, medications intended to facilitate sleep are acceptable for brief durations, but they are rarely useful on a chronic basis. We do not like to rely on medications for sleep, as they do not follow the important principle of making the patient responsible for change.

Drug Misuse

Drug misuse is extremely common in chronic pain patients. Both excessive use of drugs that are not beneficial and failure to utilize drugs that might be helpful are routinely found when an adequate history is obtained. To address this problem, it is essential to obtain an accurate history from the patient, corroborated by significant others, by physician and pharmacy records, and, if any ambiguities remain, by urinalysis. The most common finding in patients referred to a multidisciplinary pain center is the use of multiple opioids, antidepressants, anticonvulsants, anti-inflammatories, and a variety of sedative-hypnotics as well as over-the-counter nostrums. As the patient has been referred because of persistent pain and disability, we can assume that the existing medicinal regimen is a failure and can begin a program to eliminate drugs that are not helping and can even be deleterious. The "pain cocktail technique" is useful for cleaning up opioids and sedative-hypnotics [4]. All opioids are converted to an equivalent dose of methadone, which is given four times a day in 10 cc of a liquid masking vehicle (usually cherry syrup), along with any other drugs that are deemed appropriate. Anticonvulsants can be rapidly tapered. Antidepressants are usually maintained, but dosage, timing, and drug may be altered to get a better effect. Other medications are just discontinued or rapidly tapered. This elimination of non-useful drugs can be accomplished in a week for most patients; opioid tapers may require more time but are readily accomplished at 10% of the existing dose each day. Eliminating polypharmacy often has a dramatic effect upon mood, energy level, and cognition. Of course, if a chronic pain patient has never been exposed to opioids (which is very rare in our experience), a trial of opioids can be initiated prior to implementation of a multidisciplinary approach to pain management. It is important to realize that the prescribing physician is often just as much at fault as the patient when inappropriate drug use is identified.

The use of illicit drugs and excessive alcohol intake are usually contraindications to treating a patient in a multidisciplinary pain program. Cognitive/behavioral strategies as used in a pain management setting are not effective tools for dealing with addiction. Nicotine is also a problem for many chronic pain patients, but focusing on reduction of smoking can take energies away from rehabilitating the chronic pain patient. The issues surrounding opioid prescription for chronic pain patients loom large in the United States at present. Although some patients seem to do well on reasonable doses (below 60 mg of morphine or its equivalent), there is just not sufficient data to answer the question as to whether high-dose opioids are ever indicated for a chronic pain patient. My own experience has been that lower opioid dosages may be beneficial for some patients, but I have never seen a chronic pain patient taking over 100 mg of morphine or its equivalent per day who reported good pain relief. Certainly, the mere fact of referral to a multidisciplinary pain clinic indicates that the patient's pain has not been adequately alleviated by the high dose of opioid, and tapering is appropriate. If an opioid is to be used, a long-acting form is always preferable to a short-acting drug. Careful monitoring of all patients with opioid prescriptions to minimize the risks of drug diversion is always essential.

There are medications that can be helpful for the chronic pain patient. These include antidepressants, anxiolytics, and sleep enhancers, as well as drugs specific to the underlying cause of the pain; for example, anticonvulsants for those with a neuropathic pain problem. However, it must be remembered that one of the goals of multidisciplinary pain management is to place the locus of control within the patient. Reliance on medications tends to have the reverse effect, and there should always be a very good reason to keep the patient on any medication. The exception to this general rule has been antidepressants, which are helpful in many chronic pain patients, because of the ubiquity of depression in those with chronic pain. All medications should be given on a time-contingent basis. Medications taken on a p.r.n. basis ("as needed") are likely to result in increasing drug use. Patients and their families must be fully informed of the goals and risks of long-term drug therapy, especially when opioids are prescribed. It must sometimes be emphasized for the chronic pain patient that there is no legal or moral right to the use of opioids.

Disability

It is impossible to overestimate the importance of work in the life of a normal adult. Work has economic, personal, and social importance to the worker and his or her family. Failure to work can be considered an illness in itself. All too many chronic pain patients have removed themselves or have been removed from the workforce. Successful treatment of chronic pain patients in their working years must include return to work as an essential outcome; otherwise, this can be a major barrier to success. It is not only the absence from work but also the enmeshment in a disability system that so often leads to treatment failure. It is wise to remember that Franz Kafka was a clerk in the worker's compensation bureau in Prague.

A properly designed treatment program for chronic pain patients will establish a relationship between the patient, the workplace, and the disability system. The patient needs to learn the rules of the system and how to relate to the claims manager. A vocational counselor or occupational medicine physician who is skilled in the rules about disability and return to work is a key ingredient in the treatment team. Impediments to return to work need to be characterized, and treatments must be focused upon them. The obligatory paperwork needs to be completed on a timely basis to direct the patient into work status. Rapid return to work has been shown to reduce long-term disability and costs of both care and compensation; therefore, it should be a treatment goal. Unfortunately, patients have often been referred for multidisciplinary pain management after years of disability, thereby making return to work very unlikely. The longer one is on disability, the less likely one is ever to return to work. The things that health care providers do or do not do can have major impact on return to work [12]. Social factors not inherent in the patient may play a large role in the issues of return to work [8]. For example, the availability of jobs is strongly related to economic factors. Some injured workers lack the skills and attitudes that will permit them to be gainfully employed. Nonetheless, return to work is the single most important outcome for the chronic pain patient.

Catastrophizing

Dreaming about the worst things that could happen makes them much more likely and paralyzes the patient's abilities to effectively problem-solve. Pain catastrophizing has been characterized as having at least three maladaptive aspects: magnification of symptoms, rumination on the pain itself, and helplessness to control the symptoms [16]. It has been repeatedly demonstrated that patients who are fixated upon the negative aspects of chronic pain and its comorbidities have a poorer outcome than those who have better adaptation skills. Strategies for reducing catastrophizing have been described, and dealing with this maladaptive trait can improve outcomes. The optimal management of the catastrophizing patient starts with assessment by the Pain Catastrophizing Scale, which uses a 13-item self-report test [15]. Then, a multifaceted approach seems to produce the best results in terms of pain report and disability reduction. Such an approach includes cognitive/behavioral interventions, physical activity, stress reduction, emotional disclosure, reassurance, and encouragement of activities, as well as educational programs designed to increase knowledge about the functions of the body, in general, and the nervous system, more specifically. Reducing disability plays a large role in determining the outcomes in patients with chronic pain.

Misinformation from Advertising and Providers

Many of the problems manifested by chronic pain patients stem from erroneous beliefs about their bodies, disease processes, prognoses, and disability status. Some of the misinformation that leads to such problems comes from the public press, radio and television, and recently, the Internet. Belief in the freedom of communication has permitted the promulgation of advertisements and narratives that are not based upon reality or scientific observations. Advertising obviously works, or companies would not spend so much money producing it. Direct-to-consumer advertising is designed to influence the patient while bypassing the role of the provider in judging the likelihood of the product being successful. Family and friends of the patient are also capable of influencing treatment choices on the basis of the advertising that they have been exposed to. Finally, and most importantly, health care providers are an integral part of the misinformation process. Some of this is accidental, in that the provider has been misinformed by a drug or device manufacturer, and some is deliberate, designed to facilitate the implementation of the type of treatment offered by the provider. Another type of problem in this area is the interpretation of imaging studies; patients can read a report that describes in great detail the abnormalities that can be seen, without any comment on the fact that most people of the patient's age have similar changes without any symptoms. For such comorbidities originating from erroneous beliefs, the educational aspect of multidisciplinary pain management is essential. Patient imaging studies are reviewed, and the meaning of the changes that have been identified is explained to the patient. Topics are discussed in a seminar format to counteract the inappropriate beliefs that adversely affect the patient's well-being. Common topics are illustrated in Table I. An overall goal of the educational aspect of the treatment program is to make the chronic pain patient a more intelligent health care consumer and to place the patient firmly in control of his or her life. This can be a challenge, given the widespread lack of understanding of science and scientific methodology. Patients often lack understanding of how the body works; they can be nonreceptive of a different way of understanding human physiology and psychology. Concepts of how the body works seem to be matters of faith for some chronic pain patients; change may be difficult for them.

Table I
Patient education topics

Pain mechanisms	Depression
Gate theory	Effects of exercise and inactivity
Headaches	Low back pain
Biomechanics	Role of surgery for pain
Drugs: use and abuse	Dealing with doctors
Workers' compensation	Program orientation
Hurt and harm	Maintenance of gains
Acute versus chronic pain	Discharge planning
Healing and disuse	Sleep disorders

Conclusion

Relief of pain is only one aspect of treating a chronic pain patient. Alleviating the comorbidities is also essential for a good outcome. In a patient with acute pain, it is reasonable to expect that the patient will return to normal activities once the injury has healed and the pain has ceased, and this is indeed the outcome for the overwhelming proportion of those who experience an episode of acute pain. In a patient with chronic pain, one cannot expect symptom relief to resolve all of the impediments to a normal lifestyle that have been generated by the comorbidities. Since the health care system has already demonstrated that it is not capable of alleviating the symptom of pain in such patients, multidisciplinary pain centers focus upon reducing the impact of the associated comorbidities. This approach often results in a significant diminution of pain complaints and dramatic improvements in functional activities, including return to work. To reach this endpoint, all aspects of the patient's illness must be assessed, and treatments must be provided that are aimed at the achievement of multiple goals. The successes of such treatment programs have been demonstrated in 30 years of outcomes studies and multiple reviews [2,11]. It has proven impossible to identify the relative importance of each of the components of a treatment program; we believe that the entire process is greater than the sum of its parts. Providers who work together as a team and who express their concerns for the well-being of the patient are critical ingredients in a multidisciplinary pain center. The complaint of pain and its associated comorbidities can be successfully addressed in a multidisciplinary pain center.

References

[1] Bortz WM. The disuse syndrome. West J Med 1984;141:691-694.
[2] Flor H, Fydrich T, Turk DC. Efficacy of multidisciplinary pain treatment centers: a meta-analytic review. Pain 1992;49:221–30.
[3] Fordyce WE. Behavioral methods for chronic pain and illness. St. Louis: Mosby; 1976.
[4] Halpern L. Psychotropic drugs and the management of chronic pain. In: Bonica JJ, editor. Advances in neurology: International Symposium on Pain, Vol. 4. New York: Raven Press; 1974.
[5] International Association for the Study of Pain. Recommendations for pain treatment services. Seattle: IASP; 2009. Available at: www.iasp-pain.org/guidelines/services.
[6] Jensen MP. Hypnosis for chronic pain management: patient workbook. New York: Oxford University Press; 2011.
[7] Loeser J, Egan K. Managing the chronic pain patient: theory and practice at the University of Washington Pain Clinic. New York: Raven Press; 1989.
[8] Loeser JD. Basic consideration of pain: multidisciplinary pain programs. In: Loeser JD, editor. Bonica's management of pain. Philadelphia: Lippincott; 2000. p. 255–64.
[9] Loeser JD. Evaluation of the pain patient: multidisciplinary pain assessment. In: Loeser JD, editor. Bonica's management of pain. Philadelphia: Lippincott; 2000. p. 363–8.
[10] Loeser JD, Fordyce WE. Chronic pain. In: Carr JE, Dengerink HA, editors. Behavioral sciences in the practice of medicine. Amsterdam: Elsevier; 1983. p. 331–45.
[11] Loeser JD, Seres JL, Newman RJ. Interdisciplinary, multimodal management of chronic pain. In: Bonica JJ, editor. The management of pain. Philadelphia: Lee and Febiger; 1990. p. 2107–20.
[12] Loeser JD, Sullivan M. Disability in the chronic pain patient may be iatrogenic. Pain Forum 1995;4:114–21.
[13] Melzack R, Wall PD. Pain mechanisms: a new theory. Science 1965;150:971–9.
[14] Mystakidou K, Clark AJ, Fischer J, Lam A, Pappert K, Richarz U. Treatment of chronic pain by long-acting opioids and the effects on sleep. Pain Pract 2011;11:282–9.
[15] Sullivan M, Bishop S, Pivik J. The pain catastrophizing scale: development and validation. Psychol Assess 1995;7:524–32.
[16] Sullivan MJ, Thorn B, Haythornthwaite JA, Keefe F, Martin M, Bradley LA, Lefebvre JC. Theoretical perspectives on the relation between catastrophizing and pain. Clin J Pain 2001;17:52–64.
[17] Turk DC, Loeser JD. Methods for symptomatic control: multidisciplinary pain management. In: Loeser JD, editor. Bonica's management of pain. Philadelphia: Lippincott; 2000. p. 2069–79.
[18] Waddell G, Aylward M, Sawney P. Back pain, incapacity for work and social security benefits. London: Royal Society Medical Press; 2002.
[19] Wright AR, Gatchel RJ. Occupational musculoskeletal pain and disability. In: Turk DC, Gatchel RJ, editors. Psychological approaches to pain management. New York: Guilford Press; 2002. p. 349–64.

Correspondence to: John D. Loeser, MD, Department of Neurological Surgery, University of Washington 356470, Seattle, WA 98195, USA. Email: jdloeser@u.washington.edu.

Pharmacological Approaches to Pain and Its Comorbidities

20

Lucy A. Bee, Leonor Gonçalves, and Anthony H. Dickenson

*Department of Neuroscience, Physiology and Pharmacology,
University College London, London, United Kingdom*

Patients with pain can present with complaints or symptoms that go beyond what is otherwise expected from their specific pathological process; the term "comorbidities" thus refers to the presence of one or more ailments that align with the pain, either in a concomitant but unrelated fashion, or (and perhaps more commonly) in a related fashion. From the perspective of the physician or scientist, it is important to gain a good understanding of these comorbidities—which can include depression, anxiety, and sleep disorders, for example—to prevent the unnecessary progression of pain that has an identifiable physiological and temporal cause to chronic pain, which can lack both. It is well documented that central sensitization is a feature of many pain states, and thus if the spinal cord (which sends messages to supraspinal areas) is primed by an existing pain state, changes might occur in areas of the brain that are responsible for comorbid symptoms.

Various risk factors for the development of chronic pain have been identified and are highlighted in Table I [49]; these factors are divided into those that have a psychosocial basis, and those that have a medical

Table I
Psychosocial and medical risk factors for the
development of chronic pain

Psychosocial	Medical
Past experiences	Genotype
Beliefs and expectations	Medical history
Anxiety and depression	Intensity
Catastrophizing	Surgery
Social circumstances	Medications/anesthesia

basis. Psychosocial risk factors include comorbidities of pain that have a strong neurobiological basis, such as anxiety and depression, with which the pathways of pain overlap, both anatomically and pharmacologically.

The extent of comorbidities is illustrated by a recent study showing that a fifth of elderly patients with cancer reported co-occurrence of any two and almost a third had co-occurrence of any three of the following symptoms: pain, fatigue, insomnia, and mood disturbance [16]. In addition to this clustering of comorbidities, there can also be different types of pain coexisting in a single patient, such as somatic pain, headache, and visceral pain. Are there links between these types of pain?

A pharmacological approach is key to understanding putative links between pain and comorbidities, since it reveals common pathways and substrates underpinning both; to draw on an example mentioned above, there are many anatomical structures, circuits, and transmitters that are similarly activated or altered in depression and chronic pain. For example, in patients with either or indeed both of these disorders, there is a dysregulated hypothalamo-pituitary-adrenal (HPA) axis that can be normalized with antidepressants [33]. This dysregulation can be predictive as to which individuals among psychologically at-risk patients will develop chronic pain or have poor pain-related outcomes (i.e., elevated pain intensity, functional limitations, and failure to recover) where pain is present already [4].

Monoamines, Pain, and Comorbidities

Depression and pain are also associated with abnormalities in the monoaminergic system [13,82]. The neurotransmitters norepinephrine and serotonin (5-HT) are particularly prevalent in midbrain and brainstem areas, including the periaqueductal grey (PAG), and so these areas are targets for antidepressant action with respect to both complaints. The PAG can be thought of as the depression-pain interface, because it shares affective and sensory information from the limbic forebrain and midbrain structures (including the amygdala, hypothalamus, and neocortex) with brainstem structures, most notably the rostral ventromedial medulla (RVM). The position of the RVM at the base of the brain (close to the pontomedullary junction) ideally allows it to filter inhibitory or excitatory neuronal signals that pass through it down to the spinal cord to alter the level of sensory gain in the dorsal horn. Therefore, nociceptive information synapsing in the spinal cord from the periphery is subjected to supraspinal modulation as a matter of course. Put simply, this feed-forward loop that extends from the spinal cord to the brain, and then back down to the spinal cord again, provides a physical substrate through which "mind" (under the direction of forebrain motivational, cognitive, and affective systems) can influence "matter," or pain [94], and by the same continuum, allows pain to influence the mind. This robust reciprocal interaction goes some way toward explaining why many psychiatric disorders feature pain as part of the illness or can influence chronic pain.

Descending modulation, which includes the capacity of emotions to influence the amplitude of spinal nociceptive responses and reflexes [66], is partly a function of the abovementioned monoamine neurotransmitters, 5-HT and norepinephrine; 5-HT released from brainstem neurons can differentially inhibit or facilitate spinal cord activity according to the type of receptor subtype that it activates. It may therefore inhibit nociception through $5-HT_1$ receptors, or enhance nociception through $5-HT_{2A}$ and $5-HT_3$ receptors, for example [44,70,80]. The location of the receptors is also key to 5-HT's effects, because despite their excitatory cation-gated mechanics, stimulation of spinal $5-HT_3$ receptors has been reported to promote hypoalgesia [20,31]. Given that γ-aminobutyric acid (GABA) receptor antagonists block these inhibitory responses, the underlying antinociceptive mechanism is likely to involve the $5-HT_3$-receptor-mediated release of GABA from inhibitory interneurons. The inhibitory actions of 5-HT in the spinal cord have also been demonstrated in experiments in naive mice, which showed that tramadol, an agent whose actions include blocking the reuptake of released 5-HT [65], engages descending serotonergic neurons to evoke antinociception in various measures of acute pain [96]. Notwithstanding this evidence of inhibitory actions, it is thought that the more enduring effects of enhanced serotonergic output from the brainstem (i.e., those that would prevail during chronic pain) are spinal facilitations. This line of reasoning adds a time-dependent element to 5-HT's spinal actions, which may be indicative of developing plasticity in the brainstem [12].

Diffuse Pain States

With respect to clinical modulation of the serotonergic system in pain relief, 5-HT$_{1B/1D}$ receptor agonists are used to relieve migraine [32], whereas antidepressants, which variably modulate norepinephrine and 5-HT activity in the central nervous system (CNS), are used in the mainline treatment of neuropathic pain [28]. Furthermore, 5-HT$_3$-receptor modulators have been used in clinical trials to treat irritable bowel syndrome (IBS) [77], a functional disorder that is partly characterized by chronic abdominal pain [85], but of course includes affective changes too. These agents, which include alosetron and cilansetron, reduce visceral pain in patients with IBS, yet alosetron also decreases activity in various limbic structures in response to colorectal distension, which may be integral to its analgesic efficacy [51]. This finding is noteworthy because abnormal supraspinal activity may partly explain some diffuse pain states, including IBS and fibromyalgia syndrome (FMS), a disorder associated with tenderness and pain in all quadrants of the body [95], with excessive tenderness on pressure application in at least 11 out of 18 specific muscle-tendon sites. Patients with FMS commonly experience depression, sleep problems, and fatigue. The signs and symptoms of FMS do not relate to any apparent peripheral pathology; instead, the pathogenesis is thought to be centrally based. Several features of the presentation and treatment of FMS support this supposition: widespread allodynia is symmetrically distributed to the rostrocaudal axis, and patients have a high level of temporal summation of responses to repetitive thermal stimulation, which suggests that central sensitization is at play [78]. Moreover, central disruptions in FMS are indicated by elevated levels of substance P (a nociceptive neurotransmitter) in the cerebrospinal fluid of affected patients, in addition to altered

5-HT metabolism [91]. The alterations in 5-HT in particular may underlie the rationale for using tricyclic antidepressants (TCAs) to relieve painful symptoms of FMS [18], and this practice may unwittingly reflect the current understanding of this disorder as a dynamic and individualized interplay of biological and psychological factors that additionally involves mood disturbances and sleep problems [79].

The three main mechanisms of sensitization (in peripheral, spinal cord, and brain areas) act in parallel and allow "bottom-up" and "top-down" modulation. Peripheral sensitization is accompanied by signs of inflammation and is localized to anatomical areas of tissue related to the peripheral damage. In the absence of a clear peripheral process, the spinal and supraspinal mechanisms can still be active, as has been shown in animals and in a human study of opioid-induced hyperalgesia. Thus, in FMS, abnormal brain processing could potentially drive diffuse descending facilitations of spinal circuits, producing a diffuse pain state in the absence of peripheral pathology. Normal pain modulation as a process is widely recognized to be mediated by 5-HT and norepinephrine, the very transmitters involved in the descending systems from brain to spinal cord. These pathways are nonsegmental, diffuse, and bilateral and so would not be anatomically focused; they could thus produce a widespread pain syndrome. A shift from modulation to facilitation would enhance weak sensory inputs and ultimately result in sensitization. A study that used spinal nociceptive flexion reflex responses as an objective measure of spinal nociception suggests a state of central sensory hyperexcitability in patients with FMS [2]. Since, as discussed, there is an overlap between areas and transmitters implicated in pain, sleep, mood, and fear, the coexistence of these problems in FMS patients suggests that pathophysiological abnormalities in these systems could not only alter affective function and sleep, but also change descending pathways, and may explain why patients with FMS have increased sensitization to painful stimuli and diffuse pain.

Visceral Pain

Irritable bowel syndrome is a functional gastrointestinal disorder that is characterized by abdominal pain, discomfort, and altered bowel habits, with an estimated prevalence in the general population of 10–15%.

There are important negative impacts on quality of life, with psychological distress, disturbance of work and sleep, and sexual dysfunction being common in this disorder [42]. In general, visceral pain typically presents as a vague, diffuse, and poorly defined sensation usually perceived in the midline of the body at the level of the lower sternum or upper abdomen, regardless of the visceral structure forming the origin of pain. This presentation is due to a low density of sensory innervation of the viscera compared to somatic areas and extensive divergence of visceral input within the CNS. Visceral pain is therefore perceived more diffusely than noxious cutaneous stimulation with respect to location and timing [61].

Spatial discrimination of visceral pain is therefore typically referred to superficial structures (a distant cutaneous or musculoskeletal site). Secondary hyperalgesia of superficial or deep body wall tissues often occurs because of viscerosomatic convergence, which refers to the neurophysiological convergence of visceral and somatic afferent inputs to the CNS. This situation is thought to underlie the basis of phenomena such as referred visceral pain, where noxious stimulation of viscera triggers pain referred to somatic sites, which is generally attributed to viscerosomatic convergence at the level of the spinal cord [15]. Thus one could imagine that any central changes, including central sensitization arising from a somatic inflammatory or neuropathic condition, could produce a latent visceral hyperalgesia because of this convergence. It is already established that it is difficult to differentiate visceral pain from pain arising in somatic structures.

The "brain-gut axis" is a theoretical model describing the manifestation of different pathologies leading to visceral pain [52]. It entails bidirectional neural pathways linking cognitive, emotional, and autonomic centers in the brain to neuroendocrine centers, the enteric nervous system, and the immune system. Thus, the overlap with somatic processing continues, and any central changes in limbic brain areas could alter both cutaneous and visceral events.

The activity of visceral organs and their autonomic regulations are not normally influenced by higher centers of the CNS and are not perceived as conscious sensations except in pathophysiological conditions. Many visceral signals are relayed to the parabrachial area, and the ensuing projections of this nucleus to limbic and cognitive higher centers are thought to be involved in autonomic and emotional (including aversive) reactions to painful stimuli [9]. Several studies have demonstrated that the parabrachial area plays a primary role in the flow of visceral information to the forebrain and cortex, as well as to the autonomic and limbic centers of the hypothalamus and amygdala, respectively [14].

Descending modulation from the RVM has also been described in models of acute visceral pain. Electrical stimulation of the RVM produces biphasic modulation of spinal neuronal responses to colorectal distension [98,99], as it does with cutaneous events. Low doses of neurotensin administered to the RVM facilitate, whereas higher doses inhibit, acute visceral reflexes [90], and N-methyl-D-aspartate (NMDA) antagonists injected in the RVM block facilitation of visceral reflexes, whereas non-NMDA antagonists injected in the RVM block descending inhibition [19]. In a chronic model of visceral pain such as pancreatitis in the rat, selective ablation of RVM cells prevented the maintenance, but not expression, of pancreatitis-associated abdominal hypersensitivity. Therefore, the RVM may play an important role in mediating central plasticity to maintain chronic visceral pain [93].

Moreover, functional magnetic resonance imaging (fMRI) studies illustrate how subliminal visceral stimulation in humans leads to cortical activation [45]. Cortical and subcortical circuitry can modulate pain in brainstem centers such as the RVM and PAG in a top-down fashion, and this central control of nociception can either increase or decrease both the intensity and affective components of the pain experience [5,53]. Further studies have also demonstrated that visceral stimulation activates brainstem structures, some of which, like the PAG and RVM, are neural areas altered by evoked somatic pain [26]. This overlap of visceral and somatic processing may explain the coexistence of somatic and visceral pains. There is also a considerable preclinical series of studies pointing to a pronociceptive role of descending 5-HT$_3$-receptor-mediated processes, and there are positive clinical data on analgesia resulting from the use of antagonists at this receptor. Furthermore, a recent human imaging study revealed an attenuation of experimental visceral pain by pregabalin acting through subcortical mechanisms [55]. This finding agrees very well with animal data showing a reduction in both spinal and RVM neuronal activity by the same drug on visceral responses [73]. But, importantly, the three classes of neurons within the RVM, on-cells, off-cells, and neutral cells, as determined by somatic stimuli, do not display the same responses when visceral stimuli are applied, suggesting a complex interplay between descending controls and somatic and visceral pain.

Sleep, Endogenous Pain Modulation, and Mood

Individuals with primary insomnia have recently been tested for their pain responses [36]. During testing, they had lower thresholds than healthy controls for heat and pressure pain detection. Surprisingly, temporal summation of pain responses was reduced in insomnia subjects when compared to healthy controls. The authors propose that pain-inhibitory circuits in persons with insomnia are fully active in an ongoing fashion in an attempt to control subclinical pain. When challenged, this system cannot further increase its activity.

The contribution of antidepressants to chronic pain pharmacotherapy is clear from clinical studies, clinical experience, and meta-analyses of published data, where the "number needed to treat" for these drugs with respect to pain is approximately 1–4 [28,74]. The initial use of antidepressants for the treatment of pain was based not on any clear mechanistic rationale, but rather on the pragmatic recognition that depression is a treatable comorbidity in many pain states. However, it then became clear that antidepressants confer analgesic efficacy in the absence of depressive symptoms, with the necessary doses and time-courses required to achieve efficacy in each setting often differing. Topping the antidepressant efficacy table are the TCAs, followed by serotonin and norepinephrine reuptake inhibitors (SNRIs), with selective serotonin reuptake inhibitors (SSRIs) lagging behind. Indeed, with respect to SSRIs, studies have questioned their capacity to relieve pain [50], with equivocal responses being described as "moderate" at best and "clinically insufficient" [69,75]. The apparent analgesic superiority of SNRIs over SSRIs is likely to be a function of norepinephrine's inhibitory actions in many pain states. Ordinarily, this inhibition is mediated through spinal α_{2A}-adrenoceptors that are expressed on the central terminals of C fibers, and also through α_{2C}-adrenoceptors expressed on the axons of spinal projection neurons. However, in neuropathic pain, this inhibition is downregulated in conjunction with the upregulated activity of 5-HT acting at spinal 5-HT$_3$ receptors [62,63]. Thus, increasing the synaptic availability of norepinephrine in the spinal cord by preventing its reuptake could be key to the effectiveness of antidepressants, above and beyond any manipulation of 5-HT activity. Accordingly, the antihyperalgesic action of the SNRI milnacipran in neuropathic mice is principally mediated by activation of the spinal noradrenergic system, since its actions are lost after noradrenergic denervation but not after serotonergic denervation [83]. Taken together with the pronociceptive actions of 5-HT in chronic pain, this evidence provides a strong argument in favor of separating the noradrenergic reuptake inhibitory actions of antidepressants from their serotonergic effects. This ideology is reflected in the actions of tapentadol, a novel analgesic agent that enhances central inhibitions by activating mu-opioid receptors and preventing the reuptake of released norepinephrine [7].

Tapentadol's actions represent a move toward mimicking descending inhibitions in analgesia, and indeed the analgesic capacity of opioids and gabapentinoid drugs has been suggested to be partly the result of engaging these inhibitions [39]. Furthermore, the importance of descending inhibitory output in determining the propensity for the development of chronic pain has recently been demonstrated in rodents. The investigators demonstrated that inhibitory neurons projecting from the RVM to the spinal cord, in addition to providing a descending noradrenergic inhibitory output, protect against spontaneous and mechanically evoked pain. They concluded that a key component of this protection is an α_2-adrenoceptor-mediated inhibition [21]. In humans too, a type of endogenous modulation known as diffuse noxious inhibitory control (DNIC) has been described, whereby noxious stimuli activate inhibitory controls to sharpen the contrast between the stimulus zone and adjacent areas, having a net enhancing effect on the perceived intensity of the painful stimulus, and an analgesic effect in other areas [24]. Reduced DNIC is thought to be a factor in a number of pain states including FMS, chronic tension-type headache, and osteoarthritis and may possibly be predictive of subsequent pain problems [92]. Interestingly, reduced DNIC has also been noted in patients who have IBS, and these same individuals have greater comorbid presentations such as anxiety, depression, and catastrophizing relative to controls [41]. Therefore, agents that activate spinal inhibitions, such as the α_2-adrenoceptor agonist clonidine, TCAs, SNRIs, or indeed tapentadol, may theoretically protect against pain chronicity and comorbidities [23].

Shared Mechanisms, Shared Treatments?

Shared pathophysiological mechanisms are often indicated by shared treatments, as has been demonstrated for pain and depression, which both respond to antidepressants in an independent, yet also interdependent way—if an agent alleviates pain, it may have a corollary effect of lifting depression, and vice versa. Similarities in disease processes are also evident when one compares epilepsy and neuropathic pain. Although the two conditions are not comorbidly linked, a key and common feature of both is deregulated ion channel activity in neurons, hence both can be managed by drugs that block voltage-gated sodium or calcium channels, such as lamotrigine, carbamazepine, lacosamide, gabapentin, and pregabalin. There is also a growing body of genetic, molecular, physiological, and pharmacological evidence heralding the potential of voltage-gated potassium channels as novel targets in pain and epilepsy management [57,86]. In contrast to voltage-gated sodium channels, potassium channels act as brakes in the nervous system, repolarizing active neurons back to their resting states. This process reduces electrical excitability and therefore the likelihood of inappropriate or excessive neuronal firing such as that which often happens during epileptic episodes or neuropathic pain.

Interestingly, there seems to be some specificity between the mode of action of anticonvulsants and their efficacy in different types of pain. For example, carbamazepine, lamotrigine, and phenytoin reduce neuronal hyperexcitability associated with seizures by blocking sodium channels [76]; these drugs are effective in the treatment of trigeminal neuralgia. On the other hand, gabapentin and pregabalin are mostly effective in postherpetic neuralgia and painful diabetic neuropathy.

To precisely illustrate how knowledge of shared mechanisms can be instructive for the understanding and treatment of different pathophysiologies, we will focus on the example of gabapentin, an antiepileptic agent that was shown by serendipitous discovery to have efficacy in neuropathic pain [71]. Gabapentin, and also pregabalin, binds to the $\alpha_2\delta$ subunit of voltage-gated calcium channels to impede the trafficking of these subunits from inside the cell, where they are made, to the cell membrane, where they are assembled into channels [40]. Thus, Ca^{2+} ions do not enter the neuron as readily, which limits neurotransmitter release from, and synaptic transmission of, targeted (excitable) neurons, where turnover of voltage-gated calcium channels would otherwise be high. This may be the rationale behind the application of gabapentin for tinnitus (the perception of sound in the absence of acoustic stimulation) [6]. Tinnitus may be thought of as a phantom auditory phenomenon, or even an auditory "pain." As such, it too is associated with comorbidities that include anxiety, depression, and insomnia, and as with pain, there is a dichotomy of coexisting positive ("sensory gain") and negative ("sensory loss") symptoms because tinnitus often accompanies hearing loss within an aging population [3]. Tinnitus can often be traced to a peripheral nervous system lesion, most commonly a result of a sensitizing signal ("noise") that is maintained by neuroplastic changes, facilitatory drive, and loss of inhibition, yet like pain, it may exist idiopathically in the absence of any apparent pathology [10]. In both cases, there is a range of responsivity, since similar levels of tinnitus may be described as intolerable by one patient, yet barely noticeable by another. Together with the knowledge that gabapentin is not uniformly efficacious in an otherwise heterogenous population of people with tinnitus (just as in the neuropathic pain population), this range of responsivity suggests that there is a supraspinal (cognitive/affective) component to the pathology, which may contribute to comorbidities. Accordingly, limbic and auditory signals are thought to interact in the thalamus, which enables noise-sensitizing signals to be ordinarily tuned out by feedback connections from limbic neurons [64]. Thus, variations in limbic activity may alter this level of inhibition, giving rise to a spectrum of tinnitus responses following the same inciting injury, and may furthermore account for the comorbidities associated with this disorder.

Gabapentin may also be of benefit in the treatment of nausea associated with chemotherapy, pregnancy, and cholecystectomy [35]. This possible indication is interesting, given the involvement of the serotonergic system (particularly 5-HT_3 receptors) in emesis (as typified by ondansetron's antiemetic application), as well as in gabapentin's inhibitory actions in neuropathic pain [81]. Furthermore, as with pain and depression, altered central serotonergic activity can lead to disturbances in the gastrointestinal (GI) tract, resetting the threshold of various receptors (for example mechanoreceptors). As a result, normally innocuous stimuli such as gut distension, food in the stomach, or nutrients in the small intestine, can trigger abnormal afferent input analogous to that conveyed by nociceptive fibers during ongoing pain, leading to altered GI function and distortion of GI perception. The GI, pain, and affective systems seem to form a triad to the extent that a disturbance in one can have a bearing on the others, with stress and psychological factors able to trigger a range of dyspeptic symptoms that include pain and loss of appetite [17].

Gabapentin may also confer an anxiolytic effect [27], and research into its therapeutic application as a controller of mood and emotional processing is ongoing [56,68]. Less is known about the circuits, structures, and transmitters that overlap in pain and anxiety (relative to those that are known to link depression and pain). However, it is well documented that anticipation of a painful stimulus can produce a state of anxiety that will increase the perception of pain in a feed-forward manner in humans [60] and in rodents [67,68]. Functional MRI studies have looked at attentional modulation of pain and the contribution of anticipation and anxiety to pain perception; investigators have shown, for example, that pain-related activation in the entorhinal cortex increases with expectation-induced anticipatory anxiety of a highly painful stimulus [59]. More recently, fMRI studies have demonstrated the role of the midbrain and brainstem in nociceptive processing [89]. Following this seminal work, numerous studies have highlighted activity in specific areas that are consistent with the PAG, the nucleus cuneiformis, the ventral tegmentum area, and the parabrachial area during the processing of different types of pain, central sensitization, and anxiety [25,97]. In particular, cold allodynia has been shown to produce a pattern of activity that is similar (in terms of intensity and location) to that of cold pain, yet it additionally recruits neural activity in limbic areas [72]. Together with diffusion tractography work that has confirmed anatomical pathways that mediate top-down control of spinal sensory activity in humans [37], this work provides a clear picture of the midbrain and brainstem correlates of pain perception and anxiety, and delineates a clear anatomical route for brain-directed control of nociceptive processing.

Higher Brain Processing of Pain

The brain's ability to influence pain is the principle that underlies the placebo effect, which in this context refers to the capacity of an inert substance to produce analgesia. The success of placebo crucially depends on the subject's conscious perception of the "therapeutic intervention" that is being administered; hence, improvement in pain outcomes is attributed to expectation of relief. Imaging studies have identified common neural mechanisms shared by placebo analgesia and opioid analgesia, and activity in these areas can be suppressed in both circumstances by naloxone [8]. Furthermore, tests and imaging studies have shown that the analgesic placebo effect is partly mediated by descending systems that use endogenous opioids as neuromodulators [58], and covariant activity between different brainstem areas during placebo analgesia further emphasizes the role of the descending system in pain control.

The emotional component of pain has a key role in its protective function. The fact that pain is unpleasant for most people makes us not want to feel it again and therefore avoid its cause. This only happens because the circuit that processes and modulates pain is cleverly designed and includes the areas of the brain that are mainly responsible for emotions, especially unpleasant ones. These brain areas, including the thalamus, amygdala, anterior cingulate cortex (ACC), and insular cortex (IC), have their own specific functions, regardless of the presence or absence of pain.

In normal conditions, some of the functions of the thalamus include regulating sleep, consciousness, and appetite, as well as working as a relay between subcortical areas and the cerebral cortex. Pathologically, when a stroke happens in the thalamus, it results in thalamic syndrome, or central pain, characterized by steady burning or sharp pain, mood swings, and worsening of pain with touch, movement, and emotions. Although central pain does not respond to conventional pain medication, TCAs and anticonvulsants such as gabapentin can provide some relief. Notably, thalamic volumes are increased in patients with obsessive-compulsive disorder (OCD), but decrease to normal levels following treatment with the SSRI antidepressant paroxetine [30].

The ACC has a prominent role in cognitive functions such as error detection, attention, motivation, and modulation of emotional responses.

Additionally, the ACC, especially its rostral part (rACC), is involved in avoidance behavior, the process of learning to avoid noxious stimulation. Lesions to the ACC result in symptoms such as apathy, lack of attention, dysregulation of autonomic functions, emotional instability, and blockage of the aversive aspects of pain resulting from peripheral nerve injury. Curiously, although the rACC has a high density of mu-opioid receptors, and is activated during placebo analgesia [58], its activity is also increased in neuropathic pain patients. Although this finding might seem contradictory, it is in agreement with the idea that control of the ACC can reduce pain intensity and unpleasantness [22] by activating descending mechanisms of pain control. Incidentally, patients with major depressive disorder (MDD) and bipolar disorder have shown abnormal reductions of the amount of gray matter in the ACC, which cannot be reversed by antidepressants [46].

The amygdala, classically known for its role in fear, has a key function in assessing the emotional significance of sensory stimuli, in emotional learning and memory, and in anxiety, depression, and stress responses. Information enters the amygdala mainly through its basolateral and lateral nuclei, which in turn project to the central nucleus, the major output of information from the amygdala. The central nucleus of the amygdala also receives input from prefrontal, insular, temporal and olfactory cortices, from brainstem viscero-sensory and nociceptive centers, and from parts of the caudal thalamus that transmit auditory and somatosensory information [84]. Central nucleus projection fibers containing mainly glutamate are directed to different brain regions, such as the PAG, the lateral hypothalamus, the paraventricular nucleus of the hypothalamus, and several monoaminergic nuclei that are important for fear and anxiety-like behavioral responses. The basolateral nucleus, specifically, modulates memory consolidation by interacting with brain areas such as the hippocampus, entorhinal cortex, medial prefrontal cortex, insular cortex, and nucleus accumbens.

Direct stimulation of the amygdala in awake healthy humans results in complex sensory and emotional states, including fear, anxiety, and hallucinations. Klüver-Bucy syndrome occurs when there are lesions or malfunctions of both the left and right halves of the amygdala [48]. Klüver-Bucy patients develop visual agnosia (loss of ability to recognize common objects), loss of fear, hyperorality, hypersexuality, and inability to acknowledge threats. Lesions or inactivation of the amygdala can also decrease emotional pain reactions.

Nociceptive information reaches the amygdala through the spino-parabrachio-amygdaloid pain pathway, which originates from lamina I neurons in the spinal cord, and through the caudal trigeminal nucleus, which provides nociceptive input to the central nucleus of the amygdala (which also receives nociceptive information from thalamic and cortical areas through connections with the lateral and basolateral nuclei of the amygdala) [11]. The content of nociceptive neurons in the laterocapsular part of the central nucleus is so high that this nucleus is now called the "nociceptive amygdala" [54]. The central nucleus projects to several brainstem centers such as the PAG, the RVM, and the nucleus of the solitary tract, which modulate pain through descending projections to the spinal dorsal horn.

Although the normal fear reaction elicited by the amygdala is healthy and physiologically important, if the fear or anxiety reaction is prolonged for a long time, the amygdala changes, and will overreact to normal situations, eliciting high levels of anxiety. This overreaction occurs in anxiety disorders such as generalized anxiety disorder, panic disorder, social anxiety disorder, post-traumatic stress disorder, and OCD. Different anxiety disorders have in common enhanced activity not only in the amygdala, but also in the hippocampus, thalamus, and cingulate cortex.

Patients with depressive disorders [29], temporal lobe epilepsy [88], or bipolar disorder [1] may present with increased amygdala volume. Curiously, neuronal excitability of neurons of the central nucleus of the amygdala is greater in models of arthritic [38], visceral [87] and neuropathic pain [43], and a higher number of central nucleus neurons is associated with depressive-like behaviors in neuropathic pain [34].

It is to be expected that if one brain area has two functions, then if one of them is affected, the other area will also probably be affected. In the same way, when a drug is administered to improve a condition in function one, function two will probably also be altered. Although pregabalin is an anticonvulsant, and therefore effective in treating epileptic seizures, it is also one of the most successful drugs in the treatment of neuropathic pain, and it has also been used in the treatment of bipolar disorder. Although different anticonvulsants act in different ways (changing the activity of voltage-gated ion channels, enhancing the effect of GABA, or inhibiting the effect of glutamate [47]), the aim of all of them is to suppress rapid and excessive firing of neurons that may start a seizure; neuropathic pain and bipolar disorder are also associated with increased activation of the amygdala.

As mentioned previously, paroxetine improves OCD symptoms at the same time that it decreases thalamic volumes to healthy ones. Additionally, social phobia responds to the antidepressant trazodone, a serotonin antagonist and reuptake inhibitor. Trazodone seems to cause decreased blood flow to the ventral and dorsal anterior cingulate cortex and prefrontal cortex, along with increased cerebral blood flow to the middle cingulate cortex, left hippocampus, and parahippocampal gyrus. The SNRI antidepressant venlafaxine seems to decrease amygdala activity while increasing activity in the ACC. Essentially, drugs traditionally described as antidepressants are effective in treating anxiety (trazodone) and neuropathy (venlafaxine), and they result in changes in brain areas that are involved in depression and pain.

Final Comments

Understanding the circuits and pharmacology that link pain with its co-morbidities and appreciating their shared pathophysiologies and similar "signatures" should promote cross-fertilization between researchers from different fields, advancing the treatment of pain and other disorders. Here we return to two recent examples, one in patients and one in preclinical models; in the first case, patients with insomnia have an enhanced pain sensitivity that appears to be held in check by descending inhibitory controls [36]. As previously discussed, these same inhibitions (DNIC) can fail in a number of pain conditions. However, in studies of animals with neuropathy, descending inhibitory controls can protect against pain [21]. The sharing of mechanistic knowledge has been successfully demonstrated with respect to epilepsy and pain and also depression and pain. There are many further examples of the similar pathophysiologies and mechanisms that link pain with other disorders—anxiety, cough, itch, and tinnitus to name just a few—where understanding of one could prove instructive for understanding and ultimately treating the other.

Acknowledgments

The authors were funded by the Biotechnology and Biological Sciences Research Council and by the Wellcome Trust London Pain Consortium.

References

[1]   Altshuler LL, Bartzokis G, Grieder T, Curran J, Mintz J. Amygdala enlargement in bipolar disorder and hippocampal reduction in schizophrenia: an MRI study demonstrating neuroanatomic specificity. Arch Gen Psychiatry 1998;55:663–4.
[2]   Ang DC, Chakr R, France CR, Mazzuca SA, Stump TE, Hilligoss J, Lengerich A. Association of nociceptive responsivity with clinical pain and the moderating effect of depression. J Pain 2011;1:384–9.
[3]   Baigi A, Oden A, Almlid-Larsen V, Barrenas ML, Holgers KM. Tinnitus in the general population with a focus on noise and stress: a public health study. Ear Hear 2011;32:787–9.
[4]   Bair MJ, Robinson RL, Katon W, Kroenke K. Depression and pain comorbidity: a literature review. Arch Intern Med 2003;163:2433–45.
[5]   Bantick SJ, Wise RG, Ploghaus A, Clare S, Smith SM, Tracey I. Imaging how attention modulates pain in humans using functional MRI. Brain 2002;125(Pt 2):310–9.
[6]   Bauer CA, Brozoski TJ. Effect of gabapentin on the sensation and impact of tinnitus. Laryngoscope 2006;116:675–81.
[7]   Bee LA, Bannister K, Rahman W, Dickenson AH. Mu-opioid and noradrenergic alpha(2)-adrenoceptor contributions to the effects of tapentadol on spinal electrophysiological measures of nociception in nerve-injured rats. Pain 2011;152:131–9.
[8]   Benedetti F, Amanzio M, Baldi S, Casadio C, Maggi G. Inducing placebo respiratory depressant responses in humans via opioid receptors. Eur J Neurosci 1999;11:625–31.
[9]   Bester H, Menendez L, Besson JM, Bernard JF. Spino (trigemino) parabrachiohypothalamic pathway: electrophysiological evidence for an involvement in pain processes. J Neurophysiol 1995;73:568–85.
[10] Billue JS. Subjective idiopathic tinnitus. Clin Excell Nurse Pract 1998;2:73–82.
[11] Bourgeais L, Gauriau C, Bernard JF. Projections from the nociceptive area of the central nucleus of the amygdala to the forebrain: a PHA-L study in the rat. Eur J Neurosci 2001;14:229–55.
[12] Burgess SE, Gardell LR, Ossipov MH, Malan TP Jr, Vanderah TW, Lai J, Porreca F. Time-dependent facilitation from the rostral ventromedial medulla maintains, but does not initiate, neuropathic pain. J Neurosci 2002;22:5129–36.
[13] Burke NN, Hayes E, Calpin P, Kerr DM, Moriarty O, Finn DP, Roche M. Enhanced nociceptive responding in two rat models of depression is associated with alterations in monoamine levels in discrete brain regions. Neuroscience 2010;171:1300–13.
[14] Cechetto CD. Supraspinal mechanisms. In: Gebhart GF, editor. Visceral pain. Progress in pain research and management, Vol. 5. Seattle: IASP Press; 1995. p. 261–90.
[15] Cervero F. Somatic and visceral inputs to the thoracic spinal cord of the cat: effects of noxious stimulation of the biliary system. J Physiol 1983;337:51–67.
[16] Cheng KK, Lee DT. Effects of pain, fatigue, insomnia, and mood disturbance on functional status and quality of life of elderly patients with cancer. Crit Rev Oncol Hematol 2011;78:127–37.
[17] Chua AS, Keeling PW, Dinan TG. Role of cholecystokinin and central serotonergic receptors in functional dyspepsia. World J Gastroenterol 2006;12:1329–35.
[18] Clauw DJ, Crofford LJ. Chronic widespread pain and fibromyalgia: what we know, and what we need to know. Best Pract Res Clin Rheumatol 2003;17:685–701.
[19] Coutinho SV, Urban MO, Gebhart GF. Role of glutamate receptors and nitric oxide in the rostral ventromedial medulla in visceral hyperalgesia. Pain 1998;78:59–69.
[20] Crisp T, Stafinsky JL, Spanos LJ, Uram M, Perni VC, Donepudi HB. Analgesic effects of serotonin and receptor-selective serotonin agonists in the rat spinal cord. Gen Pharmacol 1991;22:247–51.

[21] De Felice M, Sanoja R, Wang R, Vera-Portocarrero L, Oyarzo J, King T, Ossipov MH, Vanderah TW, Lai J, Dussor GO, Fields HL, Price TJ, Porreca F. Engagement of descending inhibition from the rostral ventromedial medulla protects against chronic neuropathic pain. Pain 2011;152:2701–9.

[22] deCharms RC, Maeda F, Glover GH, Ludlow D, Pauly JM, Soneji D, Gabrieli JD, Mackey SC. Control over brain activation and pain learned by using real-time functional MRI. Proc Natl Acad Sci USA 2005;102:18626–31.

[23] Dickenson AH, Baron R. Descending controls: insurance against pain? Pain 2011;152:2677–8.

[24] Dickenson AH, Rivot JP, Chaouch A, Besson JM, Le Bars D. Diffuse noxious inhibitory controls (DNIC) in the rat with or without pCPA pretreatment. Brain Res 1981;216:313–21.

[25] Dunckley P, Aziz Q, Wise RG, Brooks J, Tracey I, Chang L. Attentional modulation of visceral and somatic pain. Neurogastroenterol Motil 2007;19:569–77.

[26] Dunckley P, Wise RG, Fairhurst M, Hobden P, Aziz Q, Chang L, Tracey I. A comparison of visceral and somatic pain processing in the human brainstem using functional magnetic resonance imaging. J Neurosci 2005;25:7333–41.

[27] Field MJ, Oles RJ, Singh L. Pregabalin may represent a novel class of anxiolytic agents with a broad spectrum of activity. Br J Pharmacol 2001;132:1–4.

[28] Finnerup NB, Sindrup SH, Jensen TS. The evidence for pharmacological treatment of neuropathic pain. Pain 2010;150:573–81.

[29] Frodl T, Meisenzahl EM, Zetzsche T, Born C, Jager M, Groll C, Bottlender R, Leinsinger G, Moller HJ. Larger amygdala volumes in first depressive episode as compared to recurrent major depression and healthy control subjects. Biol Psychiatry 2003;53:338–44.

[30] Gilbert AR, Moore GJ, Keshavan MS, Paulson LA, Narula V, Mac Master FP, Stewart CM, Rosenberg DR. Decrease in thalamic volumes of pediatric patients with obsessive-compulsive disorder who are taking paroxetine. Arch Gen Psychiatry 2000;57:449–56.

[31] Glaum SR, Proudfit HK, Anderson EG. 5-HT3 receptors modulate spinal nociceptive reflexes. Brain Res 1990;510:12–6.

[32] Goadsby PJ. Serotonin receptors and the acute attack of migraine. Clin Neurosci 1998;5:18–23.

[33] Gold PW, Licinio J, Wong ML, Chrousos GP. Corticotropin releasing hormone in the pathophysiology of melancholic and atypical depression and in the mechanism of action of antidepressant drugs. Ann NY Acad Sci 1995;771:716–29.

[34] Goncalves L, Silva R, Pinto-Ribeiro F, Pego JM, Bessa JM, Pertovaara A, Sousa N, Almeida A. Neuropathic pain is associated with depressive behaviour and induces neuroplasticity in the amygdala of the rat. Exp Neurol 2008;213:48–56.

[35] Guttuso T Jr, Roscoe J, Griggs J. Effect of gabapentin on nausea induced by chemotherapy in patients with breast cancer. Lancet 2003;361:1703–5.

[36] Haack M, Scott-Sutherland J, Santangelo G, Simpson NS, Sethna N, Mullington JM. Pain sensitivity and modulation in primary insomnia. Eur J Pain 2011; Epub Aug 23.

[37] Hadjipavlou G, Dunckley P, Behrens TE, Tracey I. Determining anatomical connectivities between cortical and brainstem pain processing regions in humans: a diffusion tensor imaging study in healthy controls. Pain 2006;123:169–78.

[38] Han JS, Neugebauer V. mGluR1 and mGluR5 antagonists in the amygdala inhibit different components of audible and ultrasonic vocalizations in a model of arthritic pain. Pain 2005;113:211–22.

[39] Hayashida K, DeGoes S, Curry R, Eisenach JC. Gabapentin activates spinal noradrenergic activity in rats and humans and reduces hypersensitivity after surgery. Anesthesiology 2007;106:557–62.

[40] Hendrich J, Van Minh AT, Heblich F, Nieto-Rostro M, Watschinger K, Striessnig J, Wratten J, Davies A, Dolphin AC. Pharmacological disruption of calcium channel trafficking by the alpha2delta ligand gabapentin. Proc Natl Acad Sci USA 2008;105:3628–33.

[41] Heymen S, Maixner W, Whitehead WE, Klatzkin RR, Mechlin B, Light KC. Central processing of noxious somatic stimuli in patients with irritable bowel syndrome compared with healthy controls. Clin J Pain 2010;26:104–9.

[42] Hungin AP, Whorwell PJ, Tack J, Mearin F. The prevalence, patterns and impact of irritable bowel syndrome: an international survey of 40,000 subjects. Aliment Pharmacol Ther 2003;17:643–50.

[43] Ikeda R, Takahashi Y, Inoue K, Kato F. NMDA receptor-independent synaptic plasticity in the central amygdala in the rat model of neuropathic pain. Pain 2007;127:161–72.

[44] Kayser V, Elfassi IE, Aubel B, Melfort M, Julius D, Gingrich JA, Hamon M, Bourgoin S. Mechanical, thermal and formalin-induced nociception is differentially altered in 5-HT1A-/-, 5-HT1B-/-, 5-HT2A-/-, 5-HT3A-/- and 5-HTT-/- knock-out male mice. Pain 2007;130:235–48.

[45] Kern MK, Shaker R. Cerebral cortical registration of subliminal visceral stimulation. Gastroenterology 2002;122:290–8.

[46] Korb AS, Hunter AM, Cook IA, Leuchter AF. Rostral anterior cingulate cortex theta current density and response to antidepressants and placebo in major depression. Clin Neurophysiol 2009;120:1313–9.

[47] Lason W, Dudra-Jastrzebska M, Rejdak K, Czuczwar SJ. Basic mechanisms of antiepileptic drugs and their pharmacokinetic/pharmacodynamic interactions: an update. Pharmacol Rep 2011;63:271–92.

[48] Lilly R, Cummings JL, Benson DF, Frankel M. The human Kluver-Bucy syndrome. Neurology 1983;33:1141–5.

[49] Macrae WA. Chronic post-surgical pain: 10 years on. Br J Anaesth 2008;101:77–86.

[50] Max MB, Lynch SA, Muir J, Shoaf SE, Smoller B, Dubner R. Effects of desipramine, amitriptyline, and fluoxetine on pain in diabetic neuropathy. N Engl J Med 1992;326:1250–6.

[51] Mayer EA, Berman S, Derbyshire SW, Suyenobu B, Chang L, Fitzgerald L, Mandelkern M, Hamm L, Vogt B, Naliboff BD. The effect of the 5-HT3 receptor antagonist, alosetron, on brain responses to visceral stimulation in irritable bowel syndrome patients. Aliment Pharmacol Ther 2002;16:1357–66.

[52] Mayer EA, Gebhart GF. Basic and clinical aspects of visceral hyperalgesia. Gastroenterology 1994;107:271–93.

[53] Miron D, Duncan GH, Bushnell MC. Effects of attention on the intensity and unpleasantness of thermal pain. Pain 1989;39:345–52.

[54] Neugebauer V, Li W, Bird GC, Han JS. The amygdala and persistent pain. Neuroscientist 2004;10:221–34.

[55] Olesen SS, Graversen C, Olesen AE, Frokjaer JB, Wilder-Smith O, van Goor H, Valeriani M, Drewes AM. Randomised clinical trial: pregabalin attenuates experimental visceral pain through sub-cortical mechanisms in patients with painful chronic pancreatitis. Aliment Pharmacol Ther 2011;34:878–87.

[56] O'Mahony SM, Coelho AM, Fitzgerald P, Lee K, Winchester W, Dinan TG, Cryan JF. The effects of gabapentin in two animal models of co-morbid anxiety and visceral hypersensitivity. Eur J Pharmacol 2011;667:169–74.

[57] Passmore GM, Selyanko AA, Mistry M, Al-Qatari M, Marsh SJ, Matthews EA, Dickenson AH, Brown TA, Burbidge SA, Main M, Brown DA. KCNQ/M currents in sensory neurons: significance for pain therapy. J Neurosci 2003;23:7227–36.

[58] Petrovic P, Kalso E, Petersson KM, Ingvar M. Placebo and opioid analgesia: imaging a shared neuronal network. Science 2002;295:1737–40.

[59] Ploghaus A, Narain C, Beckmann CF, Clare S, Bantick S, Wise R, Matthews PM, Rawlins JN, Tracey I. Exacerbation of pain by anxiety is associated with activity in a hippocampal network. J Neurosci 2001;21:9896–903.

[60] Ploghaus A, Tracey I, Gati JS, Clare S, Menon RS, Matthews PM, Rawlins JN. Dissociating pain from its anticipation in the human brain. Science 1999;284:1979–81.

[61] Procacci P, Zoppi M, Maresca M. Clinical approach to visceral sensation. Prog Brain Res 1986;67:21–8.

[62] Rahman W, D'Mello R, Dickenson AH. Peripheral nerve injury-induced changes in spinal alpha(2)-adrenoceptor-mediated modulation of mechanically evoked dorsal horn neuronal responses. J Pain 2008;9:350–9.

[63] Rahman W, Suzuki R, Rygh LJ, Dickenson AH. Descending serotonergic facilitation mediated through rat spinal 5HT3 receptors is unaltered following carrageenan inflammation. Neurosci Lett 2004;361:229–31.

[64] Rauschecker JP, Leaver AM, Muhlau M. Tuning out the noise: limbic-auditory interactions in tinnitus. Neuron 2010;66:819–26.

[65] Reeves RR, Burke RS. Tramadol: basic pharmacology and emerging concepts. Drugs Today (Barc) 2008;44:827–36.

[66] Rhudy JL, Williams AE, McCabe KM, Nguyen MA, Rambo P. Affective modulation of nociception at spinal and supraspinal levels. Psychophysiology 2005;42:579–87.

[67] Roeska K, Ceci A, Treede RD, Doods H. Effect of high trait anxiety on mechanical hypersensitivity in male rats. Neurosci Lett 2009;464:160–4.

[68] Roeska K, Doods H, Arndt K, Treede RD, Ceci A. Anxiety-like behaviour in rats with mononeuropathy is reduced by the analgesic drugs morphine and gabapentin. Pain 2008;139:349–57.

[69] Saarto T, Wiffen PJ. Antidepressants for neuropathic pain. Cochrane Database Syst Rev 2005;3:CD005454.

[70] Sasaki M, Obata H, Kawahara K, Saito S, Goto F. Peripheral 5-HT2A receptor antagonism attenuates primary thermal hyperalgesia and secondary mechanical allodynia after thermal injury in rats. Pain 2006;122:130–6.

[71] Segal AZ, Rordorf G. Gabapentin as a novel treatment for postherpetic neuralgia. Neurology 1996;46:1175–6.

[72] Seifert F, Maihofner C. Representation of cold allodynia in the human brain: a functional MRI study. Neuroimage 2007;35:1168–80.

[73] Sikandar S, Dickenson AH. Pregabalin modulation of spinal and brainstem visceral nociceptive processing. Pain 2011;152:2312–22.

[74] Sindrup SH, Jensen TS. Pharmacologic treatment of pain in polyneuropathy. Neurology 2000;55:915–20.

[75] Sindrup SH, Otto M, Finnerup NB, Jensen TS. Antidepressants in the treatment of neuropathic pain. Basic Clin Pharmacol Toxicol 2005;96:399–409.

[76] Sitges M, Chiu LM, Guarneros A, Nekrassov V. Effects of carbamazepine, phenytoin, lamotrigine, oxcarbazepine, topiramate and vinpocetine on Na$^+$ channel-mediated release of [3H]glutamate in hippocampal nerve endings. Neuropharmacology 2007;52:598–605.

[77] Spiller RC. Targeting the 5-HT$_3$ receptor in the treatment of irritable bowel syndrome. Curr Opin Pharmacol 2011;11:68–74.

[78] Staud R, Vierck CJ, Robinson ME, Price DD. Spatial summation of heat pain within and across dermatomes in fibromyalgia patients and pain-free subjects. Pain 2004;111:342–50.

[79] Suzuki R, Dickenson AH. Neuropharmacologic targets and agents in fibromyalgia. Curr Pain Headache Rep 2002;6:267–73.

[80] Suzuki R, Rahman W, Hunt SP, Dickenson AH. Descending facilitatory control of mechanically evoked responses is enhanced in deep dorsal horn neurones following peripheral nerve injury. Brain Res 2004;1019:68–76.

[81] Suzuki R, Rahman W, Rygh LJ, Webber M, Hunt SP, Dickenson AH. Spinal-supraspinal serotonergic circuits regulating neuropathic pain and its treatment with gabapentin. Pain 2005;117:292–303.

[82] Suzuki R, Rygh LJ, Dickenson AH. Bad news from the brain: descending 5-HT pathways that control spinal pain processing. Trends Pharmacol Sci 2004;25:613–7.

[83] Suzuki R, Ueta K, Tamagaki S, Mashimo T. Antiallodynic and antihyperalgesic effect of milnacipran in mice with spinal nerve ligation. Anesth Analg 2008;106:1309–15.

[84] Swanson LW, Petrovich GD. What is the amygdala? Trends Neurosci 1998;21:323–31.

[85] Swarbrick ET, Hegarty JE, Bat L, Williams CB, Dawson AM. Site of pain from the irritable bowel. Lancet 1980;2:443–6.

[86] Takeda M, Tsuboi Y, Kitagawa J, Nakagawa K, Iwata K, Matsumoto S. Potassium channels as a potential therapeutic target for trigeminal neuropathic and inflammatory pain. Mol Pain 2011;7:5.

[87] Tanimoto S, Nakagawa T, Yamauchi Y, Minami M, Satoh M. Differential contributions of the basolateral and central nuclei of the amygdala in the negative affective component of chemical somatic and visceral pains in rats. Eur J Neurosci 2003;18:2343–50.

[88] Tebartz van Elst L, Woermann FG, Lemieux L, Trimble MR. Amygdala enlargement in dysthymia: a volumetric study of patients with temporal lobe epilepsy. Biol Psychiatry 1999;46:1614–23.

[89] Tracey I, Ploghaus A, Gati JS, Clare S, Smith S, Menon RS, Matthews PM. Imaging attentional modulation of pain in the periaqueductal gray in humans. J Neurosci 2002;22:2748–52.

[90] Urban MO, Coutinho SV, Gebhart GF. Biphasic modulation of visceral nociception by neurotensin in rat rostral ventromedial medulla. J Pharmacol Exp Ther 1999;290:207–13.

[91] Vaeroy H, Helle R, Forre O, Kass E, Terenius L. Elevated CSF levels of substance P and high incidence of Raynaud phenomenon in patients with fibromyalgia: new features for diagnosis. Pain 1988;32:21–6.

[92] van Wijk G, Veldhuijzen DS. Perspective on diffuse noxious inhibitory controls as a model of endogenous pain modulation in clinical pain syndromes. J Pain 2010;11:408–19.

[93] Vera-Portocarrero LP, Xie JY, Kowal J, Ossipov MH, King T, Porreca F. Descending facilitation from the rostral ventromedial medulla maintains visceral pain in rats with experimental pancreatitis. Gastroenterology 2006;130:2155–64.

[94] Villemure C, Bushnell MC. Cognitive modulation of pain: how do attention and emotion influence pain processing? Pain 2002;95:195–9.

[95] Wolfe F, Smythe HA, Yunus MB, Bennett RM, Bombardier C, Goldenberg DL, Tugwell P, Campbell SM, Abeles M, Clark P, et al. The American College of Rheumatology 1990 criteria for the classification of fibromyalgia. Report of the Multicenter Criteria Committee. Arthritis Rheum 1990;33:160–72.

[96] Yanarates O, Dogrul A, Yildirim V, Sahin A, Sizlan A, Seyrek M, Akgul O, Kozak O, Kurt E, Aypar U. Spinal 5-HT7 receptors play an important role in the antinociceptive and antihyperalgesic effects of tramadol and its metabolite, O-desmethyltramadol, via activation of descending serotonergic pathways. Anesthesiology 2010;112:696–710.

[97] Zambreanu L, Wise RG, Brooks JC, Iannetti GD, Tracey I. A role for the brainstem in central sensitisation in humans. Evidence from functional magnetic resonance imaging. Pain 2005;114:397–407.

[98] Zhuo M, Gebhart GF. Facilitation and attenuation of a visceral nociceptive reflex from the rostroventral medulla in the rat. Gastroenterology 2002;122:1007–19.

[99] Zhuo M, Sengupta JN, Gebhart GF. Biphasic modulation of spinal visceral nociceptive transmission from the rostroventral medial medulla in the rat. J Neurophysiol 2002;87:2225–36.

Correspondence to: Lucy Bee, PhD, Department of Neuroscience, Physiology and Pharmacology, University College London, Gower Street, London WC1E 6BT, United Kingdom. Email: l.bee@ucl.ac.uk.

21

Antidepressants in Pain, Anxiety, and Depression

Nicole Gellings Lowe[a] and Stephen M. Stahl[a,b]

[a]Arbor Scientia, Carlsbad, California, USA; [b]Department of Psychiatry, University of California, San Diego, California, USA

Painful physical symptoms are important concomitant features of depression and anxiety [38]. Pain is not a formally recognized symptom of major depressive disorder (MDD) or generalized anxiety disorder (GAD); however, it is often prevalent. For example, 70% of patients with depression report only physical symptoms as the reason for their visit to a physician [39]. In addition, in the primary care setting, pain is reported by 35% of GAD patients and is one of the most common reasons these patients initially seek medical care [49]. It follows that relief from pain is essential for complete remission of these disorders.

At the other end of the spectrum, several disorders that have pain as a central and formal diagnostic feature also have symptoms of depression and anxiety (Fig. 1). These disorders include fibromyalgia syndrome (FMS), irritable bowel syndrome (IBS), and headache, among others. In fact, as the number of painful symptoms increases, so does the likelihood of MDD and GAD (Fig. 2).

Given the complex interactions of pain, anxiety, and depression, modern clinicians cannot ignore pain symptoms in MDD and GAD or

Pain Comorbidities: Understanding and Treating the Complex Patient
edited by Maria Adele Giamberardino and Troels Staehelin Jensen
IASP Press, Seattle, © 2012

depression and anxiety symptoms in pain disorders. Thus, practitioners must choose treatments aimed at alleviating all symptoms associated with a particular disorder to achieve remission across this spectrum (Fig. 1).

This chapter will review the use of antidepressants for the treatment of pain and comorbid depression and anxiety. The drugs reviewed are tricyclic antidepressants (TCAs); serotonin norepinephrine reuptake inhibitors (SNRIs); selective serotonin reuptake inhibitors (SSRIs); mirtazapine, which is considered a serotonin norepinephrine disinhibitor; and trazodone, a serotonin antagonist/reuptake inhibitor. It should be noted that a single drug is unlikely to relieve all pain. As a result, combinations of drugs, not just those discussed here, with complementary mechanisms of action will have the greatest analgesic effect [39].

Tricyclic Antidepressants

In the 1950s and 1960s, tricyclic antidepressants (TCAs) were synthesized and tested as treatments for schizophrenia. Despite their lack of efficacy in psychosis, they were discovered to have antidepressant effects. Much later, these effects were attributed to their ability to block reuptake pumps

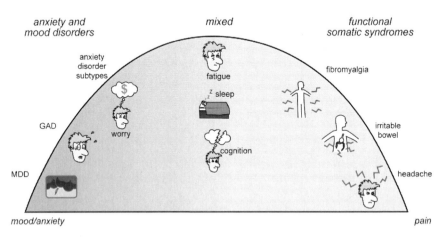

Fig. 1. The spectrum from mood and anxiety disorders to painful functional somatic symptoms. Pain is not a formally recognized symptom of major depressive disorder (MDD) or generalized anxiety disorder (GAD); however, it is prevalent in patients with those disorders. At the other end of the spectrum, several disorders that have pain as a central and formal diagnostic feature also have symptoms of depression and anxiety. Taken from Stahl [38], with permission.

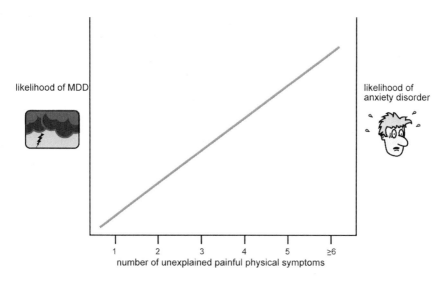

Fig. 2. Dose response for painful symptoms and the likelihood for major depressive disorder (MDD) or anxiety disorder. Clinical observations suggest that the higher the number of painful physical symptoms a patient has, the greater the likelihood that he or she has a mood or anxiety disorder. Taken from Stahl [38], with permission.

for both serotonin (5-HT) and norepinephrine (NE) [38] (Fig. 3A). The same mechanism affords TCAs the ability to decrease pain [39]. Under normal circumstances, descending spinal noradrenergic and serotonergic neurons release NE and 5-HT, which inhibits the activity of dorsal horn neurons. In turn, bodily input (e.g., input regarding muscles and joints or digestion) is prevented from reaching the brain and being interpreted as pain. In instances of chronic pain, there is a lack of both 5-HT and NE release from descending spinal neurons, as well as a lack of inhibition of the primary afferent neurons in the dorsal horn, resulting in the perception of pain (Fig. 4). Therefore, increasing the accumulation of NE and 5-HT from descending spinal neurons by blocking their reuptake pumps is thought to decrease the perception of pain.

In addition to blocking 5-HT and NE reuptake pumps, TCAs have numerous other actions (Fig. 3A). These include antagonistic effects at serotonin 2A and 2C ($5\text{-}HT_{2A}$ and $5\text{-}HT_{2C}$) receptors; and blockade of histamine 1 (H_1) receptors, muscarinic receptors, alpha 1 (α_1) adrenergic receptors, and voltage-sensitive sodium channels [38]. While antagonism at $5\text{-}HT_{2A}$ and $5\text{-}HT_{2C}$ receptors is thought to aid in the antidepressive

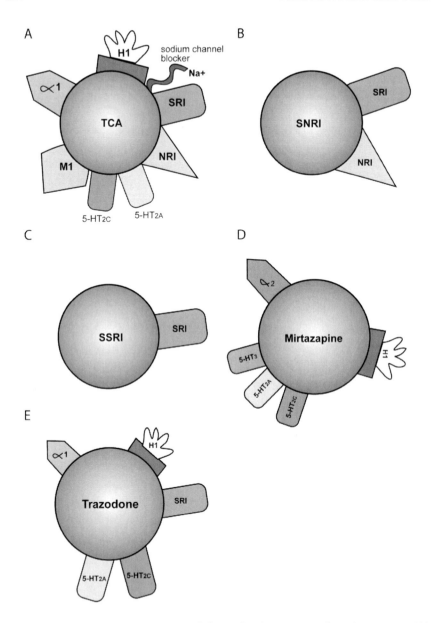

Fig. 3. Diagrammatic representations of the molecular actions of antidepressants. (A) Tricyclic antidepressants (TCAs). (B) Serotonin norepinephrine reuptake inhibitors (SNRIs). (C) Selective serotonin reuptake inhibitors (SSRIs). (D) Mirtazapine, which is considered a serotonin and norepinephrine disinhibitor. (E) Trazodone, a serotonin antagonist/reuptake inhibitor. Other abbreviations: α_1, alpha-1 adrenoceptor; H_1, histamine receptor 1; M_1, muscarinic receptor 1; NRI, norepinephrine reuptake inhibitor; SRI, serotonin reuptake inhibitor. Taken from Stahl [38], with permission.

efficacy of TCAs, other additional mechanisms contribute to a series of unwanted effects. Blockade of H_1 receptors causes sedation and may lead to weight gain; muscarinic receptor 1 (M_1) blockade is linked to blurred vision, dry mouth, urinary retention, constipation, and interference with insulin action; α_1-adrenergic receptor blockade can cause orthostatic hypotension and dizziness; and in some cases, blockade of voltage-sensitive sodium channels in the heart and brain may be the cause of coma and seizures [39].

Studies evaluating the efficacy of TCAs in the treatment of pain comorbid with depression and/or anxiety date back to the 1960s. For example, an early study of amitriptyline (30–75 mg/day) evaluated patients with chronic tension headache with or without depression [23]. Lance and Curran found the drug to be effective in treating the headache regardless of the presence of depression. As a result, they concluded that the effects of this TCA on pain were not the secondary result of the antidepressant

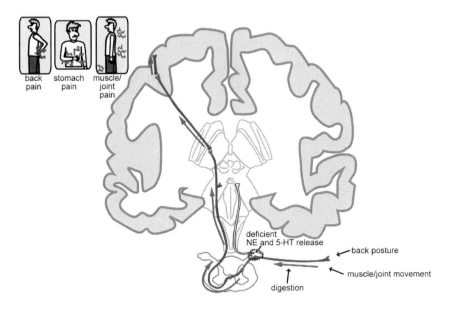

Fig. 4. Deficient norepinephrine (NE) and serotonin (5-HT) inhibition leads to pain. In instances of chronic pain, there is a lack of both 5-HT and NE release from descending spinal neurons, a lack of inhibition of the primary afferent neurons in the dorsal horn, and, in turn, the perception of pain. Therefore, increasing the accumulation of NE and 5-HT from descending spinal neurons by blocking their reuptake pumps is thought to decrease the perception of pain. Taken from Stahl [38], with permission.

effect. The putative mechanism of action of TCAs has been the theme of multiple studies over the years seeking to understand how these drugs can treat pain and depression or anxiety. Although different authors have come to various conclusions, the overwhelming majority have determined that TCAs effectively treat pain comorbid with depression and/or anxiety, noting that these effects are not reliant on one another [24,26,33,41,45,46]. In fact, TCAs have successfully relieved depression and anxiety along with comorbid pain in patients with IBS [33], postherpetic neuralgia [47], and rheumatoid arthritis [5].

Despite the notable number of studies demonstrating their efficacy, TCAs have numerous side effects, which may contribute to a lack of adherence. In fact, when amitriptyline was compared to an SSRI (paroxetine) for the treatment of depression and pain in rheumatoid arthritis, patients preferred the SSRI because of the TCA's lack of tolerability. A more recent study of amitriptyline found that the drug was effective when used alone in the treatment of migraine and concomitant depression; however, patients preferred it in combination with topiramate due to a reduction in side effects [21].

Serotonin Norepinephrine Reuptake Inhibitors

Serotonin norepinephrine reuptake inhibitors (SNRIs) have two molecular actions: inhibition of 5-HT reuptake pumps and inhibition of NE reuptake pumps [38] (Fig. 3B). Therefore, SNRIs have the same effects as TCAs without many of the unpleasant side effects.

There are three basic SNRIs: duloxetine, venlafaxine, and milnacipran. A fourth compound, desvenlafaxine, is the active metabolite of venlafaxine. These compounds vary considerably in their affinities and selectivities for 5-HT and NE transporters [40]. Venlafaxine has the highest affinity for the 5-HT transporter. As a result, it may act as a selective serotonin reuptake inhibitor (SSRI) at low doses. Desvenlafaxine has greater NE transporter inhibition and reduced 5-HT transporter inhibition compared to venlafaxine [39]. Duloxetine has more balanced affinities, and milnacipran is the most evenly balanced. Thus, at all doses, duloxetine and milnacipran will act at both transporters.

All SNRIs are generally well tolerated [40]. The most common adverse event, as with SSRIs, is nausea. Weight gain is unusual, but there can be some sedation [39]. All SNRIs should be used with caution in patients with cardiac impairment due to their potential to increase blood pressure through stimulation of catecholaminergic and noradrenergic neurotransmission. In addition, no SNRI should be coadministered with monoamine oxidase inhibitors. Duloxetine and venlafaxine are metabolized by CYP450 2D6, and therefore inhibitors of this enzyme will alter the effects of these drugs.

Duloxetine

Duloxetine has proven effective for GAD and MDD with comorbid pain in several studies. First, a 12-week, open-label study of comorbid MDD and chronic low back pain in older adults revealed the antidepressant efficacy of up to 120 mg/day duloxetine in 47% of patients, as measured by the Montgomery Åsberg Depression Rating Scale (MADRS), and a reduction in pain in 93% of patients, as measured by the McGill Pain Questionnaire-Short Form (MPQ-SF) [20]. Similarly, patients age 65 and over with MDD and comorbid arthritis had a significant reduction in depression, as measured by the Hamilton Depression Rating Scale (HAM-D), and pain, as measured on a visual analog scale (VAS), when treated with 60 mg/day duloxetine in a double-blind study [50]. In addition, duloxetine at a dose of 60 mg/day reduced both depression (measured by the MADRS) and pain (measured by the Brief Pain Inventory Short Form) when it was assessed for efficacy in patients with MDD and associated painful physical symptoms in a double-blind study over 8 weeks [15]. Lastly, a post hoc analysis of duloxetine's effects on GAD with comorbid pain indicated similarly efficacious results when dosed between 60 and 120 mg/day [17].

Evidence suggests that duloxetine is fast acting in the treatment of pain and depression. After just 1 week of 60 mg/day duloxetine in an open-label trial, patients with MDD and concurrent primary chronic headache experienced relief from both, measured by MADRS and VAS, respectively [44].

The efficacy of duloxetine on pain may be independent from its antidepressive and anxiolytic effects. Doses of 60 or 120 mg/day were studied in five trials for their effectiveness in the treatment of FMS [2,3,9,34].

In all five studies, duloxetine demonstrated a significant analgesic effect; moreover, this effect was independent of the drug's effects on depression and anxiety. These findings suggest that duloxetine has a direct effect on pain that is greater than any indirect effect due to improvement in depressive symptoms. Moreover, when several 9-week studies assessing the efficacy of duloxetine at doses ranging from 40 to 120 mg/day in the treatment of depression with comorbid pain were evaluated together, investigators found that the onset of relief from pain consistently occurred sooner than antidepressive effects [13]. Together, these analyses suggest that duloxetine's effects on pain are independent of its efficacy in depression.

Venlafaxine

Venlafaxine also appears to be efficacious in treating pain associated with MDD and GAD, although there are fewer studies compared to the more popular duloxetine [4,6,22]. Perhaps investigators have overlooked venlafaxine as a result of its lack of significant NE reuptake inhibition at lower doses. In a double-blind, 12-week study, patients presenting with multisomatoform disorder with GAD or MDD were effectively treated with 75 to 225 mg/day venlafaxine for anxiety and pain measured by the Hamilton Rating Scale for Anxiety (HAM-A) and the 15-item Patient Health Questionnaire pain subscale, respectively [22]. Effects on MDD in this study were not significant. In contrast, Bradley and colleagues found venlafaxine to have long-term efficacy in MDD with associated pain. In an open-label study, once-daily 150 mg venlafaxine successfully reduced depression and chronic pain for up to 1 year [6]. In this case, depression was measured by HAM-D and pain by VAS.

Venlafaxine has also been found to improve depression associated with painful diseases [12,35]. For example, venlafaxine improved depression and pain associated with FMS when administered at 75 mg/day for 12 weeks [35]. Although pain (measured by the Fibromyalgia Impact Questionnaire), depression (measured by the Beck Depression Inventory [BDI] and HAM-D), and anxiety (measured by the Beck Anxiety Inventory and HAM-A) all improved, the authors found no correlation between the improvements. This study further validates the hypothesis that improvement in pain by an SNRI is not a secondary effect of improved mood. Similarly, Eardley and Toth conducted a 6-month study of depression and anxiety comorbid with neuropathic pain due to polyneuropathy, using venlafaxine at a mean dose of 220 mg/day [12]. They found significant decreases in pain measured by VAS and anxiety measured by the Hospital Anxiety and Depression Scale (HADS).

Desvenlafaxine

Desvenlafaxine is the active metabolite of venlafaxine. It has greater NE re-uptake inhibitor activities than its parent compound [38]. Desvenlafaxine decreased depression and associated pain in multiple studies [11,25,36]. When investigated for its efficacy in MDD by DeMartinis and colleagues, 100 mg/day desvenlafaxine significantly decreased depression, measured by HAM-D, and associated pain symptoms, measured by VAS. However, while 200 and 400 mg/day decreased depressive symptoms, these doses did not have significant effects on pain [11]. This result was surprising, but the authors suggest that it may be explained by the fact that pain was not an inclusion criterion in this study. Therefore, the authors' ability to detect pain improvements was limited. In contrast, Septien-Velez and colleagues found significant decreases in pain (evaluated using VAS) and depression (evaluated using HAM-D) in patients suffering from MDD when treated with 200 or 400 mg/day desvenlafaxine [36]. Similar to the previous study, pain was not used as an inclusion criterion. Desvenlafaxine does not ap-pear to have been studied for its efficacy in pain associated with anxiety.

Milnacipran

There are limited data on the efficacy of milnacipran in the treatment of comorbid pain with depression or anxiety. A meta-analysis comparing the efficacy of milnacipran with duloxetine and amitriptyline in FMS found milnacipran to be inferior to the other two drugs in the treatment of pain [18]. Despite this potential limitation, there are a few studies of milnacip-ran on patients affected by depression and pain. Curiously, they focus on pain in the orofacial region such as burning mouth syndrome (BMS) and atypical odontalgia. First, after 12 weeks of use at 100 mg/day, milnacipran decreased pain (measured by VAS) and depression (measured by HAM-D) [19]. In contrast, a study using 60 mg/day milnacipran in BMS saw a decrease in depression measured by HAM-D starting 2 weeks after initia-tion of treatment, but the authors did not detect a significant change in pain during the 12 weeks of treatment [42]. The different results may be explained by varying doses. In addition, both studies are limited by a small sample size, so further analysis may be warranted.

Although milnacipran is approved in the United States for the treatment of FMS, no direct evaluation of the drug's effects on depression or anxiety associated with this condition has been performed.

Selective Serotonin Reuptake Inhibitors

Selective serotonin reuptake inhibitors (SSRIs) bear mentioning as candidates for pain treatment because of their extreme popularity in psychiatry, mental health, and general practice. It has been said that up to six prescriptions for SSRIs are written per second, 24 hours a day, 7 days a week [38]. There are seven agents in the SSRI class: citalopram, escitalopram, fluoxetine, fluvoxamine, paroxetine, sertraline, and the newly approved vilazodone.

As their name suggests, SSRIs block the reuptake of 5-HT, allowing for its accumulation (Fig. 3C). In pain, the increase of serotonin accumulation from descending serotonergic neurons is able to suppress bodily input (e.g., regarding muscles/joints or digestion) from reaching the brain and being interpreted as pain. In depression and anxiety, SSRIs increase 5-HT in key brain areas in which 5-HT deficiency results in symptoms of the diseases [39].

This popular class of drugs has a good tolerability profile, but limited efficacy in the treatment of pain, probably because concurrent increases in NE are necessary for best efficacy. In addition, SSRIs, acting via different sets of receptors in the dorsal horn, may have opposing effects on the perception of pain [38]. For example, in a study comparing fluoxetine to two TCAs (amitriptyline and desipramine) in the treatment of diabetic neuropathy [27], only the TCAs were significantly superior to placebo. Interestingly, the TCAs were effective in treating pain in patients who had diabetic neuropathy alone or in combination with depression, but fluoxetine was effective only in patients classified as depressed. This finding may suggest that fluoxetine's effects on pain were secondary to its effects on depression. There has been no observable analgesic benefit for SSRIs in low back pain [48], rheumatoid arthritis [32], or tension-type headache

[28]. Results for the treatment of FMS are mixed, with varying outcomes depending on the SSRI and the study design [1,10,30,31].

Mirtazapine

Mirtazapine treats pain, depression, and anxiety by increasing 5-HT and NE accumulation, an effect that is similar overall to that of SNRIs. However, it achieves this effect with a much different mechanism [38]. This mechanism is twofold. First, mirtazapine blocks α_2-adrenergic receptors, which disinhibits 5-HT and NE release and leads to accumulation of 5-HT and NE. Second, the increased NE can activate α_1-adrenergic receptors and further increase 5-HT release (Fig. 3D).

Mirtazapine acts at several other receptors, contributing both to its therapeutic effects and its side effects [38]. By blocking 5-HT$_{1A}$ and 5-HT$_{2A}$ receptors, mirtazapine theoretically improves cognition and restores sleep while contributing to its anxiolytic and antidepressant properties. By inhibiting 5-HT$_3$ receptors, it may counteract the gastrointestinal problems caused by increased 5-HT. At 5-HT$_{2C}$ receptors, mirtazapine may also add to its anxiolytic and antidepressant effects; however, it may also contribute to weight gain. Mirtazapine also blocks H$_1$ receptors. This effect has been associated with anxiolytic effects and reduced nighttime insomnia, but it is also linked to weight gain and daytime drowsiness.

Mirtazapine is marginally effective in treating both depression and anxiety comorbid with pain. In patients with cancer pain, 15 or 30 mg/day mirtazapine produced nonsignificant trends toward reductions in pain and anxiety, as measured by the Memorial Pain Assessment Card. Results were similar for depression, evaluated with the Zung Self-Rating Depression Scale [43]. Another study of cancer patients did not detect significant effects on pain (measured on a single-symptom scale rated by a physician) when 12 to 19 mg/day mirtazapine was administered. Depression and anxiety, as measured by the HADS, however, were effectively reduced [8].

An open-label trial studied the effects of 15–45 mg/day mirtazapine in patients diagnosed with at least one chronic pain syndrome and concomitant MDD [14]. The mean daily dose of 34.5 mg mirtazapine over 6 weeks significantly reduced pain measured on a faces scale, with no difference between depressed and nondepressed individuals. In addition, depression, as rated on a clinical global impressions scale, was significantly improved. The authors noted that it is unclear whether reduction in pain, improvement in mood, or a combination of these effects leads to the overall patient improvement.

A case study on the effects of mirtazapine on a patient with IBS and concomitant anxiety suggests a potential role for mirtazapine in treatment of these diseases [37]. This patient had previously been taking an SSRI for her anxiety. However, the SSRI exacerbated her IBS, most likely through excessive activation of $5\text{-}HT_3$ receptors. Mirtazapine, in contrast, served as an analgesic, had anxiolytic actions, and did not increase IBS symptoms.

Trazodone

Trazodone is considered a serotonin antagonist/reuptake inhibitor [38]. In other words, it inhibits 5-HT reuptake pumps, similar to SSRIs, allowing for the accumulation of 5-HT. This effect contributes in theory to the relief of depression, anxiety, and pain. In addition, antagonism at $5\text{-}HT_{2A}$ and $5\text{-}HT_{2C}$ receptors collectively increases activity of postsynaptic noradrenergic and dopaminergic neurons, thus augmenting the therapeutic effects (Fig. 3E).

Trazodone has additional molecular properties that contribute to its side-effect profile (Fig. 3E). First, trazodone is an H_1-receptor antagonist. This effect may lead to weight gain and daytime drowsiness. In addition, trazodone blocks α_1-adrenergic receptors, which can contribute to dizziness, sedation, and hypotension.

A small trial in 1990 for the effects of 201 mg/day trazodone on back pain with concomitant depression did not suggest any effect on pain or depression [16]. However, average BDI scores before onset of treatment were low enough to indicate only mild depression. Therefore, it may not have been possible to see an effect.

In an open-label, 12-week study in FMS, flexible doses of trazodone (50–300 mg/day) modestly decreased pain-related interference with daily activity, as measured by the Brief Pain Inventory [29]. In addition, both depression and anxiety were significantly reduced, especially in patients with clinically relevant depression or anxiety at baseline. The most notable effects in this study were improvements in sleep. In an extension of this study, the authors tested an additional 12-week treatment of pregabalin [7]. They found further improvements in depression and lessening of pain-related interference with daily activities.

Conclusion

There are several options for the treatment of pain in patients with MDD and/or GAD. Likewise, there are many effective treatments for patients with pain as a primary diagnosis who also have depression and/or anxiety. We have reviewed the tolerability and efficacy of various antidepressants for these types of patients. Overall, the dual-mechanism antidepressants that increase accumulation of NE and 5-HT seem to be the most efficacious. SSRIs may effectively treat depression and/or anxiety, but they appear to have little effect on concomitant pain symptoms. TCAs, mirtazapine, and trazodone appear efficacious, most likely due to their effects on 5-HT and NE; however, all three drugs have been associated with significant side effects. SNRIs as a group appear to also be highly efficacious in patients with dual diagnoses, and their overall tolerability profile is generally more acceptable. However, even when all of these facts are taken into consideration, we must remember that each patient is unique. Therefore, treatment must be individually tailored to each patient.

References

[1]   Arnold LM, Hess EV, Hudson JI, Welge JA, Berno SE, Keck PE Jr. A randomized, placebo-controlled, double-blind, flexible-dose study of fluoxetine in the treatment of women with fibromyalgia. Am J Med 2002;112:191–7.
[2]   Arnold LM, Lu Y, Crofford LJ, Wohlreich M, Detke MJ, Iyengar S, Goldstein DJ. A double-blind, multicenter trial comparing duloxetine with placebo in the treatment of fibromyalgia patients with or without major depressive disorder. Arthritis Rheum 2004;50:2974–84.
[3]   Arnold LM, Rosen A, Pritchett YL, D'Souza DN, Goldstein DJ, Iyengar S, Wernicke JF. A randomized, double-blind, placebo-controlled trial of duloxetine in the treatment of women with fibromyalgia with or without major depressive disorder. Pain 2005;119:5–15.
[4]   Begre S, Traber M, Gerber M, von Kanel R. Physician speciality and pain reduction in patients with depressive symptoms under treatment with venlafaxine. Eur Psychiatry 2010;25:455–60.
[5]   Bird H, Broggini M. Paroxetine versus amitriptyline for treatment of depression associated with rheumatoid arthritis: a randomized, double blind, parallel group study. J Rheumatol 2000;27:2791–7.
[6]   Bradley RH, Barkin RL, Jerome J, DeYoung K, Dodge CW. Efficacy of venlafaxine for the long term treatment of chronic pain with associated major depressive disorder. Am J Ther 2003;10:318–23.

[7]   Calandre EP, Morillas-Arques P, Molina-Barea R, Rodriguez-Lopez CM, Rico-Villademoros F.
      Trazodone plus pregabalin combination in the treatment of fibromyalgia: a two-phase, 24-week,
      open-label uncontrolled study. BMC Musculoskelet Disord 2011;12:95.
[8]   Cankurtaran ES, Ozalp E, Soygur H, Akbiyik DI, Turhan L, Alkis N. Mirtazapine improves sleep
      and lowers anxiety and depression in cancer patients: superiority over imipramine. Support Care
      Cancer 2008;16:1291–8.
[9]   Chappell AS, Littlejohn G, Kajdasz DK, Scheinberg M, D'Souza DN, Moldofsky H. A 1-year
      safety and efficacy study of duloxetine in patients with fibromyalgia. Clin J Pain 2009;25:365–75.
[10] Cortet B, Houvenagel E, Forzy G, Vincent G, Delcambre B. [Evaluation of the effectiveness of
      serotonin (fluoxetine hydrochloride) treatment. Open study in fibromyalgia.] Rev Rhum Mal
      Osteoartic 1992;59:497–500.
[11] DeMartinis NA, Yeung PP, Entsuah R, Manley AL. A double-blind, placebo-controlled study of
      the efficacy and safety of desvenlafaxine succinate in the treatment of major depressive disorder.
      J Clin Psychiatry 2007;68:677–88.
[12] Eardley W, Toth C. An open-label, non-randomized comparison of venlafaxine and gabapentin
      as monotherapy or adjuvant therapy in the management of neuropathic pain in patients with
      peripheral neuropathy. J Pain Res 2010;3:33–49.
[13] Fishbain DA, Detke MJ, Wernicke J, Chappell AS, Kajdasz DK. The relationship between antide-
      pressant and analgesic responses: findings from six placebo-controlled trials assessing the efficacy
      of duloxetine in patients with major depressive disorder. Curr Med Res Opin 2008;24:3105–15.
[14] Freynhagen R, Muth-Selbach U, Lipfert P, Stevens MF, Zacharowski K, Tolle TR, von Giesen HJ.
      The effect of mirtazapine in patients with chronic pain and concomitant depression. Curr Med
      Res Opin 2006;22:257–64.
[15] Gaynor PJ, Gopal M, Zheng W, Martinez JM, Robinson MJ, Marangell LB. A randomized pla-
      cebo-controlled trial of duloxetine in patients with major depressive disorder and associated
      painful physical symptoms. Curr Med Res Opin 2011;27:1849–58.
[16] Goodkin K, Gullion CM, Agras WS. A randomized, double-blind, placebo-controlled trial of trazo-
      done hydrochloride in chronic low back pain syndrome. J Clin Psychopharmacol 1990;10:269–78.
[17] Hartford JT, Endicott J, Kornstein SG, Allgulander C, Wohlreich MM, Russell JM, Perahia DG,
      Erickson JS. Implications of pain in generalized anxiety disorder: efficacy of duloxetine. Prim
      Care Companion J Clin Psychiatry 2008;10:197–204.
[18] Hauser W, Petzke F, Uceyler N, Sommer C. Comparative efficacy and acceptability of amitrip-
      tyline, duloxetine and milnacipran in fibromyalgia syndrome: a systematic review with meta-
      analysis. Rheumatology (Oxford) 2011;50:532–43.
[19] Ito M, Kimura H, Yoshida K, Kimura Y, Ozaki N, Kurita K. Effectiveness of milnacipran for the
      treatment of chronic pain in the orofacial region. Clin Neuropharmacol 2010;33:79–83.
[20] Karp JF, Weiner DK, Dew MA, Begley A, Miller MD, Reynolds CF 3rd. Duloxetine and care
      management treatment of older adults with comorbid major depressive disorder and chronic
      low back pain: results of an open-label pilot study. Int J Geriatr Psychiatry 2010;25:633–42.
[21] Keskinbora K, Aydinli I. A double-blind randomized controlled trial of topiramate and amitrip-
      tyline either alone or in combination for the prevention of migraine. Clin Neurol Neurosurg
      2008;110:979–84.
[22] Kroenke K, Messina N 3rd, Benattia I, Graepel J, Musgnung J. Venlafaxine extended release in
      the short-term treatment of depressed and anxious primary care patients with multisomatoform
      disorder. J Clin Psychiatry 2006;67:72–80.
[23] Lance JW, Curran DA. Treatment of chronic tension headache. Lancet 1964;1:1236–9.
[24] Leijon G, Boivie J. Central post-stroke pain: a controlled trial of amitriptyline and carbamaze-
      pine. Pain 1989;36:27–36.
[25] Liebowitz MR, Yeung PP, Entsuah R. A randomized, double-blind, placebo-controlled trial of
      desvenlafaxine succinate in adult outpatients with major depressive disorder. J Clin Psychiatry
      2007;68:1663–72.
[26] Max MB, Culnane M, Schafer SC, Gracely RH, Walther DJ, Smoller B, Dubner R. Amitripty-
      line relieves diabetic neuropathy pain in patients with normal or depressed mood. Neurology
      1987;37:589–96.
[27] Max MB, Lynch SA, Muir J, Shoaf SE, Smoller B, Dubner R. Effects of desipramine, amitripty-
      line, and fluoxetine on pain in diabetic neuropathy. N Engl J Med 1992;326:1250–6.
[28] Moja PL, Cusi C, Sterzi RR, Canepari C. Selective serotonin re-uptake inhibitors (SSRIs) for pre-
      venting migraine and tension-type headaches. Cochrane Database Syst Rev 2005;3:CD002919.

[29] Morillas-Arques P, Rodriguez-Lopez CM, Molina-Barea R, Rico-Villademoros F, Calandre EP. Trazodone for the treatment of fibromyalgia: an open-label, 12-week study. BMC Musculoskelet Disord 2010;11:204.
[30] Norregaard J, Volkmann H, Danneskiold-Samsoe B. A randomized controlled trial of citalopram in the treatment of fibromyalgia. Pain 1995;61:445–9.
[31] Patkar AA, Masand PS, Krulewicz S, Mannelli P, Peindl K, Beebe KL, Jiang W. A randomized, controlled, trial of controlled release paroxetine in fibromyalgia. Am J Med 2007;120:448–54.
[32] Perrot S, Javier RM, Marty M, Le Jeunne C, Laroche F. Is there any evidence to support the use of anti-depressants in painful rheumatological conditions? Systematic review of pharmacological and clinical studies. Rheumatology (Oxford) 2008;47:1117–23.
[33] Rajagopalan M, Kurian G, John J. Symptom relief with amitriptyline in the irritable bowel syndrome. J Gastroenterol Hepatol 1998;13:738–41.
[34] Russell IJ, Mease PJ, Smith TR, Kajdasz DK, Wohlreich MM, Detke MJ, Walker DJ, Chappell AS, Arnold LM. Efficacy and safety of duloxetine for treatment of fibromyalgia in patients with or without major depressive disorder: Results from a 6-month, randomized, double-blind, placebo-controlled, fixed-dose trial. Pain 2008;136:432–44.
[35] Sayar K, Aksu G, Ak I, Tosun M. Venlafaxine treatment of fibromyalgia. Ann Pharmacother 2003;37:1561–5.
[36] Septien-Velez L, Pitrosky B, Padmanabhan SK, Germain JM, Tourian KA. A randomized, double-blind, placebo-controlled trial of desvenlafaxine succinate in the treatment of major depressive disorder. Int Clin Psychopharmacol 2007;22:338–47.
[37] Spiegel DR, Kolb R. Treatment of irritable bowel syndrome with comorbid anxiety symptoms with mirtazapine. Clin Neuropharmacol 2011;34:36–8.
[38] Stahl SM. Stahl's essential psychopharmacology. New York: Cambridge University Press; 2008.
[39] Stahl SM. Stahl's illustrated chronic pain and fibromyalgia. New York: Cambridge University Press; 2009.
[40] Stahl SM, Grady MM, Moret C, Briley M. SNRIs: their pharmacology, clinical efficacy, and tolerability in comparison with other classes of antidepressants. CNS Spectr 2005;10:732–47.
[41] Stein D, Peri T, Edelstein E, Elizur A, Floman Y. The efficacy of amitriptyline and acetaminophen in the management of acute low back pain. Psychosomatics 1996;37:63–70.
[42] Sugimoto K. The dubious effect of milnacipran for the treatment of burning mouth syndrome. Clin Neuropharmacol 2011;34:170–3.
[43] Theobald DE, Kirsh KL, Holtsclaw E, Donaghy K, Passik SD. An open-label, crossover trial of mirtazapine (15 and 30 mg) in cancer patients with pain and other distressing symptoms. J Pain Symptom Manage 2002;23:442–7.
[44] Volpe FM. An 8-week, open-label trial of duloxetine for comorbid major depressive disorder and chronic headache. J Clin Psychiatry 2008;69:1449–54.
[45] Ward N, Bokan JA, Phillips M, Benedetti C, Butler S, Spengler D. Antidepressants in concomitant chronic back pain and depression: doxepin and desipramine compared. J Clin Psychiatry 1984;45:54–9.
[46] Ward NG. Tricyclic antidepressants for chronic low-back pain. Mechanisms of action and predictors of response. Spine (Phila Pa 1976) 1986;11:661–5.
[47] Watson CP, Evans RJ, Reed K, Merskey H, Goldsmith L, Warsh J. Amitriptyline versus placebo in postherpetic neuralgia. Neurology 1982;32:671–3.
[48] Wernicke JF, Pritchett YL, D'Souza DN, Waninger A, Tran P, Iyengar S, Raskin J. A randomized controlled trial of duloxetine in diabetic peripheral neuropathic pain. Neurology 2006;67:1411–20.
[49] Wittchen HU, Kessler RC, Beesdo K, Krause P, Hofler M, Hoyer J. Generalized anxiety and depression in primary care: prevalence, recognition, and management. J Clin Psychiatry 2002;63(Suppl 8):24–34.
[50] Wohlreich MM, Sullivan MD, Mallinckrodt CH, Chappell AS, Oakes TM, Watkin JG, Raskin J. Duloxetine for the treatment of recurrent major depressive disorder in elderly patients: treatment outcomes in patients with comorbid arthritis. Psychosomatics 2009;50:402–12.

Correspondence to: Nicole Gellings Lowe, PhD, Arbor Scientia, 1930 Palomar Point Way, Suite 103, Carlsbad, CA 92008, USA. Email: nlowe@arborscientia.com.

Physical Training and Rehabilitation in Patients with Pain Comorbidities

Harriet M. Wittink[a] and Jeanine Verbunt[b]

[a]Lifestyle and Health Research Group, Faculty of Health Care, Utrecht University of Applied Research, Utrecht, The Netherlands; [b]Department of Rehabilitation Medicine, Maastricht University Medical Center, Maastricht, The Netherlands

Exercise therapy is one key management strategy used in patients with pain to address impairments (problems with body function or structure, such as pain or weakness), activity limitations (difficulties in activities such as walking, sitting, and standing), and participation restrictions (problems in everyday life situations such as working, playing sports, or socializing) [91]. Exercise is a subcategory of physical activity that may be defined as "physical activity that is planned, structured, repetitive, and purposive in the sense that improvement or maintenance of one or more components of physical fitness is the objective" [7]. Multiple meta-analyses on the effects of exercise therapy on various painful conditions report that exercise reduces pain and increases aerobic capacity and physical function. The mechanisms behind these effects are not completely clear and are most likely due to multiple factors [88]. Systematic reviews and meta-analyses have provided strong evidence for the efficacy of therapeutic exercise for patients with conditions such as multiple sclerosis, osteoarthritis of the knee, chronic low back pain, coronary heart disease, chronic heart failure, chronic obstructive pulmonary disease, cystic fibrosis, and chronic and

Pain Comorbidities: Understanding and Treating the Complex Patient
edited by Maria Adele Giamberardino and Troels Staehelin Jensen
IASP Press, Seattle, © 2012

intermittent claudication [46,47,59,68,75]. Furthermore, there are indications that exercise therapy is effective in reducing symptoms, increasing physical fitness, and enhancing physical and social functioning for patients with ankylosing spondylitis, hip osteoarthritis, or Parkinson's disease, and for patients who have suffered a stroke [46,47,59,68,75]. Therapeutic exercise is more likely to be effective if it is relatively intense, and there are indications that more targeted and individualized exercise programs might be more beneficial than standardized programs [75]. Aerobic capacity and muscle strength can be improved by exercise training among patients with different diseases without having detrimental effects on disease progression [46,47]. Few adverse events are reported for exercise therapy [47,75].

Traditionally, most exercise therapy programs for patients with pain have focused on increasing physical fitness to enhance physical performance in order to improve patients' ability to perform activities of daily life. People with disabilities, because they are more sedentary, seem to be more susceptible than the general population to conditions such as heart disease, diabetes, and obesity [26], although research is lacking in this area. Therefore, we also need to exercise for health, although Haskell and Kiernan [34] suggest that a distinction between exercising for performance and exercising for health is not always possible, as exercise training will contribute to both (see Fig. 1).

A regimen of regular physical activity can play a role in the management of many conditions. It is important, however, to recognize the

Contribution to health	Components of fitness	Contribution to performance
High Medium Low		Low Medium High
←——————————————→	Cardiorespiratory endurance	←——————————————→
←——————————————→	Skeletal muscle endurance	←——————————————→
←—————————	Skeletal muscle strength	—————————→
←—————	Speed	——————→
←—————	Flexibility	——————→
←—————	Agility	——————→
←—————————	Balance	—————————→
←———	Reaction time	——————————→
←——————————————→	Body composition	←——————————————→

Fig. 1. Components of physical fitness and their relation to physical performance and health (redrawn after [36]).

specific characteristics of a pain problem. Further diagnostics are important in order to be able to make predictions about the potentially positive role of regular physical activity, to determine an exercise prescription for people with a specific pain condition, and to decide whether management of this particular problem needs a behavioral approach in addition. Exercise prescriptions should include specific recommendations about the type, intensity, frequency, and duration of exercise.

Physical Activity

Our environment has changed drastically during the last few decades, leading to changes in behavior, unhealthy dietary habits, and low physical activity. In developed countries, physical inactivity causes a considerable socioeconomic burden, with 1.5–3.0% of total direct health care costs accounted for by physical inactivity [56]. Physical inactivity has become the biggest public health problem of the 21st century [3], with at least 60% of the global population failing to achieve the minimum recommendation of 30 minutes of moderate-intensity physical activity daily [90].

Numerous well-conducted prospective observational studies have demonstrated that the least active and most unfit (deconditioned) people are at the greatest risk for developing chronic diseases. This increased risk occurs independent of ethnicity, income, education, or body size and shape, and there is a dose response across a wide range of activity and fitness levels [33,80].

A recent review [82] was unable to establish evidence for deconditioning in patients with chronic low back pain. The association of spinal musculoskeletal pain with comorbidities is unclear. One study found an association with other chronic painful conditions, chronic physical conditions, and mental disorders, but not with diabetes, heart disease, or cancer [83]. Others found common comorbidities associated with low back pain to include cardiovascular and cerebrovascular disease [37,64] For degenerative back disorders, however, there is clearer evidence for the association between low back pain and cardiovascular risk factors. A systematic review found an association between aortic atherosclerosis and stenosis of the feeding arteries of the lumbar spine with degenerative disk disease and low back pain [42]. A large-scale case-control study found a positive association between weight and lumbar disk herniation as well as lumbar disk narrowing among both men and women [65].

Evidence for a cause-and-effect relationship between chronic pain conditions in general, insufficient physical exercise, and comorbidities is lacking. This lack of evidence can be explained by the fact that most exercise studies in patients with chronic pain have either excluded patients with comorbidities or have not reported on the effect of exercise therapy on comorbidity. For evidence on the effect of exercise therapy in patients with pain and comorbidities, we must, therefore, rely on studies that have been performed in other groups of patients or in healthy subjects.

Over the past decades we have seen an increase in strong evidence for the health benefits of physical activity and physical fitness. Being physically active has beneficial effects on the body, helps prevent the development of many chronic diseases, and is a useful complement to drug treatment in numerous diseases [22]. Physical activity protects against many chronic health conditions by improving glucose uptake and insulin sensitivity, improving blood lipid profiles, lowering blood pressure, improving the health of blood vessels, and protecting against obesity [8,59]. Even a single session of physical activity lowers serum triglycerides, increases serum high-density lipoprotein (HDL, often called "good cholesterol"), decreases blood pressure, and lowers blood glucose [43]. Regular physical activity has an inverse and generally linear relationship with the rates of mortality from all causes; with total cardiovascular disease (CVD); with the incidence of, and mortalities due to, coronary heart disease; and with the incidence of type 2 diabetes mellitus. It is also associated with a reduction in the incidence of obesity and an improvement in the metabolic control of individuals with established type 2 diabetes. Physical activity is also associated with a reduction in the incidence of colon cancer and osteoporosis. Further benefits of regular physical activity include improved physical function and independent living in the elderly. Individuals with higher levels of physical activity are less likely to develop depressive illness than those with lower levels. Moreover, in those with mild-to-moderate depression and anxiety, prescribed physical activity is associated with an improvement in such symptoms. Physical activity also has a favorable impact on several cardiovascular risk factors, including a reduction in blood pressure, an improvement in plasma lipid profile, and alterations in coagulation and hemostatic factors [43].

Although the beneficial effect of exercise has been reported to be "dose related, " increasing in proportion to the duration and amount of energy expended, even a modest increase in the levels of moderate physical activity (3–6 metabolic equivalents), such as 30 minutes at least 5 days per week, has been found to reduce risk for cardiovascular events and mortality from all causes [84]. For sedentary and overweight people, evidence is emerging that "even a little is more," and half the recommended amount of activity can still produce health benefits [12]. Avoiding a sedentary lifestyle during adulthood not only prevents cardiovascular disease independently of other risk factors but also substantially expands total life expectancy and the CVD-free life expectancy for both men and women. This effect is already seen at moderate levels of physical activity, and the gains in CVD-free life expectancy are twice as great at higher activity levels [25].

Physical activity, though not a medicine, can act as one. The evidence suggests that the benefits of regular physical activity on health, longevity, and well-being easily surpass the effectiveness of any drugs or other medical treatment [9,59]. Despite this evidence, reaching the goal of 30 minutes of moderate physical activity a day has not been an important outcome parameter in exercise programs for patients with pain. A Cochrane review of interventions that promote physical activity concluded that a mixture of professional guidance, self-direction, and ongoing professional support can encourage adults to be more physically active [38]. One type of intervention that incorporates these aspects and is effective in increasing physical activity is pedometer-driven walking. The use of a pedometer is associated with significant increases in activity and significant decreases in body mass index and blood pressure [6]. An important predictor of increased physical activity was having a goal of reaching a target number of steps, such as 10,000 steps, per day.

In order to stimulate patients with back pain to reach the goal of 30 minutes of moderate physical activity a day, a pedometer-driven walking program has now been introduced in the United Kingdom [52]. Unfortunately, no results are available yet on the effects of this intervention.

Exercise Therapy for Comorbidities

Evidence on how to effectively treat patients with chronic pain and concomitant medical conditions is mostly absent. There is, however, evidence for the efficacy of exercise training in a number of common chronic diseases. For instance, the finding that aerobic exercise training consistently increases maximal oxygen uptake and physical capacity in patients with chronic diseases [47] is important, because aerobic capacity is inversely related to the clustering of CVD risk factors associated with the metabolic syndrome [63]. There is strong evidence of the positive effect of exercise therapy on the pathogenesis and symptoms of disease and on physical fitness and quality of life in patients with insulin resistance, hypertension, obesity, and dyslipidemia [59]. Exercise therapy, however, encompasses a heterogeneous group of interventions. Although studies have found that exercise can have beneficial effects on pain, function, and health, there continues to be uncertainty about the most effective exercise approach. Most studies have yielded insufficient data to provide useful guidelines on optimal exercise frequency, intensity, type, and time (duration) (FITT) parameters.

Evidence on FITT Parameters

F: Exercise Frequency

According to the Guidelines of the American College of Sports Medicine (ACSM), exercise training should be done 3 to 5 days per week to improve cardiorespiratory fitness and body composition [1]. For patients, a minimum of two sessions per week on nonconsecutive days is regarded as the lowest level that could be effective. One session per week or less is not effective for improving cardiorespiratory fitness [1].

I: Exercise Intensity

Intensity refers to the speed with which an action is performed, the power or strength required to achieve an activity (watts, level, or incline), or the effort put forth by the participant during the activity (exertion).

The "220 minus your age" prediction equation is probably the most commonly used method to estimate maximum heart rate (HR_{max}) and seems to have originally been reported by Fox et al. [24]. Inquiry into the history of this formula reveals that it was not developed from original research, but resulted from observation based on data from approximately 11 references consisting of published research or unpublished scientific compilations. Consequently, the formula HR_{max} = 220 – age (in years) has no scientific merit for use in exercise prescription [62,74]. Tanaka's formula of 208 – (0.7 × age) [74] has scientific merit, but he too reported substantial variation in HR_{max} across the entire age range, with standard deviations ranging from 7 to 11 beats/minute for HR_{max} during exercise, close to the standard deviation of 10 beats/minutes reported by Åstrand et al. [2]. HR_{max} is therefore a personal characteristic that is impossible to predict [81] and should be measured, preferably with a maximal exercise test. Respiratory gas exchange variables can help determine if a person has actually given a true maximal effort.

To determine aerobic exercise intensity, the percentage of heart rate reserve (%HRR) is widely used for prescription purposes. Although a number of studies have shown that %HRR is more closely equivalent to percentage of reserve oxygen consumption ($\%VO_2R$) than to percentage of maximal oxygen consumption ($\%VO_{2max}$), a recent review challenges these findings [18]. The authors of this review recommend that exercise should be prescribed using the ($\%HRR – \%VO_{2max}$) relationship and that VO_{2max} be determined using a ramp protocol. To calculate %HRR, the Karvonen formula [41] is used, where HR_{rest} denotes heart rate at rest:

$$\%HRR = (X\% \, {}^{*}[HR_{max} – HR_{rest}]) + HR_{rest}$$

A rule of thumb for an effective endurance training program is an intensity above 60% of HRR, as calculated using the Karvonen formula. In severely deconditioned patients, the intensity of the training can be reduced to 40–50% of HRR [60], but the intensity should increase gradually toward 60% of HRR. It is clear that for patients who take medications that influence heart rate, such as β-blockers or calcium channel blockers, the Karvonen formula cannot be used. And, since such medications are often used in patients with CVD comorbidity, this restriction limits planning of treatment for those patients. In this case, the rating of perceived exertion (RPE) [4] can be helpful. There are two versions of this scale: the Borg 6–20, the original scale as developed by Borg, with ratings between 6 and 20, and the Borg 0–10, an updated combined category and ratio scale developed by Borg, with ratings between 0 (nothing at all) and 10 (very,

very hard). Either scale can be used. RPE values corresponding with HRR intensities are shown in Table I.

Table I
Training guidelines based on heart rate, oxygen uptake, or rating of perceived exertion

Intensity of Exertion	%HRR	%HR$_{max}$	RPE 6–20	RPE 0–10
Very light	<20	<35	<10	<2
Light	20–39	35–54	10–11	3
Moderate	40–59	55–69	12–13	4–5
Heavy	60–84	70–89	14–16	6–7
Very heavy	>85	>90	17–19	8–9
Maximal	100	100	20	10

Source: Data from the American College of Sports Medicine [60].
Abbreviations: %HRR, percentage of heart rate reserve; %HR$_{max}$, percentage of maximal heart rate; RPE, rating of perceived exertion.
Notes: Percentage of reserve oxygen consumption (VO$_2$R) and HRR can be calculated by subtracting the resting value from the maximal value during exercise. There are two versions of the RPE scale: the Borg 6–20 (the original scale as developed by Borg, with ratings between 6 and 20) and the Borg 0–10 (an updated combined category and ratio scale, with ratings between 0 [nothing at all] and 10 [very, very hard]).

In general, exercise does not provoke cardiovascular events in healthy individuals with normal cardiovascular systems. The risk of cardiac arrest or myocardial infarction is very low in healthy individuals performing activities of moderate intensity. However, there is an acute and transient increase in the risk of sudden cardiac death and myocardial infarction in individuals performing vigorous exercise with either diagnosed or occult CVD [1]. Higher-risk patients (such as those with coronary artery disease or chronic heart failure) should start at a low-intensity training program. For risk stratification, see the American College of Sports Medicine (ACSM) guidelines [1].

It is good clinical practice to take blood pressure measurements before and during exercise. If systolic blood pressure exceeds 250 mm Hg or if it fails to rise or drops by >10 mm Hg during exercise, exercise should be discontinued, and the patient must be referred to a physician.

T: Types of Exercise

Types of exercise include aerobic, strength, and high-intensity interval training (HIT), as well as flexibility and coordination exercises. Aerobic or endurance training improves performance during tasks that rely mainly on aerobic energy metabolism, in large part by increasing the body's ability to transport and utilize oxygen and by altering substrate metabolism in working skeletal muscles. A number of authors have reported that higher aerobic capacity is associated with lower risk of mortality from any cause and with reduced cardiovascular risk factors [44].

Strength or resistance training aims to increase the size and strength of skeletal muscle using isometric, concentric, or eccentric contractions. It is used to improve performance on tasks that require strength and to prevent sarcopenia and osteoporosis. Resistance training may also positively influence metabolic health [86].

HIT is characterized by repeated sessions of relatively brief, intermittent exercise, often performed with an "all-out" effort or an intensity close to that which elicits peak oxygen uptake. HIT tends to improve "sprint" type performance, but it has also been shown to improve markers of aerobic energy metabolism, such as maximal aerobic capacity and mitochondrial activity [49].

T: Exercise Time (Duration)

The minimum duration of training should be 20 minutes per session. For deconditioned patients the session might be divided into two 10-minute sessions over the course of the day [28]. The duration of a session is dependent on the intensity of the activity; thus, lower-intensity activity should be conducted over a longer period of time, and individuals training at higher levels of intensity should train for at least 20 minutes [60].

Comorbidities

Hypertension

Hypertension is a major risk factor for stroke (ischemic and hemorrhagic), myocardial infarction, heart failure, chronic kidney disease, peripheral vascular disease, cognitive decline, and premature death. The diagnostic threshold for defining hypertension has been progressively lowered over the past 50 years, as treatment of hypertension has been shown to be beneficial at reducing cardiovascular morbidity and mortality when initiated at progressively lower blood pressure thresholds. During that time, the focus has also shifted from hypertension diagnosed purely on the basis of diastolic blood pressure (DBP) toward systolic blood pressure (SBP) thresholds being the most common indication for treatment. This trend reflects the increased prevalence of hypertension with aging and the usual progressive rise in systolic pressure with age [55]. Optimal blood pressure (BP) is defined as SBP ≤120 mm Hg and DBP ≤80 mm Hg, prehypertension as SBP between 120 and 139 mm Hg and/or DBP between 80 and 89 mm Hg, and hypertension as SBP ≥140 mm Hg and/ or DBP ≥90 mm Hg.

Evaluation and clearance by a physician is necessary for those with very high or uncontrolled BP prior to beginning an exercise program [1]. For patients with documented CVD, vigorous exercise training should only be conducted under the supervision of qualified personnel. Patients with a resting SBP of >200 mm Hg and/or a resting DBP of >110 mm Hg should not exercise [1].

A meta-analysis [15] of the effects of aerobic training programs (an average of 40 minutes per session, 3 times per week, at an intensity of 65% of HRR, and lasting 16 weeks), on resting and ambulatory blood pressure involving 72 trials, 105 study groups, and 3936 participants, found that training induced significant net reductions of resting and daytime ambulatory BP of 3.0/2.4 mm Hg ($P < 0.001$) and 3.3/3.5 mm Hg ($P < 0.01$), respectively. The reduction of resting BP was more pronounced in the 30 hypertensive study groups (6.9/4.9 mm Hg) than in the others (1.9/1.6 mm Hg; $P < 0.001$ for all). It has been estimated that a 2-mm Hg reduction of SBP results in a 6% reduction in stroke mortality and a 4% reduction in mortality attributable to coronary heart disease; the reductions amount to 14% and 9%, respectively, for a 5-mm Hg decrease in BP [10]. Whereas time per session and training frequency, intensity, and mode were not significantly related to the BP response, the BP decrease was more pronounced with greater increases in VO_2max ($r = 0.24$, $P < 0.05$ for SBP; $r = 0.40$, $P < 0.001$ for DBP). Finally, the BP reduction became smaller with longer total study duration ($P < 0.05$).

Cornelissen et al. [16] reviewed the effect of resistance training on resting BP and other cardiovascular risk factors in adults. They included 28 randomized, controlled trials (RCTs) in their meta-analysis, involving 33 study groups and 1012 participants. Overall, resistance training induced a significant BP mean reduction of almost 4 mm Hg in 28 normotensive or prehypertensive study groups whereas the mean reduction in SBP or DBP was not significant for the 5 hypertensive study groups. When study groups were divided according to the mode of training, isometric handgrip training in 3 groups resulted in a larger mean decrease in SBP (13.5 mm Hg) and DBP (6.1 mm Hg) than dynamic resistance training in 30 groups (SBP 2.8 mm Hg; DBP 2.7 mm Hg). The large decrease in resting BP with isometric exercise is confirmed by another meta-analysis [57] including 5 studies and 122 participants, which concluded that isometric exercise for <1 hour per week reduced SBP by 10.4 mm Hg and DBP by 6.7 mm Hg. These changes are similar to those achieved with a single pharmacological agent.

Changes in BP were not significantly related to weekly training frequency, number of sets, number of repetitions, duration of the intervention, the number of exercises per session, or total exercise volume (frequency × sets × repetitions × number of exercises) ($P > 0.10$ for all). The clinical importance of these BP reductions was estimated from large, prospective intervention studies investigating morbidity and mortality outcomes that suggest that small reductions in resting SBP and DBP of 3 mm Hg can reduce coronary heart disease risk by 5%, stroke by 8%, and all-cause mortality by 4%. Only 4 of the 30 dynamic resistance training programs included hypertensive patients, warranting some caution when prescribing this type of training for hypertensives. No serious adverse effects were reported for resistance training.

The Canadian Hypertension Education Program [30] recommends prescribing a total of 30–60 minutes of moderate-intensity dynamic exercise (such as walking, jogging, cycling, or swimming) four to seven days a week in addition to the routine activities of daily living.

Recommendation

Both aerobic training and dynamic and static resistance training have a beneficial effect on BP in subjects with optimal pressure or prehypertension.

It appears that for hypertensive patients, aerobic exercise is the exercise therapy of choice. Resistance exercise warrants further investigation in hypertensive patients.

Diabetes Mellitus Type 2

Increased physical activity and exercise are usually prescribed for people with type 2 diabetes mellitus, especially in the early stages. Unfortunately, type 2 diabetes has nearly always been present for several years before the diagnosis is made and more than half of newly diagnosed patients exhibit signs of late diabetic complications, including macrovascular diseases, such as hypertension, or microvascular complications, such as nephropathy and painful diabetic neuropathy, which may limit exercise [59]. Even major adverse effects such as stroke or coronary heart disease can be the result of type 2 diabetes. Possible adverse effects of exercise in people with type 2 diabetes may include an abnormal cardiovascular response to exercise, including silent ischemia, or problems related to foot care. Clinical guidelines [5] recommend examination of patients' feet that includes testing of foot sensation using a 10-g monofilament or vibration, palpation of foot pulses, inspection for any foot deformity, and inspection of footwear. Patients with decreased sensibility due to diabetic neuropathy should inspect their feet regularly as part of their self-care routine, especially when they start to increase their level of physical activity. In addition, the general practitioner needs to inspect the patient's feet regularly to prevent diabetic foot ulcers.

Physical activity, such as walking, can be undertaken safely and will lead to a lower risk for foot ulcers. A study that investigated the risk of diabetic foot ulcers with daily weight bearing found that moderately active participants (4.5–7.4 weight-bearing hours/day) were at substantially but nonsignificantly reduced risk of foot ulcer compared with "least active" participants (<4.5 weight-bearing hours/day). "Most active" participants (≥7.5 weight-bearing hours/day) were at significantly reduced risk (odds ratio [OR]: 0.20). Weight-bearing activity exerted similar effects on foot ulcer risk in participants with insensate or sensate feet [48].

Cardiac screening, including a stress test, is recommended for previously sedentary patients with additional cardiovascular risk factors, especially for those attempting to undergo more than brisk walking, although clinical judgment should prevail [13]. ECG exercise stress testing is not recommended for asymptomatic individuals at low risk of coronary artery disease but may be indicated for those at higher risk [14].

Beneficial effects have been shown with exercise, including both aerobic [67] and resistance [20,67] training or a combination of both modes of training, which yields greater results than either form of exercise alone [11,67]. The magnitude of HbA_{1c} (glycated hemoglobin) reduction appears dissimilar across the three exercise modalities. Church et al. [11] found that combined training, but not aerobic training alone, reduced HbA_{1c} to lower levels compared with controls, and combined training also resulted in greater decreases in body fat and increases in strength. Sigal et al. [67] found that combined exercise resulted in a significantly greater decrease in HbA_{1c} than aerobic training or resistance training alone, with reductions of 0.97%, 0.51%, and 0.38% vs. controls, respectively. More studies are needed, however, to determine whether total caloric expenditure, exercise duration, or exercise mode is responsible [14].

Meta-analyses have reported exercise related reductions of HbA_{1c} of 0.8 ± 0.3% [69] and 0.6% (−0.6% HbA_{1c}; 95% confidence interval [CI] −0.9 to −0.3; $P < 0.05$) [76] compared to control. This result is both statistically and clinically significant and comparable to medication management. A 1% absolute decrease in HbA_{1c} represents a 21% decrease in risk for any diabetes-related endpoint, a 21% decrease in risk for any diabetes-related death, a 14% decreased risk for myocardial infarction, and a 37% decreased risk for microvascular complications [72].

These improvements in glycemic control commonly result in reductions in type 2 diabetes medications. Further, there are data to suggest that the greatest benefits occur in patients with the poorest metabolic control. Importantly, studies that failed to show improvements in glycemic control have commonly reported poor exercise compliance or prescribed a low volume or intensity of exercise [39]. The mechanisms responsible for these exercise-induced benefits are complex. There are two well-defined pathways that stimulate glucose uptake by the muscles. At rest and postprandially, glucose uptake by muscle tissue is insulin dependent and serves primarily to replenish muscle glycogen stores. During exercise, contractions increase blood glucose uptake to supplement intramuscular glycogenolysis. As the two pathways are distinct, blood glucose uptake into working muscles is normal even when insulin-mediated uptake is impaired in type 2 diabetes. Muscular blood glucose uptake remains elevated after exercise, with the contraction-mediated pathway persisting for several hours and insulin-mediated uptake for longer [14]. Both aerobic and resistance exercise increase the number and function of glucose transporter 4 (GLUT4) molecules and raise blood glucose uptake, even in the presence of type 2 diabetes.

Guidelines and positions statements [13,51] recommend specific FITT (frequency, intensity, type, and time) parameters for exercise in type 2 diabetes, as shown in Table II. Exercise intervention studies showing the greatest effect on blood glucose control have all involved supervision of exercise sessions by qualified exercise trainers. A systematic review of 20 resistance training studies on type 2 diabetes found that supervised training of varying volume, frequency, and intensity improved blood glucose control and insulin sensitivity, but that when supervision was removed, exercise compliance and blood glucose control both deteriorated [28].

A meta-analysis [79] on the association of physical activity advice only or structured exercise training with HbA_{1c} levels in type 2 diabetes found that physical activity advice alone had no effect. Structured exercise training that consists of aerobic exercise, resistance training, or both combined was associated with HbA_{1c} reduction in patients type 2 diabetes. Structured exercise training of more than 150 minutes per week was associated with greater HbA_{1c} declines than training of 150 minutes or less per week.

Recommendation

Physical activity and exercise training have a positive effect on insulin sensitivity, increase GLUT4 number and function, and improve blood glucose uptake in patients with type 2 diabetes. As increased insulin sensitivity as a result of an exercise bout disappears within about 48 hours, patients with type 2 diabetes should exercise on a regular basis to improve glycemic control. It is necessary to exercise at least three times/week with one recovery day in between to maintain increased insulin sensitivity. Exercise should consist of a combination of aerobic and strength training, consistent with physical activity guidelines. Exercise of longer duration appears to have greater effects.

Table II
FITT parameters for exercise in type 2 diabetes

Type of Exercise	Intensity of Exertion	Time (Duration)	Frequency
Aerobic exercise	i) 40–60% VO$_{2max}$ or 50–70% HR$_{max}$	150 min/ week	5–7 times/week (minimum 3 times/week)
	ii) >60% VO$_{2max}$ or >70% HR$_{max}$	90 min/ week	3 times/week
Resistance exercise	3 sets, 8-10 repetitions, at a weight that cannot be lifted more than 8–10 times, with 1–2 min rest between sets		3 times/week

Abbreviations: FITT, frequency, intensity, time, and type; HR$_{max}$, maximal heart rate; VO$_{2max}$, maximum oxygen consumption.

Overweight and Obesity

Overweight and obesity are characterized by excess body weight, with body mass index (BMI) commonly used as the criterion to define these conditions. People are classified as overweight if BMI ≥ 25 kg/m, obese if BMI ≥ 30 kg/m, or extremely obese if BMI ≥ 40 kg/m.

A systematic review and meta-analysis determined statistically significant associations for being overweight with the incidence of type 2 diabetes, all cancers (except esophageal cancer [in females], pancreatic cancer, and prostate cancer), all cardiovascular diseases (except congestive heart failure), asthma, gallbladder disease, osteoarthritis, and chronic back pain. Statistically significant associations with obesity were found with the incidence of type 2 diabetes, all cancers except esophageal and prostate cancer, all types of CVD, asthma, gallbladder disease, osteoarthritis, and chronic back pain [29]. Both overweight and obesity defined by BMI were most strongly associated with the incidence of type 2 diabetes in females. Furthermore, a large recent cross-sectional trial [92] found that adults with abdominal obesity were significantly more likely to have major depressive symptoms (OR: 2.18, 95% CI: 1.35–3.59) or have moderate to severe depressive symptoms (OR: 2.56, 95% CI: 1.34–4.90) than those without.

Effective weight management for individuals and groups with overweight and obesity involves a range of strategies including reducing energy intake through dietary change and increasing energy expenditure by increasing physical activity [89]. The presence of other comorbidities may increase the risk stratification for overweight and obese individuals, resulting in the need for additional medical screening prior to engaging in an exercise program. Appropriate cuff size should be used to measure blood pressure to minimize the potential for inaccurate measurement [1].

A review [77] including aerobic exercise as a sole intervention for weight loss found that moderate-intensity aerobic exercise programs of 12 weeks to 12 months in length resulted in modest weight and waist circumference reduction and modest benefits to blood pressure and lipid levels. This review included 14 RCTs, with a total of 1847 patients. Six-month programs were associated with a modest reduction in weight (weighted mean difference [WMD] −1.6 kg; 95% CI, −1.64 to −1.56) and waist circumference (WMD, −2.12 cm; 95% CI, −2.81 to −1.44).

A Cochrane review [66] (43 studies including 3476 participants) reported a weight reduction effect size of −2.03 kg for exercise versus no treatment. Exercise combined with diet resulted in a 1 kg greater weight reduction than diet alone. In the high versus low intensity exercise without dietary change group weight loss data from four trials involving 317 participants were pooled. All trials favored high intensity exercise for weight loss. The pooled effect for interventions with a follow-up between 3.5 and 12 months was a 1.5 kg greater reduction in weight in the high intensity exercise group compared with the low intensity exercise group. The review also reported that exercise is associated with a small decrease in SBP and DBP.

Non-adherence may be a particular problem in long-term (unsupervised) programs and aerobic exercise may be under-prescribed in terms of duration and intensity. It has been reported that increasing exercise intensity stimulates the magnitude of weight loss [66].

A systematic review [23] studied the relative health risks of poor cardiorespiratory fitness (or physical inactivity) in normal-weight people vs. obesity in individuals with good cardio-respiratory fitness (or high physical activity). The data indicated that the risk for all-cause and cardiovascular mortality was lower in individuals with high BMI and good aerobic fitness, compared with individuals with normal BMI and poor fitness. In contrast, having high BMI even with high physical activity was a greater risk for the incidence of type 2 diabetes and the prevalence of cardiovascular and diabetes risk factors, compared with normal BMI with low physical activity.

The Scottish Intercollegiate Guidelines Network (SIGN) [50] guideline for the management of obesity recommends basing weight loss targets on comorbidities and risks, rather than on weight alone. Their exercise recommendations for overweight and obese people are to prescribe a volume of physical activity equal to 7.5–10.45 MJ (1800–2500 kcal) a week. This corresponds to 225–300 minutes/week of moderate intensity physical activity. Studies that have compared continuous low versus high intensity training programs with matched energy expenditure between trials report no difference in weight loss [32,78].

According to the ACSM position stand, the evidence supports moderate-intensity physical activity between 150 and 250 minutes/week to be effective in preventing weight gain. Moderate-intensity physical activity between 150 and 250 minutes/week will provide only modest weight loss. Greater amounts of physical activity (>250 minutes/week) have been associated with clinically significant weight loss. Moderate-intensity physical activity between 150 and 250 minutes/week will improve weight loss in studies that use moderate, but not severe, diet restriction. Cross-sectional and prospective studies indicate that after weight loss, weight maintenance is improved with physical activity for >250 minutes/week. However, no evidence from well-designed RCTs exists to judge the effectiveness of physical activity for prevention of weight regain after weight loss. Resistance training does not enhance weight loss but may increase fat-free mass and loss of fat mass and is associated with reductions in health risk. Existing evidence indicates that endurance training or resistance training without weight loss improves health risks [19].

Recommendation

Volume, but not intensity, of exercise forms the main factor through which weight loss is achieved. Exercise is associated with improved cardiovascular disease risk factors even if no weight is lost (see the discussion of metabolic syndrome below). Weight loss through exercise alone is not substantial, and therefore a combination of increased expenditure with decreased caloric intake is recommended. For many people a low-intensity program might be easier to adhere to than a high-intensity program. The potential for low exercise capacity in overweight and obese individuals may necessitate starting at low or very low intensities (Table III).

Table III
FITT parameters for exercise in overweight and obese individuals

Type of Exercise	Intensity of Exertion	Time (Duration)	Frequency
Aerobic exercise (weight loss and maintenance)	40–60% VO_{2max} or 50–70% HR_{max}	>250 min/ week	5–7 times week (minimum 3 times/week)

Abbreviations: FITT, frequency, intensity, time, and type; HR_{max}, maximal heart rate; VO_{2max}, maximum oxygen consumption.

Metabolic Syndrome

The metabolic syndrome is typically defined as a clustering of abnormal levels of lipids (HDL and triglycerides), glucose, blood pressure, and excess abdominal fat. Based on the National Cholesterol Education Program (NCEP) guidelines for adults, a diagnosis of metabolic syndrome is made when three of the CVD risk factors are present [54]. Even a short period of inactivity can induce metabolic changes. Numerous studies have shown that bed rest reduces the sensitivity of muscles to insulin [58]. Other metabolic and functional changes occur as well. In a study, 10 healthy young men decreased their daily activity level from a mean (SD) of 10, 501 (± 808) to 1344 (± 33) steps/day for 2 weeks. After these 2 weeks, peripheral insulin sensitivity was significantly reduced, as was cardiovascular fitness (a reduction of 7%) and lean leg mass [45]. In another study, bed rest for 5 days was associated with the development of insulin resistance, dyslipidemia, increased blood pressure, and impaired microvascular function in 20 healthy volunteers [31].

The treatment guidelines for metabolic syndrome recommended by the NCEP focus on three interventions: weight control, physical activity, and treatment of the associated CVD risk factors (which may include pharmacotherapy). Risk stratification in patients with metabolic syndrome may result in the need for additional medical screening before exercise testing and exercise prescription [1], especially when high-intensity physical activity or exercise training is being considered.

Numerous studies have investigated the effect of exercise therapy on individual CVD risk factors, yet few studies have focused on the effects of exercise on clustered CVD risk. Several studies have shown that increased physical activity and cardiovascular capacity contribute separately to reducing CVD risk. Higher-intensity physical activity, and especially higher cardiovascular capacity (VO_{2max}), are independently associated with lower risk of individual risk factors as well as clustered CVD risk [21,63]. High levels of physical activity are associated with an additional reduced risk among fit participants. In addition, an excess risk of interaction was found for waist circumference, triglycerides, and the clustered CVD risk for individuals who were neither sufficiently active nor fit [21]. A pilot RCT compared equal volumes of either continuous moderate exercise (70% of HR_{max}) or high-intensity aerobic training (90% of HR_{max}) three times a week for 16 weeks. High-intensity aerobic training was superior to continuous moderate exercise in enhancing endothelial function (9% versus 5%; $P < 0.001$), insulin signaling in fat and skeletal muscle, skeletal muscle biogenesis, and excitation-contraction coupling and in reducing blood glucose and lipogenesis in adipose tissue. The two exercise programs were equally effective at lowering mean arterial blood pressure and reducing body weight (by 2.3 and 3.6 kg with high-intensity aerobic training and continuous moderate exercise, respectively) and fat [78]. In another small study, 43 participants with metabolic syndrome were randomized to one of the following groups: aerobic interval training ($n = 11$), strength training ($n = 11$), a combination of both ($n = 10$) 3 times/week for 12 weeks, or a control group ($n = 11$). All three training groups had significant reductions in waist circumference and improvements in endothelial function. There were no changes in body weight, fasting plasma glucose, or HDL levels within or between the groups [70].

A large study [40] randomized patients with metabolic syndrome to three exercise training groups: (1) low amount/moderate intensity (caloric equivalent of approximately 19 km [12 miles]/week) at 40–55% of peak oxygen consumption (VO_{2peak}), (2) low amount/vigorous intensity (caloric equivalent of 19 km [12 miles]/week) at 65–80% VO_{2peak}, and (3) high amount/vigorous intensity (caloric equivalent of 32 km [20 miles]/week) at 65–80% VO_{2peak}. Each group exercised for 8 months. The high-amount/vigorous-intensity group had the greatest number of metabolic variables improvement. Waist circumference significantly improved for all three exercise groups. Triglycerides were significantly lower in the low-amount/moderate-intensity group, but not in the low-amount/vigorous-intensity group. According to the authors, the mechanisms responsible for this result are not yet clear, but it seems likely that either lipoprotein lipase activity was increased more (resulting in increased triglyceride clearance) or that overall production of very low-density lipoprotein by the liver was reduced more by moderate-intensity exercise than by vigorous-intensity exercise.

The authors concluded that the physical activity guideline of moderate intensity activity of 30 min/day is sufficient to obtain significant health benefits. With a higher amount of more vigorous physical activity more generalized and widespread benefits were obtained. The frequency and duration of exercise might matter, as the same amount of exercise at a more vigorous intensity (shorter duration of exercise) was not significantly different from the inactive.

One meta-analysis [71] investigated resistance training in the treatment of metabolic syndrome and included 13 RCTs and 513 subjects. Resistance training reduced HbA1c by 0.48% (95% CI, −0.76, −0.21; $P = 0.0005$), fat mass by 2.33 kg (95% CI, −4.71, 0.04; $P = 0.05$), and SBP by 6.19 mm Hg (95% CI, 1.00, 11.38; $P = 0.02$). There was no statistically significant effect of resistance training on total cholesterol, HDL, LDL, triglycerides, or DBP.

Recommendations

Exercise has beneficial effects on metabolic health. Interventions for reducing clustered metabolic risk should focus on both increasing physical activity and cardiovascular capacity. Significant benefits are already obtained with moderate-intensity physical activity for 30 minutes/day. Cardiovascular capacity can be increased through high-intensity physical activity, continuous aerobic training (at >60% HRR), or high-intensity interval training. Strength training appears to have beneficial effects as well. More studies need to be done to guide optimal exercise prescription.

Affective Disorders

Depression

Depressed patients with chronic pain report greater pain intensity, less life control, and more use of passive or avoidant coping strategies. They also describe greater interference from pain and exhibit more pain behaviors than do chronic pain patients without depression [36]. The prevalence of major depression in patients with chronic low back pain is 3–4 times greater than in the general population [17,73]. A Cochrane review on exercise for depression included 23 trials (907 participants) comparing exercise with no treatment or a control intervention. The pooled standardized mean difference (SMD) was −0.82 (95% CI, −1.12, −0.51), indicating a large clinical effect. Moderate effects were found in the long-term follow-up. When compared with cognitive therapy or antidepressants, exercise was found to be as effective as either of these treatments. However, when only the three trials with adequate allocation concealment and intention-to-treat analysis and blinded outcome assessment were included, the pooled SMD was −0.42 (95% CI, −0.88, 0.03), showing a moderate, nonsignificant effect. The effect of exercise was not significantly different from that of cognitive therapy [53]. Mixed and resistance exercise showed larger effect sizes (but also larger confidence intervals) than aerobic exercise. In general, high exercise intensities (e.g., the public health recommended dose) seemed more effective than lower doses for both exercise types. Another meta-analysis examined the effects of exercise on depressive symptoms in 58 randomized trials (n = 2982) [61]. The overall effect size indicated an improvement in depression scores of 0.80 standard deviation units following an exercise program. Analysis of moderating variables indicated that aerobic exercise and resistance exercise are equally effective, but exercise interventions that combined aerobic and resistance exercise resulted in larger effects than aerobic or resistance exercise alone. Within the clinically depressed population, exercise bouts of 45–49 minutes resulted in larger effects than bouts of 30–44 minutes or ≥60 minutes.

All studies that reported exercise intensity used intensities ranging from 50% to 85%. No significant relationship between energy expenditure and changes in depression score was found for the clinically depressed population. Significant differences in effects were found for exercise frequency within the clinically depressed population; exercising five times per week resulted in a significantly larger effect than exercise two to four times per week. However, only one study utilized a protocol of five exercise sessions per week.

Anxiety

A meta-analysis, including only RCTs, was conducted to examine the effects of exercise on anxiety. Results from 49 studies show an overall effect size of −0.48, indicating larger reductions in anxiety among exercise groups than no-treatment control groups. Exercise groups also showed greater reductions in anxiety compared with groups that received other forms of anxiety-reducing treatment (effect size = −0.19) [87]. In chronic pain, depression and anxiety can be present as comorbidities, but they can both appear as a reaction to the pain problem itself. Exercise, when included in this multidimensional treatment, can have a beneficial effect, but a multidimensional approach is necessary for long-term effects.

Severe Mental Illnesses

People with severe mental illnesses, such as schizophrenia or bipolar disorder, have worse physical health and a reduced life expectancy compared to the general population [85]. Evidence shows that they have a 2–3-fold increased mortality rate and that the mortality gap associated with mental illness compared to the general population has widened in recent decades. People with serious mental illness have an increased risk of mortality associated with physical illness, with the most common cause of death being cardiovascular disease (CVD). The etiology of this excess CVD risk is multifactorial and includes genetic, socioeconomic, and lifestyle factors, as well as disease-specific and treatment effects. People with serious mental illness are more likely to be sedentary, to be overweight, to smoke, and to have diabetes, hypertension, and dyslipidemia [85].

A Cochrane review examined the effects of exercise on physical and mental health in patients with schizophrenia [27].Three RCTs met the inclusion criteria. Out of two RCTs comparing exercise to standard care, one study found stronger (but nonsignificant) reductions in body fat, BMI, and scores on the Positive and Negative Symptoms Scale (PANSS) after 16 weeks of aerobic exercise, whereas the other study reported improvements in the Mental Health Inventory score after 12 weeks of combined aerobic and strength training. The third RCT found that 4 months of light exercise was less effective than yoga therapy in reducing negative symptoms and depression and increasing social and occupational functioning and quality of life. A recent RCT allocated 25 inpatients to either high-intensity interval training (HIT) or playing computer games, 3 days per week for 8 weeks. Although VO_{2peak} improved in the HIT group, the psychiatric symptoms, expressed as scores on the PANSS and the Calgary Depression Scale for Schizophrenia, did not improve in either group [35].

Recommendation

Exercise therapy appears to have no effect or to significantly reduce depressive symptoms, depending on the methods and interpretation used in meta-analyses. Higher frequency, a combination of aerobic and resistance exercise, and a duration of 45 minutes appear to have positive effects on depressive symptoms. More research is needed for optimal intensity. Exercise training also appears to have a positive effect on anxiety. In patients with serious mental illness, more research is needed.

Conclusions

It is important to take exercise restrictions due to comorbidity in mind when planning exercise treatment for pain problems. Safety precautions should be observed prior to engaging patients with comorbidities in exercise, especially high-intensity exercise. However, for most comorbidities, exercise will be beneficial. Physical activity and exercise training have beneficial effects on a number of common comorbidities.

Different FITT training modalities appear to have different effects. A treatment plan must cover physical activity and exercise elements for both pain and comorbid conditions. A treatment goal should include achieving guideline recommendations for physical activity or 10, 000 steps per day at moderate intensity. There is evidence that pedometers might be helpful in achieving this goal.

References

[1]   American College of Sports Medicine. ACSM's guidelines for exercise testing and prescription. Philadelphia: Lippincott, Williams and Wilkins; 2009.
[2]   Astrand PO, Rodahl K, Dahl HA, Stromme SB. Textbook of work physiology. Physiological bases of exercise. Champaign, IL: Human Kinetics; 2003.
[3]   Blair SN. Physical inactivity: the biggest public health problem of the 21st century. Br J Sports Med 2009;43:1–2.
[4]   Borg G. Perceived exertion as an indicator of somatic stress. Scand J Rehabil Med 1970;2:92–8.

[5]   Boulton AJ, Armstrong DG, Albert SF, Frykberg RG, Hellman R, Kirkman MS, Lavery LA, Le-
       master JW, Mills JL Sr, Mueller MJ, Sheehan P, Wukich DK. Comprehensive foot examination
       and risk assessment. A report of the Task Force of the Foot Care Interest Group of the American
       Diabetes Association, with endorsement by the American Association of Clinical Endocrinolo-
       gists. Phys Ther 2008;88:1436–43.
[6]   Bravata DM, Smith-Spangler C, Sundaram V, Gienger AL, Lin N, Lewis R, Stave CD, Olkin I, Si-
       rard JR. Using pedometers to increase physical activity and improve health: a systematic review.
       JAMA 2007;298:2296–304.
[7]   Caspersen CJ, Powell KE, Christenson GM. Physical activity, exercise, and physical fitness: defi-
       nitions and distinctions for health-related research. Public Health Rep 1985;100:126–31.
[8]   Chakravarthy MV, Joyner MJ, Booth FW. An obligation for primary care physicians to prescribe
       physical activity to sedentary patients to reduce the risk of chronic health conditions. Mayo Clin
       Proc 2002;77:165–73.
[9]   Chief Medical Officer. On the state of the public health. Annual report of the Chief Medical Of-
       ficer; 2009. Department of Health; 2010.
[10]   Chobanian AV, Bakris GL, Black HR, Cushman WC, Green LA, Izzo JL Jr, Jones DW, Materson
       BJ, Oparil S, Wright JT Jr, Roccella EJ. The Seventh Report of the Joint National Committee on
       Prevention, Detection, Evaluation, and Treatment of High Blood Pressure: the JNC 7 report.
       JAMA 2003;289:2560–72.
[11]   Church TS, Blair SN, Cocreham S, Johannsen N, Johnson W, Kramer K, Mikus CR, Myers V,
       Nauta M, Rodarte RQ, Sparks L, Thompson A, Earnest CP. Effects of aerobic and resistance
       training on hemoglobin A1c levels in patients with type 2 diabetes: a randomized controlled trial.
       JAMA 2010;304:2253–62.
[12]   Church TS, Earnest CP, Skinner JS, Blair SN. Effects of different doses of physical activity on
       cardiorespiratory fitness among sedentary, overweight or obese postmenopausal women with
       elevated blood pressure: a randomized controlled trial. JAMA 2007;297:2081–91.
[13]   Colberg SR, Sigal RJ, Fernhall B, Regensteiner JG, Blissmer BJ, Rubin RR, Chasan-Taber L, Al-
       bright AL, Braun B. Exercise and type 2 diabetes: the American College of Sports Medicine and
       the American Diabetes Association: joint position statement. Diabetes Care 2010;33:e147–67.
[14]   Colberg SR, Sigal RJ, Fernhall B, Regensteiner JG, Blissmer BJ, Rubin RR, Chasan-Taber L, Al-
       bright AL, Braun B. Exercise and type 2 diabetes: the American College of Sports Medicine and
       the American Diabetes Association: joint position statement executive summary. Diabetes Care
       2010;33:2692–6.
[15]   Cornelissen VA, Fagard RH. Effects of endurance training on blood pressure, blood pressure-
       regulating mechanisms, and cardiovascular risk factors. Hypertension 2005;46:667–75.
[16]   Cornelissen VA, Fagard RH, Coeckelberghs E, Vanhees L. Impact of resistance training on blood
       pressure and other cardiovascular risk factors: a meta-analysis of randomized, controlled trials.
       Hypertension 2011;58:950–8.
[17]   Currie SR, Wang J. Chronic back pain and major depression in the general Canadian population.
       Pain 2004;107:54–60.
[18]   da Cunha FA, Farinatti PT, Midgley AW. Methodological and practical application issues in ex-
       ercise prescription using the heart rate reserve and oxygen uptake reserve methods. J Sci Med
       Sport 2011;14:46–57.
[19]   Donnelly JE, Blair SN, Jakicic JM, Manore MM, Rankin JW, Smith BK. American College of
       Sports Medicine Position Stand. Appropriate physical activity intervention strategies for weight
       loss and prevention of weight regain for adults. Med Sci Sports Exerc 2009;41:459–71.
[20]   Dunstan DW, Daly RM, Owen N, Jolley D, De Court, Shaw J, Zimmet P. High-intensity resis-
       tance training improves glycemic control in older patients with type 2 diabetes. Diabetes Care
       2002;25:1729–36.
[21]   Ekblom-Bak E, Hellenius ML, Ekblom O, Engstrom LM, Ekblom B. Independent associations of
       physical activity and cardiovascular fitness with cardiovascular risk in adults. Eur J Cardiovasc
       Prev Rehabil 2010;17:175–80.
[22]   Eyre H, Kahn R, Robertson RM, Clark NG, Doyle C, Hong Y, Gansler T, Glynn T, Smith RA,
       Taubert K, Thun MJ. Preventing cancer, cardiovascular disease, and diabetes: a common agenda
       for the American Cancer Society, the American Diabetes Association, and the American Heart
       Association. Stroke 2004;35:1999–2010.

[23] Fogelholm M. Physical activity, fitness and fatness: relations to mortality, morbidity and disease risk factors. A systematic review. Obes Rev 2010;11:202–21.

[24] Fox SM 3rd, Naughton JP, Haskell WL. Physical activity and the prevention of coronary heart disease. Ann Clin Res 1971;3:404–32.

[25] Franco OH, de Laet C, Peeters A, Jonker J, Mackenbach J, Nusselder W. Effects of physical activity on life expectancy with cardiovascular disease. Arch Intern Med 2005;165:2355–60.

[26] Ginis KA, Hicks AL. Considerations for the development of a physical activity guide for Canadians with physical disabilities. Can J Public Health 2007;98(Suppl 2):S135–47.

[27] Gorczynski P, Faulkner G. Exercise therapy for schizophrenia. Cochrane Database Syst Rev 2010;CD004412.

[28] Gordon BA, Benson AC, Bird SR, Fraser SF. Resistance training improves metabolic health in type 2 diabetes: a systematic review. Diabetes Res Clin Pract 2009;83:157–75.

[29] Guh DP, Zhang W, Bansback N, Amarsi Z, Birmingham CL, Anis AH. The incidence of co-morbidities related to obesity and overweight: a systematic review and meta-analysis. BMC Public Health 2009;9:88.

[30] Hackam DG, Khan NA, Hemmelgarn BR, Rabkin SW, Touyz RM, Campbell NR, Padwal R, Campbell TS, Lindsay MP, Hill MD, Quinn RR, Mahon JL, Herman RJ, Schiffrin EL, Ruzicka M, Larochelle P, Feldman RD, Lebel M, Poirier L, Arnold JM, Moe GW, Howlett JG, Trudeau L, Bacon SL, Petrella RJ, Milot A, Stone JA, Drouin D, Boulanger JM, Sharma M, Hamet P, Fodor G, Dresser GK, Carruthers SG, Pylypchuk G, Burgess ED, Burns KD, Vallee M, Prasad GV, Gilbert RE, Leiter LA, Jones C, Ogilvie RI, Woo V, McFarlane PA, Hegele RA, Tobe SW. The 2010 Canadian Hypertension Education Program recommendations for the management of hypertension. Part 2: therapy. Can J Cardiol 2010;26:249–58.

[31] Hamburg NM, McMackin CJ, Huang AL, Shenouda SM, Widlansky ME, Schulz E, Gokce N, Ruderman NB, Keaney JF Jr, Vita JA. Physical inactivity rapidly induces insulin resistance and microvascular dysfunction in healthy volunteers. Arterioscler Thromb Vasc Biol 2007;27:2650–6.

[32] Hansen D, Dendale P, van Loon LJ, Meeusen R. The impact of training modalities on the clinical benefits of exercise intervention in patients with cardiovascular disease risk or type 2 diabetes mellitus. Sports Med 2010;40:921–40.

[33] Haskell WL, Blair SN, Hill JO. Physical activity: health outcomes and importance for public health policy. Prev Med 2009;49:280–2.

[34] Haskell WL, Kiernan M. Methodologic issues in measuring physical activity and physical fitness when evaluating the role of dietary supplements for physically active people. Am J Clin Nutr 2000;72:541S–50S.

[35] Heggelund J, Nilsberg GE, Hoff J, Morken G, Helgerud J. Effects of high aerobic intensity training in patients with schizophrenia: a controlled trial. Nord J Psychiatry 2011;65:269–75.

[36] Herr KA, Mobily PR, Smith C. Depression and the experience of chronic back pain: a study of related variables and age differences. Clin J Pain 1993;9:104–14.

[37] Hestbaek L, Leboeuf-Yde C, Manniche C. Is low back pain part of a general health pattern or is it a separate and distinctive entity? A critical literature review of comorbidity with low back pain. J Manipulative Physiol Ther 2003;26:243–52.

[38] Hillsdon M, Foster C, Thorogood M. Interventions for promoting physical activity. Cochrane Database Syst Rev 2005;CD003180.

[39] Hordern MD, Dunstan DW, Prins JB, Baker MK, Singh MA, Coombes JS. Exercise prescription for patients with type 2 diabetes and pre-diabetes: a position statement from exercise and sport science Australia. J Sci Med Sport 2012;15:25–31.

[40] Johnson JL, Slentz CA, Houmard JA, Samsa GP, Duscha BD, Aiken LB, McCartney JS, Tanner CJ, Kraus WE. Exercise training amount and intensity effects on metabolic syndrome (from studies of a targeted risk reduction intervention through defined exercise). Am J Cardiol 2007;100:1759–66.

[41] Karvonen J, Vuorimaa T. Heart rate and exercise intensity during sports activities. Practical application. Sports Med 1988;5:303–11.

[42] Kauppila LI. Atherosclerosis and disc degeneration/low-back pain: a systematic review. Eur J Vasc Endovasc Surg 2009;37:661–70.

[43] Kesaniemi YK, Danforth E Jr, Jensen MD, Kopelman PG, Lefebvre P, Reeder BA. Dose-response issues concerning physical activity and health: an evidence-based symposium. Med Sci Sports Exerc 2001;33:S351–8.

[44] Kodama S, Saito K, Tanaka S, Maki M, Yachi Y, Asumi M, Sugawara A, Totsuka K, Shimano H, Ohashi Y, Yamada N, Sone H. Cardiorespiratory fitness as a quantitative predictor of all-cause mortality and cardiovascular events in healthy men and women: a meta-analysis. JAMA 2009;301:2024–35.

[45] Krogh-Madsen R, Thyfault JP, Broholm C, Mortensen OH, Olsen RH, Mounier R, Plomgaard P, Hall GV, Booth FW, Pedersen BK. A two-week reduction of ambulatory activity attenuates peripheral insulin sensitivity. J Appl Physiol 2010;108:134–40.

[46] Kujala UM. Evidence for exercise therapy in the treatment of chronic disease based on at least three randomized controlled trials: summary of published systematic reviews. Scand J Med Sci Sports 2004;14:339–45.

[47] Kujala UM. Evidence on the effects of exercise therapy in the treatment of chronic disease. Br J Sports Med 2009;43:550–5.

[48] Lemaster JW, Reiber GE, Smith DG, Heagerty PJ, Wallace C. Daily weight-bearing activity does not increase the risk of diabetic foot ulcers. Med Sci Sports Exerc 2003;35:1093–9.

[49] Little JP, Safdar A, Wilkin GP, Tarnopolsky MA, Gibala MJ. A practical model of low-volume high-intensity interval training induces mitochondrial biogenesis in human skeletal muscle: potential mechanisms. J Physiol 2010;588:1011–22.

[50] Logue J, Thompson L, Romanes F, Wilson DC, Thompson J, Sattar N. Management of obesity: summary of SIGN guideline. BMJ 2010;340:c154.

[51] Marwick TH, Hordern MD, Miller T, Chyun DA, Bertoni AG, Blumenthal RS, Philippides G, Rocchini A. Exercise training for type 2 diabetes mellitus: impact on cardiovascular risk: a scientific statement from the American Heart Association. Circulation 2009;119:3244–62.

[52] McDonough SM, Tully MA, O'Connor SR, Boyd A, Kerr DP, O'Neill SM, Delitto A, Bradbury I, Tudor-Locke C, Baxter DG, Hurley DA. The back 2 activity trial: education and advice versus education and advice plus a structured walking programme for chronic low back pain. BMC Musculoskelet Disord 2010;11:163.

[53] Mead GE, Morley W, Campbell P, Greig CA, McMurdo M, Lawlor DA. Exercise for depression. Cochrane Database Syst Rev 2009;CD004366.

[54] National Cholesterol Education Program. Third Report of the National Cholesterol Education Program (NCEP) Expert Panel on Detection, Evaluation, and Treatment of High Blood Cholesterol in Adults (Adult Treatment Panel III). Final report. Circulation 2002;106:3143–421.

[55] National Institute for Health and Clinical Excellence. Hypertension: clinical management of primary hypertension in adults. NICE Clinical Guideline. National Institute for Health and Clinical Excellence; 2011. Available at: http://guidance.nice.org.uk/CG127.

[56] Oldridge NB. Economic burden of physical inactivity: healthcare costs associated with cardiovascular disease. Eur J Cardiovasc Prev Rehabil 2008;15:130–9.

[57] Owen A, Wiles J, Swaine I. Effect of isometric exercise on resting blood pressure: a meta analysis. J Hum Hypertens 2010;24:796–800.

[58] Pavy-Le Traon A, Heer M, Narici MV, Rittweger J, Vernikos J. From space to Earth: advances in human physiology from 20 years of bed rest studies (1986–2006). Eur J Appl Physiol 2007;101:143–194.

[59] Pedersen BK, Saltin B. Evidence for prescribing exercise as therapy in chronic disease. Scand J Med Sci Sports 2006;16(Suppl 1):3–63.

[60] Pollock ML, Gaesser GA, Butcher JD, Despres J-P, Dishman RK, Franklin BA, et al. American College of Sports Medicine Position Stand. The recommended quantity and quality of exercise for developing and maintaining cardiorespiratory and muscular fitness, and flexibility in healthy adults. Med Sci Sports Exerc 1998;30:975–91.

[61] Rethorst CD, Wipfli BM, Landers DM. The antidepressive effects of exercise: a meta-analysis of randomized trials. Sports Med 2009;39:491–511.

[62] Robergs RA, Landwehr R. The surprising history of the "HRmax = 220 – age" equation. J Am Soc Exerc Physiol 2002;5:1–10.

[63] Sassen B, Cornelissen VA, Kiers H, Wittink H, Kok G, Vanhees L. Physical fitness matters more than physical activity in controlling cardiovascular disease risk factors. Eur J Cardiovasc Prev Rehabil 2009;16:677–83.

[64] Schneider S, Mohnen SM, Schiltenwolf M, Rau C. Comorbidity of low back pain: representative outcomes of a national health study in the Federal Republic of Germany. Eur J Pain 2007;11:387–97.

[65] Schumann B, Bolm-Audorff U, Bergmann A, Ellegast R, Elsner G, Grifka J, Haerting J, Jager M, Michaelis M, Seidler A. Lifestyle factors and lumbar disc disease: results of a German multi-center case-control study (EPILIFT). Arthritis Res Ther 2010;12:R193.

[66] Shaw K, Gennat H, O'Rourke P, Del Mar C. Exercise for overweight or obesity. Cochrane Database Syst Rev 2006;CD003817.

[67] Sigal RJ, Kenny GP, Boule NG, Wells GA, Prud'homme D, Fortier M, Reid RD, Tulloch H, Coyle D, Phillips P, Jennings A, Jaffey J. Effects of aerobic training, resistance training, or both on glycemic control in type 2 diabetes: a randomized trial. Ann Intern Med 2007;147:357–69.

[68] Smidt N, de Vet HC, Bouter LM, Dekker J, Arendzen JH, de Bie RA, Bierma-Zeinstra SM, Helders PJ, Keus SH, Kwakkel G, Lenssen T, Oostendorp RA, Ostelo RW, Reijman M, Terwee CB, Theunissen C, Thomas S, van Baar ME, van't Hul A, van Peppen RP, Verhagen A, van der Windt DA. Effectiveness of exercise therapy: a best-evidence summary of systematic reviews. Aust J Physiother 2005;51:71–85.

[69] Snowling NJ, Hopkins WG. Effects of different modes of exercise training on glucose control and risk factors for complications in type 2 diabetic patients: a meta-analysis. Diabetes Care 2006;29:2518–27.

[70] Stensvold D, Tjonna AE, Skaug EA, Aspenes S, Stolen T, Wisloff U, Slordahl SA. Strength training versus aerobic interval training to modify risk factors of the metabolic syndrome. J Appl Physiol 2010;108:804–10.

[71] Strasser B, Siebert U, Schobersberger W. Resistance training in the treatment of the metabolic syndrome: a systematic review and meta-analysis of the effect of resistance training on metabolic clustering in patients with abnormal glucose metabolism. Sports Med 2010;40:397–415.

[72] Stratton IM, Adler AI, Neil HA, Matthews DR, Manley SE, Cull CA, Hadden D, Turner RC, Holman RR. Association of glycaemia with macrovascular and microvascular complications of type 2 diabetes (UKPDS 35): prospective observational study. BMJ 2000;321:405–12.

[73] Sullivan MJ, Reesor K, Mikail S, Fisher R. The treatment of depression in chronic low back pain: review and recommendations. Pain 1992;50:5–13.

[74] Tanaka H, Monahan KD, Seals DR. Age-predicted maximal heart rate revisited. J Am Coll Cardiol 2001;37:153–6.

[75] Taylor NF, Dodd KJ, Shields N, Bruder A. Therapeutic exercise in physiotherapy practice is beneficial: a summary of systematic reviews 2002–2005. Aust J Physiother 2007;53:7–16.

[76] Thomas DE, Elliott EJ, Naughton GA. Exercise for type 2 diabetes mellitus. Cochrane Database Syst Rev 2006;3:CD002968.

[77] Thorogood A, Mottillo S, Shimony A, Filion KB, Joseph L, Genest J, Pilote L, Poirier P, Schiffrin EL, Eisenberg MJ. Isolated aerobic exercise and weight loss: a systematic review and meta-analysis of randomized controlled trials. Am J Med 2011;124:747–55.

[78] Tjonna AE, Lee SJ, Rognmo O, Stolen TO, Bye A, Haram PM, Loennechen JP, Al Share QY, Skogvoll E, Slordahl SA, Kemi OJ, Najjar SM, Wisloff U. Aerobic interval training versus continuous moderate exercise as a treatment for the metabolic syndrome: a pilot study. Circulation 2008;118:346–54.

[79] Umpierre D, Ribeiro PA, Kramer CK, Leitao CB, Zucatti AT, Azevedo MJ, Gross JL, Ribeiro JP, Schaan BD. Physical activity advice only or structured exercise training and association with HbA1c levels in type 2 diabetes: a systematic review and meta-analysis. JAMA 2011;305:1790–9.

[80] U.S. Department of Health and Human Services. Physical activity guidelines for Americans. U.S. Department of Health and Human Services; 2008.

[81] Vanhees L, Stevens A. Exercise intensity: a matter of measuring or of talking? J Cardiopulm Rehabil 2006;26:78–9.

[82] Verbunt JA, Smeets RJ, Wittink HM. Cause or effect? Deconditioning and chronic low back pain. Pain 2010;149:428–30.

[83] Von Korff M, Crane P, Lane M, Miglioretti DL, Simon G, Saunders K, Stang P, Brandenburg N, Kessler R. Chronic spinal pain and physical-mental comorbidity in the United States: results from the national comorbidity survey replication. Pain 2005;113:331–9.

[84] Washburn RA, Zhu W, McAuley E, Frogley M, Figoni SF. The physical activity scale for individuals with physical disabilities: development and evaluation. Arch Phys Med Rehabil 2002;83:193–200.

[85] Wildgust HJ, Beary M. Are there modifiable risk factors which will reduce the excess mortality in schizophrenia? J Psychopharmacol 2010;24:37–50.

[86] Williams MA, Haskell WL, Ades PA, Amsterdam EA, Bittner V, Franklin BA, Gulanick M, Laing
      ST, Stewart KJ. Resistance exercise in individuals with and without cardiovascular disease: 2007
      update: a scientific statement from the American Heart Association Council on Clinical Cardiol-
      ogy and Council on Nutrition, Physical Activity, and Metabolism. Circulation 2007;116:572–84.
[87] Wipfli BM, Rethorst CD, Landers DM. The anxiolytic effects of exercise: a meta-analysis of ran-
      domized trials and dose-response analysis. J Sport Exerc Psychol 2008;30:392–410.
[88] Wittink H, Verbunt JA. Physical rehabilitation in patients with chronic pain. In: Benzon HT,
      Rathmell JP, Wu CL, Turk DC, Argoff CE, editors. Raj's practical management of pain. Philadel-
      phia: Mosby Elsevier; 2008. p. 773–84.
[89] World Health Organization. Obesity: preventing and managing the global epidemic. Report of a
      WHO consultation. World Health Organ Tech Rep Ser 2000;894:i–xii, 1–253.
[90] World Health Organization. Physical activity. Geneva: World Health Organization; 2010.
[91] World Health Organization. The international classification of functioning, disability and health
      (ICF), 2nd edition. Geneva: World Health Organization; 2001.
[92] Zhao G, Ford ES, Li C, Tsai J, Dhingra S, Balluz LS. Waist circumference, abdominal obesity, and
      depression among overweight and obese U.S. adults: national health and nutrition examination
      survey 2005–2006. BMC Psychiatry 2011;11:130.

Correspondence to: Harriet M. Wittink, PT, PhD, Lifestyle and Health Research
Group, Faculty of Health Care, Utrecht University of Applied Research, PO Box
85182, 3508 AD Utrecht, The Netherlands. Email: harriet.wittink@hu.nl.

Psychological Management of Chronic Pain and Comorbidities

Lance M. McCracken

Health Psychology Section, Psychology Department, Institute of Psychiatry, King's College London; INPUT Pain Management Service, Guys' and St Thomas' NHS Foundation Trust, London, United Kingdom

Chronic pain can be associated with many problems in health and daily living. In turn, these problems can affect the pain experience, create further problems of their own, and interact with each other. Here we are calling these additional problems "comorbidities," and they include a full range of symptoms, syndromes, and conditions of mental or physical ill health. In the context of these associated problems the complexity of chronic pain increases, which can drastically reduce a person's health and functioning. Hence, it is important to understand the many comorbidities of chronic pain and how they interrelate with each other, so that they can be predicted, identified, and treated. Psychological approaches have proven effective in the treatment of chronic pain and of many of the problems associated with it. Some of these approaches will be reviewed in this chapter.

Applications of psychological approaches have a long history in physical health problems, including chronic pain. These applications also continue to develop and expand. In addition to chronic pain, the physical health problem areas include epilepsy, cancer, chronic fatigue,

Pain Comorbidities: Understanding and Treating the Complex Patient
edited by Maria Adele Giamberardino and Troels Staehelin Jensen
IASP Press, Seattle, © 2012

453

diabetes, hypertension and cardiac conditions, insomnia, obesity, and smoking cessation [27]. It is not possible to adequately review psychological applications for all emotional and physical conditions potentially comorbid with chronic pain within the scope of a single chapter. This chapter will review four problem areas that represent some of the most common collateral complaints presented by people seeking treatment for chronic pain: mood disturbance, insomnia, fatigue, and cognitive impairment.

Comorbid Mood Problems

Mood and Chronic Pain

Community and clinical studies consistently show that both emotional distress and diagnosable mood disturbance occur at high rates in conjunction with chronic pain. It is estimated that between 30% and 54% of those seeking treatment for chronic pain also meet diagnostic criteria for a depressive disorder [1]. In a sample of nearly 6,000 representative individuals with chronic pain from the United States, 20.2% of those surveyed reported an episode of depression in the last year [32], similar to the 17.5% found in another study [53]. A large household survey from Canada found that people with chronic pain were three times more likely to be depressed than those without chronic pain [5].

Dersh and colleagues [9] reported prevalence rates of between 16.5% and 28.8% for comorbid anxiety disorders, such as panic disorder and generalized anxiety disorder, in patients with chronic pain. McWilliams et al. [32] found that 35.1% of people with chronic pain also met criteria for anxiety disorders. A large-scale international survey examined comorbidities in more than 85,088 individuals across 17 countries. The odds ratios (with confidence intervals) for people with chronic pain having specific comorbid disorders were 2.8 for dysthymia (CI = 2.5–3.2), 2.7 for generalized anxiety disorder (CI = 2.4–3.1), 2.6 for post-traumatic stress disorder (CI = 2.3–3.0), 2.3 for major depression (CI = 2.1–2.5), 2.1 for agoraphobia or panic (CI = 1.9–2.4) and 1.9 for social phobia (CI = 1.7–2.2) [8].

Negative impacts of chronic pain on functioning appear to increase if significant mood problems are also present. A study of 21,425 people in Europe showed that people with both pain and depression took more than double the number of days off work per month compared with people who had only pain or depression in isolation, and people with both pain and depression reported taking more than five times as many days off work compared with those with neither pain nor depression [7].

Psychological Approaches to Anxiety and Depression in Chronic Pain

There are many ways to treat depression and anxiety, medication being perhaps the most frequent choice. Among psychological approaches, cognitive-behavioral therapy (CBT) and behavior therapy for depression are deemed to have "strong research support" from the Society of Clinical Psychology of the American Psychological Association (Division 12, APA) [47]. These approaches include a range of methods, typically used in combination. Cognitive therapy methods include exercises to monitor moods, thoughts, and behavior, aiming to identify dysfunctional thoughts and beliefs and then change them. Behavioral methods include techniques to gradually increase engagement with physical and social situations and with direct experiences, as an alternative to an inward focus on ruminative thought patterns.

Trials investigating separate components of treatment for depression show that for severe depression, therapy classified as "behavioral activation" alone is comparable in efficacy to antidepressant medication use and more efficacious than cognitive therapy methods alone [10]. Results from meta-analyses show that CBT as a package is superior to antidepressant medication in the treatment of depression [3]. Other studies suggest that both cognitive therapy methods and behavioral activation are less expensive and longer lasting than medication for depression, and treatment effects are substantial [11,20].

Research support is also strong for CBT in the treatment of several anxiety disorders, including generalized anxiety disorder, obsessive compulsive disorder, panic disorder, post-traumatic stress disorder, social phobia, and various specific phobias [47]. Cognitive therapy methods as described for depression are frequently used with anxiety disorders. Another important method is what is called "exposure." Exposure therapy consists of coordinating contact between the person with the anxiety disorder and the situations that occasion anxiety and avoidance. Either sessions including repeated graduated contact or sessions of prolonged contact are conducted to create changes in anxious responses, including avoidance, so that formerly anxiety-provoking situations no longer lead to restrictions in functioning.

As in treatment for depression, CBT produces large treatment effects for generalized anxiety disorder, panic disorder, post-traumatic stress disorder, and social phobia [3]. Once again, CBT seems to produce enduring effects, effects that are longer lasting than medication [20]. There is even evidence that medication can actually undermine the effects of CBT [20].

Results from studies of CBT for depression and anxiety in general are useful but do not answer the specific question about treatment for depression and anxiety comorbid with chronic pain. An interesting meta-analysis showed that comorbid psychiatric disorders in general do not appear to affect the magnitude of treatment effects for anxiety disorders [40]. While encouraging, this evidence also does not answer the question of the effectiveness of treatment for depression or anxiety in those with chronic pain.

There are many individual studies that show that depression and anxiety improve with treatments for chronic pain based broadly on CBT [30,44,50,57], although the evidence tends to be stronger for improvement in depression than in anxiety. Interestingly, meta-analyses of randomized controlled trials (RCTs) of CBT for chronic pain have not consistently supported a significant treatment effect on depression. A meta-analysis of these methods focusing on chronic low back pain alone showed an effect on depression [19], while similar meta-analyses that focused on general chronic pain did not [13,36]. On the other hand, newer approaches within CBT that are referred to as "acceptance-based" show small to moderate significant effects on anxiety and depression based on five controlled clinical trials and nine RCTs [51]. These treatments include mindfulness-based methods and acceptance and commitment therapy (ACT) [18]. Although promising and growing, the evidence-based support for these approaches remains relatively immature.

Chronic Pain and Comorbid Insomnia

Sleep and Chronic Pain

Pain is commonly identified as a cause of sleep disturbance, and sleep disturbance is a common complaint in people with chronic pain [33]. In a large survey of 4,839 people with chronic pain in Europe, 65% reported sleep problems [2]. Among patients receiving specialty services for chronic pain, as many as 79% meet criteria for significant insomnia [31]. The experience of sleep disturbance in people with chronic pain is associated with a wide range of adverse outcomes, including reports of more severe pain, worse anxiety and depression, and greater disability [29,45,46,49].

Psychological Approaches to Insomnia

As with treatment for depression and anxiety, medications are frequently used as treatment for insomnia. Among nonpharmacological treatments, cognitive-behavioral and behavioral therapies appear to be the most firmly established approaches for insomnia. Division 12 of the APA lists CBT, sleep restriction therapy, stimulus control therapy, relaxation, and paradoxical intention as having strong research support [47]. Many therapists would regard this entire set of methods as generally consistent with a cognitive-behavioral approach. CBT generally focuses on changing maladaptive behaviors and dysfunctional thought patterns that perpetuate sleep problems. Maladaptive behaviors can include irregular sleep patterns and daytime napping. Dysfunctional thoughts can include thoughts about how *terrible* it will be if sleep is inadequate and thoughts that one *must* get a certain amount of sleep. Sleep restriction is, just as it sounds, a process of using systematic sleep deprivation to enhance sleep efficiency (time asleep in relation to time in bed) and regularity. In a sense, stimulus control, relaxation, and paradoxical intention are each intended to reduce anxiety, tension, and arousal around bedtime. Paradoxical intention, interestingly, does so by asking patients to try to stay awake as long as they can, thus reducing pressure to sleep and related "performance anxiety."

Meta-analyses show that broadly cognitive-behavioral methods are effective for insomnia, including moderate to large effects on sleep quality, that are well sustained over time, in both middle-aged and older adults [21,35]. These methods are deemed effective for patients with insomnia that is secondary to a primary psychiatric or medical condition and can facilitate discontinuation of medication in chronic hypnotic medication users [35]. There is evidence that CBT for insomnia can improve sleep and decrease pain in patients with osteoarthritis [52].

In a trial of CBT designed specifically for insomnia secondary to chronic pain, 57% of patients showed reliable improvement in sleep quality. However, only 18% achieved full recovery from their sleeping problems (reflected in restoration of sleep quality to within a normal range) [6]. Cognitive-behavioral approaches to insomnia and chronic pain continue to develop. Promising new approaches for combinations of chronic pain and insomnia include mindfulness-based approaches [41] and ACT [25,31].

Chronic Pain and Comorbid Fatigue

Fatigue and Chronic Pain

More than 75% of people seeking treatment for chronic pain also report fatigue [22], and as many as 93% of people with chronic fatigue syndrome report headache or muscle pain [23]. Clearly, the co-occurrence of these symptoms is very high. In fact, chronic fatigue syndrome includes multiple symptoms, including severe persistent fatigue, sleep disturbance, difficulties with concentration, headaches, and muscle pain [15]. Hence, more or less, chronic pain is built into the definition of this condition. Chronic pain and chronic fatigue are similar problems in some ways, as both can defy easy medical explanation, both can lead to struggles for control over the experiences, and both can lead to reduced activities.

There is an interesting contrast in approaches to chronic pain and chronic fatigue. It tends to be more accepted in treating chronic pain that increased activity and even vigorous exercise can be beneficial, even if there is an increase in pain in the short term. In chronic fatigue there seems to be a stronger sense that limiting activity is necessary and that physical exercise can worsen the condition, at least within some approaches [55]. This situation creates a potential dilemma where appropriate management of one condition may be seen as exacerbating the other.

Psychological Approaches to Comorbid Fatigue

Evidence-based guidelines, such as those produced by the National Institute for Health and Clinical Excellence (NICE) in the United Kingdom, recommend CBT as well as other behavioral approaches, including graded exercise therapy (GET) and activity management, for chronic fatigue [39]. As usual, CBT includes validating the patients' experiences, building rapport, formulating the symptoms and the factors that influence them into a working model, and then applying methods for changing symptoms and behavior. Identifying and managing factors that exacerbate symptoms is a primary focus. Sleep and activity management methods form another focus of treatment. Both GET and activity management are specifically focused on creating healthy patterns of activity by systematically introducing changes in how daily activities are structured. Both approaches start by establishing a baseline of activity and then attempt to create steady sustainable activities that are consistent with individuals' goals.

There are several meta-analyses of treatments for chronic fatigue that include broadly psychological methods, and specifically CBT. One of these meta-analyses identified 13 studies that included random assignment to a cognitive-behavioral treatment or a control condition. These studies included 1371 participants and yielded 15 effect sizes. The average effect after treatment was close to medium-sized, but technically small (d = 0.48) [26]. These analyses found that 50% of participants were no longer in the clinical range on fatigue after completion of treatment, based on five studies that provided these data. A slightly more recent meta-analysis essentially produced the same conclusion, that CBT is effective for reducing chronic fatigue at the completion of treatment, but results at follow-up are somewhat less clear [42].

Two particular treatment trials for chronic fatigue are notable. One trial sought to determine whether CBT for chronic fatigue is also effective for pain and included adults and adolescents with chronic fatigue [24]. Their analyses showed that those participants who reached a normal range of fatigue after treatment, and were thus classed as recovered, also reported significant reductions in pain. In the other trial, what is called "adaptive pacing therapy" (APT) was compared to CBT, GET, and specialist medical care in a relatively large sample of 641 participants [55]. In this trial, both CBT and GET were superior to APT in their impact on fatigue and on physical functioning. This study is interesting because the theory behind APT would not predict this result. APT is designed around the idea that chronic fatigue syndrome is an organic disease that results in a finite amount of energy and that its core processes of pathology cannot be improved by changes in behavior. APT is essentially designed around the goal of reducing or avoiding fatigue.

Chronic Pain and Comorbid Impaired Cognitive Functioning

Cognitive Functioning and Chronic Pain

Difficulties with concentration, memory, and other aspects of cognitive functioning are very common in people seeking treatment for chronic pain. Around 54–62% of adults seeking treatment for chronic pain at a university medical center reported at least one problem with attention, concentration, or memory [28,43].

In a large population-based study of community-dwelling adults aged 50 years and older in the United Kingdom, 46.5% reported at least one cognitive complaint [54]. In this study, cognitive complaints were 50% higher for those over 80 years old compared to those in their fifties, and the frequency of complaints was about 70% higher in those reporting pain. Cognitive complaints appear to be associated with greater pain severity, anxiety, and depression [28,38,43].

Great difficulties are inherent in attempting to understand relations between chronic pain and cognitive functioning. Obviously, people with chronic pain do not experience pain in isolation. They also experience depression, anxiety, fatigue, sleeping problems, comorbid medical conditions, and the effects of medications. Any of these variables may underlie complaints of cognitive impairment or measured impairments in cognitive functioning.

Effects of Analgesic Medications on Cognitive Functioning

Among analgesic medications that raise concerns for cognitive functioning, opioids appear to be of particular concern. Current clinical guidelines from the American Pain Society and American Academy of Pain Medicine state that chronic opioid therapy can be effective for selected and monitored patients with chronic pain [4]. These guidelines also note that opioid use can lead to adverse effects, such as "transient or lasting cognitive impairment that may affect driving and work safety" (p. 122).

Opinions vary. One recent study concluded that both short-term and long-term opioid use can have broad effects on cognitive performance, including impairment in attention, concentration, visual and verbal recall, visual-spatial skills, psychomotor speed, and hand-eye coordination [17]. Long-term opioid use can affect executive functions such as the ability to adapt one's behavior and inhibit inappropriate responses. Results in this review were derived from normal subjects, heroin users, and patients in methadone maintenance, as well as some samples of pain patients. The generalizability of these results to patients with chronic pain is not clear. In another review that excluded current or recovering substance abusers, the conclusions were far more positive, deeming impairments in cognitive functioning to be minimal [14]. There are calls for further research into the mechanisms of pain- and analgesia-induced effects on cognitive functioning [37].

Psychological Approaches to Comorbid Cognitive Complaints

Rehabilitative treatments for people who have cognitive complaints as a result of head trauma appear to be reasonably effective [e.g., 34]. However, most patients with chronic pain who present with cognitive complaints have no history of head trauma [28]. The literature on treatment of cognitive complaints in people with no history of head injury or neurological disease is not very well developed.

As an approach to their clinical management, cognitive complaints must first be assessed to see if their roots lie directly in some medical condition or whether they are secondary to psychological influences, or both. People who find themselves having difficulty with cognitive functioning are likely to have many thoughts, beliefs, judgments, and emotional reactions in relation to these difficulties and their meaning [16]. Their behavior is likely to be affected by these many experiences. Essentially, ruminating, catastrophizing, or obsessing about poor memory and concentration can lead to poor memory and concentration.

The methods and processes of mindfulness and ACT appear particularly well suited to dealing with cognitive complaints that are deemed to have a psychological component. First, many of the experiences encountered with chronic pain are uncontrollable, or at least uncontrollable on the timeline desired by the patient (some of the problems may subside over a longer term). Confusing situations around pain and comorbid symptoms can create a context of needing to analyze or know what is wrong. ACT includes specific methods for promoting acceptance and "letting go" of the struggles with these experiences, when doing so enhances daily functioning. Proponents of ACT assume that people are more likely to be effective and engaged in treatment and with their goals, once their efforts are freed from analyzing and struggling with pain-related experiences. Second, experiences of pain and other symptoms are likely to distract, disrupt, or disintegrate behavior patterns that require sustained attention [12]. Again, ACT and mindfulness-based methods can promote more skillful attention and awareness, which may decrease these interruptive effects. Third, patients' thoughts about their pain and health may have a worried, ruminative, or catastrophizing quality [48]. ACT has specific methods for what is called cognitive defusion for reducing the impact of dominating and emotionally evocative thoughts. Finally, values-based methods from ACT can help patients to connect or reconnect with the directions they deem important and desirable in their lives, even if these directions include barriers or challenges that they did not encounter before, such as problems with cognitive functioning.

Summary

In this chapter, a number of particular conditions comorbid with chronic pain have been reviewed. They were selected because they are common complaints seen in clinical practice in patients with chronic pain and because they appear amenable or potentially amenable to psychological treatment methods. Depression, anxiety, insomnia, and fatigue each appear to be effectively treated with broadly cognitive-behavioral methods, even though some patients may not achieve full recovery from their symptoms, or full recovery of their functioning, from these methods.

With impaired cognitive functioning or complaints of impaired cognitive functioning, the other comorbid condition reviewed here, effective treatment is not yet clear. Another area touched on in this chapter was the effects of analgesic medication on cognitive functioning. This area is of high current interest to clinicians; however, further study will be needed before the adverse roles of analgesics on patient functioning, and ways to manage these effects, can be better understood.

The four areas discussed here—mood problems, insomnia, fatigue, and impaired cognitive functioning—represent, in combination, a significant burden of additional symptoms for those with chronic pain. They provide the potential for interacting with each other and greatly magnifying the overall burden of ill health these people experience. Crucially, each of the comorbidities presented here defies clear medical explanation, much like chronic pain itself much of the time. By implication, they also defy clear medical solutions.

All the symptoms presented here happen in the experience of thinking, feeling, reacting, and problem-solving human beings. Each of the symptoms is confusing, distressing, threatening, and can lead to losses and to ultimately unhelpful, solicitous, stressful, or rejecting interactions with others. Whatever happens with our developing knowledge and skill in the medical management of these symptoms, these psychological aspects require our continued investigation and integration into wider management strategies.

While CBT has a good evidence base for most of the conditions presented here, there is room for the methods to produce larger effects, in more outcome domains, for more people, over a longer term. Some of the developments within CBT that may help to spark this improvement include those that involve mindfulness and acceptance-based methods.

References

[1]   Banks SM, Kerns RD. Explaining high rates of depression in chronic pain: a diathesis-stress framework. Psychol Bull 1996;119:95–110.
[2]   Breivik H, Collett B, Ventafridda V, Cohen R, Gallacher D. Survey of chronic pain in Europe: prevalence, impact, on daily life, and treatment. Eur J Pain 2006;10:287–333.
[3]   Butler AC, Chapman JE, Forman EM, Beck AT. The empirical status of cognitive-behavioral therapy: a review of meta-analyses. Clin Psychol Rev 2006;26:17–31.

[4]   Chou R, Fanciullo GJ, Fine PG, Adler JA, Ballantyne JC, Davies P, Donovan MI, Fishbain DA,
      Foley KM, Fudin J, Gilson A, Kelter A, Mauskop A, O'Connor PG, Passik SD, Pasternak GW,
      Portenoy RK, Rich BA, Roberts RG, Todd KH, Miaskowski C. Opioid treatment guideline:
      clinical guidelines for the use of chronic opioids therapy in chronic noncancer pain. J Pain
      2009;10:113–30.
[5]   Currie SR, Wang J. Chronic back pain and major depression in the general Canadian population.
      Pain 2004;107:54–60.
[6]   Currie SR, Wilson KG, Curran D. Clinical significance and predictors of treatment response to
      cognitive-behavior therapy for insomnia secondary to chronic pain. J Behav Med 2002;25:135–53.
[7]   Demyttenaere K, Bonnewyn A, Bruffaerts R, Brugha T, De Graaf R, Alonso J. Comorbid pain-
      ful physical symptoms and depression: prevalence, work loss, and help seeking. J Affect Disord
      2006;92:185–93.
[8]   Demyttenaere K, Bruffaerts R, Lee S, Posada-Villa J, Kovess V, Angermeyer MC, et al. Mental
      disorders among persons with chronic back or neck pain: results from the World Mental Health
      Surveys. Pain 2007;129:332–42.
[9]   Dersh J, Polatin PB, Gatchel RJ. Chronic pain and psychopathology: research findings and theo-
      retical considerations. Psychosom Med 2002;64:773–86.
[10] Dimidjian A, Hollon SD, Dobson KS, Schmaling KB, Kohlenberg RJ, Addis ME, Gallop R, Mc-
      Glinchey JB, Markely DK, Gollan JK, Atkins DC, Dunner DL, Jacobson NS. Randomized trial of
      behavioral activation, cognitive therapy, and antidepressant medication in the acute treatment of
      adults with major depression. J Consult Clin Psychol 2006;74:658–70.
[11] Dobson KS, Hollon SD, Dimidgian S, Schmaling KB, Kohlenberg RJ, Gallop RJ, Rizvi SL, Gollan
      JK, Dunner DL, Jacobson NS. Randomized trial of behavioral activation, cognitive therapy, and
      antidepressant medication in the prevention of relapse an recurrence in major depression. J
      Consult Clin Psychol 2008;76:468–77.
[12] Eccleston C, Crombez G. Pain demands attention: a cognitive-affective model of the interruptive
      function of pain. Psychol Bull 1999;125:356–66.
[13] Eccleston C, Williams ACDC, Morley S. Psychological therapies for the management of chronic
      pain (excluding headache) in adults. Cochrane Database Syst Rev 2009;2:CD007407.
[14] Ersek M, Cherrier MM, Overman SS, Irving GA. The cognitive effects of opioids. Pain Manage
      Nursing 2004;5:75–93.
[15] Fukuda K, Straus SE, Hickie I, Sharpe MC, Dobbins JG, Kamaroff A. The chronic fatigue syn-
      drome: a comprehensive approach to its definition and study. Ann Intern Med 1994;121:953–9.
[16] Glass JM, Park DC, Minear M, Crofford LJ. Memory beliefs and function in fibromyalgia pa-
      tients. J Psychosom Res 2005;58:263–9.
[17] Gruber SA, Silveri MM, Yurgelun-Todd DA. Neuropsychological consequences of opiate use.
      Neuropsychol Rev 2007;17:299–315.
[18] Hayes SC, Strosahl K, Wilson KG. Acceptance and commitment therapy: an experiential ap-
      proach to behavior change. New York: Guilford Press; 1999.
[19] Hoffman BM, Papas RK, Chatkoff DK, Kerns RD. Meta-analysis of psychological interventions
      for chronic low back pain. Health Psychol 2007;26:1–9.
[20] Hollon SD, Stewart MO, Strunk D. Enduring effects for cognitive behavior therapy in the treat-
      ment of anxiety and depression. Annu Rev Psychol 2006;57:285–315.
[21] Irwin MR, Cole JC, Nicassio PM. Comparative meta-analysis of behavioral interventions for
      insomnia and their efficacy in middle-aged adults and in older adults 55+ years of age. Health
      Psychol 2006;25:3–14.
[22] Iverson GL, McCracken LM. "Postconcussive" symptoms in persons with chronic pain. Brain Inj
      1997;11:783–90.
[23] King C, Jason LA. Improving diagnostic criteria and procedures for chronic fatigue syndrome.
      Biol Psychol 2005;68:87–106.
[24] Knoop H, Stulemeijer M, Prins JB, van der Meer JWM, Bleijenberg G. Is cognitive behaviour
      therapy for chronic fatigue syndrome also effective form pain symptoms? Behav Res Ther
      2007;45:2034–43.
[25] Lundh LG. The role of acceptance and mindfulness in the treatment of insomnia. J Cogn Psycho-
      ther 2005;19:29–39.
[26] Malouff JM, Thorsteinsson EB, Rooke SE, Bhullar N, Schutte NS. Efficacy of cognitive behavioral
      therapy for chronic fatigue syndrome: a meta-analysis. Clin Psychol Rev 2008;28:736–45.

[27] McCracken LM, editor. Mindfulness and acceptance in behavioral medicine. Oakland, CA: New Harbinger; 2011.

[28] McCracken LM, Iverson GL. Predicting complaints of impaired cognitive functioning in patients with chronic pain. J Pain Symptom Manage 2001;21:392–6.

[29] McCracken LM, Iverson GL. Disrupted sleep patterns and daily functioning in patients with chronic pain. Pain Res Manag 2002;7:75–9.

[30] McCracken LM, Vowles KE, Eccleston C. Acceptance-based treatment for persons with complex, long standing chronic pain: a preliminary analysis of treatment outcome in comparison to a waiting phase. Behav Res Ther 2005;43:1335–46.

[31] McCracken LM, Williams JL, Tang NKY. Psychological flexibility may reduce insomnia in persons with chronic pain: a preliminary retrospective study. Pain Med 2011;12: 904–12.

[32] McWilliams LA, Cox BJ, Enns MW. Mood and anxiety disorders associated with chronic pain: an examination in a nationally representative sample. Pain 2003;106:127–33.

[33] Menefee LA, Cohen MJM, Anderson WR, Doghramji K, Frank ED, Lee H. Sleep disturbance and nonmalignant chronic pain: a comprehensive review of the literature. Pain Med 2000;1:156–72.

[34] Mittenberg W, Canyock EM, Condit D, Patton C. Treatment of post-concussion syndrome following mild head injury. J Clin Exp Neuropsych 2001;23:829–36.

[35] Morin C, Bootzin RR, Buysse DJ, Edinger JD, Espie CA, Lichstein KL. Psychological and behavioral treatment of insomnia: update of the recent evidence (1998–2004). Sleep 2006;29:1398–414.

[36] Morley SJ, Eccleston C, Williams A. Systematic review and meta-analysis of randomized controlled trials of cognitive behaviour therapy and behaviour therapy for chronic pain in adults, excluding headache. Pain 1999;80:1–13.

[37] Moriarity O, McGuire B, Finn DP. The effects of pain on cognitive functioning: a review of clinical and preclinical research. Prog Neurol 2011;93:385–404.

[38] Muñoz M, Esteve R. Reports of memory functioning by patients with chronic pain. Clin J Pain 2005;21:287–91.

[39] National Institute for Health and Clinical Excellence. Chronic fatigue syndrome/myalgic encephalomyelitis (or encephalopathy). Clinical guideline 53. National Institute for Health and Clinical Excellence; 2007. Available at: www.nice.org.uk.

[40] Olatunji BO, Cisler JM, Tolin DF. A meta-analysis of the influence of comorbidity on treatment outcome in the anxiety disorders. Clin Psychol Rev 2010;30:642–54.

[41] Ong JC, Shapiro SL, Manber R. Combining mindfulness meditation with cognitive-behavior therapy for insomnia: a treatment development study. Behav Ther 2008;39:171–82.

[42] Price JR, Mitchell E, Tidy E, Hunot V. Cognitive behaviour therapy for chronic fatigue syndrome in adults. Cochrane Database Syst Rev 2008;3:CD001027.

[43] Roth RS, Geisser ME, Theisen-Goodvich M, Dixon PJ. Cognitive complaints are associated with depression, fatigue, female sex, and pain catastrophizing in patients with chronic pain. Arch Phys Med Rehabil 2005;86:1147–54.

[44] Slater MA, Doctor JN, Pruitt SD, Atkinson JH. The clinical significance of behavioral treatment for chronic low back pain: an evaluation of effectiveness. Pain 1997;71:257–63.

[45] Smith MT, Haythornthwaite JA. How do sleep disturbance and chronic pain inter-relate? Insights from the longitudinal and cognitive-behavioral clinical trials literature. Sleep Med Rev 2004; 8:119–32.

[46] Smith MT, Perlis ML, Smith DE, Giles DE, Carmody TP. Sleep quality and presleep arousal in chronic pain. J Behav Med 2000;23:1–13.

[47] Society of Clinical Psychology, Division 12 of the American Psychological Association. Research-supported psychological therapies. Available at: http://www.div12.org/Psychological-Treatments/treatments/chronicpain_act.html. Accessed 7 August, 2011.

[48] Sullivan MJ, Thorn B, Haythornthwaite JA, Keefe F, Martin M, Bradley LA, et al. Theoretical perspectives on the relation between catastrophizing and pain. Clin J Pain 2001;17:52–64.

[49] Tang NKY, Wright K, Salkovskis PM. Prevalence and correlates of clinical insomnia co-occurring with chronic pain. J Sleep Res 2007;16:85–95.

[50] Turner JA, Mancl L, Aaron LA. Short- and long-term efficacy of brief cognitive-behavioral therapy for patients with chronic temporomandibular disorder pain: a randomized, controlled trial. Pain 2006;121:181–94.

[51] Veehof MM, Oskam MJ, Schreurs KMG, Bohlmeijer ET. Acceptance-based interventions for the treatment of chronic pain: a systematic review and meta-analysis. Pain 2011;152:533–42.

[52] Vitiello MV, Rybarczyk B, Von Korff M, Stepanski EJ. Cognitive behavioral therapy for insomnia improves sleep and decreases pain n older adults with co-morbid insomnia and osteoarthritis. J Clin Sleep Med 2009;5:355–62.

[53] Von Korff M, Crane P, Lane M, Miglioretti DL, Simon G, Saunders K, et al. Chronic spinal pain and physical-mental comorbidity in the United States: results from the national comorbidity survey replication. Pain 2005;113:331–9.

[54] Westoby CJ, Mallen CD, Thomas E. Cognitive complaints in a general population of older adults: prevalence, association with pain and the influence of concurrent affective disorders. Eur J Pain 2009;13:970–6.

[55] White PD, Goldsmith KA, Johnson AL, Potts L, Walwyn R, DeCesare JC, Baber HL, Burgess M, Clark LV, Cox DL, Bavinton J, Angus BJ, Murphy G, Murphy M, O'Dowd H, Wilkes D, McCrone P, Chalder T, Sharpe M. Comparison of adaptive pacing therapy, cognitive behaviour therapy, graded exercise therapy, and specialist medical care for chronic fatigue syndrome (PACE): a randomized trial. Lancet 2011;377:823–36.

[56] Wicksell RK, Ahlqvist J, Bring, A, Melin L, Olsson GL. Can exposure and acceptance strategies improve functioning and life satisfaction in people with chronic pain and whiplash-associated disorders (WAD)? A randomized controlled trial. Cogn Behav Ther 2008;37:169–82.

[57] Williams AC de C, Richardson PH, Nicholas MK, Pither CE, Harding VR, Ridout KL, Ralphs JA, Richardson JA, Justins DM, Chamberlain JH. Inpatient vs outpatient pain management: results of a randomized controlled trial. Pain 1996;66:13–22.

Correspondence to: Lance M. McCracken, PhD, Health Psychology Section, Psychology Department, Institute of Psychiatry, King's College London, 5th Floor, Bermondsey Wing, London SE1 9RT, United Kingdom. Email: lance.mccracken@ymail.com.

Synopsis 24

Maria Adele Giamberardino and Troels Staehelin Jensen

The first part of the book is devoted to a description of general aspects of comorbidities, their epidemiology, how such conditions can be modeled, and the role played by factors ranging from genetic to immune, hormonal, and psychosocial. In an introduction that draws on historical aspects of pain, Harold Merskey discusses the importance of the interrelationship between pain and emotions. Merskey stresses that the most common complication of chronic pain in clinical practice is probably depression or a combination of anxiety and depression. He then raises the important question about the extent to which comorbid emotional conditions could also be causative in terms of pain.

In their epidemiological chapter, Clare H. Dominick and Fiona M. Blyth continue the discussion about how chronic pain and nonpain comorbidity should be conceptualized. They emphasize that studies on the interaction between chronic pain and nonpain comorbidity throughout the human lifespan provide an opportunity to understand the possible shared causal pathways of chronic pain with some comorbid conditions.

Pain Comorbidities: Understanding and Treating the Complex Patient
edited by Maria Adele Giamberardino and Troels Staehelin Jensen
IASP Press, Seattle, © 2012

In an important chapter, Anna P. Malykhina describes various animal models of pain and comorbidity. She gives an overview of the existing models for pain and non-pain-related disorders and possible clinical implications of translating information from basic science. Most animal models are directed toward single pathophysiological conditions, and only a few are aimed at comorbid disorders. Malykhina mentions animal models of systemic dysfunctions and related comorbidities such as diabetes, hypertension, stress, and fibromyalgia. She also describes animal models of viscerosomatic and viscerovisceral comorbidities and discusses the possible neural, endocrine, and immune mechanisms behind the development of comorbid conditions. In the chapter by Lars Arendt-Nielsen and colleagues, various methods of studying the nociceptive system in health and disease are discussed. Although the influence of comorbidity on nociceptive processing is far from being clarified, the quantitative measures seem to differ for individuals with and without comorbidity to their existing pain. The problem here, as in other clinical pain conditions, is the shift in dynamics in the pain system over time as the condition changes.

In the chapter by Gordon Munro on animal models for chronic pain and comorbidities, it is acknowledged that the experience of chronic pain involves a diversity of parallel processing within somatosensory, limbic, and thalamocortical circuitries, which are responsible for the sensory-discriminative, affective-motivational, and cognitive-evaluative aspects of pain. The question is, of course, to what extent animal models can mimic such complexity. However, an analysis of different pain models indicates that affective behaviors and cognitive impairments can be observed in animal models of pain. On the other hand, animal models of chronic stress are associated with hypersensitivity in nociceptive systems. According to the author, these findings suggest that neuroplastic changes in certain neural structures, such as the hypothalamus, amygdala, and hippocampus, which are involved in affective states and in cognitive function, might persist in the absence of ongoing nociceptive input.

Dan Buskila and Antonio Collado Cruz discuss the role of genetic factors in comorbid pain conditions. They focus on fibromyalgia and review the possible etiological role of gene polymorphisms in the catecholaminergic and serotoninergic systems for these chronic pain conditions. The catecholaminergic system has been studied in most detail. Catechol-*O*-methyltransferase (COMT) is an enzyme that metabolizes catecholamines and may thereby change dopaminergic neurotransmission. A common functional polymorphism of the *COMT* gene that codes for the substitution of valine (val) by methionine (met) occurs at codon 158. Polymorphism at this site is associated with changed pain sensitivity in the temporomandibular joint, but the authors also mention other conditions, such as migraine and whiplash, where *COMT* polymorphisms might play a role in pain. The other elements of the catecholaminergic system, dopamine and epinephrine, have an effect on pain perception. Polymorphism in dopaminergic and adrenergic receptor activity is related to the risk of developing fibromyalgia. Among other candidate genes, polymorphism of the serotonin transporter is related to different functional pain syndromes as well as associated comorbidities.

Roger Fillingim's chapter deals with hormonal influences on the pain experience. Based on the fact that sex differences in the prevalence of many pain conditions vary across the lifespan, it is likely that hormonal factors may play a role. This is the case in migraine and temporomandibular pain disorders. More specifically, changes in the level of the menstrual hormones progesterone and estradiol influence both experimental and clinical pain. The mechanism by which these gonadal hormones affect pain experience is not yet fully understood, but it may be mediated by effects on the peripheral or central nervous system or by immune/inflammatory processes. Testosterone may also have an influence on pain processing. In addition to a direct effect on pain processing, hormones might also exert their effects indirectly, for example by influencing cognitive and affective processes.

The role of the immune system and inflammatory mechanisms on comorbidities such as depression, anxiety, and opioid abuse is dealt with in the chapter by Peter M. Grace and colleagues. Both experimental and clinical findings indicate that cytokines have an effect on depressive and anxiety disorders. This effect may be mediated in part by an action on serotonin and dopamine but possibly also by actions on neuroendocrine functions. The authors raise the hypothesis that chronic pain and its comorbidities might be regarded as manifestations of a maladaptive reaction to a common underlying disorder involving immunological mechanisms, rather than as a scenario in which one disease is driving another.

In the chapter by Akiko Okifuji and Dennis C. Turk, on the influence of the psychosocial environment on pain comorbidities, the authors first review psychological variables known to influence pain experience in general and then discuss how these factors may contribute to pain comorbidities. There is overwhelming evidence that psychological factors have an impact on pain. From a therapeutic point of view, it is important to know that patients vary in their psychosocial profiles, even within a single pain condition, and it is therefore unlikely that patients' psychological needs can be predicted from their pain diagnosis alone. The authors suggest that the psychological needs of each pain patient should be explored and addressed on an individual basis.

The second part of the book is devoted to describing specific pain and nonpain comorbidities, which are discussed with respect to clinical presentation, pathophysiology, diagnostic challenges, and implications for therapy.

The role of hypertension on pain—acute as well as chronic—is discussed in the chapter by Stephen Bruehl. Increased blood pressure and manifest hypertension are associated with reduced pain sensitivity both in animals and in human experimental pain. This blood-pressure-related hypoalgesia is absent in individuals experiencing chronic pain. It is suggested that changes in baroreflex function and in endogenous opioids or α_2-adrenergic systems may contribute. Clinical and epidemiological observations suggest that chronic pain plays a role in the development and maintenance of hypertension. Whether this is due to dysfunctions in a normal homeostatic cardiovascular–pain-modulatory interaction remains to be seen.

Diabetes mellitus is an almost epidemic disease, which is accompanied by neuropathic pain in nearly 20% of affected patients. Solomon Tesfaye's chapter stresses that neuropathic pain in diabetes is also accompanied by significant mood disorders and a severe reduction of the quality of life. For this reason, management of the diabetic neuropathy patient with pain must be tailored to individual needs, taking into consideration comorbidities and other factors. Most attention has been focused on pharmacological treatment, but it is important to recognize that non-pharmacological management programs may be equally important in treating the diabetic patient with neuropathic pain, although few studies have addressed this topic.

Peggy Mason's chapter is about another epidemic disorder: obesity. The author asks two major questions: does obesity cause pain, and does chronic pain give rise to obesity? There is currently no clear answer to these questions, although intuitively one can see a link between chronic pain and obesity. An important aspect is that many pharmacological treatments of chronic pain have weight gain as an important adverse effect.

Cardiovascular disease (CVD) is a major health problem in the general population, and so are headaches, because of their frequency and impact on patients' quality of life. Evidence has rapidly grown in recent years for a link between various expressions of CVD and headache symptoms. In their chapter, Paolo Martelletti and Andrea Negro examine the complex interrelationship between headache—particularly migraine—and different forms of CVD, from ischemic stroke to hypertension and various congenital defects. They highlight how CVD comorbidity in migraine is important from different perspectives: co-occurrence of diseases can complicate the diagnosis, as in the case of focal signs of migraine and stroke; one disease can remind the clinician of another, such as migraine and coronary disease; one treatment can be effective for two diseases, such as ACE inhibitors or sartans for migraine patients with hypertension; and comorbidity of illnesses can provide clues to the pathophysiology of migraine. The authors thoroughly and critically discuss all the implications of these interactions for the clinician faced with differential diagnosis and treatment of the headache patient with CVD.

Headache is also frequently comorbid with myofascial pain syndromes from trigger points (TrPs) in the craniocervical area. The chapter by César Fernández-de-las-Peñas discusses the pathophysiological mechanisms behind this association, addressing important questions such as: Can TrPs contribute to sensitization processes in chronic headache? Can TrPs be involved in the pathogenesis of headache? Can they precipitate a migraine attack? From the evidence they review, the authors conclude that in tension-type headache, pain can probably be explained, at least partially, by the referred pain elicited by active TrPs, and in migraine, TrPs may be a trigger factor for initiating or perpetuating a migraine attack. The authors report that deactivation of TrPs may be effective in reducing migraine and tension-type headache, providing the rationale for an integrated therapeutic approach to the headache patient. Effectiveness of local myofascial pain therapy for headache symptoms is probably the result of a reduction of the degree of central sensitization observed in headache, especially in forms with a high frequency of attacks or in chronic headache, through a decrease of the peripheral nociceptive input from TrPs.

In Robert D. Gerwin's chapter, the chronic and diffuse musculoskeletal pain of the devastating condition of fibromyalgia syndrome is discussed with its frequent comorbidities, here again with headache but also with dysfunctional visceral pains, such as irritable bowel syndrome, painful bladder syndrome, or chronic pelvic pain. The author underlines how fibromyalgia and these comorbidities share common dysfunctions in central pain-processing modulation that increase the likelihood of multiple pain complaints at both the somatic and visceral level. Central sensitization is thus key to fibromyalgia and to the multiple comorbid conditions considered in this chapter. The author stresses how the clinical presentation may be fibromyalgia alone, or any one of the associated conditions described, or a complex presentation of multiple conditions that require a thorough evaluation to guide a more comprehensive and effective treatment, especially because these associations appear to mutually enhance each other's symptoms in many cases. Gerwin also reports on the impact of treatment of myofascial pain syndromes from TrPs—also very frequently comorbid with fibromyalgia—on the diffuse pain and tenderness of this condition. Specific fibromyalgia symptoms are decreased by this treatment, attesting to the role of TrPs as peripheral pain generators in the syndrome, similarly to what is described for TrPs in headache.

Musculoskeletal pain is further addressed as an important comorbidity in painful joint diseases in the chapter by Thomas Graven-Nielsen and colleagues. The authors focus on various forms of primary painful joint disease (caused by trauma, infections, osteoarthritis, or rheumatoid arthritis) and their muscle pain comorbidities, such as myofascial pain syndromes. They discuss comorbid manifestations of joint pain, the potential mechanisms involved, and methods of assessment. One major aspect highlighted in the chapter is the difficulty in differentiating various forms of muscle pain that are comorbid with joint pain from muscle pains that are secondary (referred from the joint) and are thus a direct consequence of joint pain (referred pain from joints is a challenge, as it may mimic a localized source of pain). The authors report on the importance of quantitative sensory testing in assessing the various clinical combinations and discuss the pathophysiological implications of joint-muscle associations, as the pain and the sensitization of joint nociceptors are a robust source of central sensitization. They conclude, however, that at present only hypothetical models are available to explain the transition from localized pain due to joint tissue challenges to widespread pain. They call for further development of standardized sensory assessment protocols to optimize diagnostic approaches, as well as drug effects, and provide rational treatment strategies.

A number of inflammatory, infectious, and metabolic diseases can be associated with or be the cause of neuropathic pain, one of the most difficult-to-treat forms of pain that a patient can experience. In his chapter, Troels S. Jensen provides an ample overview of the neuropathic pain patterns in these conditions, from postherpetic neuralgia, Guillain-Barré syndrome, human immunodeficiency virus infection (HIV) and consequences of its treatment with antiretroviral therapy (HAART), to neuroborreliosis and various vasculitic disorders (as observed in different connective tissue diseases such as systemic lupus, Wegner's granulomatosis, polyarthritis nodosa, and sarcoidosis). The author also reports on the neuropathic pain associated with metabolic disorders—other than diabetes—such as thyroid diseases, hepatitis C, Fabry's disease, and vitamin deficiency. In addition to describing the neuropathic pain associated with each of these conditions, the author addresses the relative underlying pathophysiological mechanisms and offers a critical discussion of the therapeutic options. He underlines how causal treatment should always be attempted because there is now a strong desire in medicine to move from a simple reduction of symptoms to a disease-modifying strategy. However, such treatment may not solve the pain problem if nerve damage has already occurred, so pharmacological symptomatic treatment is needed in most cases. In describing symptomatic treatment options, Jensen emphasizes the importance of careful assessment of comorbidities, particularly heart diseases and convulsive disorders, that represent a contraindication for the use of tricyclic antidepressants, frequently used to relieve this type of pain. For anticonvulsants the contraindications are fewer, but side effects such as sedation, dizziness, tremor, and skin rashes are not uncommon and thus require particular attention in complex patients, especially the elderly.

The chapter by Maria Adele Giamberardino and colleagues deals with viscerovisceral hyperalgesia, a relatively neglected phenomenon, where noxious information from one organ spreads to another viscus with which it shares parts of its central sensory projection pathways. It is important for the clinician to look for viscerovisceral hyperalgesia, when pain symptoms from one organ are excessively intense and out of proportion to a specific pain disorder affecting a particular organ. In these cases, all the organs that share at least part of their central sensory projections should be systematically explored in order to determine the underlying pathology.

Comorbidity between pain and affective disorders is almost the rule, especially in chronic pain. Ample space has been given in this volume to the topic, although chapters by various authors have addressed it from different perspectives, providing a multifaceted insight into a complex interrelationship. The question of affective disorders being primary or secondary to chronic pain remains problematic. The philosophical "chicken-or-egg" question, already introduced by Merskey, is further developed in the chapter by Ephrem Fernandez and Robert D. Kerns. The authors review a number of studies addressing comorbidity between different types of pain and affective disorders, including anxiety, depression, and anger. The weight of evidence favors anxiety as a precipitant of pain and depression as a consequence of pain, while the evidence is inconclusive with regard to anger. Irrespective of the crucial primary-to-secondary question, the authors stress the concept that each additional affective disturbance imposes an increased burden on the mental and physical health of the pain patient. For example, in patients with musculoskeletal pain, the presence of both depression and anxiety appears to be associated with greater severity of pain and pain interference than observed for those reporting depression or anxiety alone. The authors address this phenomenon as "added morbidity," pointing out how it is strikingly similar to the increased pain and hyperalgesia observed in individuals with comorbid visceral conditions.

In their analysis of the chicken-or-egg issue, they ultimately conclude that what is more important in the association between mood disorders and pain is to ask how the chicken influences the egg it lays and how the egg influences the chicken that is hatched.

The third part of the book is devoted to specific therapeutic aspects of the comorbid patient. Pain management is undeniably complex and requires a multidisciplinary approach, especially in chronic cases, which are inevitably associated with several comorbidities. John Loeser's chapter illustrates how a multidisciplinary pain clinic might offer advantages to the management of the complex patient. He stresses that relief of pain is only one aspect of treating a chronic pain patient and that alleviating the comorbidities—such as deactivation, depression, sleep disturbance, or disability—is also essential for a good outcome. Loeser specifically states: "What has been learned in the 50 years since the birth of multidisciplinary pain centers is that the complaint of pain almost always decreases as the comorbidities are successfully managed." It has proven impossible to identify the relative importance of each of the components of a treatment program, but the author believes that the entire process is greater than the sum of its parts, which is the basis for the success of the multidisciplinary pain center.

Although treatment of pain conditions and comorbidities involves a wide range of therapies, pharmacological treatment is the mainstay. The chapter by Lucy A. Bee and colleagues focuses on the main classes of drugs employed for pain treatment, including interactions, side effects, and thus differential indications in various clinical circumstances. The authors emphasize the importance of assessing comorbidities carefully for pharmacological treatment. They brilliantly describe the rationale for use of specific classes of drugs in various types of pains and clusters of pain conditions, i.e., different comorbidities, entering into details of the various pathophysiologies of the different conditions: shared pathophysiological mechanisms are often indicated by shared treatments. They explain that an understanding of the circuits and pharmacology that link pain with its comorbidities and an appreciation of their shared pathophysiologies and similar "signatures" should promote collaboration among researchers from different fields, advancing the treatment of pain and other disorders.

The chapter by Nicole Gellings Lowe and Stephen M. Stahl focuses more specifically on pharmacological treatment with antidepressants. These drugs are commonly used for treatment of mood disorders, but they are effective analgesics as well in a number of comorbid pain conditions, such as fibromyalgia and migraine, which may have common pathophysiological mechanisms. The authors highlight the use of these compounds in pain and comorbid mood disorders; they review the tolerability and efficacy of various antidepressants for patients with these types of disorders, stressing, however, that treatment must be individually tailored to be effective and safe.

Physical training and rehabilitation are an essential component of the management of the pain patient. However, programs need to be individualized, depending on comorbid conditions. For example, recommendations for physical activity cannot be the same for a pain patient who is otherwise healthy as they would be for a pain patient with comorbid cardiovascular disease or diabetes. The chapter by Harriet M. Wittink and Jeanine Verbunt illustrates the principles that are at the basis of specific programs in various comorbid situations with pain: hypertension, diabetes, overweight and obesity, and metabolic syndrome, but also affective disorders, such as depression and anxiety, or severe mental illness. The authors stress the importance of considering exercise restrictions due to comorbidity when planning exercise treatment for pain problems and also recommend safety precautions prior to engaging patients with comorbidities in high-intensity exercise.

Management of the pain patient—especially in the case of chronic pain—inevitably requires a psychological approach along with classical drug and nondrug therapies. The chapter by Lance M. McCracken illustrates this approach to handling the comorbid patient. The author reviews a number of conditions that can be comorbid with chronic pain. Depression and anxiety, insomnia, and fatigue each appear to be effectively treated with broadly cognitive-behavioral methods, even though some patients may not achieve complete alleviation of their symptoms, or full recovery of their functioning, by using these methods. For patients with complaints of impaired cognitive functioning, the other comorbid condition reviewed, effective treatment is not yet clear. McCracken also touches on the effect of analgesic medication on cognitive functioning, a topic of high current interest to clinicians; however, further study will be needed before the adverse effects of analgesics on patient functioning, and ways to manage them, can be better understood.

In synthesis, a common thread appears to connect all the chapters in this book, where a pain or nonpain condition in one chapter is linked to another pain or nonpain condition that is dealt with in subsequent chapters, in a continuum that reflects not only the high level of multiple comorbidities in pain patients but also the multidisciplinary interconnections of these comorbidities. Complexity is the rule in the comorbid pain patient, not only for diagnosis, but also for management, which necessarily needs to be thorough and integrated among disciplines. In an era of super-specialization, where there is a risk of treating diseases specifically and separately, we must acknowledge the essential role of a unifying clinical figure, who can sum up and coordinate all the specialistic interventions for a pain patient. The key message for clinicians is to always remember that the patient with comorbidities is a whole person whose clinical picture represents a complex interaction of multiple factors and not merely the sum of symptoms of each separate condition.

Index

Page numbers followed by f refer to figures, and by t to tables.

sexual abuse and, 336
fibromyalgia and, 336–337
gastrointestinal and urinary tract
dysfunction in, 43
in women, 309
Pelvic-urethral reflex activity, 50
Peptidergic receptors, 97
Periaqueductal gray (PAG), 127, 389
Pericranial tenderness, 300–301
Peripheral cross-organ sensitization, 48–49
Peripheral nervous system, 127
Peripheral neuropathy, diabetic. *See*
Diabetic peripheral neuropathy
(DPN)
Peripheral sensitization, 391
PFO. *See* Patent foramen ovale (PFO) in
Phantom limb pain, 66
Pharmacology of pain and comorbidities,
475–476. *See also* Drugs and drug
therapy
antidepressants for pain modulation,
394–396. *See also* Antidepressants
descending inhibitions in analgesia,
395
diffuse pain states, 390–391
higher brain processing of pain,
399–402
monoaminergic system, 388–390
shared mechanisms and treatments,
396–398
visceral pain, 391–394
Phenytoin, 209, 396
PHN (postherpetic neuralgia), 267–268,
396
Phobias, 164
Phototherapy, near-infrared, 214
Physical activity. *See also* Exercise; Exercise
therapy
deactivation treatment programs,
377–379
health benefits, 428–429
inactivity and chronic disease risk, 427
life expectancy and, 429
socioeconomic burden of inactivity,
427
Physical therapy, 304–305
Physical training and rehabilitation,
425–447, 476. *See also* Exercise
therapy; Physical activity
Physicians' Health Study, 234, 242–243

Physiological pain, 262
Pinprick stimulation, cutaneous, 61
Placebo effect, 399, 400
Polyarteritis nodosa, 270
Polymyalgia, 352
Polyneuropathy, acute inflammatory, 268
Positive and Negative Symptoms Scale
(PANSS), 446
Postherpetic neuralgia (PHN), 267–268,
396
Postoperative pain
cold thresholds predicting, 63
COMT polymorphisms and intensity,
110
temporal summation and post-
thoracotomy pain, 66
Post-traumatic stress disorder (PTSD)
amygdala and, 401
as anxiety disorder, 164
back or neck pain and, 282
cognitive-behavioral therapy, 455, 456
comorbidities, 15
dopaminergic system polymorphisms
in, 113
in fibromyalgia and irritable bowel
syndrome, 341
pain prevalence in, 281, 282, 454
quantitative pain assessment, 67
rape and fibromyalgia, 336
serotonin transporter gene polymorphisms, 112
Potassium channels, voltage-gated, 396
PPT. *See* Pressure pain threshold (PPT)
Preeclampsia, 237
Prefrontal cortex, 161
Pregabalin
as calcium channel blocker, 396, 397
for diabetic neuropathies, 207,
210–211, 212
for neuropathic pain, 401
for painful diabetic neuropathy, 209,
213
visceral pain and, 393
Pregnancy
gabapentin for nausea in, 397
migraine decline in, 123
musculoskeletal pain and added
weight, 222–223
temporomandibular pain decline in,
123

Editors

Maria Adele Giamberardino, MD, is Associate Professor of Internal Medicine, Research Director of the Pathophysiology of Pain Laboratory, and Head of the Center for Fibromyalgia and Musculoskeletal Pain and the Headache Center at the Department of Medicine and Science of Aging of the "G. D'Annunzio" University of Chieti, Italy. Since her graduation in Medicine in 1984, she has conducted intensive clinical and experimental research in the fields 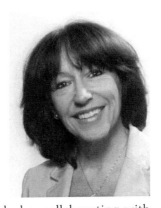 of visceral pain, musculoskeletal pain, and headache, collaborating with numerous research groups in Europe and the United States. In 2004 she was awarded the International Research Prize of the International Myopain Society for her research in musculoskeletal pain. She was a founding member and Vice-President of "EuroPain" (Brussels, 1992–98) and served as councilor (1996–99), member of the committees for Research (1993–99), Finance (2002–05), Nominations (2009–12), and Taxonomy (2010–12), and was on the ballot for Presidency (2005) for the International Association for the Study of Pain (IASP). She chaired the "European Campaign Against Fibromyalgia" (2008–09) and the Publications Committee (2008–11) for the European Federation of IASP Chapters. She was President of the Italian Chapter of IASP from 2009 to 2011. Involved in editorial activity for various national and international journals (*Pain, European Journal of Pain, Pain: Clinical Updates*), she is currently Editor-in-Chief of IASP Press (2010–15). Since 1985, she has participated in many national and international congresses on pain as speaker, chair, session organizer, and member of the scientific committee. She is author of over 200 scientific publications in international journals and books.

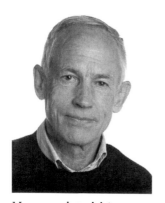

Troels Staehelin Jensen, MD, DMSc, is a Consultant in Neurology at Aarhus University Hospital and Professor of Experimental and Clinical Pain Research at Aarhus University in Aarhus, Denmark, and director of the Danish Pain Research Center and its Neuropathic Pain Clinic. He obtained his degree of Doctor of Medical Sciences from the University of Aarhus on work conducted in part at the Mayo Clinic in Rochester, Minnesota, USA. He completed his postgraduate clinical fellowship at la Salpêtrière Hospital in Paris, France, and his residency in neurology at university hospitals in Aarhus and Copenhagen. He has obtained research fellowships in the United States and guest professorships in other countries including the United States and Germany. Dr. Jensen has authored more than 300 peer-reviewed papers on various neurological and neurobiological topics, mainly related to experimental and clinical pain, and has received several awards and honors for his pain research, including the Nis-Hanssen Pain Research Award (1986), the Norwegian Monrad-Krohn Research Award (1997), the Scandinavian Pain Research Award (2001), and the P.D. Wall Medal of the British Pain Society (2009). Dr. Jensen is honorary member of several societies. In 2006 he was knighted by the Queen of Denmark. Dr. Jensen's research interests include neurophysiology, neuropharmacology, mechanisms and treatment of neuropathic pain, and translation from acute to chronic pain. He has served as section editor for the journal *PAIN* and now serves on the editorial boards of other journals. He is a reviewer for several international journals and grant committees. Dr Jensen was President of the Scandinavian Association for the Study of Pain during 1989–94. He was member of the Council of the International Association for the Study of Pain (IASP) from 1996 to 2010 and served as president for IASP from 2005 to 2010.

Contributing Authors

Giannapia Affaitati, MD, PhD, *Department of Medicine and Science of Aging, "G. D'Annunzio" University of Chieti, Italy*

Cristina Alonso-Blanco, RN, PT, Phd, *Department of Nursing, Rey Juan Carlos University, Alcorcón, Madrid, Spain*

Lars Arendt-Nielsen, DMSc, PhD, *Center for Sensory-Motor Interaction, Department of Health Science and Technology, Faculty of Medicine, Aalborg University, Aalborg, Denmark*

Lucy A. Bee, PhD, *Department of Neuroscience, Physiology and Pharmacology, University College London, London, United Kingdom*

Henning Bliddal, DMSc, MD, *The Parker Institute, Frederiksberg Hospital, Frederiksberg, Denmark*

Fiona M. Blyth, MBBS, MPH, PhD, *Pain Management Research Institute, Sydney School of Public Health, University of Sydney, Sydney, New South Wales, Australia*

Stephen Bruehl, PhD, *Vanderbilt University Medical Center, Nashville, Tennessee, USA*

Dan Buskila, MD, *Department of Medicine, Soroka Medical Center; Faculty of Health Sciences, Ben Gurion University in the Negev, Beer Sheva, Israel*

Antonio Collado Cruz, MD, PhD, *Fibromyalgia Unit, Rheumatology Service, Hospital Clinic of Barcelona, University of Barcelona, Barcelona, Spain*

Raffaele Costantini, MD, PhD, *Institute of Surgical Pathology, "G. D'Annunzio" University of Chieti, Italy*

Ana Isabel de-la-Llave-Rincón, PT, MSc, PhD, *Department of Physical Therapy, Occupational Therapy, Physical Medicine and Rehabilitation, and Esthesiology Laboratory, Rey Juan Carlos University, Alcorcón, Madrid, Spain*

Anthony H. Dickenson, PhD, *Department of Neuroscience, Physiology and Pharmacology, University College London, London, United Kingdom*

Clare H. Dominick, BA(Hons), MPH, *Pain Management Research Institute, Royal North Shore Hospital, University of Sydney, Sydney, New South Wales, Australia*

505

Ephrem Fernandez, PhD, *Department of Psychology, University of Texas at San Antonio, San Antonio, Texas, USA*

César Fernández-de-las-Peñas, PT, MSc, PhD, *Department of Physical Therapy, Occupational Therapy, Physical Medicine and Rehabilitation, and Esthesiology Laboratory, Rey Juan Carlos University, Alcorcón, Madrid, Spain; Centre for Sensory-Motor Interaction, Department of Health Science and Technology, Aalborg University, Aalborg, Denmark*

Roger B. Fillingim, PhD, *University of Florida College of Dentistry and North Florida/South Georgia Veterans Health System, Gainesville, Florida, USA*

Robert D. Gerwin, MD, *Department of Neurology, Johns Hopkins University School of Medicine, Baltimore, Maryland, USA; Pain and Rehabilitation Medicine, Bethesda, Maryland, USA*

Maria Adele Giamberardino, MD, *Department of Medicine and Science of Aging, G. D'Annunzio University of Chieti, Chieti, Italy*

Leonor Gonçalves, PhD, *Department of Neuroscience, Physiology and Pharmacology, University College London, London, United Kingdom*

Peter M. Grace, *PhD, Discipline of Pharmacology, School of Medical Sciences, University of Adelaide, Adelaide, South Australia, Australia; Department of Psychology and the Center for Neuroscience, University of Colorado at Boulder, Boulder, Colorado, USA*

Thomas Graven-Nielsen, DMSc, PhD, *Center for Sensory-Motor Interaction, Department of Health Science and Technology, Faculty of Medicine, Aalborg University, Aalborg, Denmark*

Mark R. Hutchinson, PhD, *Discipline of Physiology, School of Medical Sciences, University of Adelaide, Adelaide, South Australia, Australia*

Troels Staehelin Jensen, MD, DMSc, *Danish Pain Research Center, Department of Neurology, Aarhus University Hospital, Aarhus, Denmark*

Robert D. Kerns, PhD, *Departments of Psychiatry, Neurology, and Psychology, Yale University, New Haven, Connecticut; PRIME Center, VA Connecticut Healthcare System, West Haven, Connecticut, USA*

John D. Loeser, MD, *Department of Neurological Surgery, University of Washington, Seattle, Washington, USA*

Nicole Gellings Lowe, PhD, *Arbor Scientia, Carlsbad, California, USA*

Anna P. Malykhina, PhD, *Division of Urology, Department of Surgery, University of Pennsylvania School of Medicine, Glenolden, Pennsylvania, USA*

Paolo Martelletti, MD, *Department of Clinical and Molecular Medicine, La Sapienza University of Rome; Regional Referral Headache Center, Sant'Andrea Hospital, Rome, Italy*

Peggy Mason, PhD, *Department of Neurobiology, University of Chicago, Chicago, Illinois, USA*

Lance M. McCracken, PhD, *Health Psychology Section, Psychology Department, Institute of Psychiatry, King's College London; INPUT Pain Management Service, Guys' and St Thomas' NHS Foundation Trust, London, United Kingdom*

Harold Merskey, DM, FRCP, FRCPsych, FRCPC, *Professor Emeritus of Psychiatry, University of Western Ontario, London, Ontario, Canada*

Gordon Munro, PhD, *Neurodegeneration 2, H. Lundbeck A/S, Valby, Denmark*

Andrea Negro, MD, *Department of Clinical and Molecular Medicine, La Sapienza University of Rome; Regional Referral Headache Center, Sant'Andrea Hospital, Rome, Italy*

Akiko Okifuji, PhD, *Pain Research and Management Center, Department of Anesthesiology, University of Utah, Salt Lake City, Utah, USA*

Laura Petrini, PhD, *Center for Sensory-Motor Interaction, Department of Health Science and Technology, Faculty of Medicine, Aalborg University, Aalborg, Denmark*

Margarete Ribeiro-Dasilva, DDS, MS, PhD, *University of Florida College of Dentistry, Gainesville, Florida, USA*

Stephen M. Stahl, MD, PhD, *Arbor Scientia, Carlsbad, California, USA; Department of Psychiatry, University of California San Diego, San Diego, California, USA*

Solomon Tesfaye, MB ChB, MD, FRCP, *Consultant Physician and Honorary Professor of Diabetic Medicine, University of Sheffield, Royal Hallamshire Hospital, Sheffield, United Kingdom*

Dennis C. Turk, PhD, *Department of Anesthesiology and Pain Medicine, University of Washington, Seattle, Washington, USA*

Jeanine Verbunt, MD, PhD, *Department of Rehabilitation Medicine, Maastricht University Medical Center, Maastricht, The Netherlands*

Linda R. Watkins, PhD, *Department of Psychology and the Center for Neuroscience, University of Colorado at Boulder, Boulder, Colorado, USA*

Harriet M. Wittink, PhD, PT, *Lifestyle and Health Research Group, Faculty of Health Care, Utrecht University of Applied Research, Utrecht, The Netherlands*